AF820527

The Contest of Modern Chinese and Western Medicine

Kuoli Pi

The Contest of Modern Chinese and Western Medicine

Antibacterial History of Traditional Chinese Medicine

中華書局
ZHONGHUA BOOK COMPANY

Springer

Kuoli Pi
National Central University
Taoyuan, Taiwan

Translated by
Ma Li
East China University of Political Science
and Law
Shanghai, China

ISBN 978-981-95-2831-8 ISBN 978-981-95-2832-5 (eBook)
https://doi.org/10.1007/978-981-95-2832-5

Jointly published with Zhonghua Book Company
The print edition is not for sale in China (Mainland). Customers from China (Mainland) please order the print book from: Zhonghua Book Company.

Translation from the Chinese Simplified language edition: "《近代中西医的博弈》" by Kuoli Pi, © Zhonghua Book Company 2019. Published by Zhonghua Book Company. All Rights Reserved.

The original submitted manuscript has been translated into English. The translation was done using artificial intelligence. A subsequent revision was performed by the author(s) to further refine the work and to ensure that the translation is appropriate concerning content and scientific correctness. It may, however, read stylistically different from a conventional translation.

Sponsored by Chinese Fund of Humanities and Social Sciences

© Zhonghua Book Company 2026, corrected publication 2026

This work is subject to copyright. All rights are solely and exclusively licensed by the Publisher, whether the whole or part of the material is concerned, specifically the rights of translation, reprinting, reuse of illustrations, recitation, broadcasting, reproduction on microfilms or in any other physical way, and transmission or information storage and retrieval, electronic adaptation, computer software, or by similar or dissimilar methodology now known or hereafter developed.
The use of general descriptive names, registered names, trademarks, service marks, etc. in this publication does not imply, even in the absence of a specific statement, that such names are exempt from the relevant protective laws and regulations and therefore free for general use.
The publishers, the authors, and the editors are safe to assume that the advice and information in this book are believed to be true and accurate at the date of publication. Neither the publishers nor the authors or the editors give a warranty, express or implied, with respect to the material contained herein or for any errors or omissions that may have been made. The publishers remain neutral with regard to jurisdictional claims in published maps and institutional affiliations.

This Springer imprint is published by the registered company Springer Nature Singapore Pte Ltd.
The registered company address is: 152 Beach Road, #21-01/04 Gateway East, Singapore 189721, Singapore

If disposing of this product, please recycle the paper.

Foreword: The Gains and Losses of Anti-bacteria in Chinese Medicine History

Zhang Zhongjing's *Treatise on Typhoid Fever* is undoubtedly one of the most important classic works in the history of Chinese medicine. This medical book, which is regarded as the gold standard for all medical schools, is also deemed as the pioneering work of Chinese clinical medicine. After the Song Dynasty, this work began to be respected by many doctors and became more and more canonized. In the Ming and Qing Dynasties, with the establishment of Zhang Zhongjing's medical Saint status, *Treatise on Typhoid Fever* gradually became a medical classic similar to the four books in Confucianism. At the same time, doctors in the Ming and Qing Dynasties, especially in the Qing Dynasty, also developed the "theory of febrile diseases" on this basis. This theory is known as one of the most important achievements in the development of medicine in the Ming and Qing Dynasties. There should be no doubt that the understanding and treatment of "typhoid fever" and "febrile disease" are among the most important achievements in traditional Chinese medicine (TCM). According to today's disease classification, these diseases can be generally classified as exogenous diseases, namely infectious diseases caused by pathogens and also generalized as infectious diseases. According to the understanding by today's medicine, there are many varieties of such pathogens, mainly bacteria and viruses. Before the virus was recognized in the twentieth century, academia and the general public named it bacteria. In other words, the diagnosis and treatment of exogenous diseases caused by bacteria had not only been the focus, but also the specialty, of Chinese medicine for a long period of time.

Even though the status of Zhang Zhongjing and *Treatise on Typhoid Fever* have been continuously recognized and promoted since modern times, generations of TCM scholars have also paid great attention to "typhoid fever" and "febrile diseases" with extensive research and construction. It is paradoxical to see the fact that the treatment of exogenous diseases caused by bacteria was no longer the main battlefield of TCM. In the understandings of ordinary people, TCM has relinquished this position, being replaced by western medicine to practice its specialty. In this regard, Dr. Pi Kuoli of Zhongyuan University has grasped the key issue by exploring the development of modern TCM and the debate between TCM and Western medicine from the perspective of bacteria or antibacterial origins.

Kuoli has long been committed to the study of modern Chinese medical history. He grew up in Taiwan, where there is a strong commitment to medical history study in history circles, and has frequent contact with both sides of the Taiwan Strait. He is a young scholar with extensive influence in the field of Chinese medical history and modern history on both sides of the Taiwan Strait. Over the past ten years, Kuoli has been writing continuously with great achievements. I personally take him as one of the few scholars with the most academic achievements in the field of medical history research in China. After taking Tang Zonghai as the leading figure to explore the integration of modern Chinese and Western medicine, he locked on to this key topic to carry out the research on the evolution of modern Chinese medicine in the context of the debate between Chinese and Western medicine, which not only presents his diligence and initiative, but also shows his keen academic visions.

Whether it is the debate between TCM and Western medicine or the development of modern TCM, it is no longer a new topic. To derive new ideas and interests on this old topic, the key is to grasp the poignant facts of the problem and put forward good questions. Kuoli hopes to present and think about the process of "re canonization" of modern TCM from the influence of the bacterial theory. Both the topic and the intention are very ingenious and meaningful. In my opinion, the reason why he can make it is probably due to the following two factors:

First of all, it is attributed to his in-depth study of the many discussions by modern TCM scholars. In his early years, Kuoli studied the theory of the integration of Chinese and Western medicine in modern times, especially during the late Qing Dynasty. Later, he read a lot of works by Yun Tieqiao and many other TCM scholars during the Republic of China period. It was this systematic and intensive reading that enabled him to realize that since the 1920s and 1930s, TCM scholars turned their attention to Western medicine from physiology to bacteriology, which prompted him to take this as the starting point of his research.

Secondly, it also stems from his clear understanding of the modernity of TCM. In many people's understandings, Chinese medicine is a knowledge system for the treatment of diseases originated and developed from China. It has come down in one continuous line and has been developing since ancient times. As early as the Qin and Han Dynasties and even earlier, classic works such as *Inner Canon of the Yellow Emperor*, *Classic on Medical Problems* and *Treatise on Typhoid Fever* have taken shape, and they are still "living classics" in today's TCM education system, with Yin-Yang and the five elements, deficiency, excess cold and heat, acupuncture, moxibustion, including the old concepts and methods of "syndrome differentiation and treatment", which seem to share common ground from ancient to modern times. Although the knowledge of TCM has developed intermittently from time to time, it is fundamentally an essential existence. Its essence had been determined as early as the pre-Qin, Qin and Han Dynasties, and the changes by later generations were just some modifications based on its fundamental system. Chinese medicine is not only the essence and treasure of China's traditional culture, but also China's only "ancient science". Such a view is very popular, even conclusive, in today's Chinese medical history and TCM works. Since TCM is a long-standing tradition, it essentially comes down in one continuous line. It doesn't show any differences between the modernity of modern Chinese medicine or TCM itself.

However, this may not be the case. We might as well start with the basic understanding of modern TCM. When it comes to TCM in modern times, many would agree to regard "syndrome differentiation and treatment" and "overall concept" as the fundamental characteristics and advantages of TCM. The research so far has convincingly shown that even though the theory and method of "syndrome differentiation and treatment" and "overall concept" were not completely absent in medicine before modern times, they were rarely discussed, let alone being regarded as the fundamental feature and theory of TCM. Ever since 1949, influenced and driven by the policies of "western learning in China" and "vigorously developing TCM", a group of medical elites have developed the dual concepts and dialectical values of "scientization" and "sinology". Under the influence of materialism based on many discussions during the Republic of China period, the two theories of "syndrome differentiation and treatment" and "overall concept" were successfully constructed, which not only filled the vacancy of the TCM key theory caused by abandoning Yin-Yang and the five elements, but also constructed a TCM image different from Western medicine, and showed its uniqueness and advantage. In a word, the traditions of Chinese medicine, taken as being traditional with Western medicine as a frame of reference, are actually "modern" from the evolution context of Chinese medicine itself. As contemporary TCM has been questioned and even denied with the development of Chinese traditional culture since modern times, along with the aggressive entry and increasingly rapid development of Western medicine, generations of TCM scholars have gradually constructed a set of modern knowledge systems with modern scientific and disciplinary thinking, through the records of medical history and the screening of traditional medical knowledge. That is to say, TCM is not an essential existence as much as a traditional symbol, nor is it isolated and self-sufficient from Chinese history and culture, but a knowledge system that constantly evolves with the changes of Chinese history and culture.

Needless to say, Kuoli is knowledgeable about this. It is particularly by this understanding that he put forward the idea of "re canonization" of modern TCM. By focusing on the concepts of "bacteria", "Qi", "typhoid fever" and "warm disease", carefully combing through the discussions of many scholars, mainly in the TCM area during the Republic of China period, Kuoli presented us how modern TCM digested the Western bacterial theory and incorporated some theories and knowledge into the old concepts. In the tide of scientization and specialization, many TCM sages struggled to survive when facing the increasingly aggressive Western civilization and Western medicine, either out of surviving crisis, or out of their own cultural or national attachment, and finally endowed TCM the modernity that can be grounded in modern society in both content and form. For the reshaping of TCM by the scholars of the Republic of China period and even contemporary TCM due to the trend of scientization and specialization, it is apparent that these achievements are undoubtedly the crystallization of the civilization of the times and the wisdom of generations of TCM elites, despite the criticism by some TCM practitioners from time to time. In my opinion, their efforts are also quite fruitful on the whole. There is no doubt that

TCM can be a medical system coexisting with Western medicine in contemporary China. Their efforts are absolutely crucial. Although there are still various problems, TCM, as a science, technology, specialty and medical system in modern society, has undoubtedly integrated into modern society successfully, at least in terms of form, mechanism, academic expression, knowledge inheritance, educational mode and the operational mode of medical institutions.

Nevertheless, if we go back to the question raised at the beginning, we have to admit that since modern times, TCM has been trying to survive and constantly pursuing development, which is also a process of retreating and withdrawing from the main battlefield in the competition with Western medicine. Why? The reason for this is definitely complicated, but there is a simple fact. The overwhelming victory of Western medicine in the treatment of infectious diseases is not due to its profound theory or reasoning, but to the "magic bullet" of antibiotics against bacteria which was invented on the basis of the continuous development of bacteriological theory. Looking back at the statements of many TCM elites since modern times, it can be found that they seem to spend the most energy on how to make TCM scientific and legitimate, how to make its theory logically self-consistent, appealing and convincing, so that they can survive with the political and public support, rather than committing more resources to improving specific medical technology. In spite of the great achievements in the development of modern Chinese medicine, this fact makes us wonder: shall we question this academic orientation in retrospect?

Although Kuoli did not directly mention these concerns in his book, he stated in his preface: "In addition to historical data, readers are expected to reflect on the development and positioning of modern TCM, not to compete with Western medicine, but to treat diseases, help the world and benefit all mankind". This is exactly what I wish for! Kuoli and I both majored in history, a discipline which is undoubtedly our career path. By reading his words, I realize that he has a heartfelt concern for TCM. This may be a minority stand among the colleagues in the field of medical social history, which is often called external history. Due to this, I feel gratified and encouraged to realize our common interests. In recent years, I have always actively advocated that the research of medical history should break the barriers of internal and external history, eventually achieving the integration of both. Although Kuoli's statement is different from mine by advocating "multi-dimensional medical history", that is, he hopes to build the connection between medical academic and daily medical social discussion through the discussion of "multi-dimensional medical history", we share approximately the same purport.

To a large extent, ideal reading is the communication between the reader and the author. It is precisely by this communication that reading the book is a pleasant experience for me. The academic enlightenment from time to time is gratifying, and the common interests we share make the reading a pleasure. With this, I really feel obligated to recommend this excellent work, which is both academic and enjoyable. At the same time, I would like to say that academic research is an endless journey, especially for premature Chinese medical history research. The contributions we made are far from being enough for us to stop and enjoy the results. If we were to have the self-inspection according to some scholars' high standard in the field of TCM, we should ask ourselves: what real benefits does our research bring to the development of TCM? How does "multi-dimensional medical history" show the shaping of medical knowledge from the perspective of daily life and medical practice? For such questions, obviously the premature research on Chinese medical history in the field of history study may not be ready for the answers yet for the time being. In this case, how can we make believe that we have got into the key part of Chinese medicine?

Doubtlessly that there is still a long way to go in the future for the study of Chinese medical history. I am here to congratulate Kuoli on the publication of his new book, and to share my brief views with Kuoli and the colleagues in the academic circles, in order to jointly promote the development of this study.

Tianjin, China Yu Xinzhong
January 2019

The original version of this book has been revised: The author name has been updated from "Guoli Pi" to "Kuoli Pi" as per the author's passport and the line "Sponsored by Chinese Fund of Humanities and Social Sciences" has been included on the copyright page. The corrections to this book can be found at https://doi.org/10.1007/978-981-95-2832-5_11

Author's Preface: The "Living" Medical History

The meeting, collision and communication between TCM and Western medicine is not only an unavoidable topic in the history of modern medicine, but also a major event in the history of cultural exchange between China and the West. Here there is not much to say about my personal learning experience, but to express my gratitude. The following few words are just to show my respect to my readers.

Since the beginning of my pursuit of the master's program, I have been engaged in the research of "life and medical history", so as to have a glimpse into the mysteries of Chinese medicine, analyze the challenges it encountered in modern times, and explore the possibility of a generation of scholars to find a way out. In the late Qing Dynasty, the collision between Chinese and Western medicine was mainly in the dispute of anatomy and physiology. After the Republic of China period, TCM and Western medicine turned to compete in bacteriology and pathology. Later it involved the actual treatment and the core theoretical system of Chinese medicine, which had been dominated by "internal medicine" typhology and warm diseases. No matter on curative effect, or academic theory, it involves a wider range and more heated disputes than the previous generation. The main focus of this book is on the diseases and medical history since the Republic of China period. I am very interested in the theory of TCM. Though not being able to practice medicine to help the world, I can always put forward some observations on the development of TCM from the perspective of history. It is worth thinking that modern Chinese medicine did not yield to Western medicine in the battle of febrile disease treatment between Chinese and Western medicine. If TCM is not even qualified in "declaring a war" or "fighting in a war", with years passing by and its features being lost, it won't be long before its "life" comes to an end. There are lessons learned from history. Shouldn't the researchers of TCM be vigilant?

The contest of modern Chinese and Western medicine began in the late Qing Dynasty. At first, it mostly fought in anatomy and physiology. The debate in theory was actually greater than in curative effect. TCM therapy still had certain advantages at that time. At the beginning of the 20th century, Western medicine made a major breakthrough in the theory of bacteria. The Beiyang government and the national government, which were successively established, fully approached Western medicine in terms of health policies such as epidemic prevention, and restricted the development of TCM in terms of education policies. The focus of the game between Chinese and Western medicine was the proposal of the "TCM Abolition Act". In 1928, the Ministry of Health of the national government was established. According to the organizational law of the Ministry, the Central Health Committee was established as the decision-making organ of health decision-making. At that time, none of the members had the TCM background. The first committee was held in Nanjing on February 23, 1929. At the meeting, on the grounds of "TCM hinders national medical health", it put forward four proposals for the abolition of TCM, namely "Abolishing Old Medicine to Remove Medical Health Obstacles", "The Unified Registration Measures for Doctors", "Limitation on Time of Registration for TCM" and "Proposed Measures for Applying Regulations to Restrict TCM Doctors and TCM", which are collectively referred to as the "TCM Abolition Act". Finally, it was adopted and merged into the "Principles for Regulating the Registration of Old Medicine", which can be summarized simply as: TCM is not allowed to run schools, "non scientific" news magazines related to TCM are banned, gradually cancel the registration of TCM license, take gradual measures to restrict TCM, and finally achieve the goal of completely eliminating TCM.[1] Subsequently, newspapers in Shanghai and other media first exposed the contents of the meeting of the Central Health Commission, which caused an uproar. On March 17, the Shanghai Association of TCM organized a National Congress of medical groups in Shanghai, gathering a petition delegation in Beijing, and decided to petition various organs of the central government in Nanjing, which eventually disabled the "Medical Abolition Case" and TCM got a slight chance of survival.[2] This is the first great unity of the Chinese medicine circle in China. It is a major movement to strive for their own rights and interests with various forces and channels, which calls for strong reflection of modern Chinese medicine.[3]

The author believes that this movement is actually "the beginning of the history of modern TCM". Before this event or movement, the give and take or integration between TCM and Western medicine was only based on academic interests and written discussion, and whether it was adopted or not depended on the individual choice of TCM. However, after the occurrence of this movement, the various measures tried by the TCM community since the late Qing Dynasty, such as organizing societies, publishing medical newspapers, gathering unions, resorting to the media for public opinion or seeking political and legal equality, had become "necessary" overnight. All the problems, as how to learn Western medicine, how to be scientific, what is the efficacy, what experimental steps for TCM to take, and how to change the TCM knowledge system, had become an urgent issue for TCM to survive and to have the sustainable development in the game. This incident can be the push

---

[1] Wen Xiang, *Transplantation and Transcendence: Medical Administration of TCM during the Republic of China Period*, Beijing: China TCM Press, 2007, pp. 78–83.

[2] Unknown Author, The Preservation and Abolition of TCM, Local News, *Shen Bao*, March 21, 1929, p. 15.

[3] Unknown Author, The Forerunner in the Integration of Chinese and Western Medicine, *Shen Bao*, March 21, 1929, p. 16.

for the Chinese medicine community to make rapid changes in all aspects, resulting in huge differences and the widened gap between modern Chinese medicine and TCM.

In terms of historical research and thinking on practical problems, Lv Simian, one of the modern historians, was appreciated by the author paramountly. Lv was low-key and down-to-earth. Although his academic brilliance is not as dazzling as that of Fu Sinian, Gu Jiegang and other scholars of the Republic of China period, his writing achievements far exceeded those of most scholars during that period. He also wrote *Exploring the Medical Classics* and laid the foundation for the well-known work *On the Origin and Development of Chinese Medicine.* Lv once said: "In teaching, I disagree with the so-called 'doing academic research for the sake of pure academic studies'. Why? There are more people doing practical things than those that are good at theory. A theory can be more proved by practices than by books, which could be mistaken. All the theories have to be founded on the basis of facts, and the book knowledge can be used to make up for what is missing in practice as the support to complete the cycle".[4] Historical research must be combined with practice in order to be used in the discussion of history. Lv also said that if history is divorced from real life, it is high "drama". Historians can not be ignorant of contemporary situation, by studying indoors day and night to make the discoveries of the world. This is his practical understanding of the function of history.[5] The above is based on the author's experience. As the main body of Chinese medical history research, TCM not only continues to exist, but is filled with vitality. It is valuable in most historical relics and literature and is one of the best historical topics in exploring the outlet for modern Chinese culture. This is also what the author seeks from the readers: in addition to gaining historical knowledge, the readers are expected to reflect on the development and positioning of modern TCM, not to compete with Western medicine, but to treat diseases to help the world and benefit all mankind. Only with the above-mentioned could this book be endowed with "life"—the "life" given by Chinese medical history and culture. Under the challenge of the West, with twists and turns, it is revitalized, proudly moving forward in its own way.

Finally, I would like to express my gratitude. The old edition of this book has gained the appreciation from many scholars. Prefaces were written by Mr. Lv Fang-shang, Huang Yichao, Zhang Henghong, Zhang Zheja, Liu Shiyong, Su Yizhang separately. Other academic seniors, fellow TCM doctors and friends whom I want to thank can be found in the old self preface "Introspection of A Historian's Life and Research", which will not be repeated in this book. Upon the new publication of this simplified Chinese character version, Professor Yu Xinzhong at Nankai University wrote a new recommendation preface, which added a lot of luster to the book. In 2006, when I first published my paper on medical history in the mainland, I was

---

[4] Lv Simian, Self-portrait—Summary in the Learning of Three Oppositions and Thought Formation,*Research on Historical Theory,* 1996 (4), pp. 58–59.

[5] Lv Simian, Reading Methods of Chinese Historical Records, *Four Kinds of Historiography*, Shanghai: Shanghai People's Publishing House, 1991, pp. 46–48.

invited by Mr. Yu to publish this book in the mainland. This opportunity is also particularly meaningful at the moment. In addition to new content, the book also includes new chapters, and it is comprehensively "slimmed down" by eliminating lengthy footnotes as much as possible, so as to make it more readable. After all, the text is more concise with some new ideas. Finally, I would like to thank Mr. Yu Zuozan, the former general manager of the Zhonghua Book Company of the Shanghai Branch, and Ms. Wu Yanhong, the editor-in-chief, for all their support given to the publishing work during this period. Their enthusiasm for editorial work and their unique insight in selecting books are the important promoters for the publication of this book.

Zhengzhou, China Kuoli Pi
December 2018

Acknowledgments In presenting this translation work, I have the profound gratitude and appreciation for the author Mr. Pi Kuoli and Zhonghua Book Company. Without their invaluable support, this translation work would be impossible.

This translation project was not just a linguistic exercise, it was a collaborative effort that required the expertise, perseverance and creativity of each member of our dedicated team. Our American expert, Gregg Bellenkes, with his keen eye for details, carefully reviewed and refined the translation, ensuring that it conformed to the grammatical and stylistic norms of the target language; Fu Jiamei and Song Xiupin, the associate professors with linguistic background, were responsible for ensuring the accuracy and fluidity of the terminologies in translation. They were dedicated to the textual research of the medical classics to verify the connotations of the medical terms. The efforts they made in preserving the original intent and style of the text was commendable. Xie Quantang, our historical advisor, delved into the cultural and historical background of the original text, providing valuable insights that enriched the translation with deeper cultural nuances. My thanks also goes to the other members who were involved in the data collection and the interpretation of medical terminologies.

As a testament of the team, we are proud to present this translation to the world, believing that it will serve as a bridge between cultures, bringing the wisdom and beauty of the original text to a wider audience.

Competing Interests The author has no competing interests to declare that are relevant to the content of this manuscript.

Contents

Chapter 1
Introduction: What Is the Correlation Between the History of TCM and Bacteriology

1.1 History of Diseases in TCM—"A Sheer Fabrication"

In the study of Chinese medical history, no one has ever noticed the importance of bacteria, as it has never been in the discussion of Chinese medicine, and how can there be a historical research of it? This reflects a historiographical inversion perpetuated by lay perceptions. It comes from the fact that modern Chinese medicine does not particularly study the problem of bacteria, and modern policymakers seldom incorporate TCM principles into public health strategies, developing vaccines, antibacterial and viral drugs. Given this context, what led TCM to disregard bacteriology in its modern evolution?[1]

Even today, universal antibiotics can be seen in every hospital and clinic, but the problems of bacteria and viruses still plague the medical community. Yang Sibiao, dean of the Medical School of Taiwan University, pointed out that Western medicine today adopts the approach of targeting and eliminating pathogens, and uses stronger drugs to treat stronger bacteria. However, it is impossible to kill all the germs. With the progress of medical technology, high-tech medical treatment will only make bacteria develop drug-resistant mutations. In order to fight against the increasingly mutated bacteria, more and more toxic drugs need to be used to kill them. In recent years, the United States has found that modern medicine is more costly, new problems have been caused by antibiotics. As medical costs escalate annually, both the insurance industry and government health agencies grapple with impending financial collapse.

[1] The reflection from "modernization" to "modernity" represents a change, which reverses the past view of modernization and Westernization as a magnificent evolutionary process, and also points out the inherent limitations and repressive nature of the original modernization theory. Modernization should not be regarded as the product of monistic single line historical teleology, but should be understood in a pluralistic historical space. The author believes that the example of the history of modern Chinese medicine is a model. The development of Chinese medicine has not completely shifted to the West as expected, which is also one of the presuppositions of the general framework of this book. Xu Jilin & Chen Dakai (eds), *The History of China's Modernization, Vol. 1, (1800–1949)*, Shanghai: Xuelin Publishing House, 2006, Preface, pp. 1–6.

© Zhonghua Book Company 2026

K. Pi, *The Contest of Modern Chinese and Western Medicine*,
https://doi.org/10.1007/978-981-95-2832-5_1

Why did the dean, who had the Western medicine thinking and many years of clinical experience, make such statements? Isn't the antibacterial history of TCM worth exploring and using for reference? What alternative thinking do we have when dealing with bacteria?

Most people do not particularly think of the invisible enemy of "bacteria". What many people described is only the specific disease and its impact. In the works of Albert Camus (1913–1960), an existentialist writer who won the Nobel Prize for literature in 1957, the plague is "a cunning and tenacious enemy; it is a scheming organizer".[2] Historians rarely discussed bacteriology. Being more specialized, it can only be found in special books on medical history.[3] It is obviously of great historical significance, as according to the research of archaeological anthropologists on demography, the number of lives taken by infectious diseases in history far exceeds that in war and natural disasters, while bacteria and viruses surpass fungi and parasites,[4]which were the main cause of ancient human death.[5] It must be noted that in fact, about 75% of infectious diseases were caused by "viruses" rather than "bacteria". But the microscope in the early Republic of China period could not effectively observe the virus. Although many diseases were caused by viruses, they were still said to be caused by "bacteria". Influenza is the best example. Coupled with the problem of translation, the pathogen of fever was generally referred to as "bacteria". The term "microorganism" was also used quite often at that time. As this book does not include the discussion of parasite history, it is not used as a proposition so as to avoid misunderstandings.

Another view for the cause of diseases, based on the Chinese people's traditional cognition of TCM diseases, interprets it with "Qi". In the field of the TCM history, the treatment of "exogenous fever" (hereinafter referred to as "fever") was

---

[2] Albert Camus, translated by Meng Xiangsen, *The Plagues*, Taipei: Laurel Book Co., Ltd., 1996, p. 170.

[3] For general works, see William Bulloch, *The History of Biology,* New York: Dover Publications, 1979, c1938. As for the impact of bacteriology on history, for example, David S. Barnes discusses the historical role of bacteriology by taking the impact of bacteriology on the great progress of public health in France at the end of the nineteenth century and the changes in people's social life as examples. See David S. Barnes, *The Great Stink of Paris and the 19th Century Struggles against Filth and Germs,* Baltimore: John Hopkins University Press, 2006. As for the example in the United States in the early twentieth century, it can be found that with the strengthening of bacterial theory, it has a greater impact on the Americans' daily life and medical testing. See Nancy Tomes, *The Gospel of Germs: Men, Women, and the Microbe in American Life*, Cambridge, Mass.: Harvard University Press, 1998.

[4] Li Shunbao & Wang Zili (eds), *The Complete Book of TCM Diagnosis and Treatment of Viral Diseases*, Beijing: Xueyuan Publishing House, 2007, Preface, pp. 1–3.

[5] Western anthropologists put forward an interesting view that there were no antibiotics in ancient times, and people lacked the knowledge of correctly replenishing water when the body was dehydrated, which might lead to the higher mortality rate. In addition, the young individuals represented by a large number of minors' bones found in archaeological sites may have perished of an acute explosive infectious disease, because the bodies had not had enough time to produce observable bone pathological changes. From Charlotte Roberts & Keith Manchester, *Archaeology of Diseases*, Ji'nan: Shandong Pictorial Press, 2010, p. 179.

regarded as the beginning of the treatment of all diseases, and it was usually synonymous with infectious diseases.[6] According to medical history and clinical treatments, modern scholars have concluded that there are several diseases that can be included in the category of so-called exogenous diseases. However, the focus of this book is the history of diseases from the invasion of the human body by exogenous six pathogenic factors (including epidemic Qi) into the human body, and the history of diseases caused by the damage of viscera. Qi and blood, which are equivalent to infectious diseases in Western medicine. The history of these diseases discussed by TCM is mainly recorded in the medical books of typhoid and warm diseases.[7] Shi Yiren (1896–1966) once said: "Typhoid, warm and infectious diseases (i.e. febrile diseases in a broad sense) are not only the focus of disputes between TCM and Western medicine, but also the gateway of classical and seasonal schools of TCM. The treatment of typhoid and warm disease is the essence of TCM".[8]

This shows the importance of the fever system. If the impact of modern bacteriology on China is put into the TCM history, the exploration of the transmission and change of the fever system can not only help us understand the development context of Chinese medical history, but also further explore the historical transformation in disease interpretation in the contest between TCM and Western medicine, which is of great significance. Moreover, each era has its own unique diseases and

---

[6] With regard to exogenous febrile diseases, Chinese medicine has the following definition: "Febrile diseases refer to acute feverish diseases caused by exogenous six pathogenic factors, that is, typhoid and warm diseases (including plague) in TCM". Quoted from Shi Yiren's original work, adapted by Shi Zhensheng, *Essentials in the Treatment of Exogenous Fever*, Beijing: China Medical Science and Technology Press, 1996, p. 1. In the field of TCM, "exogenous febrile disease" includes many schools and theories spread and created in ancient times, such as "popular typhoid fever school", "warm disease school", "epidemic warm disease school" and "classic typhoid fever school". They contended with each other, but also influenced each other and integrated their findings into theory. From Shan Shujian & Chen Zihua (eds), *Clinical Demonstrations of Ancient and Modern Famous Doctors. Exogenous Fever, Vol. I,* Beijing: China TCM Press, 1999, Summary, pp. 1–19. During the SARS epidemic, more attention was once again paid to the history of exogenous febrile diseases. Many people wanted to seek practical experience in treatment from the history of febrile diseases. Microorganisms were not included in the observation of various infectious diseases in Chinese medicine, but these diseases were named after the most consistent clinical feature-"fever". Therefore, it is also called "febrile disease" (Cao Dongyi (ed.), *The Battle of TCM Heroes against SARS—SARS and the Study on the TCM Standard of Diagnosis and Treatment of Exogenous Febrile Diseases,* Beijing: Ancient Books of TCM Press, 2006, pp. 4–13). Why add the word "exogenous"? The reason is that many kinds of febrile diseases, some of which have visceral damage or inflammation (such as arthritis), and even parasitic diseases, share the same fever symptoms. It is impossible for this discussion to go across this wide borderline. Wind, cold, heat, dampness, dryness, fire (six pathogenic factors or six Qis), as well as "toxin" or "epidemic Qi", all come from the outside world. They added "exogenous" to distinguish it from other febrile diseases.

[7] Ke Xuefan, Zhao Zhangzhong & Wang Yuqun (eds), *Differentiation and Treatment of Exogenous Diseases in TCM*, Beijing: People's Health Publishing House, 2001, the definition in the preface. However, it must be emphasized that this book is still based on the traditional category of typhoid and warm diseases. Parasite disease is left aside as it involves miscellaneous diseases in internal medicine and children's diseases.

[8] Shi Yiren, *Typhoid and Warm Diseases in TCM*, Taipei: Lixing Publishing House, 1995, Preface, p. 3.

medical culture. Combing the disease history of different periods not only has practical or reference significance in medicine, but also creates a new theme for historians to explore historical issues and construct social and cultural features. As Chen Shengkun (1951–1989) said[9]: "Looking at the evolution of Chinese history from the perspective of disease history, the result will be completely different from the vision obtained by analyzing or explaining history from the perspective of political history and family history".[10]

1.2 Discussion on Medical History Research

The research of medical treatment and disease history has been well documented.[11] The context of medical history research can be divided into two systems: internal history and external history. Rough as this classification is, it is enough to highlight the distinct characteristics of the development of medical history. This classification will guide us to a new way of thinking in medical history. Strictly speaking, there were not any historians specializing in Chinese medical history initially. Chen

[9] Hong Wansheng, In Memory of Chen Shengkun, A Young Hero in the History of Science, *Science Monthly*, No. 354 (1999.6).

[10] Chen Shengkun, *History of TCM*, Taipei: Shibao Culture Publishing Co., Ltd., 1979, p. 13.

[11] Pi Kuoli, *Body View and Ideological Transformation of Modern TCM—Tang Zonghai and the Era of Convergence of TCM and Western Medicine,* Beijing: SDX Joint Publishing Company, 2008, Introduction; Exploring the Past and Discovering New Methods—A Review of the Research on the History of Modern Chinese Diseases on Both Sides of the Strait, *Journal of History of Taiwan Normal University*, No. 35, (2006.6), pp. 251–278. For more new research, see Chen Xiufen, Medical History Research in Taiwan (1990–2010)—also on Its Relationship with "New Historiography", *Sinology Research Newsletter,* No. 29, (2010.03), pp. 19–28. For the Review of the disease history of TCM, see Lin Boxin, Review of the Research on the Disease History of TCM, *Discourse in Ancient and Modern Times*, No. 14 (2006.05), pp. 98–112. In recent years, there have been quite a lot of other relevant studies from the perspective of modern health history, such as Ruth Rogaski, *Hygienic Modernity: Meanings of Health and Diseases in Treaty-port China,* Berkeley: London: University of California Press, 2004. This book has been translated into Chinese by Jiangsu People's Publishing House (Nanjing). For its book review, see Zhang Shuqing, *Proceedings of the Institute of Modern History, Academia Sinica,* No. 57 (2007), pp. 193–199. Zhang Taishan, *Infectious Diseases and Society in the Period of the Republic of China Period: Focusing on the Prevention and Control of Infectious Diseases and Public Health Construction*, Beijing: Social Science Literature Press, 2008;Liu Ronglun & Gu Yuqian, *A Brief History of Chinese Health Administration*, Guangzhou: Guangdong Science and Technology Press, 2007; Zhang Daqing, *Social History of Modern Chinese Diseases (1912–1937),* Jinan: Shandong Education Press, 2006; Deng Tietao, *History of Epidemic Prevention in China*, Nanning: Guangxi Science and Technology Press, 2006; Wang Shucheng, *Development of China's Health Service*, Beijing: Ancient Books of TCM Press, 2006; Zhu Deming, *History of Zhejiang Medicine during the Republic of China Period*, Beijing: China Social Sciences Press, 2009. However, the research from the perspective of health history is greatly influenced by the history of Western medicine and health. It is debatable how much the characteristics of Chinese society and the actual medical situation can be reflected. In addition, when talking about public health, the role of TCM is often ignored. Even if some individual studies bring it up, they can not explain the in-depth relationship between TCM theory and TCM health. Innovative research methods are definitely needed for a breakthrough. See details below.

Bangxian (1889–1976), Xie Liheng (1880–1950), Wu Liande (1879–1960), even Li Tingan (1898–1948)[12] and Ding Fubao (1874–1952) were doctors, rather than medical historians. In his translated work *History of Western Medicine* in 1914, Ding Fubao stated that "the knowledge of medical history in medical study" is to clarify the breakthrough and invention of medicine as a science in the past. Such a statement can be a progressive view of history. Although his research has the feature of "internal history", he had noticed the status of foreign medicine (for the society and the country) was also in line with the fanfare social history and environmental history today,[13] in the same way as history, geography or pathology.[14] Those are the development context of foreign medical history, which Ding just introduced without putting forward the slogan of studying medical history from the perspective of environment or society. Another example is the *Brief History of National Medicine* written by Qin Bowei (1901–1970), which is mostly to review the achievements and obstacles of medical development in previous dynasties, and provide a solution to the crisis faced by TCM at that time. "Today's medicine is a period of degradation", he said.[15] These remarks may be related to his era, "people are more likely to follow their own era than their fathers' era".[16] Back then, medical history had a striking characteristic of its time, which mostly revolved around doctors and medical development.[17]

It might be better to share Taiwan's medical history research with a wide range of mainland readers. Early scholars studying medical history in Taiwan were mainly composed of doctors or so-called scientists who were also engaged in the study of "internal history". Their ambition to write medical history or translate medical history works is "to have a deeper understanding of the developmental history of medical knowledge and pay respect to their careers",[18] stated in the preface of the *History of Western Medicine*—a book translated by doctors in early Taiwan. It shows that the readers of medical history at that time were still mainly doctors, and it is

---

[12] Li Ting'an, *Introduction to Chinese and Foreign Medical History*, Beijing: Commercial Press, 1947.

[13] The study of disease history in environmental history is also a relatively new research topic in recent years. For the results related to disease history, see Mark Elvin, Liu Ts' ui Jung (ed.), *Episodes of Time: Environment and Society in Chinese History*. New York: Cambridge University Press,1998.

[14] Ding Fubao, History of Western Medicine, *Series of the Republic of China Period, Part III. History of Science and Technology 79*, Shanghai: Shanghai Bookstore Press, 1991, pp. 1–3.

[15] Qin Bowei, *A Brief History of National Medicine*, Shanghai: Shanghai National Medical Publishing House, 1931, p. 22b.

[16] Arabic proverbs quoted by Bullocks. Marc Bloch: *Feudal Society*, translated by L. A. Manyon, Chicago: The University of Chicago Press, 1961, p. 148.

[17] Pi Kuoli, Chinese Medical History Textbooks and Medical History Education during the Republic of China Period, included in Zhang Zhongmin & Zhang Ke (eds.), *Knowledge Production and Cultural Politics in Modern China,* Shanghai: Fudan University Press, 2014, pp. 40–66.

[18] Felix Marti Ibanez, translated by Ye Songshou & Ye Songxi, *History of Western Medicine.* Taipei: Journal of Contemporary Medicine, 1978, Translation Preface, p. 1. Nearly half of the book, from page 96 to page 186, are the works or translations of several doctors, including Chen Shengkun, Ye Songxi, Lai Qiwan, Chen Dingxin and Ye Songshou, from which we can see the desire and interest of the medical community in the knowledge of medical history at that time.

the responsibility of the doctors or educators interested in medicine to write medical history. The research of Du Congming (1893–1986) and Chen Shengkun can be the representatives. Du's achievements are extraordinary. Without knowing that he had written medical history,[19] most people first take him as a scientist and a medical doctor in Taiwan.[20] Chen Shengkun is quite different. His achievements in medical history research surpass his contributions in psychiatry. He is a very special case. He majored in medicine, but loved history and humanities, which brought him a lot of pressure from his family and even finally led to his early death.[21] Being involved in modern medical history, the author was deeply intrigued by his *Modern Medicine in China,* a thin but popular book that the author read many times.[22] Chen's struggle and misfortune highlight the biggest problem in the doctors' study of medical history: being ridiculed for running an irrelevant business! Medical history could not be a tradition of doctors' academic research, which was once true in Taiwan.

From the 1970s to the mid-1980s, the works of Liu Boji, Zheng Manqing and Shi Zhongxu came out successively,[23] which mostly describes the development of medical technology, stages, drugs, major medical events of previous dynasties, biographies of doctors or diseases, for the major purpose of enhancing their confidence in the development of TCM and even Chinese culture by studying the TCM history, or inserting it in the textbooks for medical students. These authors were not all doctors. For example, Liu Ze wrote *History of Chinese Culture* and *Modern History of China*,[24] Liu wrote *Politics of the Spring and Autumn League*, *History of Politics and Religion in the Tang Dynasty*.[25] Therefore, Taiwan had long ago broken the taboo that "medical history cannot be written by non doctors". However, the problem of medical history research at that time was that medical history works written by historians were still amateur or sporadic, which could not become the

[19] Du Congming, *A Brief History of Chinese and Western Medicine.* Taipei: Chinese Canon Editing and Printing Association, 1965.

[20] Yang Yuling, *Du Congming—the Doctor of A Generation*, Taipei: Tianxia Culture Press, 2002; Zheng Zhimin, *Du Congming and the Study of Medical History in Taiwan*, Taipei: China Institute of Medicine, 2005. Recent studies include Sean Hsiang-Lin Lei, *Du Congming's Mystery of Chinese Medicine Research: also on Value-creating Integrated Medical Research*, Science & Technology, Medical Treatment and Society, 2010 (11), pp. 199–284.

[21] For relevant recollections, see Liao Yunfan et al., *A Collection of Dr. Chen Shengkun,* Taipei: Jujing Culture Co., Ltd., 1992, pp. 15–71.

[22] Chen Shengkun's other works include the *History of TCM*, Taipei: Shibao Culture Publishing Co., Ltd., 1979, and the *History of Chinese Diseases*, Taipei: Natural Science and Culture Corporation, 1981.

[23] Liu Boji, *History of Chinese Medicine Vol. I–II,* Taipei: Huagang Publishing House, 1974;Zheng Manqing, Lin Pinshi (eds.), *History of Chinese Medicine*, Taipei: Taiwan Commercial Press, 1982; Shi Zhongxu, *History of Chinese Medicine*, Taipei: Zhengzhong Publishing House, 1984.

[24] Shi Zhongxu, *History of Chinese Culture*, Taipei: Shi Zhengxin, 1991; *Modern History of China*, Taipei: Shi Zhengxin, 1995.

[25] Liu Boji, *Politics of the Spring and Autumn League*, Taipei: the Editorial Committee of the Chinese Series, 1977; *History of Politics and Religion in the Tang Dynasty*. Taipei: Taiwan Zhonghua Book Company, 1974. Liu's works, which are too diverse to be introduced here, can be consulted by the readers.

main body of the research of a generation of historians, let alone the possibility of forming a school.

From the late 1980s to late 1990s, in the field of general medical history, the works of mainland medical history scholars became popular in Taiwan,[26] and the medical history of Taiwan began to transform. It was not until the past two decades that the medical history in the field of new historiography has been dominated by historians. The most important milestone in Taiwan's history of life and medical research is the establishment of "Disease, Medical Treatment, and Culture" team at the Institute of History and Language of the Chinese Academy of Sciences (hereinafter referred to as the "Institute of History and Language") in 1992. In June 1997, the first academic seminar on "Medical Care and Chinese Society" was held. Long before the establishment of the "Disease, Medicine, and Culture" group, Academician Angela Ki Che Leung had already published many articles on medical history, which were closer to the medical history later. On the basis of extensively utilizing the local chronicles of the Ming and Qing dynasties, Leung constructed a possible image of a lower class society, in which the medical relief cause was rooted.[27] Her research covers issues such as doctors,[28] women and society,[29] the underlying medical conditions, and how medical technology is implemented.[30] The history of disease is probably the most distinctive part of Liang's research, such as her early study of smallpox and her later attention to the social and cultural transmission of leprosy and vaccination technology. In her research, she constantly stressed the importance of society and culture to the study of disease history. For example, she believed that vaccination is not derived from the idea of "orthodox medicine" and should be investigated from patients. The popularization of this technology is closely related to businessmen, gentry and local officials.[31] Vaccination is a very special example. The context of the formation and evolution of many diseases should be explored from medical books.

---

[26] Zhen Zhiya & Fu Weikang (eds), *History of Chinese Medicine*, Taipei: Zhiyin Publishing House, 1994.

[27] See Angela Ki Che Leung's early key work, *Charity and Enlightenment: Charitable Organizations in the Ming and Qing Dynasties* Taipei: Lianjing Publishing House, 1997, pp. 67, 95–96.

[28] Anglea Ki Che Leung, Medical Learning from the Song to the Ming Dynasties, included in Paul Jakov Smith & Richard Von Glahn (eds.), *The Song-Yuan-Ming Transition in Chinese History*, Cambridge, Mass.: Harvard University Asia Center, 2003, pp. 374–398.

[29] Angela Ki Che Leung, Women Practicing Medicine in Pre-modern China, included in Harriet T. Zurndorfer & Leiden (eds), *Chinese Women in the Imperial Past: New Perspectives*, Boston: Brill, 1999, pp. 101–134.

[30] Angela Ki Che Leung, A Preliminary Study of Local Medical Resources in the Song, Yuan and Ming Dynasties, *China Social History Review*, Volume III, Beijing: Zhonghua Book Company, 2001, pp. 219–237; Angela Ki Che Leung: Medicine in the Society of the Ming Dynasty, *French Sinology*, Vol. 6, Beijing: Zhonghua Book Company, 2002, pp. 346–347; Angela Ki Che Leung, The Relationship between Diseases and Regions: Views of Medical Circles from the Yuan to Qing Dynasties, in Li Jianmin (ed.), *Life and Medical Treatment,* Beijing: China Encyclopedia Press, 2005, pp. 357–389.

[31] Angela Ki Che Leung, The Evolution of Smallpox Prevention Measures in the Ming and Qing Dynasties, in Yang Liansheng, Quan Hansheng & Liu Guangjing (eds.), *Interpretation of National*

Leung also noticed this. At least in the study of leprosy, she had carried out her textual research on the "disease concept" from past dynasties. However, in her research, "the formation of 'disease concept' is obviously not only a matter of medical knowledge, but also involves complex social and cultural factors".[32] It becomes the unique feature of her research on disease history. Her later research on modern isolation of leprosy also covers the promotion of international factors (tropical medicine and colonialism) and the power of Chinese society itself (the relationship between leprosy and nationalism).[33] Recently, she called the attention of modern medical study in China for the Chinese characters and how western concepts or science take root in China, rather than looking at TCM and Western medicine from a western point of view.[34] She also pointed out that the development of Chinese medicine is the transformation of the internal system, rather than relying on the government or doctors to develop it through scientific experiments. Basically, doctors trained by the government, such as imperial physicians, could not literally lead the development of medical theory.[35] If we try to understand the "transformation" of the medical system, we may explore it from the changes of medical theory itself. She said: "Since the nineteenth century, modern Western medicine has played an important role in China. It is difficult for us to distinguish between traditional medical factors and Western medical factors in the concept of disease."[36] Perhaps, Leung started to realize the diversity of modern Chinese medicine and thus came up with a unique insight: understanding the concept of Chinese and Western medicine at the same time will be a more arduous task in medical history.

Some scholars held that the research of Chinese medical history has always been focusing on medical theory, symptoms, prescriptions, medical records and doctors. In the sense of new social history, the topics of medical history should turn to: the understanding to the cultural significance of the body, the classification of doctors (the relationship with witchcraft, Taoism and Confucianism), the family history of men, women, old and young, the public mentality reflected by medical cultural exchange and medical treatment. This medical history must be "organic and comprehensive" and can become a colorant for the study of ideological history or folk customs. These are significantly different from the medical history study done by doctors in the past. They focus on exploring the problem of where "people" are in history, obviously following the exploration at the level of "people" and "life realization" in

---

History: A Collection of Essays by Mr. Tao Xisheng on Celebrating His Birthday, Taipei: Shihuo Publishing House, Vol. I, 1987, pp. 239–253.

[32] Angela Ki Che Leung, The History of the Evolution of Leprosy Concept, *Proceedings of the Institute of Historical Language, Academia Sinica*, 1999 (70.2), pp. 399–438.

[33] Angela Ki Che Leung, Leprosy Isolation and Modern China, *Historical Studies*, 2003 (5), pp. 3–14.

[34] Angela Ki Che Leung, Medical History and China's "Modernity", *Chinese Social History Review*, Vol. 8, 2007, pp. 1–18.

[35] Angela Ki Che Leung, The History of Disease in Pre-modern China, Kenneth F. Kiple (ed.), *The Cambridge History and Geography of Human Diseases*, Cambridge University Press, 1993, p. 360.

[36] Angela Ki Che Leung, The History of the Evolution of Leprosy Concept, *Proceedings of the Institute of Historical Language, Academia Sinica*, 1999 (70.2), p. 401.

the "new social history". From this point of view, the academic community first saw medical treatment at a social level, and now it has added more topics and implications such as human life and body. On this premise, in addition to Fu Sinian's proposal to apply new tools and new materials, more fields can be explored. The establishment of several "Special Research Laboratories", including Life and Medical History Research Laboratory in the Institute of History and Language, was just the beginning of this attempt.

Li Jianmin stated that what impressed him most about the "disease, medical treatment and culture" seminar group was not the specific research, but the "academic team" formed among his peers. It is unlikely to have a lasting and influential academic tradition without a long-term academic team, plus academic journals were run on and off, the research had to be conducted in isolation, the arguments would be "gone when the person is gone", just like what Gu Jiegang had experienced (1893–1980).[37] At the beginning, medical history study was completely alien in the Institute of History and Language. Take the early seminar on "pure history" as an example. At that time, Lin Fuji wrote an article referring to the question of predecessors in the history circle: how could the Institute of History and Language organize such an "anthropological" seminar? Even anthropologists disapproved of the historical study of this topic. Lin believed that we should break the boundaries of various disciplines and be a "hybrid" in academic studies.[38]

It can be seen that it is never easy for a new field and topic to gain a firm foothold in the academic circles. After all, the scientific and technological integration between disciplines is very important. At the beginning, the institute could carry out the team cooperations based on the "common" topics among different disciplines, such as population, society and culture, and the academic teams could only survive on the premise of mutual assistance. If the central subject was lost, all disciplines would be bound to go their separate ways, which would affect the development of academia. Now, the research of the next generation is more mature and gradually present themselves in public with their monographs.[39]

1.3 Differences Between Internal and External History

In mainland China, it was mostly doctors who wrote history after 1949, rather than historians who even didn't considered themselves being capable of dealing with such a special subject. But mainland scholars gradually saw the shortcomings of "internal

[37] Wang Xuedian, *Li Mei, Sun Yanjie: Gu Jiegang and His Disciples* (Updated Edition), Beijing: Zhonghua Book Company, 2011, pp. 134–142.

[38] Lin Fuji, The "Pure" History, *Discourse in Ancient and Modern Times*, No. 2 (1999.06), pp. 78–82.

[39] Li Shangren (ed.), *Empire and Modern Medicine*, Taipei: Lianjing Publishing House, 2008; Li Zhende (ed.), *Gender, Body and Medicine,* Taipei: Lianjing Publishing House, 2008. Both have been published in simplified Chinese.

history" written by some doctors.[40] Liao Yuqun questioned that with so much research of medical history in the mainland, how can new scholars find the "key spot" in their study? He got the inspiration from the research approach of the Japanese scholar Yamada Kiyoshi: departing from the routine of "achievement" and "scientificity" as that of internal history, focusing on the rational analysis of historical phenomena and ideological context.[41] Is it true that historians have no ability to delve into medical history? Both Chen Yuan (1880–1971) and Chen Yinke (1890–1969) have published articles on medical history. It is not fair to say that they have no medical literacy or what they did is the "external history" of historians, for the reason that they had been exposed to medical theories.[42] Chen Yuan studied Western medicine at Boji Medical College run by the American church in 1907, and then transferred to Guanghua Higher Medical School (later renamed as Guanghua Medical School). He was not only a director of the school, but also the first graduate. After graduation, he published many medical history articles, and then gradually turned to historical research.[43] At that time, people's mastery of medical knowledge was different from today, and even everyone was more or less knowledgeable of medical theory. However, there is no doubt that historians will encounter many problems in the history of medical treatment. The same is true of the topic discussed in this book—the history of febrile diseases of TCM. Li Jianmin maintained that the number of internal medicine documents of TCM is huge, especially the documents of fever.[44] Among the traditional "external pathogenic factors", heat disease is also emphasized.[45] No matter what kind of medical history documents have been discussed, historians will encounter

---

[40] The medical history research in mainland China generally does not discuss "internal history" (except for the medical history research done by doctors), but defines the so-called medical history as the history of "medical treatment and society", which is in line with the general direction of research in Taiwan. For reference, see Yu Xinzhong, *Epidemics and Society in the South of the Yangtze River in the Qing Dynasty—A Study of Medical Social History (Revised)*, Beijing: Beijing Normal University Press, 2013; Yu Xinzhong, Past, Reality and Possibility of the Exploration of Chinese Diseases and Medical History, *Historical Research*, 2003 (4), pp. 158–168. In recent years, more and more attention has been paid to the overview of foreign and the latest research on medical and health history. See Yu Xinzhong, Problems and Prospects of Medical History Research in China Today, *Historical Research*, 2015 (2), pp. 22–27. (This issue is a special number of medical history research).

[41] Liao Yuqun, Mr. Yamada I know, *Discourse in Ancient and Modern Times*, No. 2 (1999.06), pp. 112–113.

[42] Chen Yinque's medical history articles and views on TCM are included in his *A Collection of the Cold Willow Hall*, Beijing: SDX Joint Publishing Company, 2001, pp. 157–160, 176–181, 188–190.

[43] Chen Yuan's greatest contribution is generally considered to be in historical research, including religious history, the Yuan (Dynasty) history, philology, Chinese and western communication history and so on. After graduating from medical school, he was about 28 to 33 years old. He successively published many articles on the history of Chinese medicine in *Medical and Health News*, *Guanghua Medical* and *Health Journal and Chinese and Western Medicine News*. See Liu Naihe, Zhou Shaochuan, et al. *The Complete Compilation of Chen Yuan's Chronology with Pictures*, Shenyang: Liaohai Publishing House, 2000, pp. 39–61.

[44] Li Jianmin, *Hua Tuo's Hidden Surgery—Chinese Medical History of Surgery*, Taipei: Dongda Book Company, 2011, pp. 204–205.

[45] Li Jianmin, *Viewing Chinese Culture from TCM*, Beijing: Commercial Press, 2016, pp. 66–67.

many medical terms. Just for "definition" itself, including clarifying the language changes behind these terms, and their physical meanings, or even theoretical interpretations, many difficulties were involved. For example, when discussing infectious diseases, the terms "plague", "epidemic", "disease", "epidemic disease" and "severe epidemics" are often used in historical documents. TCM uses more professional terms such as "typhoid", "warm", "heat disease", "seasonal Qi (disease)" to explain a common disease with similar symptoms during the same period. It is difficult for these terms to be explained or named with today's certain disease, and modern scholars generally refer to these diseases as "infectious diseases" or "exogenous fever". If we don't dig into the world of medical classics and theories when thinking about the definition of a disease and the meaning of the expressions, we can't interpret a certain disease at all. From the perspective of medical books, the earliest infectious diseases with modern significance were represented by "fever" or "typhoid fever". Therefore, according to the internal classic, "today's febrile is also typhoid".[46] In fact, this classification is very general, because there are no actual prescriptions and discussions. Literally, it only describes the feeling of "fever" when the human body is sick. It was not until Zhang Zhongjing (150–219) wrote *Treatise on Typhoid Fever*, combined with the syndrome differentiation of actual diseases and the treatment of classical prescriptions, that the foundation of clinical medicine was laid.[47] By the end of the Ming Dynasty, after the publication of the *Theory of Warm Epidemics* (1642) by Wu Youxing (1592–1672, style name Youke), the study of warm diseases began to develop rapidly.[48] Qing Dynasty witnessed the best development of febrile diseases. Ye Gui (1667–1746, style name Tianshi), Xue Xue (1681–1770, style name Shengbai), Wu Tang (1758–1836, style name Jutong) and Wang Shixiong (1808–1868, style name Mengying) were known as the "four masters of warm disease school",[49] symbolizing the era of febrile diseases. Febrile disease has its own system in theory, method, prescription and medicine, forming a relatively complete theory of febrile disease, which is slightly different from the theory of prototyphoid fever.[50]

---

46 Guo Aichun (ed.), No. 31 of Heat Theory, *Interpretations to the Inner Canon of the Yellow Emperor*, Beijing: People's Health Publishing House, 1996, p. 192.

47 Lin Fuji, *The Terminator of Diseases—Taoist Medicine in Early China*, Taipei: Sanmin Publishing House, 2001, p. 53.

48 Meng Shujiang (ed.) *Febrile Diseases*, Beijing: People's Health Publishing House, 1997, pp. 4–5.

49 Sheng Zengxiu (ed.), *On the Four Masters of Warm Disease School*, Beijing: China TCM Press, 2000, p. 1.

50 Marta Hanson once combed the causes of the warm disease school. In addition to the local conditions, Ye Tianshi's own legends and the spread of medical books are also important factors in the formation of this school. She also pointed out an important fact: no matter how the warm disease school explains it, they have always been deeply influenced by the view of "typhoid being caused by cold". This can be seen in many works claiming to be warm disease studies. However, the author believes that most studies only emphasize the "differences" of the cold and heat theory, but ignore their "commonness "and the relationship between the inheritance of the theories. See Marta Hanson: *Inventing A Tradition in Chinese Medicine: from Universal Canon to Local Medical Knowledge in South China, from the 17th to the 19th Century,* (Ph.D Dissertation, University of Pennsylvania, 1997), pp. 268–301. Marta Hanson later rewrote her published papers and doctoral theories into a book, which mainly discusses the cognition of Chinese doctors in school, disease and plague under

It must be noted that they are not two completely opposite and conflicting systems. Febrile diseases not only supplement the deficiency of typhoid theory, but also serve as an assistant to the typhoid theory, so that the theory, diagnosis and prevention of exogenous febrile diseases in Chinese medicine continue to develop in a better direction.[51] Some discussed medicine in the Ming and Qing Dynasties by bringing up the debate of febrile and typhoid, but the summary started from the Ming Dynasty. Doctors began to reorganize the old knowledge system, trying to separate them from the theory of warm diseases. Meanwhile, they also made various textual research and textual exegesis to reconstruct classics.[52] The author does not think that typhoid and warm diseases have become two independent and irrelevant systems. There is another inheritance relationship between the two theories.[53]

If we want to separate typhoid and warm diseases with a clear concept or the concept of today's classification of infectious diseases, it would be difficult to find the common ground at least before the beginning of the Republic of China period. In fact, people differed in their views and preferences. Even the issue of whether typhology or febrile disease system can cover all exogenous febrile diseases or become the orthodoxy of the theoretical system had been a controversial issue among doctors in the Ming and Qing Dynasties.[54] Zhu Peiwen, a famous doctor of TCM and Western medicine (born in the middle of the nineteenth century), said: "The forefather Zhang Zhongjing wrote *Treatise on Febrile Diseases*, based on the essence of *Interpretations* and *Classics on Medical Problems, a*s well as the prescriptions of Yi Yin, to elaborate on the prescriptions of exogenous diseases".[55] "It is either external or internal for all kinds of personal diseases. There are many external symptoms, and the doctor should

the influence of geospatial factors. However, she mainly focused on the theory of warm diseases and seldom analyzed in detail the relationship between the development of typhoid fever school and Western medicine theory. See Marta Hanson: *On Epidemics in Chinese Medicine: Disease and the Geographic Imagination in Late Imperial China* (Abingdon, Oxon: Routldge, 2001. Especially Part III about "early model medical transformations", and also" Northern Purgatives, Southern Restoratives: Ming Medical Regionalism" in *Asia Medicine*, Vol. 2, 2006 (2), pp. 115–170.

[51] Yang Yiye (ed.), *History of Chinese Medicine*, Shijiazhuang: Hebei Science and Technology Press, 1996, p. 140.

[52] Ouyang Bing, The Influence of the Study of Typhoid Fever Theory in the Ming Dynasty on Later Generations, *Journal of Chinese Medical History,* 1995 (25.2), pp. 92–94.

[53] The relationship between the two can also be referred to Zhu Pingyi, Medicine or Buddha: the Medical Market, Medical Knowledge and the Relationship between Medicine and Disease in the Ming and Qing Dynasties, *Collection of the Institute of Modern History, Academia Sinica,* No. 57 (2007), pp. 193–199.

[54] The relationship between the two can also be referred to Zhu Pingyi, Medicine or Buddha: the Medical Market, Medical Knowledge and the Relationship between Medicine and Disease in the Ming and Qing Dynasties, *Collection of the Institute of Modern History, Academia Sinica,* No. 57 (2007), pp. 193–199.

[55] Liu Boji, *History of Chinese Medicine, Vol. II*, Taipei: Huagang Publishing House, 1974, pp. 604–606; Shi Zhongxu, *History of Chinese Medicine,* Taipei: Zhengzhong Publishing House, 1997, pp. 121–122. For a general introduction to the debates of previous dynasties in *Treatise on Typhoid Fever*, see Li Shunbao, *Complete Editions of Treatise on Typhoid Fever*, Beijing: Xueyuan Publishing House, 2000, pp. 1–9.

study them in detail".[56] It can be seen that typhoid fever had often been interpreted as "exogenous disease" in the category of TCM, which was generally referred to as infectious diseases in a broad sense. Febrile diseases and epidemics were regarded as "the feeling of filth, and toxin is the serious syndrome of external infection".[57] The scope of "exogenous disease" is very wide, and doctors in the past had never made a unified definition of it. Instead, all the observed fever, heat and some febrile diseases similar to cold symptoms were summarized, resulting in the continuous expansion of the whole system.

"Typhoid fever" and "febrile disease" are all inclusive concepts. Both are exogenous febrile diseases, which belong to the category of infectious diseases, rather than being referred to as one disease only. They should be regarded as the whole of the "febrile disease" discipline. When discussing the disease history of TCM, we should note that the diagnosis of ancient Chinese medicine is based on "syndrome differentiation". Different people and different diseases use different drugs. Relatively speaking, it is also very likely that the symptoms of the two diseases are the same, that is, the "disease symptoms" are the same, and they were categorized as similar diseases.[58] This is the formation of a system, which is to classify a series of diseases with common principles.

Before modern times, the subject of febrile disease was broad and complex. Scholars mainly focused on the disputes between the "old study of typhoid fever" and the "new study of febrile disease", as well as their differences in theory, development and medication. Fan Xingzhun, in the discussion on the development of febrile diseases in his *A Brief History of Chinese Medicine,* distinguished himself in this area. Liao Yuqun's *The Healing Art of Qi Huang* has the most clear organization of the theories and syndromes. In addition, there are other monographs of the overall research including Zhao Hongjun's *History of Comparative Analysis on Febrile Diseases Between TCM and Western Medicine* and *Cao Dongyi's History of Exogenous Febrile Diseases in TCM*. The latter is more detailed than the former,[59] but the intersection of traditional Chinese and Western febrile diseases was rarely touched since modern times. In other words, "the modern history of fever" has not been explored, which is the original proposition of this book. The author aims to find a feasible and new interpretation of the internal logic of disease theory by combing the modern (historical) transformation of TCM in this discipline.

---

[56] (Qing) Zhu Peiwen, The Ways of Reading, *Compilation of Images of Chinese and Western Viscera* (Lithography of Hongwen Press 1897, collected in the library of Shanghai University of TCM), Vol. 1, pp. 34a–b.

[57] (Qing) Zhu Peiwen, The Ways of Reading, *Compilation of Images of Chinese and Western Viscera,* Volume I, p. 36b.

[58] Ma Jianzhong, *Diagnostics of TCM*, Taipei: Zhengzhong Publishing House, 1999, pp. 1–2.

[59] Zhao Hongjun, History of Comparative Analysis on Febrile Diseases Between TCM and Western Medicine and Cao Dongyi's History of Exogenous Febrile Diseases in TCM, Shijiazhuang: Department of Medical History, Hebei University of TCM, 1987; Cao Dongyi, History of Exogenous Fever in TCM, Beijing: Ancient Books of TCM Press, 2004.

1.4 From the Modern Transformation of Fever

McNeil believed that doctors deal with secular affairs. No matter where they are, doctors cherish these methods that can treat specific diseases. The difference is that doctors in Asia can not innovate once their medical theory and skills meet the requirements of "classics". This may be too arbitrary. McNeil probably wanted to make a comparison: Western doctors would gain more benefits and higher social status when they develop new treatment methods, which motivates Western medicine to actively develop more new treatment technologies and replace the old organizations with the new medical and health system. On the contrary, TCM before modern times never practiced medicine in a modern hospital environment, but only adhered to the ancient authority to obtain the clinical experience.[60] Similarly, Li Jianmin once mentioned the process of "canonization" of classical medicine. "Canon" means that a discipline has some beliefs and ideas. If it is to be reliable knowledge, it must be proved, with the premise that the "foundation" is not to be verified, but to provide a basis for alternative beliefs.[61] Li further believed that "canonization" is a principle of "exclusion", and the so-called parallel theory can be at different levels, and they are by no means equal.[62] The author would still like to ask: since modern times, has TCM been sticking to the "canon" or is it on its way of "re canonization" by absorbing the knowledge of Western medicine (passively or actively) so as to confirm or eliminate some knowledge?[63]

Ever since modern times, Western medicine and its study of infectious diseases have been further introduced, and the gap between China and the West widened. The author believes that the first stage of the integration of TCM and Western medicine should be the dispute over the body and physiological concepts of TCM and Western medicine. This part of history has been discussed in the book *Body View and Ideological Transformation of Modern TCM—Tang Zonghai and the Era of Convergence of TCM and Western Medicine*. Zhang Zhongmin also studied the physiology textbooks in the late Qing Dynasty and believed that physiology was the main body of health knowledge in the late Qing Dynasty.[64] At that time, the translated Western medicine books were mainly physiology, not microbiology.[65] In the second stage, the conflict between Chinese and Western medicine increased day by day because of the dispute of bacteriology after the Republic of China period, Western medicine

[60] William H. McNeill, translated by Yang Yuling, Plague and Man—the Impact of Infectious Diseases on Human History Impact, pp. 276–278.

[61] Li Jianmin, Pursuing the Passion of Chinese Medicine, *Thought 4: the 1970s in Taiwan*, p. 254.

[62] Li Jianmin, Pursuing the Passion of Chinese Medicine, *Thought 4: the 1970s in Taiwan*, pp. 254–255.

[63] See Chapter 2 for details.

[64] Zhang Zhongmin, *Publication and Cultural Politics: A Study of "Health" Books in the Late Qing Dynasty*, Shanghai: Shanghai Bookstore Press, 2009, Chapter 2.

[65] Yuan Yuan, *Modern Physiology in China (1851–1926)*, Shanghai: Shanghai People's Publishing House, 2010.

had gradually completed the unification of medical term translations in China.[66] On the other hand, China's medical universities had also successively set up bacteriology courses, and some had also set up bacteriology research departments. Most of the teaching materials were in foreign languages such as English. Regarding the conditions of the country and teaching needs at that time, some microbiology books compiled or translated by themselves gradually came out. These translated medical books further expanded the theory and knowledge of Western medicine to the whole country. The core of medical discourse kept on changing, and eventually became the way of defining diseases. In this context, the voice for a precise definition of national diseases was also growing. Yu Yunxiu (i.e. Yu Yan), who was strongly opposed to the traditional theory of TCM, said: "In ancient times, there was no theory of infectious diseases. They were all taken as miasma, the action of heaven, and the sneakiness of ghosts. Therefore, when an epidemic arises, there must be a spell of using prayers to the gods". "As for today, except for China, few people in the civilized society of the world are not aware of bacteria, nor the fact that the pathogens of infectious diseases are caused by bacteria. All public health practices were generic and were improved as time went by. Looking around China, it is still the same as before. Whenever there was a disease, ghosts and gods would be brought up before medicine. There was no idea how to take preventative measures to avoid it, and thousands of people died of epidemics."[67] Yu's words reflect that classical medicine had neither the study of infectious diseases, nor the knowledge of bacterial pathogens and preventive measures, and its concepts were inaccurate and primitive. Different from the dispute between Chinese and Western physiology and body view in the initial stage of modern times, TCM then could stick to its own theory and keep a dialogue with Western medicine, and the overall pressure was relatively small. However, after the Republic of China period, the guiding ideology and foundation behind health work was actually bacteriology. The knowledge of Western medicine was fully recognized by the whole nation. The pressure of "abolition" of TCM theory became a surging tide. The conflict was inevitable, and TCM circle was also engaged in a comprehensive debate.

Sean Hsiang-Lin specialized in studying the transformation of TCM in all aspects during the Republic of China period. He believed that what TCM should be more responsible for is the patients rather than the definition of the disease itself.[68] When bacteriological knowledge was introduced into China, the causes of the disease were discovered one after another, thus the major responsibility of doctors shifted from

---

[66] Zhang Daqing, Gao Xilan-The Promoter of the Standardization in the Translation of Medical Terms, *Historical Materials of Chinese Science and Technology*, 22.4 (2001), pp. 324–330; The Unification of Early Medical Terms: the Efforts and Influence of the Medical Expo, *Journal of Chinese Medical History*, 1994 (24.1), pp. 15–19.

[67] Yu Yunxiu, *Infectious Diseases*, Shanghai: Commercial Press, 1929, Preface, p. 1.

[68] Sean Hsiang-Lin Lei, Responsible Doctors and Patients with Faith—the Debate between Chinese and Western Medicine and the Transformation of the Relationship between Doctors and Patients during the Period of the Republic of China, *New Historiography* 14.1 (2003), pp. 62–69.

patients to the disease itself.[69] TCM must gradually recognize and pursue the new trend of a single cause of a disease.[70] However, there was still much room for discussion as whether this trend had an impact on the interpretation of diseases by TCM, or how to urge TCM to reinterpret the impact of bacteria and infectious diseases. By using the example of the statement of Patrick Manson (1844–1922) on reversing the western "malaria theory" and his establishment of the etiology of malaria caused by microorganism—plasmodium, Li Shangren tried to explain that the formation of scientific research or theory actually involves highly complex microscope operation technology, the acquisition of research materials, the publication and establishment of research results, which can not be solved from the ancient medical books of TCM.[71] In the monographs on febrile diseases written by Cao Dongyi in recent years, the summary of this period only cites Zhang Xichun's effective use of Chinese and Western medicine (aspirin gypsum decoction) in treating febrile diseases, affirms the support of some Western medicine to TCM, and says that this is "the combination of TCM and Western medicine". This conclusion and analysis are too presumptous based on the fact that the problems encountered by TCM during the Republic of China period were obviously more complex.

If we examine it from the perspective of disease classification in today's Western medicine (most of today's disease concepts are also western), the classification method of traditional medicine is rough and inaccurate. For example, the so-called "typhoid fever" in Western medicine is a systemic acute infectious disease caused by typhoid bacillus. Its clinical symptoms include a prolonged fever, relatively slow pulse, splenomegaly, rosette, abdominal distension, special toxified symptoms, leucopenia, and a few cases can be complicated with intestinal bleeding or perforation. Typhoid bacilli are excreted with wastes and spread through contaminated hands, tableware, food, beverages, flies or cockroaches. Daily contact is the major way to spread pathogens.[72] This includes the patient's physical symptoms, etiology, infectious agents and routes of infection. This is the classification and interpretation of disease knowledge brought by the introduction of modern Western medicine, which is very different from the body views of TCM such as "typhoid fever" or "febrile disease", "six meridians" or "Wei, Qi, Ying, Blood" and "three energizers". If modern doctors put forward the terms "typhoid fever" and "febrile disease", most

[69] That is, the research transformation from "individual" to "object" in Western medical cosmology. See N.D. Jewson, The Disappearance of the Sick-man from Medical Cosmology, 1770, 1870, *Sociology*, 1976 (10): pp. 225, 244; Li Shangren, From Patient's Story to Medical Case Record—the Turning Point of Western medicine from the Middle of the 18th Century to the End of the 19th Century, Ancient and Modern, *Discourse in Ancient and Modern Times*, No. 5 (2000), pp. 139–146.

[70] Bridie Andrews, Tuberculosis and the Assimilation of Germ Theory in China, *Journal of the History of Medicine and Allied Sciences*, 1997(52), pp. 114–115.

[71] Li Shangren, Manson, Ross and the Material Culture of British Tropical Medical Research at the End of the 19th Century, *New Historiography* 17.4 (2006), pp. 145–194; *The Parasite—Scientific Practice in the Study of S. Mansoni Filariasis*, Collection of Institute of History and Language, Academia Sinica 78.2 (2007), pp. 225–259.

[72] Huang Gaobin, Xie Xianchen & Chen Yinglin (ed.), *An Overview of Infectious Diseases in the Mainland*, Taipei: Mainland Affairs Council, 1996, p. 27.

patients would be confused, as it pertains to our acquired knowledge, the names of the diseases have been standardized by the terms of Western medicine. This process began during the Republic of China period.[73] Then, from the standpoint of TCM, how can they resolve the past academic disputes or differences between "typhoid fever" and "febrile disease", and appropriately integrate the western theory in the theory of body cognition to establish a new and convincing knowledge pedigree?

Since modern times, what changes have taken place in exogenous fever, including typhoid and warm diseases in TCM? Fan Xingzhun believed that: "Throughout this century, the works of febrile diseases were numerous, but most of them copied Chen Yan or described one or two new diseases as a cover. Soon their studies gradually diminished, and were replaced by the study of new diseases derived from febrile diseases. The writings of febrile diseases, like the general theory, no longer had its heyday as in the past. Also, the general theory in the name of febrile diseases, as a matter of fact, just focused on one infectious disease". Fan held that either "typhology" or "febrile disease" in modern times is a weak notion, with the only "general theory" left.[74] If the two representatives of febrile diseases are only "general", how can they keep their practicability in modern times and even after the Republic of China period? Fan's inference is debatable. However, the definition of various diseases in modern Chinese medicine febrile diseases has obviously been greatly impacted. The current research cannot explain the relationship between TCM febrile diseases and infectious diseases. Instead of repeating the understandings of TCM on individual infectious diseases, this book would directly explore the disputes between "pathogenic Qi" and "bacteria", the theoretical core for the definition of "infectious diseases" in TCM and Western medicine, and examine the impact of these disputes on the TCM development in febrile diseases, as well as the historical context of changes represented by these discussions.

As for the interpretation of terms, take Chinese society as an example, it is understandable that influenza was regarded as "pathogenic cold". The "scientific term" and "common term" still coexist today.[75] However, the exogenous diseases of TCM can also be taken as "the sniffles", "cold" or "catching cold", which are too complex and difficult to distinguish. For example, Yu Yunxiu said, "typhoid fever and ordinary wind pathogen cannot be separated at the beginning of a fever". It is true that what is called exogenous diseases in Chinese medicine is also called febrile diseases, but the scope is so wide that it turned out to be "completely indistinguishable".[76] In the autumn of 1918, the outbreak of influenza, which described by Yu Yunhou as "very rampant, causing many deaths, spreading all over the world, such as Britain,

[73] For a preliminary introduction, see Deng Tietao (ed.), *Modern History of TCM*, Guangzhou: Guangdong Higher Education Press, 1999, pp. 93–100; Zhao Hongjun, *The History of Modern Debates between TCM and Western Medicine*, Shijiazhuang: Hebei Branch of Integrated TCM and Western Medicine Research Association, 1983, pp. 236–242.

[74] Fan Xingzhun, *A Brief History of Chinese Medicine*, p. 240.

[75] Yu Yunxiu, *Influenza, Infectious Diseases*, p. 35.

[76] Pi Kuoli, Epidemic Diseases and Social Response during the Republic of China Period—A Regional Comparative Study of the 1918 Pandemic in Beijing, Tianjin, Shanghai and Shaoxing, *New Historiography* 27.4 (2016), pp. 57–107.

the United States, Germany, France and Japan, besides China". When infectious diseases become the common enemy of mankind, there must be a unified model of a disease term, prevention law and diagnostic rules among the international community with frequent exchanges, so as to prevent their spread. Ever since the end of the nineteenth century, it has been compulsory world widely for most infectious diseases to be defined, and China was no exception. Human body itself was interpreted as the most critical factor in maintaining healthy. In the competition between the two disease interpretation systems of Chinese and Western medicine, there would also be a transformation in the view of some disease processes (such as infection) and the response of daily care such as the technology of recuperation (TCM style nourishment).

Generally speaking, with a few exceptions (such as surgical leprosy, tuberculosis, etc.), the vast majority of infectious diseases can be classified as febrile diseases. As for the syndrome differentiation theory of TCM, it is impossible to analyze the etiology and causes of infectious diseases in modern ways. TCM adopts another theoretical framework. Like the theory of typhoid fever, febrile diseases were first aimed at epidemic infectious diseases, but their clinical application was not completely limited to the treatment of epidemic diseases and exogenous diseases. In fact, they both developed and expanded in response to the further understanding of diseases in the medical system. When Western medicine was introduced, TCM still adhered to its own principles in the treatment of epidemic diseases. This tendency further increased the differences between Chinese and Western medical systems in disease cognition. In 1880, Karl Eberth found typhoid bacteria in the bodies of typhoid patients. By 1900, paratyphus was further confirmed.[77] In modern times, infectious diseases were regarded as a "living organism" that "cannot exist without living beings".[78] However, before the Republic of China period, TCM had attached importance to abstract philosophical thinking. Instead of intersecting with external microorganisms, the body view of disease was related to climate (such as six Qis), environment (such as North and South) and invisible "Qi". In the early years of the Republic of China period, even though the TCM technology of treating diseases was no less than that of Western medicine, the pressure of uncertain definitions of diseases, due to the different views on diseases, would be directly passed on to the bewildered patients. Therefore, how to face the major changes in disease interpretation brought about by the prosperity of bacteriology was an unavoidable problem for TCM during the Republic of China period.

At the beginning of the Republic of China period, Xie Liheng said: "There are different theories of TCM and Western medicine, the terms of physiology are different, and the inference of pathology are different– from bacteria to six pathogenic factors. Therefore, the diseases can differ in terms of their names, causes and pathology. If there is no profound research on TCM and Western medicine, how

---

[77] Hiroshi Ishikawa, translated by Mu Liang, *Medical History*, Taipei: Taiwan Commercial Press, 1968, pp. 171–172.

[78] Sigerist, Henry S., translated by Gu Qianji, reviewed by Hu Shi, *People and Medicine*, Taipei: Taiwan Business Press Museum, 1967, p. 101.

can there be the convergence!"[79] Whoever understands some of TCM and Western medicine would know that the unification of the disease names of TCM and Western medicine would cause big trouble in communication. Ma Guangya (1914–2005), a famous TCM expert in Taiwan, once said: "There are dozens of treatment methods for a disease in TCM. It is really difficult to integrate and unify the disease names". "If we want to unify the disease names of Chinese and Western medicine, how can Western medicine cooperate with the unification of the disease names of the six meridians in *Treatise on Typhoid Fever*?"[80] Yes, unifying disease names is an ideal and a goal, but what achievements did modern Chinese medicine have in dealing with this? The "dispute of unifying disease names" that arose in 1931 was actually a push to the traditional academic of TCM by the forces of policy, Western medicine and patients. What we focus on and want to pursue is: how doctors change their statements, or how to convince TCM that the inherent thinking mode is trustworthy. If not, what have they changed and defended? This is an intriguing topic of medical history. Moreover, we should not only look at the pressure from Western medicine, but also look at the disease names of Western medicine or the mode discussed by bacteriological definition, the responding mode of TCM, and how TCM fought against bacteria.

1.5 The New Medical History—"Multi-dimensional Medical History Research"

"TCM antibacterial history" seems to be a topic that had never been attended to. The exploration of what TCM had neglected in the past and more research topics in medical history reminds the author of what Fu Sinian once said:

> When an area of knowledge is not established as science, it must have a wide range and it cannot be distinguished from other knowledge. When it first becomes science, it must try to merge with other types of knowledge. As learning is always related to each other, they are integrated from all directions, since learning can not be established in isolation. Gradually, other types of knowledge became science, each has its own territory, and it is more specified. As a result, to excel in learning, it is better to use Monroe Doctrine than imperialism by having specialized areas of studies, so as to narrow the scope and explore each in more depth. The narrower, the deeper.

In fact, it is generally recognized that social history, cultural history and even medical history are closely related to the influence of western academia. From the beginning of the Republic of China period, scholars have been engaged in western research. Even if the "Western tide" had become a part of China, the trend continued for a hundred years in the twinkling of an eye. No one knows when it will stop. Fu Sinian, who studied abroad and founded the Institute of Historical Language, admired Westernization, for the purpose of "serving the needs of China" as other scholars at the beginning of the Republic of China period. He even felt that it

[79] Wang Mimi & Li Lin (eds.), Research on Tang Rongchuan's Academic Thoughts of Medicine, *Complete Work of Tang Rongchuan's Medicine*, Beijing: TCM Press of China, 1999, p. 640.

[80] Ma Guangya, compiled by Liang Mingda, The Difficulties in Unifying the Names of Chinese and Western Diseases", *A Series of Chinese Medicine Clinicians for A Century. Ma Guangya*, Beijing: China TCM Press, 2001, pp. 287–288.

> was a big shame for Chinese Studies and East Asian studies to be undertaken by Europeans.[81] Even when Gu Jiegang went to teach at Yanjing University hosted by foreigners, Fu Sinian denounced him as "ungrateful" and attacked Gu's academic services for foreigners. It can be seen that Fu hoped to establish the research of Chinese subjectivity. Chen Yinke even resented that Japan was entitled to interpret Chinese history. "People inquired about the history of China to the East Neighbor, which is a humiliation for Chinese scholars."[82]

Li Jianmin believed that in the field of historical studies, medical history has long been regarded as a branch of folk custom, the history of lower class or society, which does not belong to the "upper" gradation of political history and institutional history. However, the ancient medical mentality and its way of thinking are actually inseparable from the literature work of the elite. Medical doctors are also a part of the scholar sect. It is hard to say that they are only a reflection of the life of the lower class.[83] The medical history is also a theoretical component of the upper level. The discussion of the new social history can not be separated from the influence of the so-called "politics" of the upper class, just like what is presented in Sean Hsiang-Lin Lei's doctoral thesis, which highlights the changes of TCM in modern times, along with the fact that TCM communities were committed to obtaining the power conferred to them by the state. Especially after the TCM Abolition Act, TCM actively organized itself, spoke moderately, fought for their status and finally survived.[84] In order to piece together a complete medical history picture between the upper and lower levels, the author believes that it is advisable to discuss the TCM antibacterial history from the perspective of "multi-dimensional medical history research". In addition to studying the TCM special books, we should also see how the people resisted bacteria and try to explain how these interesting cognition took place in modern Chinese history. "Multi-dimensional medical history research" is a method and a perspective, rather than a rigid model. Instead of being a framework, it should be flexibly set to study the specific history of TCM. However, the design of the whole framework structure and the arrangement of chapters should be presented into the following parts: (1) it must be based on the interpretation of literature (medical books, newspapers and periodicals). (2) Regarding literature, there must be a wide range, which can be comprehensive and must be related to politics or society. (3) On the basis of literature, we should sort out the discussion of "internal history". For example, in discussing Qi and bacteria, we should sort out the technical aspects of sterilization and epidemic prevention. (4) There must be a role of "people". In addition to discussing medical classics, we should also pay attention to the characteristics of the era and the contribution of the doctors in its research. (5) Analysis from the perspective of cultural history: in terms of medical history research, the focus is on the relevant

---

81 Liang Qichao, *Methodologies of Chinese History Research*, Taipei: Liren Book Company, 1994, p. 356.

82 For the influence of some western theories on Fu, see Wang Fansen, *Fu Sinian: An Individual in Modern Chinese History and Politics*, Beijing: SDX Joint Publishing Company, 2012, esp. Chapter 2.

83 Li Jianmin, Pursuing the Passion of Chinese Medicine, *Thought 4: the 1970s in Taiwan*, pp. 248–250.

84 Sean Hsiang-Lin Lei, *Neither Donkey Nor Horse: Medicine in the Struggle over China's Modernity*, Chicago: University of Chicago Press, 2014, pp. 67–120.

perspectives of daily life history and body history. In short, the multi-dimensional medical history research is a comprehensive perspective research method, including internal history (literature publication, literature analysis, academic trend analysis) and external history (daily life, society, politics and culture).

The major concern of this new medical history should be the attention to the impact of medical knowledge on people (not only patients in a narrow sense). The interpretation of classical medical knowledge by doctors and patients is a dynamic analysis, sometimes even extended to the expectation of national development.[85] Data from the late Qing Dynasty and the early Republic of China period show that patients at that time often actively participated in the discussion of the diagnosis process, and even questioned doctors with their TCM knowledge. Edward H. Hume (1876–1957), a missionary doctor who came to China in the late Qing Dynasty, found that his Chinese patients would question him from their knowledge of medical books, and even women could use the knowledge of classical medical books to communicate with him about recuperation, including drawing TCM viscera diagrams to explain their condition.[86] It can be seen that the knowledge of classical medicine that we do not understand today may had been familiar to patients in the early Republic of China period, and were even used as a tool to question doctors.

For Chinese people, all theories, such as religion, philosophy, body view, medicine, natural history, martial arts, physiognomy and Feng Shui, are all related to the philosophy of "Qi", and the role of "Qi" is everywhere in the traditional knowledge system.[87] Modern scholars such as Kang Youwei, Liang Qichao and Tan Si also constantly use "Qi" to explain the "foundation" of everything. In fact, there is a corresponding concept of "Qi" in Western vocabulary,[88] which constitutes the basis of the dialogue between TCM and Western medicine in early modern times. In terms of the Chinese view of the universe, the sense of form and Qi can transform all things. As far as the viscera of the body are concerned, its function is the life expression of "Qi".[89] The concept of Qi is based on the theory of Yin and Yang, which regards the human body as an organism. Yin and Yang can divide the internal and external of viscera organs and meridians, physiological function (mutual promotion and restraint between the five elements), position (outside, inside, up and down), etc. It is the basic theory of visceral image theory of TCM. In the late Qing Dynasty, Tang

---

85 The focuses of this book is more on the nation than on the history of TCM knowledge. See Pi Kuoli, *Nation, National Medicine and Patients: Medical Treatment and Body in Modern China*, Taipei: Wunan Publishing House, 2016, pp. 2–15.

86 Edward H. Hume, translated by Du Lihong, *The Common Ground: 30 Years of An American Doctor Living in China*, Beijing: Zhonghua Book Company, 2011, pp. 39–40, 86.

87 For these discussions, see Yang Rubin, *Qi Theory and Body View in Ancient Chinese Thought*, Taipei: Juliu Publishing House, 1993.

88 Seiichi Onozawa, et al., *The Thought of Qi: the Development of China's View of Nature and Human Concept*, Shanghai: Shanghai People's Publishing House, 1999, pp. 512–537.

89 A lot of research is done on Qi in Chinese (medical) culture. See Qu Feng, *Discussion on Clinical Theoretical Thinking of TCM*, Beijing: China Medical Science and Technology Press, 1992, pp. 21–30; Elisabeth Hsu, *The Transmission of Chinese Medicine*. New York: Cambridge University Press, 1999, pp. 58–87.

Zonghai (style name Rongchuan) quoted openly the *The Inner Canon of the Yellow Emperor Interpretations Path of Qi to Heaven* at the beginning of the chapter *Essence of Medical Classics*: "What connects heaven, since ancient times, is the foundation of life, which is based on Yin and Yang".[90] He explained: "Yin and Yang of heaven and earth produce the five movements and six Qis, and the human body develops its viscera on the basis of Yin and Yang".[91] Qi is the foundation of TCM theory of human physiology and viscera, and it is also the principle on which life is created. Although Tang doesn't think that the knowledge of Western medicine based on anatomical methods is wrong, he maintained that Western medicine "can't separate Yin from Yang, knowing the shape but not Qi. Opening the viscera can only examine the shape of dead bodies but not the movement of Qi function of the body".[92] It shows that the TCM Qi theory is very extensive and completely dominates the core of TCM theory. It is not only the basis for static expression, but also a dynamic and flowing material. In addition, Qi is combined with natural views such as climate and geography to become a type of knowledge to discuss and speculate about diseases or famine. It was based on the view that "exogenous fever is no more than six pathogenic factors, and common diseases are normally caused by four Qis". Exogenous fever was also based on this set of variable Qi knowledge.

Qi theory of TCM has the characteristics of being open and explanatory to natural phenomena, and its influence can be seen in almost every system. During the Republic of China period, the TCM Qi theory was frequently challenged, as the West during modern times prevailed with their advanced ships and artillery, as well as their science. The discussion of "Qi" could neither make China prosperous nor solve the problems relating to infectious diseases or health policies. In the *Spring and Autumn of Medical World*, Chen Huangxi attacked those claiming to be "knowledgeable of Qi", who mocked others for their being "superstitious of materials and addicted to machines". Chen believed that the mechanism of the internal organs of the human body is originally a natural machine. He ridiculed TCM by urging it to "take immediate action of inventing your own diagnostic instruments", with the intention to reassure that ancient Chinese doctors did use the devices such as a stone needle, measuring cup, moxibustion needle, decoction and bronze manikin. This is the weapon to compete against Western medicine, rather than the "Authoritative Qi Theory".[93]

Science is to be developed by research, so does bacteriology. It doesn't help in talking about metaphysics. Hu Shi once regarded the success of Pasteur's study of bacteriology as an example of "saving the country through science". In his article *To the College Graduates of This Year* in 1932, he said:

> After being defeated by Prussia, France cut off two provinces and paid 500,000 francs. At this time, Pasteur, a hard-working scientist, stayed in his laboratory all day, doing his chemical

[90] Guo Aichun (ed.), 31. Heat Theory, *Interpretations to the Inner Canon of the Yellow Emperor*, Beijing: People's Health Publishing House, 1996, p. 14.

[91] (Qing) Tang Zonghai, *Essence of Medical Classics*, p. 1.

[92] (Qing) Tang Zonghai, *Essence of Medical Classics*, pp. 2–3.

[93] Chen Huangxi, Qi and Materials, *Spring and Autumn of Medical World*, 1936 (115), pp. 6–7.

> experiments and microbiological research. He was very patriotic, but he was convinced that only science can save the country. He used his whole life to prove three scientific problems: (1) All fermentation is due to the development of a microbe; (2) All infectious disease are caused by the development of a microbe in the organism; (3) The microbe of infectious diseases can reduce its virulence under special cultures and turn it from a pathogen into a drug vaccine for disease prevention. On the surface, these three problems do not seem to have much to do with the great cause of saving the country... Huxley, a British scientist, highly praised Pasteur's achievements in the Royal Society by commenting that the yields from this one person can easily pay off the 500,000 francs indemnity to Germany. Pasteur had all the confidence in science, so he refused to take off from his microscope and laboratory when the country was facing great humiliation. He never thought of being able to pay an indemnity of 500,000 francs by working with his microscope, but before he could see or think of it, he had reaped the miracle of saving the country by science.[94]

Pasteur's miracle was not only to pay an indemnity, but his major discoveries made under the microscope in the laboratory had won worldwide prestige for France. This is called saving the country by science. Another example is the historian Fu Sinian, who was well known in the field of historical study, as well as in the field of medicine for his anti TCM position. It is written in his *On the So-called National Medicine*:

> I remember what Mr. Jiang Menglin told me about himself when he was in middle school. In the late Qing Dynasty, when he was a student in Nanyang public school, the TCM school doctors tried a new medical improvement method at school, that is, to test the body temperature with a thermometer. He didn't know sterilization -- originally, there was no anti quintessence term "pathogen" in the TCM dictionary -- so it was taken out of one person's mouth and sent directly to the mouth of another. During the prevalence of diphtheria, the number of deaths at that school was above that of ordinary citizens. This caused a big chaos. The school doctor was expelled and the school had to be closed by taking a break! Obviously, this is an extreme example, but the danger of plagiarizing something unknown is just like having a grid installed on a wall by someone who doesn't know what the electric current is.[95]

This means that he believed that it is just like building a castle in the air if TCM tries to learn new medical science. There is no term as "pathogen" in TCM. To accept Western medicine and improve Chinese medicine, we must "completely westernize".[96] However, TCM had a set of rejecting rhetoric. Although it recognized the importance of bacteriology and Western medicine material science, it still believed that TCM is more suitable for the constitution of the Chinese people. For example, Lu Shige said in his *Review of TCM and Western Medicine* (1930):

---

[94] Hu Shi, *To the College Graduates of This Year, Narration in My 40,* Haikou: Hainan Publishing House, 1997, pp. 261–262.

[95] Fu Sinian, On the So-called National Medicine, *Fu Sinian's Complete Works, Vol. 6,* Taipei: Lianjing Publishing House, 1980, p. 323.

[96] Fu Sinian said: "All improvement must be based on feasibility. Artemisia can be grafted with chrysanthemums, and wild peaches can be grafted with refined peaches, because they belong to the same species. We can't transplant a person's head to a wood! The progress of Western medicine, up until now, is a systematic knowledge, not a piecemeal irrelevant thing. Its pathological judgment and treatment are consistent. If it is accepted, it should be accepted as a whole. Just plagiarizing some parts would make things worse." Fu Sinian, On the So-called National Medicine, *Fu Sinian's Complete Works, Vol. 6,* Taipei: Lianjing Publishing House, p. 323.

> Chinese and Western medicine are strikingly different. TCM advocates six Qis, while Western medicine advocates micro bacteria. One uses experience as a weapon and the other takes science as a shield, each has its clear-cut stand and won't give in. In terms of form, Western medicine is superior. In terms of treatment, TCM is better. In terms of instruments, Western medicine is the best. In terms of efficacy, TCM gains the upper hand. To meet the world trend, use Western medicine; to match the physique of Chinese people, use TCM.[97]

This theory is fairly flat, but some TCM doctors believe that we should continue to advocate "Qi Theory" and study it from the perspective of science. Shen Lin even said in his *Interpretations of Febrile Diseases*: "The invention of pathology of Qi theory in the human body spread the thoughts of the ancient sages, which brightened the world".[98] This reflects the consistency of the discussion of "Qi" in TCM. On the contrary, the anti TCM Qi theorists say that "Qi" is difficult to explain with specific material concepts. Even the "air" that can be studied also conflicts with it. In 1936, Chen Huangxi published an article in the *Spring and Autumn of Medical World*, saying: "The Qi theory in *Internal Canon of Medicine* can be summarized by the following, that is, 'the sky controls the five positions with five elements, resulting in cold, heat, dryness and dampness. People change the five Qis with five internal organs, resulting in joy, anger, sadness and fear'". All of the above are still "materials" under today's scientific verification. Chen cited the example of modern scientists' classification and discriminated the natural substances into various elements, which delve deeper into the science of "materials". He said, "It's funny to hear 'six Qis, Qi theory' from one or two TCM doctors. If he is asked what are' six Qis? 'He would reply:' air is the Qi that is static, cold and hot are the Qis of relevance; heat, dryness and fire are all hot Qis, dampness is the dense Qi of Yin and Yang, dampness and wind are variable. 'Let's try to count, how many Qis here?" He asked sarcastically: can the air stay motionless? Even children who read the *Textbook of Nature for Primary School* would know that air flows. These "Qi" defenders still insist on their own views, which is truly the "domestic disgrace that can not be publicized". To Chen's bewilderment, the opponents also scolded: "It is the behaviors of abolishing Yin and Yang, pounding six Qis, overthrowing Qi theory, blindly worshiping materials, turning the world into a place of barbarism and perversion". Chen thinks that Chinese medicine should be based on the facts and develop a material science, instead of being linked with Confucius and Mencius.[99]

Some TCM doctors believed that the debate between Chinese and Western medicine has shifted from physiology to bacteriology, and the dispute over the Qi of the body had gradually shifted to the "six Qis" and "epidemic miasma" to the outside world. Lu Jinsheng, a TCM doctor, complained in his *Collection of Medical Manuscripts in Jingjing*:

---

[97] Lu Shige, *Review of TCM and Western Medicine,* 1930. Quoted from Tian Ruohong, Lu Shige's Medical Works and Medical Literature Review (Continued), *TCM Literature Journal*, 2003 (1), p. 24.

[98] Shen Lin, Interpretations of Febrile Diseases, included in Cao Bingzhang's collection: *Great Achievements in Chinese Medicine*, Vol. 18, Shanghai: Shanghai Science and Technology Press, 1990, Shen Lin's preface, p. 2.

[99] Chen Huangxi, Qi and Materials, *Spring and Autumn of Medical World*, 1936 (115), p. 7.

> For diseases, TCM is divided into internal injury and external infection. Wind, cold, heat, dampness, dryness and fire, all those bringing in the disease from the outside, are called six pathogenic factors. Happiness, anger, sorrow, joy, melancholy, shock and panic, which bring in the disease from the inside, are called seven emotions. It is necessary to distinguish between cold and heat, exterior and interior deficiency and excess. Nowadays they are no longer discussed, except for the Western medicine terms like certain inflammations, certain membrane or bacteria. Average Chinese people tend to think that the theory of TCM is unreliable, so they abandoned it and let themselves down.[100]

Lu's rebuttal is not aimless. Zhu Weiju once believed, in his *The Play of Pathology*, that even if the bacteriology of Western medicine is too "universally recognized" for TCM compete with, and the so-called bacterial protozoa is unable to explain the occurrence of diseases.

> The so-called bacterial protozoa can be identified by microscopic examination. It's undeniable that it is indeed of considerable value in the history of the invention of medicine, and his denial that six Qis and seven emotions are one of the pathogens is also too paranoid and it is regrettably incomplete. Why? The reason is bacteria protozoa are pathogens. Without the inducement of six Qis and seven emotions, they have a strong resistance and are strongly anti-virus. Although there are bacterial protozoa, it is difficult to develop.[101]

This attitude of not recognizing bacteriology angered some scholars who believed bacteriology is the base in their support of health modernity. Fu Sinian said, "China is a country with the largest number of infectious bacteria worldwide, and the types of diseases outnumbered those in the rest of the world, so the mortality rate is higher than any civilized and semi civilized human races". Therefore, we must rely on "the intelligence of people who study public health". The so-called national medicine can by no means fulfil this responsibility.[102] Although TCM still claims to be able to treat diseases, Hu Shi held that it is just the countless "old ghosts" in the "pile of papers", who "can eat people, put them under a spell, which would do more harm to people than any kinds of bacteria found by Pasteur". With this believe, it can "catch demons" and "beat ghosts",[103] though not being able to kill bacteria. If TCM is an "old ghost" that can't kill bacteria, it makes people wonder what attitude TCM holds toward the bacteriology of Western medicine, and how will it explain and respond to the sterilization problem?

The purpose of this book is to explore the process of the prosperity, declination or transformation of a discipline in modern times. Looking back on the paradox that still exists today, on the one hand, we are no longer confused about the definition of diseases. In our common health knowledge, terms and concepts such as cold,

[100] Lu Jinsheng, On the Harm of Blindly Following Western Medicine, *Collection of Medical Manuscripts in Jingjing*, included in Shen Hongrui & Liang Xiuqing (eds), *General Views on Chinese Medicine in China*, Taiyuan: Shanxi Science and Technology Press, 1996, pp. 2063–2064.

[101] Zhu Weiju, The Play of Pathology, included in Xing Bin & Huang Li (ed.), *Five Book Reviews of Zhu Weiju's Medicine*, Beijing: Chinese Traditional Medicine Publishing House, 2008, p. 259.

[102] Fu Sinian, On the So-called National Medicine, *Complete Works of Fu Sinian*, Vol. 6, pp. 305–306.

[103] Hu Shi, Sorting out National Heritage and "Beating Ghosts"—A Letter to Mr. Hao Xu, *Narration in My 40,* p. 136.

influenza and infectious diseases have replaced traditional disease classifications or names such as “typhoid”, “febrile” and “plague”. On the other hand, in terms of academic life, typhoid and warm diseases in TCM theory did not perish. In addition to research and teaching, TCM doctors rarely mentioned to patients whether they were suffering from typhoid or febrile diseases. It can be seen that TCM knowledge often presented itself differently. The author expects to take into account both the upper knowledge theory of TCM and the daily care experience of many patients in history, to find out the less known TCM antibacterial knowledge and methods.

Chapter 2
The Convergence of Modern Chinese and Western Medicine Before the Antibacterial Discussion

2.1 Fever Issue at the First Encounter of TCM and Western Medicine

When it comes to the role of infectious diseases in modern society, it can be easily found that whether it is SARS, influenza or avian influenza, modern medical treatments have been able to formulate countermeasures according to the types of pathogens and disease prevention methods, including personal hygiene, vaccine application, research and development of specific drugs, so as to continuously fight against the diseases. However, the diagnosis of the diseases in different periods is often closely related to the doctor's cognition and the development of medical theory, and even to the patient's body cognition, combined with the social environment. Therefore, when describing the diseases, the historical research method is of great significance.[1]

The medical technology displayed by modern Western medicine in China depends on the development of Western medicine. We should first examine the exposition of Western Medicine on febrile Diseases in the nineteenth century. British doctors believed that corrupt substances gave birth to fever through "zymosis". The primitive environment of China became the target of accusation for many Western doctors.[2] However, Western medicine was not very optimistic about the clinical technology of treating fever then. Although various sera and vaccines have been manufactured and applied in Western medicine as early as the end of the nineteenth century, there had been little progress in the drug treatment after the onset of some infectious diseases. Paul Ehrlich developed arsenic based chemotherapy, once known as the "magic bullet", but it was only effective for syphilis, and even if improved, it can only deal with very few germs.

---

[1] This chapter was published in Yu Xinzhong (ed.), *Diseases, Medical Treatment and Health since the Qing Dynasty*, Beijing: SDX Joint Publishing Company, 2009, pp. 189–215.

[2] Li Shangren, *Healthy Moral Economy: Dezhen's View on Chinese People's Living Habits and Health*, Collection of Institute of History and Language, Academia Sinica, 76.3 (2005), pp. 467–509.

© Zhonghua Book Company 2026

K. Pi, *The Contest of Modern Chinese and Western Medicine*,
https://doi.org/10.1007/978-981-95-2832-5_2

It was not until the emergence and efficacy of sulfonamides and antibiotics (penicillin) in 1935 and 1940s that Western medicine could effectively treat many infectious diseases.[3] William Osier said, "Today's young doctors can use more than 20 kinds of drugs to deal with any disease; while doctors in the past could use one drug to treat more than 20 diseases."[4] Many years before the introduction of antibiotics and other drugs, the effect of Western medicine in the treatment of acute fever was relatively low. Most doctors could only remove infected limbs or internal organs, which most patients didn't need, as they would have been dead before the removal unless their immune system could luckily overcome the disease.[5]

Since modern times, Western medicine has been definitely more optimistic in the technology of identifying pathogens than its practical treatment. In the study of infectious diseases, Hippokrates (about 460–377 BC), the father of early Western medicine, only attributed the pathogenic factors to air infection, but what substances in the air caused the disease was still an unsolved mystery at that time.[6] The "germ hunt" of the West after the 1880s exposed more germs that caused tetanus, cholera, pneumonia and diphtheria, all popping up "like fried corn in a pan".[7] Later, the immunological research of Western medicine began to change with each passing day. When Pasteur (1822–1895) put forward the observation of "streptococcus" in 1879, some people still ignored the statement that microorganisms can cause diseases. Robert Koch (1843–1910) demonstrated that bacillus anthracis had caused anthrax in 1876. However, medical talents still refused to accept that microorganisms were the main cause of diseases, and even described this theory as being "unworthy".[8] So, how to describe fever before the official presence of microorganisms?

The physical sickness is one's personal experience. Whether they are the TCM typhoid, febrile or other infectious diseases, the body will go through a process of fever, which makes the patient extremely uncomfortable. Therefore, the "fever" has long been used in the literature of TCM to summarize these infectious diseases.[9] Yun Tieqiao, a TCM doctor in the early Republic of China period, said: "One can not avoid illness, especially fever. This statement is almost irrefutable". "Other diseases are just as common. Febrile diseases are the most acute and changeable. If it is not

---

[3] Roy Porter, *Cambridge Medical History*, Changchun: Jilin People's Publishing House, 2000, pp. 424–425.

[4] For the history of Western immunology, see Chen Dingxin, The History of Immunology, included in Felix Martin Ibanez, translated byYe Songshou, compiled by Ye Songxi, *The History of Western Medicine*, Taipei: Journal of Contemporary Medicine, 1978, p. 93.

[5] Meyer Friedman & Gerald W. Friedland, translated by Zhao Sanxian, *Geeks, Chances and Medical Discoveries,* Taipei: Shang and Zhou Publishing House, 2004, p. 253.

[6] Du Congming, *A Brief History of Chinese and Western Medicine.* Taipei: Chinese Canon Editing and Printing Association, 1965. p. 16.

[7] Bettman. Otto L, translated by Li Shizheng, *History of World Medicine.* Taipei: Minsheng Daily, 1980, p. 553.

[8] Meyer Friedman & Gerald W. Friedland, translated by Zhao Sanxian, *Geeks, Chances and Medical Discoveries,* Taipei: Shang and Zhou Publishing House, 2004, pp. 78–92.

[9] Yun Tieqiao, Narration, Febrile Diseases, included in *The Wisdom of Experts*, Taipei: Huading Publishing House, 1988, p. 1.

properly controlled, the risk is absolutely high. Isn't this the most important fact for everyone to learn?" It can be seen that fever has always been one of the common diseases for Chinese. Modern Western medicine also paid equal attention to fever. For example, Li Shangren indicated that during the First Opium War, the greatest harm to British soldiers was not the war itself, but the diseases, especially the harm of "fevers" and dysentery.[10]

Benjamin Hobson (1816–1873), a British doctor, was the most valued by TCM since modern Western medicine was introduced into China.[11] He set the tone for the fever theory of Western medicine in his medical books. First of all, the term "febrile disease" is a unified noun covering several diseases. In translation, it may be influenced by the "syndrome" of TCM and summarizes the same symptoms of several diseases. Western medicine used to subdivide their symptoms with "heat syndrome" instead of "heat disease". In view of this, Hobson first defined it in his *A Survey of Western Medicine* (1857): "Heat syndrome, which is called fever in foreign language, means heat syndrome in Chinese, is divided into toxic and non-toxic, and the treatment methods are the same".[12] Then he added in *New Theories of Internal Medicine* (1858): "The toxic are epidemic diseases, and the non-toxic are collectively referred to as heat syndrome". Being toxic might mean infectious, and "heat syndrome" should generally refer to all febrile, infectious and non-infectious diseases. Hobson explained: "If fever is caused by other diseases, it can be divided into different kinds, but there is also a syndrome of fever from oneself".[13] The heat caused by lung and kidney diseases belongs to "other (organ) disease", while fever caused from a disease should be a specifical indication of infectious diseases. As for why the fever occurred, Western medicine could not find the definite cause at that time. Hobson said: "The cause of the disease is either internal and external inflammation, or typhoid fever, heat stroke, lack of proper diet, excessive work, panic, and sun exposure".[14] All these are different, and Western medicine also admitted: "It is hard to know the cause of the diseases. "Maybe being caused by infection" means "infection" may only be one of the answers to the question "why do people have a fever". It was based on the description of the symptoms of fever in Western

[10] Li Shangren, British Military Medical Treatment in the Battle of the British and French Coalition Forces, *Collection of Institute of History and Language, Academia Sinica*, 82.3 (2011), pp. 533–575.

[11] Almost all doctors "integrating TCM and Western medicine" have read his book. See Pi Kuoli, Body View and Ideological Transformation of Modern TCM—Tang Zonghai and the Era of Convergence of TCM and Western Medicine, Chapter 2.

[12] Hobson, On Heat Syndrome, *A Survey of Western Medicine*, Jiangsu Shanghai Renji Medical School Collection, Xianfeng 7th Annual, p. 45A.

[13] Hobson, On Heat Syndrome, *New Theories of Internal Medicine*, Jiangsu Shanghai Renji Medical School Collection, Xianfeng 8th Annual, p. 17b.

[14] For detailed description of disease symptoms and signs of gradual recovery, see On Heat Syndrome, *A Survey of Western Medicine*, p. 45a–b and Hobson, On Heat Syndrome, *A Survey of Western Medicine,* pp. 18b–19a. In addition, "sexual indulgence" is also a possible cause of fever.

medicine, which was basically the same as that in TCM then.[15] It is particularly worth mentioning that Western medicine took heat syndrome as a single symptom, and heat syndrome became the general name of several diseases. For example, typhus and dysentery are now commonly referred to as a kind of fever, but Western medicine attributed their individual symptoms to the fever itself, "extending to large and small intestines" and ending up in dysentery; or "two or three days of high fever" was diagnosed as "rash" or "early onset of hemp pox".[16] As stated in *New Theories of Internal Medicine*: "Generally, if it (heat syndrome) gets to a certain part of the body, you can see the symptom in that part".[17] According to current analysis, it may be due to the reason that the pathogen of a single disease was not clearly understood yet. So we have to use the common symptom of "fever" to define several fever diseases and their development.

In addition, the concept of "inflammation" was not found in TCM. Hobson believed that the word "Yan (inflammation)" had the same meaning as the Chinese word "Shao (burn)".[18] In other words, the fever state in exogenous fever was actually similar to "inflammatory syndrome". However, Hobson believed that the names of TCM diseases were mixed and unclear, and "inflammation" was not completely equivalent to heat. Hobson said: "In Chinese medical books, some names do not match the reality.... Some mistakenly refer to the syndrome as the name of a disease. The heat has the inflammation syndrome and heat syndrome, which were both generalized as "heat" in Chinese medicine. Such confusion must be clarified".[19] In Western medicine, "heat" is a physical feeling and a representation of diseases. Hobson recorded in *A Survey of Western Medicine—On Inflammatory Syndrome*: "Heat, pain, redness and swelling are called inflammation... The four syndromes need not be complete. It is possible that reddish heat comes with swelling and pain, one or the other. When there is just one symptom and it dissipates quickly, it is not to be regarded as inflammation".[20] Therefore, the symptom of "inflammation" also includes the component of "heat". The only difference between "inflammation" and heat syndrome is: "it is referred to as 'inflammation' because it covers one part of the body while ' heat' covers the whole body."[21] In other words, the feeling of heat is also likely to be an inflammation, but the area of the inflammatory heat is small, different from heat, which refers to the encompassing of the whole body. It is very confusing if they are not compared in detail. The comparison between the heat syndrome of TCM and the inflammation syndrome of Western medicine continued till the Republic of

---

[15] Hobson, On Heat Syndrome, *A Survey of Western Medicine*, Jiangsu Shanghai Renji Medical Collection School, Xianfeng 7th Annual, p. 45A.

[16] Hobson, On Heat Syndrome, *New Theories of Internal Medicine*, Jiangsu Shanghai Renji Medical Collection School, Xianfeng 8th Annual, p. 17b.

[17] Hobson, On Heat Syndrome, *A Survey of Western Medicine*, Jiangsu Shanghai Renji Medical Collection School, Xianfeng 7th Annual, p. 45A.

[18] Hobson, On Inflammatory Syndrome, *New Theories of Internal Medicine*, p. 12a.

[19] Hobson, *A Survey of Western Medicine,* Introduction, p. 1a.

[20] Hobson, On Heat Syndrome, *A Survey of Western Medicine,* p. 12 A–B.

[21] Hobson, On Heat Syndrome, *A Survey of Western Medicine,* p. 45A.

China period, and became a convergence of Chinese and Western pathology. For example, Qiu Qingyuan (1879–1948) said in the *Collection of Medical Talks*: "For the reference of a disease, TCM would say it's the heat of a certain syndrome, while Western medicine would say it's the inflammation of a certain part".[22]

In fact, according to Hobson, inflammatory syndromes covers many specific diseases, including organ and internal diseases, such as encephalitis and heart inflammation, as well as traumatic inflammation.[23] In this way, "inflammation" itself is the induction of a disease name, and diseases are classified according to the context of "syndrome (redness, heat) presenting diseases (encephalitis, heart inflammation)". John Dudgeon (1837–1901) believed that Eastern people seem to have strong resistance to epidemic diseases such as fever, inflammatory diseases, typhoid or acute respiratory organs. However, Europeans have an "inflammatory constitutions"[24] because they eat more meat. From the literature of modern Western medicine translation, it seems that there could still be a dialogue between Chinese and Western medicine. At the end of the Qing Dynasty, Tang Zonghai took "inflammation" as "fire". If the fire in the human body does not settle its position according to the nature of the viscera, the inflammation syndrome will occur in where it flows.[25] Both the TCM "fire" and the "inflammation" of Western medicine produce fever. A large part of the so-called "heat syndrome" in Western medicine can be used to explain infectious diseases, that is, it can be understood according to the category of exogenous heat disease in TCM. Hobson said: "One kind of toxins can be infectious. The warmth in spring turned to be epidemic in summer. Should there be a discord between times, one sick can infect the people of the whole area".[26] The "warmth" and "epidemic" of TCM can be regarded as the integration of Chinese and Western medicine theories. Though not accurate enough in today's view, the diseases referred to in TCM and Western medicine at that time should be similar.

2.2 Where Did the Epidemic Originate From?

TCM has a long history of treating epidemic diseases. In terms of relevant written records, "epidemic" first appeared in the Yin and Shang Dynasties. The oracle bone inscriptions have the records of "疒 (disease) 伇 (epidemic)". With textual research, scholars believe that the Yin people may judge the severity of the epidemic through divination. *The Classic of Mountains and Rivers* records: "The sight of certain

---

[22] Qiu Qingyuan (ed.), Medicine Chat with A Friend, Collection of Medical Talks, included in *Collection of Rare Modern TCM. Medical Talks,* Lu Zheng (ed.), Hangzhou: Zhejiang Science and Technology Press, 1994, p. 327.

[23] Hobson, On Inflammatory Syndrome, *A Survey of Western Medicine,* Vol. 1, pp. 8B–9A.

[24] Li Shangren, *Healthy Moral Economy: Dezhen's View on Chinese People's Living Habits and Health,* pp. 476–477, 480.

[25] (Qing) Tang Zonghai, Three Character Formula for Dysentery, included in Wang Mimi, Li Lin (ed.), *The Complete Book of Tang Rongchuan Medicine,* pp. 633–634.

[26] Hobson, On Heat Syndrome, *A Survey of Western Medicine,* p. 45B.

animals... Would cause a major epidemic". In the "Le Wei Leaf Emblem" of *Lost Book of Yuhan Mountain House, Vol. 54,* there are five species of "phoenix birds" (phoenix genus). One of them had the "round eyes with a turtle beak", which were followed by epidemics as soon as it made its appearance.[27]

The causes for the occurrence of infectious diseases may be due to social politics, geographical environment, famine, transportation and other factors. Research in China's epidemic history indicates that many infectious diseases were caused by political and military factors before the Sui and Tang Dynasties. After the Sui and Tang Dynasties, geographical environment and transportation were developed, and the frequent exchanges between China and foreign countries led to more infectious diseases.[28] After the Song and Yuan Dynasties, China's political and economic development center gradually moved south. Due to differences in climate and geographical environment,[29] the first infectious disease showed up was mainly related to parasites,[30] and many diseases began to show differences between the North and South regions. These factors indirectly promoted the development and reform of the TCM theory.[31] As the ancients were unaware of bacteria, they could only describe the etiology with the invasion of various "Qis". In addition to "heat", it is believed in TCM that wind, cold, summer heat, dampness, dryness and fire (six pathogenic factors) may lead to infectious diseases. For example, according to *Records of the Grand Historian Records of Money and Commerce*: "It's damp in the south of the Yangtze River, and people died early".[32] This is the combination of environment (natural factors, biological environment and humanistic social environment) and disease causality, which is closely related to the development of TCM. "Dampness" is one of the important factors leading to human diseases. The original meaning of "疫 epidemic" should be related to "役service". Zhang Gang explained in his *An Examination of the Origins of 100 Diseases in TCM:*" In ancient times, those who served in the army were the most hard-working suffering from hunger and cold. Epidemic diseases were most likely to occur among people in service.[33] The ancients also believed that epidemic diseases were brought by ghosts, so there was a saying

[27] Zhang Gang, *An Examination of the Origins of 100 Diseases in TCM*, p. 49.

[28] Zhang Zhibin, Preliminary Study on Various Factors of Ancient Epidemic Diseases, *Journal of Chinese Medical History,* 1990 (20.1), p. 34.

[29] For example, the concept of endemic disease originally was a general term for diseases that were limited to one region without spreading all over. Chen Shengkun, Song's Migration to the South and Endemic Diseases, *History of TCM*, Taipei: Shibao Culture Publishing Co., Ltd., 1979, p. 137.

[30] Saburo Miyazawa, Medical Treatment in the Song and Yuan Dynasties, included in Yabuuti Kiyosi, *History of Science and Technology in the Song and Yuan Dynasties*, Kyoto: Institute of Humanities, Kyoto University, 1967, p. 130.

[31] Angela Ki Che Leung, *Facing Diseases: Medical Concepts and Organizations in Traditional Chinese Society*, Beijing: China Renmin University Press, 2012, pp. 217–251.

[32] Sima Qian, *Records of the Grand Historian*, Taipei: Jianhong Publishing House, 1978, p. 3268.

[33] Zhang Gang, *An Examination of the Origins of 100 Diseases in TCM*, pp. 49–50.

that "epidemic disease, namely service, service of ghosts".[34] These are the superficial understanding of diseases when ancient medicine was still at its primitive stage. Not until the medical discussion based on "Qi", there came a significant change in view of epidemic diseases.[35] As for other pathogenic factors, there has been relatively little discussion on febrile diseases in *Treatise on Typhoid Fever*.[36] Only a few concepts have been passed down, such as "taiyang disease, fever caused by thirst without feeling much cold are febrile diseases", "sweating before feeling hot on the body is wind febrile disease", etc.[37] It was not until the publication of Wu Youxing's *Theory of Warm Epidemics* (1642) in the late Ming Dynasty that another system for treating fever, febrile diseases, found its way into medicine. However, not all doctors believed that the discussion of febrile diseases in *Treatise on Typhoid Fever* was insufficient. For example, Lu Maoxiu (style name Jiuzhi, 1818–1886) in the Qing Dynasty held that typhoid fever was the general name of all febrile diseases in ancient times. The methods of treating febrile diseases were also included in the treatment of typhoid fever.[38] He explained in his *Differentiation of Pueraria and Cinnamomum Branches* and *On Febrile Diseases* that clues for all aspects of diagnosis, syndrome differentiations and treatments for febrile diseases can be found from the "Yangming disease" system in *Treatise on Typhoid Fever*.[39]

Another theory to explain the system of the epidemics is Wu Youxing's *Theory of Warm Epidemics*. He had a similar experience of going through the major epidemics with Zhang Zhongjing. He saw that doctors only used Zhang Zhongjing's prescription to treat the disease at that time, resulting in a large number of deaths. Wu Youxing said: "Of the medical discussions among dozens of authors, they were all about typhoid fever, with much less of febrile disease. All that the medical practitioners

---

[34] Zhang Gang, *An Examination of the Origins of 100 Diseases in TCM*, p. 48; Paul R. Katz, *Demon Hordes and Burning Boats: the Culture of Marshall Wen in Late Imperial Chekiang*, Albany: State University of New York Press, c1995.The research results on epidemics, gods and ghosts.

[35] For example, the concept of "infection" before the Wei and Jin Dynasties involved various ideas of the transfer between Qi, ghosts, rituals and dead bodies. For details, see Chienmin Li, *Contagion and Its Consequences: the Problem of Death Aggregation in Ancient China*, in Yasuo Otsuka & Shizu Sakai (ed.), *Medicine and the History of the Body*, Tokyo: Ishiyaku EuroAmerica, 1999, pp. 201–222.

[36] As for this study, some people explain it by the different climate in Zhang Zhongjing's era, while others explain the omissions in *Treatise on Typhoid Fever* by the differences between the northern and southern regions. For the former, see Lai Wen & Li Yongchen, *History of Epidemics in Lingnan*, pp. 1–26.

[37] Meng Shujiang (ed.), *Febrile Diseases*, p. 5. Marta Hanson also combed the causes of the epidemic warm disease school in On Epidemiology in Chinese Medicine: Disease and the Geographic Imaging in Late Imperial China.

[38] Lu Jiuzhi said: "In ancient times, all diseases caused by wind, coldness, warmth, heat and dampness were called 'typhoid'.... in case of a warm disease, no prescription for typhoid fever was used, and no one knew that warm diseases were originally included in the *Treatise on Typhoid Fever*, the prescription for warm diseases were no other than that for typhoid fever". (Qing) Lu Jiuzhi, Fu Qingzhu & Dai tianzhang, Five Theories on Typhoid Fever, *Complete Collection of Medical Books in Shibu Room*, p. 36.

[39] (Qing) Lu Jiuzhi, Differentiation of Pueraria and Cinnamomum Branches, On Febrile Diseases, *Complete Collection of Medical Books in Shibu Room*, pp. 71–72, 80–81.

recorded and recited were based on typhoid fever and its clinical symptoms. It was rare for the warm diseases to be discovered and distinguished from typhoid fever".[40] Wu recorded the epidemic he had witnessed:

> Since Xinsi year in Chongzhen's reign (1641—translator's note), the epidemic had been spreading, especially in Shandong and Zhejiang Provinces, from north to south. It became worse in May and June and could even get through closed doors. At the beginning, doctors mistreated it as typhoid fever, which had no effect. Or some patients mistook it as being able to heal by itself in 7-14 days and they missed the time for treatment. Some died of delayed treatment, some of the abusive use of severe drugs and some of the disordered intake of drugs. Still some other deaths were caused by poor medical skills of the doctors who used palliative drugs for sever diseases. Though not deadly, the treatment was delayed, which eventually caused death.[41]

Although the experiences of the epidemics were similar, it was quite a long time span from the end of the Eastern Han Dynasty to the end of the Ming Dynasty. The prescriptions for the treatment of infectious diseases in the original *Treatise on Typhoid Fever* were not up-to-date, so Wu wrote *On Warm Epidemics* to present a new thinking on the treatment of febrile diseases. As recorded in *On Warm Epidemics. Miscellaneous Qi*:

> It is difficult to enumerate all kinds of diseases. If the disease is limited in a certain region with shared symptoms, in the open air or in doors, it is due to the current of Qi, that is, miscellaneous Qi. Different diseases are caused by different Qis. Certain Qi can enter into certain viscera and meridians, causing a certain specific disease. Therefore, if a disease is contracted by all people, it is due to a certain Qi, rather than the problems in the viscera and meridians. A disease is not limited to a certain age nor due to luck, but it can happen anytime, in the cities or in the villages. Where there is no disease, it is that the Qi can not settle. Epidemic Qi is also one of the miscellaneous Qis, but it is more than regular Qis. As the diseases it caused are rather serious, it is called epidemic Qi.[42]

Wu believed that all kinds of Qis, collectively referred to as miscellaneous Qi, may lead to epidemic diseases, but "epidemic Qi" is the most serious cause. This theory officially set the tone for the identity of the epidemic and overturned the cognitive system of "being caused by cold" in the past. However, the Qing Dynasty was the most developed era of febrile disease theory.[43] Wu's statement just opened a different way of thinking from *Treatise on Typhoid Fever*, but did not become the only model. His so-called theory of "miscellaneous Qi", which is different from epidemic Qi, was replaced by the theory of "pathogenic Qis" derived from the concept of six Qis by most febrile disease scholars in the Qing Dynasty. Since then, the warm disease system has become more diverse and complex.

---

[40] (Ming) Wu Youxing, annotated by (Qing) Zheng Zhongguang, *Additional Annotations On Warm Epidemics,* Taipei: Xinwenfeng Publishing Company, 1985, Original Preface, p. 1.

[41] (Ming)Wu Youxing, annotated by (Qing) Zheng Zhengguang, *Supplemented Annotations On Warm Epidemics*, Beijing: People's Health Publishing House, 1995, Original Preface, pp. 3–4.

[42] (Ming) Wu Youxing, annotated by (Qing) Zheng Zhongguang, *Additional Annotations On Warm Epidemics*, Volume II, p. 42.

[43] Sheng Zengxiu (ed.), *On the Four Masters of Warm Disease School*, Beijing: China TCM Press, 2000, p. 1.

The chaos of war during the Ming and Qing Dynasties, coupled with foreign trade since the Qing Dynasty, had led to the rapid growth of the population in southern China, quickly turning febrile disease into the synonym of the particular disease in southern China.[44] Among them, Wu Tang divided febrile diseases into wind warmth, warm heat, warm epidemic, warm toxin, summer heat, damp warmth, autumn dryness, winter warmth, warm malaria, and so on.[45] Among them, warmth, heat, summer heat and dryness were generalized as unhealthy Qis, "warm toxin" and "warm epidemic" were caused by the toxic Qis of pandemics and filth.[46] Now these "disease Qis" were all classified as febrile diseases, which dominate the feelings of the body. For example, "dampness" will cause bone and joint pain, as well as stagnation. As Ye Gui said, "cold and fever, body weight, joint pain, are all due to dampness in muscles".[47] This refers to the "hot" feeling of febrile disease and "damp" Qi, because "heat" and "dampness" are both pathogenic Qis and factors of disease occurrence, while headache, body pain and fever can be the symptoms of either. If the former is more serious, the fever will be worse; if the latter is more serious, the body pain will increase. The symptoms of patients became the treatment criterion. In his *Essays of Chongqing Hall*, Wang Shixiong said: "Heat is also damp, which is one of the five Qis. Heat belongs to fire, and dampness belongs to soil, each has the position as one of the five elements. Fire and soil are compatible by nature, so the convergence of heat and dampness makes good sense".[48] Generally speaking, miscellaneous Qi is not only the cause of disease, but also that its attribute dominates the source of body feelings. The fevers described in febrile diseases of TCM are not only symptoms, but also a collection of patients' body feelings, which can not be treated according to its disease name. In TCM theory, there are shared symptoms for some diseases, but rarely a fixed definition for a certain disease name.

Xie Liheng, a medical historian, said in *On the Origin and Development of Chinese Medicine*: "*Treatise on Typhoid Fever* is an ancient book of the Han Dynasty, and febrile disease is a special disease today. It is said that there is no way to cure febrile disease in *Treatise on Typhoid Fever.* It is too pedantic to demand people in the Han Dynasty for curing all kinds of diseases such as febrile disease in later generations."[49] Although ancient books are classic, today's diseases are ever-changing. Interestingly this theory of "being caused by the cold" still exists in the system of treating febrile diseases, and has not been labeled as "being untimely" nor forgotten. For example, Wu Tang held that "cold" was still the main cause of all exogenous fevers, and it was

---

[44] Liao Yuqun, *Qi Huang Medical Knowledge*, Shenyang: Liaoning Education Press, 1991, p. 178.

[45] (Qing) Wu Tang, edited by Yang Dongxi, *Upper Body, A Study on the Analysis of Febrile Diseases*, Xinzhu: Guoxing Publishing House, 1999, p. 32.

[46] (Qing) Wu Tang, edited by Yang Dongxi, *Upper Body, A Study on the Systematic Differentiation of Warm Diseases*, p. 33.

[47] (Qing) Wang Shixiong (ed.), annotated by Chen Hui, *A Survey of Febrile Diseases*, Beijing: Xueyuan Publishing House, 1997, p. 88.

[48] (Qing) Wang Shixiong, Essays of Chongqing Hall, Vol. 1, p. 4. included in *10 Kinds of Reclusive Room Medical Series*, Taipei: Natural Therapy Magazine, 1987.

[49] Xie Liheng & You Zaijing, *On the Origin and Development of Chinese Medicine· Notes of Corrected Medicine*, Taipei: Xinwenfeng Publishing House, 1997, p. 28B.

hidden in the body until spring when it was activated, eventually causing diseases. "Being caused by the cold" was still an important inducement of febrile diseases. When criticizing *Epidemic Febrile Diseases*, Wu Tang said: "without knowing that the underlying Qi is the cause of the disease, nor being able to distinguish between typhoid fever and warm diseases which occurs in spring, he directly cuts off the source of febrile fever, claiming it is not caused by the wind nor cold. Rather than blaming himself for his ignorance, he criticized the fallacy of the classics." "In the severe famine and war period during Emperor Chongzhen, Wu witnessed the blast of the epidemics and he directly criticized the statement 'contracting cold in winter would definitely lead to febrile disease in spring' from the classics. All held their own prejudices rather than the understandings based on the context".[50] From this point of view, most febrile pathologists may still respect Zhongjing's theory. The barriers between typhoid fever and warm disease schools were not as big as we think.[51]

Not to mention the doctors advocating *Treatise on Typhoid Fever*. They mostly held that the difference between the typhoid fever and warm disease school was just an excuse for doctors who were not knowledgeable about *Treatise on Typhoid Fever*. For example, Tang Zonghai thought that *Treatise on Typhoid Fever* contained "the hidden inclusion of all diseases".[52] He refuted many doubts that "all books of later generations followed Zhongjing by only discussing typhoid fever, regardless of febrile diseases". Tang believed that "syndrome differentiation of six meridians" was the outline of Zhongjing's theory of diseases. Zhongjing took into account the Qi of wind, cold and warmth. More importantly, *Treatise on Typhoid Fever* took meridian diseases as the system[53] to classify the symptoms and treatment system of exogenous fever. It did not only take "cold" as the only basis, so that it could be independent of "miscellaneous Qi" and "epidemic Qi". This is the primary condition for the clinical and academic value of the "typhoid" system to continue the treatment of fever. Therefore, in modern times, the TCM disease theory of typhoid verses febrile system could still carry a dialogue with Western epidemiology.

---

[50] (Qing) Wu Tang, edited by Yang Dongxi, *Original Diseases, A Study on the Systematic Differentiation of Warm Diseases*, Hsinchu: Guoxing Publishing House, 1999, pp. 3–4.

[51] For the development of warm diseases in the Qing Dynasty and the debate of the typhoid Vs. warm schools, see Pi Kuoli, The History of Exogenous Febrile Diseases in the Qing Dynasty—the Typhoid Fever Vs. Warm Disease Debate and the Interpretation of the TCM History, included in the Office of Life and Medical History Research (ed.), *A New Theory of Chinese History. Medical History*, Taipei: Lianjing Publishing House, 2015, pp. 475–526.

[52] For Tang Zonghai's thoughts, see Pi Kuoli, *Body View and Ideological Transformation of Modern TCM—Tang Zonghai and the Era of Convergence of TCM and Western Medicine*, esp. Chapter 2 and Conclusion.

[53] Cao Dongyi, *History of Exogenous Fever in TCM*, pp. 10–15.

2.3 The Internal and External of the Human Body in Chinese and Western Medicine—Feelings and Diseases

Fever or heat are the pioneering symptoms of most infectious diseases, which have been discussed for a long time in the history of TCM. *Treatise on Typhoid Fever* records: "taiyang disease accompanied with fever, sweating, pathogenic wind and slow pulse are the symptoms of apoplexy".[54] "taiyang disease, with or without fever, being accompanied with the cold, body pain, nausea, intense pulse in both Yin and Yang, is called typhoid fever."[55] "Fever" is one of the obvious "sensations" of the body. *Epidemic Febrile Diseases* states: "At the beginning of epidemic febrile diseases, one might first feel cold before fever, and then the cold stays until the fever is gone."[56] It describes a physical feeling of more heat than chills. It is said in *Inner Canon of the Yellow Emperor*: "The fever causes sweat, breathlessness and repeated heat, as well as pricking on the skin. The shortage of breath would cause death".[57] It shows the fatal symptoms of fever and the time to prohibit acupuncture. On the whole, the "fever" in febrile diseases in TCM does not just refer to Qi, but a physical feeling of the disease, which is quite similar to modern Western medicine. For example, in *New Theories of Internal Medicine*, Hobson divided fever into three categories: one is "feeling the heat but not cold, day and night"; the second is "feeling both heat and cold, getting worse at times, more serious at night than in the morning"; third, it is similar to "malaria syndrome", presented by "the turns of feeling cold and heat".[58] Like TCM, they all describe the physical feelings of fever and the classification of diseases.

In particular, TCM believes that excessive heat is bad, while Western medicine believes that "heat", as a disease, is harmful to human health, but "heat", as a normal Qi, is an indispensable health element for human function, which is slightly different from TCM. According to *Lessons in Elementary Physiology* (1884) by the British doctor Huxley, it was recorded that the fever of the human body is peaceful at all times, from morning till night, and the limbs are not different from the body.[59] Moreover, the fever is by nature evenly distributed in the human body constantly. The dead become

---

[54] (Han) Zhang Zhongjing, Distinguishing the Pulse Syndrome of Taiyang Disease and Its Treatment, Part I, *Treatise on Typhoid Fever* (Gold Mirror of Medical Forbears Edition), Taipei: Lixing Publishing House, 1985, p. 2.

[55] (Han) Zhang Zhongjing, Distinguishing the Pulse Syndrome of Taiyang Disease and Its Treatment, Part II, *Treatise on Typhoid Fever* (Gold Mirror of Medical Forbears Edition), Taipei: Lixing Publishing House, 1985, pp. 51–52.

[56] (Ming) Wu Youxing, annotated by (Qing) Zheng Zhongguang, The Beginning of the Epidemics, *Additional Annotations On Warm Epidemics*, Taipei: Xinwenfeng Publishing Company, 1985, p. 12.

[57] (Qing) Wu Tang, edited by Yang Dongxi, *Original Diseases, A Study on the Analysis in Febrile Diseases*, p. 14.

[58] Hobson, On Heat Syndrome, *A Survey of Western Medicine*, p. 17b.

[59] Huxley, translated by (Qing) Kong Qinggao, On the Heat of Human Body, *Lessons in Elementary Physiology, Vol. 2*, The original engraving of Boji Medical Bureau, in Yangcheng, Guangxu 10th year, p. 48A.

frozen cold. People will get cold due to wind cold, because the cold stimulates blood vessels, leading to vasoconstriction, and blood cannot transport enough heat to the skin of the human body.[60] In other words, the increase or decrease of heat depends on the amount of blood flow (heat), which is the normal operation of the human body.[61] Therefore, the feeling of fever also has its physiological value. Fever is not only a kind of Qi, but also a standard for judging pathological and physiological conditions, as well as a measure of one's health. Before the bacteria theory was introduced and flourished, it played an important role in Western pathology.

The infectious power of fever is also one of the most important part of medical history. Infectious disease has long been part of TCM. For example, *Origin of Chinese Characters* includes the terms "epidemic, causing a lot of sickness" and "a disease that is epidemic", which shows the infectivity of "epidemic disease".[62] The expression "heavenly disease (i.e. infectious disease) is variable"[63] indicates that the ancients have also learned that the evolution of infectious diseases advanced at a tremendous pace, which explains particularly why many RNA viruses now have high mutation rates and ever-changing characteristics. Over the past 10,000 years, human beings have gone through 300 generations to strengthen their immune system, but for bacteria and viruses, it would take only one or two weeks to complete this process. The efficiency difference between them is as far apart as heaven and earth.[64] There are many methods of classifying diseases in TCM. Although some studies show that the "epidemic" discussed in TCM does not necessarily take "infection" as the only standard of classification,[65] no one believed that the "typhoid fever" mentioned by TCM was about diseases other than infectious diseases. Therefore, using the concept of "infection" to discuss the symptoms of fever is a feasible and appropriate approach. On the contrary, before the theory of bacterial pathogenicity was confirmed, Western medicine used "fermentation" to understand fever. For example, *New Theories of Internal Medicine* recorded: "Rotten grass, rotten wood, moldy gas, which are toxic and infectious to people, can bring the toxin into the blood and cause diseases".[66] In addition, Western medicine at that time believed that the experiments proved that animals would gradually die if they breathe in too much carbon dioxide, so that one major reason for diseases (including infectious diseases)

---

[60] Huxley, translated by (Qing) Kong Qinggao, On the Difference between Winter and Summer on the Outside and Inside of Heat, *Lessons in Elementary Physiology, Vol. 2*, p. 50A.

[61] Huxley, translated by (Qing) Kong Qinggao, On Blood Heat Being Originated from Body Heat, *Lessons in Elementary Physiology*, p. 49A.

[62] Yu Yunxiu, *Meanings of Ancient Disease Names*, Taipei: Free Press, 1972, pp. 148–149.

[63] Xie Liheng & You Zaijing, On the Origin and Development of Chinese Medicine· Notes of Corrected Medicine, p. 26A.

[64] Nesse & Williams, translated by Liao Yuejuan, *Why Do We Get Sick-the New Science of Darwinian Medicine*, Taipei: World Vision Publishing Company, 2001, pp. 14, 72, 82, 86 and 88.

[65] Zhang Jiafeng, *Epidemics and Infections—on the Disease Views in the Medical Books from Wei, Jin to Sui and Tang Dynasties Based on the 'General Treatise on the Cause and Symptoms of Diseases'*, pp. 46–61.

[66] Hobson, A General Introduction to Pathogens and Their Treatments, *New Theories of Internal Medicine*, p. 2A.

is inhaling the toxins of "Qi".[67] There are many toxins in the air, and the dirty environment is more toxic in the air. Hobson pointed out that toxic diseases, which are caused by heat, road pollution and ditch congestion, can be infectious.[68] In fact, at least in the Southern Song Dynasty, Chinese people realized that ditch pollution could cause disease,[69] which share the common ground with the environmental discussion of modern Western medicine, making the dialogue between Chinese and Western medicine possible. Like TCM, the literature of Western medicine also takes fever as "toxin" and associates it with the environmental factors at the same time.

It is very surprising that Hobson explained a lot about the relationship between natural customs and diseases in medical books. In terms of the combination of climate change and environmental factors during the four seasons, Hobson said: "The disease is weather-related, such as febrile disease occurs in spring and summer, malaria and dysentery in autumn and lung disease in winter".[70] This is to summarize the law of the disease occurrences according to the seasonal characteristics. However, according to the opinions of "feeling cold and heat, or facing the east wind", "attacked by cold wind, or living in a dirty and wet place" in *New Theories of Internal Medicine,*[71] its context is quite similar to that of TCM, that is, the cold, heat, wind and wet Qi of nature may lead to fever. In terms of the interaction between personal constitution and environment, Hobson believed that those born in cold areas in the north tend to have cold syndrome; those born in hot areas in the south tend to have hot syndrome. Countries with 40°E to 60°E have moderate temperatures, people there are healthier and livelier than other countries.[72] The environment dominates the occurrence of diseases. With different environments, the human body is also different in their adaptability. Hobson said:

> It is common to consume meat in cold places in the north, as there are more animals. There's an abundance of cereals, fruits and vegetables in the southern tropical countries, which are all the benevolence of God. The adaption of the natural environment and climate would keep diseases away. A lot of death and sickness are caused by dislocation. There are also those who are so used to the life of an alien land and later feel themselves alien to the life of their homeland. Therefore, the adaptability to a place should be the first factor to be examined for a doctor when giving treatment.[73]

---

[67] Hobson, Miscellaneous Descriptions of Medical Science, *New Theories of Internal Medicine*, p. 11A.

[68] For the detailed description of his physical symptoms, see Hobson, Theory of Yellow Syndrome Fever, *New Theories of Internal Medicine*, pp. 19b–20a.

[69] Liang Gengyao, Public Health Problems in the Cities of the Southern Song Dynasty, *Collection of Institute of History and Language*, Academia Sinica 70.1 (1999.3), pp. 119–163.

[70] Hobson, Miscellaneous Descriptions of Medical Science, *New Theories of Internal Medicine*, p. 8B; Hobson, On Heat Syndrome, *A Survey of Western Medicine*, p. 45B.

[71] Hobson, A General Introduction to Pathogens and Their Treatments, *New Theories of Internal Medicine*, Vol. 1, pp. 1B–2A.

[72] Hobson, Miscellaneous Descriptions of Medical Science, *New Theories of Internal Medicine*, pp. 11B–12A.

[73] Hobson, Miscellaneous Descriptions of Medical Science, *New Theories of Internal Medicine*, p. 11B.

When doctors give diagnosis to patients, they need to examine the natural environment of where they live. It was first discussed in *Inner Canon of the Yellow Emperor On the Adaptability to a Different Environment,* such as: "The East is where the world started. The ocean side is the land of fish and salt, where people live on fish and are fond of salt, a style suitable for them. Fish increases heat in one's body, and salt causes blood stagnation. People with dark skin tend to have carbuncle and ulcer". Attaching importance to the relationship between environment and disease occurrence is quite similar to the discussion of modern Western medicine. The British doctor Dudge said in the *Physical Description* (1869): "In the 11th year of Xianfeng's reign (1861), epidemic and yellow fever prevailed, and Doctor Luo treated 370 people. The infections were few in the beginning and then a lot more later, with the symptoms of body pain and fever. It was incurable if delayed. The disease was caused by irregular cold and warmth in spring and autumn. With the sudden cold and heat, blood flew inward and accumulated in the liver which was overloaded".[74] In addition to the season and environment, the condition of the human body itself will also affect the occurrence of fever. Hobson even pointed out that sophistication and poor psychological feelings may lead to fever. The above examples show the diverse discussions from Western medicine before bacteriology was introduced into China before the late Qing Dynasty.

In terms of the treatment of Chinese people by foreign doctors at that time, malaria and cholera were the most serious infectious diseases. As for the infection of cholera, Dudge said: "The diseases occur where there is the most filth in the streets and ditches".[75] The infection of malaria is caused by "the rain falling on the streets and the odor fumigation of the ditch water".[76] These descriptions are consistent with the causes of "heat syndrome" described by Western medicine. In addition, Hobson discussed the cold and heat of the malaria epidemic: "It is possible that it is infected by the toxic Qi, or transmitted due to Feng Shui, or people, or houses and clothes. The toxic Qi enters the blood from the lung, and the blood gradually becomes toxic. This is also the origin of these diseases".[77] It is very similar to the discussion of fever in TCM, which might sound very familiar to Chinese readers, but these diseases were classified as "fever". In a word, there are still many arguments that can be cross referenced between Chinese and Western medicine in terms of the causes of diseases.

---

[74] Hobson, Miscellaneous Descriptions of Medical Science, *New Theories of Internal Medicine*, p. 11B.

[75] Hobson, Cholera, *Physical Description*, p. 3B.

[76] Hobson, Malaria, *Physical Description*, p. 9B.

[77] Hobson, Miscellaneous Descriptions of Medical Science, *New Theories of Internal Medicine*, pp: 10B–11A.

2.4 Chinese Versus Western Treatment and the First Encounter of Disease Prevention

When China first faced a large number of Western medical theories, the relationship between Chinese and Western medicine was not as tense as presented in the political history and diplomatic history, but there were many deja vu occurrences. In fact, there are similarities in the understanding of modern Chinese and Western medicine in the treatment of fever. For example, Hobson stated in *A Survey of Western Medicine*: "It is better for fever to release at the beginning, and the forced sweating method should be applied if the sweat doesn't come out".[78] Compared with Western medicine, "sweating" is an important means of eliminating diseases, whether from the system of typhoid fever or warm disease in TCM. In his *Theory of Warm Epidemics,* Wu Youxing also talked about the "re-occurred fever" after the treatment of the epidemic disease, also known as "re-gathering of pathogenic Qis". The "re-occurred fever" must use the sweating method to force pathogenic Qis out of the body, which is an important method to treat an epidemic.[79] According to Ye Gui in his *A Survey of Febrile Diseases*, when febrile disease begins, "sweat would work and then Qis can be cleared out when they are gathered".[80] In other words, the sweating method can be used for mild diseases at the early stage. There were different treatments during different periods. Sweating methods are like the initial defense against fever, which has been generally approved in Chinese medical circle.

In terms of practical treatment methods, there had been only slight differences between China and the West. TCM is based on a variety of prescriptions, while Western medicine has a wide variety of specific methods. For example, *A Survey of Western Medicine* records the sweating methods of "soaking the feet in hot water" or wrapping the body in several layers of bedding. In addition, the "vomit method" is used to expel the pathogenic elements. "Laxatives" or "diuretics" can be used to treat individual symptoms such as short and astringent urination.[81] Even sweating itself can "cure without medicine", which is quite similar to the traditional treatment of TCM.[82] In terms of drugs, Western medicine uses "vomit medicine"—croton oil, mercury powder, rhubarb and even opium for treatment. Just like the treatment for "fever", "warm water bath" or "sour and vinegar water bath" are also applicable.

If it is "head heat", one can put "ice on top of the head", "pour cold water on the head", "swallow ice" or "drink ice' water" to assist the treatment. TCM must see whether there is "cold aversion" and fever. If there is a cold aversion syndrome with

---

78 Hobson, On Heat Syndrome, *A Survey of Western Medicine*, p. 45B.

79 (Ming)Wu Youxing, annotated by (Qing) Zheng Zhengguang, *Supplemented Annotations On Warm Epidemics*, Vol. I, p. 8.

80 (Qing) Zheng Zhengguang's supplementary annotations, *Supplementary Annotations On Warm Epidemics*, Vol. 1, p. 8; Wang Shixiong (ed.), annotated by Chen Hui, *A Survey of Febrile Diseases*, p. 50.

81 For the above discussion, see Hobson, On Heat Syndrome, *A Survey of Western Medicine*, pp. 45B-46A.

82 Hobson, On Heat Syndrome, *A Survey of Western Medicine*, p. 45A.

the intake of ice, the consequences will be unimaginable. As for the treatment of using ice to alleviate fever in Western medicine, Tang Zonghai at the end of the Qing Dynasty stated, in his *Essence of Medical Classics,* that it is absolutely forbidden. He criticized:

> When a fever occurs, a Western medicine doctor would put ice on patient's chest. The ice can be removed as soon as the fever drops. If the fever is severe and the outside is blocked by ice, the fever will counteract the internal attack and the sick would die of heat toxin. At present, the epidemic in Hong Kong is being treated with Western medicine but many ended with death. For this reason, Hong Kong people fled. However, Western medicine should also be knowledgeable of the alternative plans.[83]

Tang criticized the idea of Western medicine by using "ice" to fight against "heat", which is related to "inhibiting" patients' pain. According to the characteristics of the five elements of internal organs, Tang believed that heat was closely related to the "heart". Suppressing heat with ice would lead to a heart attack and death of heat toxin, so we can't treat fever diseases by only inhibiting "heat".[84] TCM pays attention to the use of drugs to reduce heat, which should be excreted from the body, rather than suppressing heat. In Tang's view, the technology of Western medicine for epidemic treatment is very problematic. In terms of adjuvant therapy, Hobson maintained that it could also be improved by taking drugs for "tonifying the stomach" and "tonifying the spirit", and having more drinks such as vinegar and the juices of sour fruit, like grapes, lemons or oranges. They are all acidity, which have the function of "regulating blood"[85] to help resist diseases.[86] All the above show that there was no one-to-one symptomatic drug in Western medicine but just a general direction for the treatment and recuperation of warm diseases, and most of them were adjuvant treatments and recuperation.

As for the course of fever in Western medicine, in terms of written narrations, Chinese and Western medicine can also be well integrated. Going through the symptoms described in detail by Hobson in the *Theory of Yellow Syndrome Fever*, we can find that "fever", "aversion to cold", "pulse number", "severe thirst for water", "vomiting", "hair blemish",[87] as well as critical symptoms such as "disordered speech" and "unconsciously touching the bed or clothing" are consistent with the TCM terms which can find their equivalents in a foreign language. In addition, it is worth mentioning that the most serious syndrome of warm disease in TCM is called "the entry of heat into the pericardium".[88] There are pericardial syndromes

---

[83] (Qing) Tang Zonghai, The Damage to the Five Internal Organs, Vol. II, *Essence of Medical Classics*, Taipei: Lixing Publishing House, 1998, p. 114.

[84] TCM also focuses on releasing "heat" out of the body, which is to expel heat toxin from the body rather than to inhibit it, and it is one of the important arguments of modern TCM against bacteriology.

[85] Hobson, On Heat Syndrome, *A Survey of Western Medicine*, p. 46A.

[86] The above information is quoted from Hobson: Theory of Yellow Syndrome Fever, *New Theories of Internal Medicine*, pp. 20A–B.

[87] Hobson, Theory of Yellow Syndrome Fever, *New Theories of Internal Medicine*, p. 20A.

[88] Ye Tianshi said in the chapter of Febrile Disease: "When febrile pathogenic factor is in the body, it first invades the lung and reversely transmits to the pericardium". Wu Tang also said,

such as clinical high fever, dizziness and delirium, which Western medicine refers as "brain involvement".[89] Although there are differences in the perception of heart and brain, it might all related to the main viscera that manage human life,[90] which can still be regarded as a similar description of the last stage symptoms of fever in both TCM and Western medicine. However, there were still differences. If Western doctors believed that suffering from fever will lead to weakness, "chicken porridge, beef broth" should be the right food.[91] But, he also said: "it is better to control the diet and eat healthily, which is the way to prevent the disease from coming back".[92] "In the Arctic countries, it is appropriate to eat meat only, as meat can generate blood and heat. It would be deadly for Africans and Indians in the Southern part of the world to have the same kind of fat and greasy food every day".[93] Therefore, it is no good to have excessive food as it would aggravate the febrile disease. TCM believes that "tonic" is absolutely taboo in most cases of febrile disease. *On Warm Epidemics* records that a patient named Shen Yinlai in Wujiang, Jiangsu Province, had a bad temper and suffered from hematemesis. As a result, he was infected with the disease, and had the symptoms like fever, body pain and hematemesis, which was quite severe. The doctor gave him ginseng for more nutrition, only to find out that what he had was the epidemic. He was vomiting blood and ended in death.[94] The discussion of related dietary issues will be continued in Chapter 8 of this book.

In terms of prevention thoughts, ancient China had its own set of health care methods, and the thought of avoiding and preventing epidemics has been established for a long time. During the Ming and Qing Dynasties, the scientist Fang Yizhi (1611–1671) said in his *A Little Knowledge of Physics* that "when the epidemic arises, the whole family would be infected. The patient's door should be filled in with ropes to fit in the gaps along the walls, which is a way to prevent infection." Doctor He in Dantu said: "When entering the house of epidemic patients, one preventative measure is to smear sesame oil in the nose, then burn the paper to make one sneeze, or wear the Jade Pivot Elixir." Even a fire attack is used to eliminate the pathogenic spirit of the epidemic.[95] The rulers of the past dynasties in China also set the policy to

"If the lung disease spreads inversely, it is the pericardium disease." When the febrile disease is not treated, the febrile pathogenic factor is directly trapped in the hand-foot-pericardium from the lung meridian. Clinically, there are high fever, dizziness and delirium for pericardial syndrome. See (Qing) Wu Jutong, Li Shunbao (ed.), *Collected Annotations and New Theories on the Differentiation of Epidemic Warm Diseases,* Vol. 2, Beijing: Xueyuan Press, 2005, p. 338.

89 Hobson, On Heat Syndrome, *A Survey of Western Medicine*, p. 18A.

90 Pi Kuoli, Body View and Ideological Transformation of Modern TCM—Tang Zonghai and the Era of Convergence of TCM and Western Medicine, Chapter 8.

91 Hobson, On Heat Syndrome, *A Survey of Western Medicine*, p. 19A.

92 Hobson, On Heat Syndrome, *A Survey of Western Medicine*, p. 19B.

93 Hobson, Miscellaneous Descriptions of Medical Science, *New Theories of Internal Medicine*, p. 11B.

94 (Ming) Wu Youxing, further annotated by (Qing) Zheng Zhengguang, *Supplementary Annotations On Warm Epidemics*, Vol. 1, p. 33.

95 (Ming) Fang Yizhi, Epidemic Prevention, Vol. 5, *A Little Knowledge of Physics*, Taipei: Taiwan Commercial Press, 1978, p. 123.

fight against the epidemic, which was what happened in the Han Dynasty. It was recorded, "those suffering from the epidemic spent all their money for treatment. Money was given by the government to the family of the deceased, five thousand for the burial of more than six corpses, three thousand for four corpses and two thousand for two corpses".[96] There are countless other examples of epidemic prevention and rescue.[97] For example, before the Yuan Dynasty, there were preventive and therapeutic drugs such as "golden boiled water for coffin breaking", "powder of Holy Lord" and "tiger-head ghost killing therapy".[98] In the Qing Dynasty, there were quite a lot of preventive drugs similar to "anti-plague pill" and "sacred anti-plague pill". It is said in the *Supplementary Clinical Guide*: "The burning of the herbal medicine can stop the epidemic from spreading. Burning it in an empty room could exorcise pathogenic spirits".[99] Therefore, TCM has long had its methods of preventing and treating diseases. Today we are trying to solve the problem of how to integrate Chinese and Western cultures. Hobson once said: "(Fever) is being infected, probably for the patient's insanitary clothes, and the pathogenic Qi in where they were sitting and lying".[100] Such views, combined with the vigorous development of western public health since the early nineteenth century, promoted the requirements of clean environment, proper residence and personal hygiene being introduced into China with the knowledge of Western medicine at the time.[101] For example, in *A Survey of Western Medicine*, the methods to prevent infection are described as the following:

> No weak nor people suffering from hunger are to be in the room of the sick. When feeling the pulse, the doctor should also be full and avoid the breath of the patient, so as to prevent infection. Those around the sick should be old rather than young, as it's easier for younger people to be infected. Don't wear the clothes of the sick, and don't taste the leftover food of the sick. The house should be open, and household utensils, clothes, urinals should be cleaned frequently.[102]

This knowledge of hygiene and disease prevention is a two-way reminder to doctors and patients. The requirements of a clean environment and the cultivation of personal hygiene habits are the best guarantee to keep away from diseases. Seeing the poor living environment in modern China, Hobson put forward many ideas: "The small and thick curtains in China are most likely to accumulate toxic air".[103] He told

---

[96] (Han) Ban Gu, annotated by (Tang) Yan Shigu, Yang Jialuo (ed.), *The New Revised Collection of Han History with Two Kinds Sets Annotations*, Taipei: Ding Wen Book Company, 1983, p. 353.

[97] Fan Xingzhun, *History of Chinese Preventive Medicine Thought*, Beijing: People's Health Publishing House, 1955.

[98] (Jin) Ge Hongzhuan, supplemented by (Liang) Tao Hongjing, further supplemented by (Jin) Yang Yongdao, edited by Shang Zhijun, *Supplement to Zhou Hou Prescriptions*, Hefei: Anhui Science and Technology Press, 1996, pp. 54, 78, 79.

[99] (Qing) Ye Tianshi, *Supplementary Clinical Guide,* p. 605.

[100] Hobson, On Heat Syndrome, *A Survey of Western Medicine*, p. 46A.

[101] Ackerknecht, translated by Dai Rongling, *Introduction to Medical History,* Xindian: China Medical Research Institute, 1983, pp. 108–112.

[102] Hobson, On Heat Syndrome, *A Survey of Western Medicine*, p. 46A.

[103] Hobson, On Heat Syndrome, *The New Theory of Internal Medicine*, p. 19B.

Chinese readers: "Rotten grass and leaves, steamy and soaked in the rain every day, will turn toxic air into the lungs and blood, particularly at night. So it is easy for people to get sick in filthy places".[104] The importance of environmental sanitation has been pinpointed. Once febrile diseases are unfortunately around, "quarantine is critical. According to Hobson, there were special vacant rooms in British hospitals to accommodate febrile disease patients, respectively. The reason was "to stop people from gathering in one place so as to avoid infection".[105] It can be seen that the knowledge of western "quarantine" was introduced into China very early. Of course, many of Hobson's theories are questionable. For example, it is stated in *A Survey of Western Medicine*: "After the death of the epidemic disease patient, it is better to burn nardostachys, sulfur, atractylodes rhizome and firecrackers in the room to avoid the epidemic, and the room is not to be inhabited till after a few months".[106] Such methods are susceptible of the partial absorption of TCM and they might even be folk remedies in China. An example cited in *The New Theory of Internal Medicine* is to sprinkle the floor with "vinegar"[107] for disinfection to prevent fever, a way nobody knows why it would work.

As time went on, the new European ideas of epidemic prevention and health preservation were gradually introduced into China after the 1890s. What was the "new" part? When Western medicine was introduced into China in early modern times, the terms of "bacteria" and "microorganisms" were not used. It mostly explained the causes of infectious diseases as the "transpiration of filth and toxin" and the "stuffy air".[108] An article entitled "On the Battle between Man and Microorganisms" in the *Journal of Science* (1876–1892) records: "Most human diseases are caused by extremely fine and micro creatures. How can humans fight against such invisible micro objects?"[109] This new concept of microorganism is different from the Chinese people's traditional concept that the occurrence of disease is due to deficiency, pathogenic Qi, miscellaneous Qi, epidemic Qi and even epidemic ghosts.[110] As far as cholera is concerned, Western medicine could discover its pathogen at the time.

It is recorded in *On the Battle between Man and Microorganisms*: "The proof is to be discovered by carefully examining the cause of the diseases. The related microorganism is called a tail point microorganism as it has the shape like a point of a tail described in Western books, which is actually similar to the shape of a screw drill. Cholera patients tend to vomit and have diarrhea like thin rice slurry, in which

---

[104] Hobson, Miscellaneous Descriptions of Medical Science, *The New Theory of Internal Medicine*, p. 10B.

[105] Hobson, On Heat Syndrome, *The New Theory of Internal Medicine*, p. 18B.

[106] Hobson, On Heat Syndrome, *A Survey of Western Medicine*, p. 46B.

[107] Hobson, On Heat Syndrome, *The New Theory of Internal Medicine*, pp. 19A–B.

[108] Hobson, On the Cause of Disease, *A Survey of Western Medicine*, pp. 7A–B.

[109] Fryer (ed.), On the Battle between Man and Microorganisms, *Journal of Science*, Vol. 6, Guangxu 2nd year, photocopy of Shanghai Library in 1992,the spring of Guangxu 18th year, p. 76.

[110] Lin Fuji, The Terminator of Diseases—Taoist Medicine in Early China, pp. 18–22; Yu Yunxiu, Infectious Diseases, Preface, p. 1.

there are a lot of microorganisms".[111] With the knowledge of pathogens, measures must be taken to prevent the diseases. So the discussion then turns to hygiene: "The walls, floor, beds, bedding and all the rest of the house should be cleaned by killing microorganisms".[112] Attention should be called on in daily life. Other diseases such as tuberculosis, silkworm epidemic, rabies, scarlet fever and smallpox were also discussed. Moreover, an American doctor pointed out, in his *The General Theory on Longevity,* that the flying powder dust in the air contains "toxic organisms". All diseases such as pox rash, tuberculosis, and cholera are "caused by microorganisms".[113] In addition, these diseases "can be infectious, which are also based on this toxin. The extent of infection depends on the number of such microorganisms".[114] So far, the theory of microbial pathogenicity has been established and gradually became the main body of medical knowledge dissemination in China. However, it must be noted that as early as 1910, some TCM doctors maintained that the so-called pathogenic Qis (six pathogenic factors) was what Western medicine called "bacteria", which is carried in the atmosphere or the dust.[115] But at that time, the TCM Qi theory was not yet replaced by the bacteria theory of Western medicine.

Back then, China did not have a clear idea of epidemic prevention, and the government did not pay much attention to environmental sanitation.[116] An article in *Journal of Science* in 1881 criticized: "Health preservation depends on the principles of chemistry. With little knowledge of hygiene, the ordinary people ignored the principles of chemistry".[117] Through the introduction of Westerners, Chinese people gradually understood the commonality of environmental health, chemistry and medicine—health was not just a matter of medicine! On this basis, Westerners also brought Chinese health preservation into the theory of epidemic prevention. The article "On Disease Prevention" published in *Journal of Science* says that "the Qi absorbed by people should be clean", emphasizing the importance of health preservation. In this context, the impact of the environment on human health is discussed again: "In Liverpool, a big city in England, the sewers were blocked, releasing a lot of stench and causing more than 10,000 deaths every year".[118] Therefore, systematical approaches and special attention to the concept of environmental sanitation and

---

[111] Fryer (ed.), On the Battle of Man and Microorganism, *Journal of Science*, Vol. 6, p. 68.

[112] Fryer (ed.), On the Battle of Man and Microorganism, *Journal of Science*, Vol. 6, p. 71. It is said, "Microorganisms of pneumonia and tuberculosis mostly live in the lung, which is the more stabilized area of human body, to do their damage".

[113] J.H. Kellogg, translated by M.C. Wilcox, How to Avoid the Danger from the Air, *The General Theory on Longevity*, Shanghai: Shanghai Meihua Book Company, 1910, p. 101.

[114] J.H. Kellogg, translated by M.C. Wilcox, Microbe in Particles, *The General Theory on Longevity,* pp. 102–103.

[115] He Xichen, Pathogenic Qis in TCM and Microorganisms in Western Medicine, *Journal of TCM and Western Medicine,* 1910 (2), p. 27.

[116] Lai Wen & Li Yongchen, *History of Epidemics in Lingnan*, pp. 560–562.

[117] On the Principles of Health Preservation, *Journal of Science (3),* September, Guangxu 7th Year, p. 535.

[118] Xu Xuecun, On Diseases Prevention, *Journal of Science* (1), March, 1876, pp. 70–71.

health also advanced the old theory owing to the discovery of pathogens. In addition, it also introduces the methods of preventing diseases, eliminating the cause of diseases, treating symptoms and self-recovery of Western medicine. Among them, the health preservation concept of "compliance with the four seasons" in TCM was often discussed in *Journal of Science*.[119]

The westerners' attention to food hygiene was based on the existence of bacteria and microorganisms and led to the discussion about the relationship between people and the health system, which was the early prototype of Western medicine epidemic prevention thought in the late Qing Dynasty and the early Republic of China period. For example, *Journal of Science* in 1881 recorded: "Western medicine says that there are many small and micro sized worms in pork. The meat eaters might carry the worms in them". "When the worms first enter the body, it would cause sudden vomiting and diarrhea or white dysentery for most people. When the worms enter the whole body, the symptoms would be rheumatism or deficiency fever". For food parasite problems, the actual practice of westerners is: "Inspectors were sent to major cities and towns. If the pork sold was discovered to carry the disease, it was to be confiscated so as not to cause harm".[120] This should be a considerable enlightenment for the concept of preventing diseases at that time. Perhaps we eventually found out how this concept was put into action in the progress of several major epidemic prevention campaigns since the late Qing Dynasty and the early Republic of China period. Of course, in *The General Theory on Longevity*, we can still see the discussion emphasizing the "danger of air". The existence of microorganisms is due to a lot of "toxins" in the air, including dust, turbid gas, microorganisms and other substances. The next is the "cold" in the air, which will lead to flu.[121] However, western doctors explained that the cause of flue is not the "wind", but the "cold" in the air, and the cold itself alone will not lead to disease, as is recorded in *The General Theory on Longevity*: "Flu is caused by the sudden heat and sweat of the body, which is invaded by the cold".[122] The cold itself has to be coupled with adverse factors to a cause disease. If the adverse factors are removed by maintaining the environment and keeping the residence clean, the disease can be prevented, which is in line with the emphasis on disease prevention since Hobson. However, the implication is: "The origin of disease is due to the weakness of one's constitution".[123] This is much like today's concept of physical resistance. When microorganisms invade the body, the blood can "clean up" microorganisms. However, when they have bad food or bad sleep, their "cleansing power" will be weakened, leading to the "proliferation of toxic bodies" of

119 Translated by Yin Duanmo, revised by John Glasgow Kerr, A Survey of Medical Theory, *Journal of Science* (5), March, 1891, p. 81.

120 Questions and Answers, *Journal of Science* (3), 1891, pp. 548–549.

121 J.H. Kellogg, translated by M.C. Wilcox, How to Avoid the Danger from the Air, *The General Theory on Longevity*, pp. 98–100.

122 J.H. Kellogg, translated by M.C. Wilcox, How to Avoid the Danger from the Air, *The General Theory on Longevity*, p. 101.

123 J.H. Kellogg, translated by M.C. Wilcox, Microbe in Particles, *The General Theory on Longevity*, p. 104.

microorganisms, which will eventually get out of control, and the disease will arise.[124] At this time, microorganisms have been included in the discussion of health, along with the cold, showing a transitional stage of the development of Western medical theory.

At this time, patients were not only informed of the need for hygiene and tidiness, but also the care of their own physical health, which is similar to the traditional concept of "health preservation". For example, in *The General Theory on Longevity,* the patient with lung disease is instructed to "do the exercise of breathing, which is also the most important part of hygiene".[125] Skin cleaning is another part of "hygiene". Western medicine suggests taking a cold bath to increase blood circulation, with the reminder of using the water with moderate temperature, and that "warm bath should be taken at night and the best time is before going to bed",[126] which is obviously not entirely the requirement of basic hygiene. This "hygiene" is different from what we understand today. It seems that it is also appropriate to translate this term into "health" and "health preservation". In addition, "mental hygiene" belongs to the "method of keeping fit", which should avoid toxifying the mental health with tobacco or alcohol.[127] In this case, various "hygienic" actions were meant to pursue physical health. Furthermore, the relationship among the thickness or the material of clothing and the physical health, along with the concept of doing exercises to fight against disease had also been introduced to Chinese people before the founding of the Republic of China. Namely Western medicine had discussions at more dimensions on "health" besides the mode of public health.[128]

So why didn't TCM actively participate in the public health system of modern countries?[129] This question can't be fully answered in a few words. However, from the above analysis, we can see that TCM, even though with many epidemic prevention practices in history, was still fighting individually with no systematic guidelines.

Fan Xingzhun believed that the Chinese people have all the negative personal health thoughts, which is related to the historical character of TCM.[130] There are two aspects of the concern: one is that various measures for epidemic prevention had never been implemented at the grass-roots level. For example, there was quarantine

---

[124] J.H.Kellogg, translated by M.C. Wilcox, Qi Production and Breathing, *The General Theory on Longevity*, p. 92.

[125] J.H. Kellogg, translated by M.C. Wilcox, Qi Production and Breathing, *The General Theory on Longevity*, p. 92.

[126] J.H. Kellogg, translated by M.C. Wilcox, Skin Hygiene, *The General Theory on Longevity*, pp. 110–112.

[127] J.H. Kellogg, translated by M.C. Wilcox, Mental Health, *The General Theory on Longevity*, pp. 129–130.

[128] J.H. Kellogg, translated by M.C. Wilcox, The Gain and Loss of Clothing, The Effect of Exercises, *The General Theory on Longevity*, pp. 115–118 and 121–123.

[129] The term "public health" is not applicable to explain the concept of health preservation in the TCM theory. Owing to the development after 1949, TCM started to play an important role in the modern public health system. For this history, see Kim Taylor, *Chinese Medicine in Early Communist China, 1945–63: A Medicine of Revolution*, New York: Routledge Curzon,2005.

[130] Fan Xingzhun, *History of Chinese Preventive Medicine Thought*, p. 10.

in ancient China, though far from being popularized. It was also pointed out by the westerners: "In fact, we found that the Chinese people do not know how to isolate infectious patients from normal people".[131] It shows that the basic health knowledge in modern China has not been established at all. Second, the classical exposition at the top of the TCM academic circle had never set the tone for the overall work and direction of epidemic prevention. Except for supplementing the words of saints and therapeutic prescriptions, what the new theory offered at most was just the speculations about the epidemic.[132] Various kinds of pills for epidemic prevention were not fully summarized and collected. They were just folk prescriptions, which were difficult to popularize and spread. As Fan Xingzhun said, this is only "individual behavior" and "fragment experience".[133] For another example, the *Book of Rites·the Later Han Dynasty* recorded the theory of "changing water" and "changing fire" to prevent "febrile disease", which was retained until the Song Dynasty.[134] However, these were all the living rites and customs without any empirical basis and were even superstitious, not being at the level of conversing with the scientific experiments of modern Western medicine. The only statement that can be related to personal hygiene and health was within the scope of health preservation, such as the exhortations to ventilation, spaciousness and moderate temperature in the residence in the *Common Sayings of Lao Lao* in the Qing Dynasty.[135] Even this was still generally intended for the longevity and disease prevention, rather than for infectious disease prevention and control. So it is still far from the health system in the modern sense.[136]

---

[131] I.T. Hedland, translated by Wu Zixuan & Li Xin, *The Courts in the Late Qing Dynasty in the Eyes of An American*, Tianjin: Baihua Literature and Art Publishing House, 2002, p. 158.

[132] To speculate on the law of the epidemic diseases, Wu Tang said: "Seasonal change is the cause of febrile disease". It can not play a positive role in the real epidemic prevention work. See (Qing) Wu Tang, edited by Yang Dongxi: *Original Diseases, A Study on the Analysis in Febrile Diseases*, p. 1.

[133] Fan Xingzhun, History of Chinese Preventive Medicine Thought, Preface, p. 1.

[134] Yu Shenchu, *A Brief History of Chinese Medicine*, Fuzhou: Fujian Science and Technology Press, 1983, p. 140.

[135] Yu Shenchu, *A Brief History of Chinese Medicine*, Fuzhou: Fujian Science and Technology Press, 1983, p. 140.

[136] With the passage of the times, the concept of the word "health" has been constantly transformed. Among them, there are definitely many integrated details between Chinese and Western medicine, presenting a different scene. For more information on the concept of "hygiene" and physical health during the Republic of China period, see Sean Hsiang-Lin Lei, Why Hygiene Is Not Protecting Life—Alternative Understandings of Hygiene, Self and Disease in the Republic of China Period, *Taiwan Social Research Quarterly*, No. 54 (2004.06), pp. 17–59.

2.5 From the Initial Meeting to Being Fake Friends

From the perspective of treating diseases, the "syndrome differentiation and treatment" of TCM focuses on the elimination of human disease symptoms, rather than the accurate identification of disease names.[137] However, Western medicine focuses on the unity and precise definitions of the names of the diseases. "Each disease has its own origin", which can not be explained freely.[138] However, from the significance of the above descriptions of fever, it can be seen that there was a surprising coincidence in the disease discussion of TCM and Western medicine before the Republic of China period. Even if the West used a microscope to confirm the existence of "pathogens" in 1880, it could not be completely resolved in the explanation of epidemic diseases and the dispute between the so-called schools of "miasma" and "contagion".[139] Hobson still explained febrile diseases in terms of climate, seasons, soil, filth, toxins, law of nature, heat sensation and so on. In fact, it is similar to the TCM theory of diseases. The meeting of Chinese and Western medicine at this time was just like deja vu.

It is recorded in the *Confucian Medicine* (1876) in the late Qing Dynasty: "There are many disease names in the western countries, which are not consistent with those in China".[140] However, in terms of fever, the description of various symptoms in TCM and Western medicine is very similar. For example, in the induction of disease knowledge, Western medicine also named the diseases after their "symptoms" in *Internal Medicine Elucidation*, rather than using the name of a disease to summarize the external symptoms. In addition, the compendium of diseases—"On Cough", "On Sneezing", "On Pain" and "On Delirium"—all refer to symptoms,[141] just like "cold" is classified under "sneezing".[142] These examples show that Western medicine also has the purport of "classifying diseases with symptoms" as in modern China, which is not as accurate as names given after the discovery of pathogens. Even with different names for some diseases, there were not too many misunderstandings between Chinese and the West. At least in these translated works, TCM can find the common ground and the familiar knowledge system of "Qi Theory". Moreover, before the invention of antibiotics, the treatment of fever in Western medicine was not much better than that of TCM. At the beginning of the Republic of China period, Chen Cunren (1899–1976) recalled his experience of switching from Western medicine study to TCM in his *Life History of the Silver Dollar Era*:

---

[137] Volker Scheid, *Chinese Medicine in Contemporary China: Plurality and Synthesis*, Durham: Duke University Press, 2002, pp. 200–237.

[138] Yu Yunxiu, *Infectious Diseases*, Preface, p. 1.

[139] Willim H. McNeill, translated by Yang Yuling *Plague and Man—the Impact of Infectious Diseases on Human History Impact*, Taipei: Tianxia Culture Press, 1998, pp. 311–308, 334.

[140] Frederic Willim Headland, interpreted by John Fryer, narrated by (Qing) Zhao Yuanyi, *Confucian Medicine,* Shanghai Jiangnan Manufacturing Administration, Guangxu Reign of the Qing Dynasty, Preface, p. 1A.

[141] John Glasgow Kerr, *Internal Medicine Elucidation*, Original Copy of Yangcheng Boji Medical Bureau, Tongzhi 12th year, Contents, pp. 1A-3A.

[142] John Glasgow Kerr, *Internal Medicine Elucidation*, p. 16A.

> After one year's hard work at Nanyang Medical University, I gradually learned the basics of medicine. Unfortunately, during the summer vacation, I suffered from typhoid fever, and I went to a teacher in the university for treatment. Western medicine had no drugs for typhoid fever and I was asked to lie still for four weeks, taking glucose and vitamin C. However, it was getting worse. Later, my family urged me to see Dr. Ding Ganren in Menghe. After taking his Chinese medicine for five days, the fever was gone. My fourth uncle said: the Western medicine you are learning failed to cure your disease, but Chinese medicine did. You might as well learn TCM instead.[143]

It can be seen that in terms of the efficacy of treatment alone, TCM is backed with its clinical experience and effect in fever treatment. Therefore, TCM in the late Qing Dynasty did not argue with Western medicine, especially with disease treatment. This is an important mentality. As time went by, some changes took place in the understanding of diseases in Western medicine, and the discussion of cleanliness, hygiene and self-healthcare caught more attention with the discovery of pathogens. To some extent, TCM tended to blend into and adapt to the natural environment, while Western medicine tended to control and improve the environment through a set of theories and mechanisms. So far, in addition to drugs, the concept of health and hygienism of Western medicine had been shaped into a magic recipe in fighting against infectious diseases. The ultimate thought of "treating a disease upon discovering what it is" stressed by TCM had been implemented in the mode of public health through the power of Western medicine and the state. This is exactly the start of the critical period for the power growth of TCM or Western medicine.

When modern Western medicine was introduced, it did not have too much impact on TCM in terms of treatment methods, visceral physiology and cognition of pathogenic factors. In this chapter, even the public health thought of Western medicine had not destructively knocked down the statements of TCM. On the other hand, "bacteria theory prevails in human health issues"[144] over time. After the establishment of the Republic of China period, the ruling class was faced with the problem of reshaping the nation and it comprehensively adopted the Western health management system. Under this influence, the discussion of infectious diseases supported by bacterial pathology in Western medicine and a series of knowledge behind it, such as body views, disease definitions and disease prevention concepts, have gradually been accepted by Chinese people and become the standard and common sense for the knowledge of health management. TCM was being openly challenged. After Western Medicine established its specialized and institutionalized epidemic prevention system, the epidemic prevention efforts of TCM were put into the category of "folk prescriptions" for the lack of expertise in modern sense. Chen Bangxian, a famous medical historian (1889–1976), called those who believed folk prescriptions "people lacking common sense",[145] which reflects the unbearable pressure on

[143] Chen Cunren, *Life History of the Silver Dollar Era,* Shanghai: Shanghai People's Publishing House, 2000, p. 16.

[144] Edward S. Golub, *The Limits of Medicine: How Science Shapes Our Hope of the Cure*, New York: Times Books, c1994, pp. 85–108.

[145] Chen Hangxian, The Danger of Lacking Common Sense, *Essays of Zimian Study*, Shanghai: Shanghai Bookstore Press, 1997, p. 64.

modern Chinese medicine then. Did TCM ever think of establishing a set of special study on infectious diseases of itself? This will be discussed later.

What followed was that TCM was facing the challenge of new theories. Even though many TCM doctors upheld the concept of "convergence", Chinese and Western medicine remain friendly in appearance but estranged at heart after all. Once the "honeymoon period" with transitional significance was over, the gap between Chinese and Western medicine gradually expanded, with the difference as that between water and fire, ending in heated debates which was probably the general trend after the beginning of the Republic of China period.

Chapter 3
History of Antibacterial Books: Literature on Exogenous Fevers of TCM During the Republic of China Period

3.1 Preface

TCM treatment of diseases infected by microorganisms has been based on the ancient books of TCM exogenous fevers retained in previous dynasties. In specialized categorizations, they are mentioned in the medical books including the study of typhoid fever and warm diseases (as epidemics). No one has ever studied the publications of these classics since 1840. There had been great coincidences in the discussion of fevers between Modern Chinese and Western medicine, but the influence of the microbial pathogenesis theory didn't occur until the Republic of China period. Gu Jiegang's thoughts on sorting out the catalogue of books are very enlightening: he took the academic development trend of the era as the main body in general, and then selected his own subject from an organized category (febrile disease in this chapter). Of course, Gu's statement that "Chinese knowledge has always been a generalized view without divisions"[1] is not entirely correct, because TCM not only has divisions, but also had the detailed classifications in the same division. Currently, literature on the publications between 1912 and 1949 were mostly obtained, and the preliminary analysis were made in regard to its contents, based on the *National Joint Catalogue of TCM Books* compiled by the library of the Chinese Academy of TCM (hereinafter referred to as the *Catalogue*).[2] So far, the mainland has updated the statistical data, such as the *General Catalogue of Ancient Chinese Traditional Medicine Books* (2008), which is open for further supplementation. The author tends to inform the

---

[1] Gu Jiegang, *Walking on the Road of History—the Author's Own Account*, Nanjing: Jiangsu Education Press, 2005, p. 31.

[2] Library of the Chinese Academy of TCM (ed.), *National Joint Catalogue of TCM Books*, Beijing: TCM Classics Publishing House, 1991.

© Zhonghua Book Company 2026

K. Pi, *The Contest of Modern Chinese and Western Medicine*,
https://doi.org/10.1007/978-981-95-2832-5_3

readers of how TCM treated their inherent "antibacterial" assets at that time, and what new assertions they made.[3]

3.2 Republication of Classical Medical Books

The study of history can not be carried out without discussing inheritance and innovation, which often coexist and sometimes conflict with each other. The former involves continuity, while the latter involves the so-called "change". Qian Mu once said in *The Methodologies on the Study of Chinese History* that "the study of history enlightens the understanding of changes", "there is nothing to add into this history if there are no changes of the times", which is absolutely true.[4] One of the characteristics of Chinese medical history is to emphasize the inheritance of medical classics. The accumulated experience and clinical thinking of doctors can not be completely separated from medical classics.[5] Before discussing changes, we must understand the historical trend of its inheritance in order to obtain a clearer panorama in history.

Let's first talk about the inheritance of classical medicine. The so-called inheritance orientation here refers to the publication and engraving of traditional classical medical books, or the use of traditional methods of interpreting scriptures to explain and study of classical medical literature. The theory of Western medicine was rarely used, that is, there was no forum for the dialogue with Western medicine. It is impossible for Chinese medicine during the Republic of China period not to know nor ignore the challenges of Western medicine. Some of them chose to continue the textual research and exegesis of doctors in the Qing Dynasty by annotating medical books and publishing them. There were even cases that the ancient versions were published with no annotations at all. For example, there were as many as 8 editions of *Annotation on Treatise on Typhoid Fever* of the Song Dynasty version. There were also 9 editions of *The Ancient Treatise on Typhoid Fev*er *and Miscellaneous Diseases* in Nanyang Medical Saint Temple, which shows that TCM attached great importance to the medical classics at that time.

Yun Tieqiao was a famous doctor of the typhoid fever school during the Republic of China period. He not only used the theory of Western medicine bacteriology to interpret the provisions of typhoid fever theory, but also published 7 editions of *Treatise on Typhoid Fever* according to the original engraved by Zhao Kaimei in the Wanli reign. It is worth noting that the versions of *Treatise on Typhoid Fever*

---

[3] For the statistical tables sorted out, see Pi Kuoli, TCM Literature and Academic Transformation—An Investigation Centered on the Medical Books of Febrile Fever (1912–1949), Han Jianping et al. (eds), *Technological Heritage and Scientific Tradition*, Beijing: China Science and Technology Press, 2013, pp. 276–314.

[4] Qian Mu, *The Methodologies on the Study of Chinese History*, Beijing: SDX Joint Publishing Company, 2001, p. 4.

[5] Li Jianmin, Knowledge Form of Classical Medicine, Zhu Pingyi (ed.), *A New Theory of Chinese History. Science, Technology and Chinese Society*, Taipei: Lianjing Publishing House, Academia Sinica, 2010, pp. 125–179.

with annotations by the doctors in the Song Dynasty and the Qing Dynasty were still marketable. According to the statistics, those in the Song Dynasty include 5 editions (times) of Pang Anshi's *Treatise on the General Disease of Typhoid Fever*, 6 editions of Xu Shuwei's *Song of 100 Syndromes of Typhoid Fever*, 3 editions of Zhu Gong"s *Book of Living People with Typhoid Fever Syndrome,* and Qian Wenli's *Song of 100 Questions of Typhoid Fever.* The typhoid medical books of the Ming Dynasty include 4 editions of Tao Hua's *Six Books on Typhoid Fever*, which were more popular. Tao Huazhi's *Complete Collection of Typhoid Fever* were printed at least 5 editions in the Ming Dynasty and 10 editions during the Qing Dynasty, which shows its influence on the people of the Qing Dynasty. During the Republic of China period, only Shanghai Jiangdong Book Company engraved a version in 1912. *Six Books on Typhoid Fever* had 4 editions during the Republic of China period, which seemed to be popular, but it was published more than 10 times in the Ming Dynasty and 15 times in the Qing Dynasty. Compared with the relatively developed printing technology and the circulation demand of medical books during the Republic of China period, the number of these engraved books was quite limited.[6]

In terms of the works by doctors on typhoid fever in the Qing Dynasty, Chen Xiuyuan's works were extremely popular. In addition to the 6 editions of *Therapies to Typhoid Fever*, there were also 4 editions of *Changsha Prescription Songs of Typhoid Fever*. The most popular is the *Brief Annotations on Typhoid Fever*, which was published 7 times during the Republic of China period. Furthermore, with the supplementary annotations and revisions of Tang Zonghai in the late Qing Dynasty, *Supplemented Brief Annotations on Typhoid Fever* was introduced. The book had 10 editions during the Republic of China period, which shows that it was quite well received. Tang's medical book was published 5 times between 1900 and 1911 and more editions came out during the Republic of China period, proving itself as a book of overwhelming popularity. Tang was a leading doctor of the typhoid fever school, holding high the banner of "integration of TCM and Western medicine". Other notable typhoid medical books include Zhang Zhicong's *Annotation and the Collection of Notes on Typhoid Fever* compiled and annotated by Gao Shixuan, which had been published in 13 editions; Ke Qin's *Collection of Typhoid Fever Therapies* had 7 editions. The next is Yu Chang's *Commentaries of the Classics* (5 editions), Lv Zhenming's *The Sources of Typhoid Fever* and *The First Book of Typhoid Fever* compiled by Che Zongyu and Hu Xianshu (each 4 editions), and Wang Mengzu's *Compendium of Typhoid Fever* (3 editions).

The new medical books written by doctors after 1912 tend to use traditional ways of interpreting the classics and are less involved in the discussion of Western medicine. There are as many as 3 editions of *The Adaptions of Treatise on Typhoid Fever* compiled by Bao Yuhua and Bao Shisheng (also known as Yixu, style name Dedai), *The Ancient Writings on Typhoid Fever* written by Liao Ping and *The Interpretations of Typhoid Fever Prescriptions* compiled and annotated by He Zhonggao. Among them, the Bao family had treated typhoid fever for three generations and

---

[6] Library of the Chinese Academy of TCM (ed.), *National Joint Catalogue of TCM Books*, Beijing: TCM Classics Publishing House, pp. 68–69.

formed its own school during the Republic of China period. It's a pity Bao Shisheng "never talked about Western medicine". Although he had published medical books such as the *Handouts on Typhoid Fever, Handouts on Typhoid Prescription* and *The Table of Typhoid Fever*, such personal views limited his understandings of Western learning, and his annotations were not novel, which impaired his influence.[7] However, he once taught at the Shanghai Special School of TCM and also ran the Shenzhou Special School of Medicine, having Shenzhou Hospital attached for medical students' internship. Ding Jiwan, Cheng Menxue, Zhang Zanchen and others were all known as his disciples. In 1914, Bao and Yu Botao (1868–1944) initiated and organized the first "National Medical Salvation Petition Group" to unite with their counterparts all over the country to fight for the survival of TCM, the influence of which were incomparable with the publication of medical books.[8] Bao had another 3 volumes of *Bao's Medicine*, the first of which includes all typhoid works that were referred to as "internal infectious diseases".[9] Though he never talked about Western medicine, he still used the disease classifications of Western medicine, such as "infectious diseases", which is the product of the era when the academic study of infectious diseases in TCM was established in the early Republic of China period.

In addition, *A Record of Classical Prescription Experiments* by Cao Yingfu (1866–1938) is not contained, as it should be, in the typhoid medical books like the *Catalogue.* Cao wrote *A Record of Classical Prescription Experiments* in the hope of "melting warmth and heat into typhoid fever", so as to end the debate between typhoid fever and warm diseases.[10] *Catalogue* only lists Cao's *Exploring Typhoid Fever*, which has not been reprinted since its publication in 1931. The book annotates typhoid fever in a traditional way, but also refers to the theory of Western physiology. Cao said: "Visceral anatomy should take the western theory as the standard rather than adhering to the old theory".[11] However, comparing with the other TCM doctors at the time, he was more conserved in discussing the new knowledge of bacteria. This may be related to Cao's literary temperament. Although Cao had a lot more students than other famous doctors in Shanghai at that time, his "medical business was stagnant", which might be another reason why his medical books were not repeatedly published during the Republic of China period.[12] As a doctor of the pure typhoid

---

[7] The table shows that his son Bao Tianbai rewrote *Exploring Typhoid Fever* in 1937, which is a handout and had not been widely spread. However, Bao Tianbai had also taught in many Chinese medicine colleges and universities in Shanghai, which shows that Bao's traditional treatise on typhoid fever still was passed down. Zhao Hongjun: *The History of Modern Debate between TCM and Western Medicine*, Hefei: Anhui Science and Technology Press, 1989, pp. 223–224.

[8] Bao Shisheng, The Adaptions of Treatise on Typhoid Fever, *Bao's Medicine, Vol. 1* Shanghai: Bao's Medical School Publishing Department, 1930, Forward, pp. 4–5.

[9] Bao Shisheng, The Quintessence of Chinese Medicine, *Bao's Medicine Vol. 3,* Shanghai: Bao's Medical School Publishing Department, 1936, Forward, p. 1.

[10] Cao Yingfu, *A Record of Classical Prescription Experiments*, Fuzhou: Fujian Science and Technology Press, 2004, Yao Shichen's preface, Introduction, pp. 20, 29.

[11] Cao Yingfu, *Cao's Golden Collection of Exploring Typhoid Fever*, Shanghai: Qianqing Hall Publishing House, 1956, Introduction, p. 5.

[12] Cao Yingfu, Cao's *Golden Collection of Exploring Typhoid Fever*, Qin Bowei's preface, p. 2.

fever school, Cao once said: "Watching out the mouths of warm disease school and make sure they hold the sage in awe and veneration".[13]

In 1955, Qin Bowei (1901–1970) recalled that before his clinical practice with his teacher Ding Ganren (1865–1926), he had studied in the Shanghai Special School of TCM.[14] Cao Yingfu made a connection with Ding, co-chaired the medical school and often exchanged medical skills with each other. Qin followed Cao Xueyi, who was a lecturer at that time. His classmates included Xu Banlong, Yan Cangshan, Zhang Cigong. Qin recalled: "Master Cao is a typical example of the classic school. The prescription and medication are in accordance with the laws of *Treatise on Febrile Diseases* and *Synopsis of the Golden Treatise*, emphasizing that the prescriptions after Zhongjing are insignificant". Zhang Cigong, another student, said: "The dispute between classic school and modern school is only the distinction between ephedra and mulberry chrysanthemum in the eyes of Master Cao".[15] It can be seen that Cao hated the drugs of the warm disease school. Cao believed that with all the symptoms of typhoid fever, sweat should be discharged from the pores of the human body at first. "If air from the lung is unblocked, the diseases will heal by themselves",[16] which can also be the cure for the plague. This is the reason why ephedra decoction had become a holy medicine for the treatment of typhoid fever. Cao took the classic prescription as the basis of all prescriptions and must be studied.[17]

Huang Handong, another student of Cao, recalled that at that time, TCM was impacted by Western medicine, and everyone was striving to prove the strength of TCM. However, many people were used to the more modern prescriptions and mild doses of medication—which could only cure minor diseases, but not the serious ones. They attacked the medicine of the classic school to protect their own reputation, which would stagnate medicine study. So Cao advocated that the classic school learn from the original scriptures.[18] Ding Ganren, Cao's friend, was a doctor of the modern school. Ding explained: "The reason why I use mild doses of medication is that it is only for those who are not seriously ill". It is said that most of his patients were well-off, some just had the occasional cold and some were just physically weak or emotionally depressed. For such patients, mild doses of medication such

---

[13] Cao Yingfu, *A Record of Classical Prescription Experiments*, p. 117.

[14] It happened between 1919 and 1923.

[15] Qin Bowei said: "The knowledge of classical prescriptions is the basis of all prescriptions, and most prescriptions of later generations have developed upon classical prescriptions. For example, a tree has branches, leaves, flowers and fruits only when it has roots. We can't appreciate one branch, leaf, flower and fruit alone and ignore its roots.... He held that the study of TCM should seek for its origin rather than abandoning the basics, which gives a clear guide for the later learning". From Cao Yingfu, *Cao's Golden Collection of Exploring Typhoid Fever,* Qin Bowei's preface, pp. 1–2. Ephedra was a drug commonly used by the classic school to induce sweat, which was feared by the modern school. The latter mostly adopted mulberry leaves and chrysanthemums commonly used by the warm disease school to deal with exogenous febrile diseases, which was the division of the two academic schools at that time.

[16] Cao Yingfu, *Exploring Typhoid Fever*, Taipei: Zhiyuan Publishing House, 2005, Sun, p. 22.

[17] Wang Zhipu et al. (eds.), Cao Yingfu's Life and Academic Thoughts.

[18] Cao Yingfu, *A Record of Classical Prescription Experiments*, p. 6; Cao Yingfu: *Cao's Golden Collection of Exploring Typhoid Fever*. Preface of the reprint, p. 2.

as Huoxiang, mulberry leaves, tangerine peel and cardamom were considered to be good enough to take effect. Cao, as his good friend, also acknowledged this and respected it. However, for the patients of severe cases, Ding did not hesitate to use the heavy dose of the classic school. This kind of open, flexible and assimilating attitude became a model for doctors during the Republic of China period.[19]

As for the statistical part of warm disease medical books, it is even more special. The warm disease medical books during the Republic of China period can be inferred from the times and coverage of its printings, which were almost entirely those of the Qing Dynasty. The doctors during the Republic of China period did not continue to cultivate this theory. This situation is not surprising, because from the perspective of typhoid fever verses warm disease debate in the Qing Dynasty, the prosperity of typhoid fever works represents that the creativity of its opponent, the warm disease school, was relatively weak. Secondly, Fan Xingzhun once said in *A Brief History of Chinese Medicine* that the science of warm diseases began to weaken after Jiaqin-Daoguang period, and those who became more popular instead mostly distinguished new diseases from warm diseases, and the writings on warm diseases based on the original "general theory" was no longer grand. In fact, the real general theory of warm diseases only focused on one infectious disease.[20] In other words, the knowledge and medical books of the "general theory" of warm disease s in this era did not need to bring forth the new through the old. The four members of the warm diseases school have had a far-reaching impact that few doctors could surpass or update the classics of warm diseases in the Qing Dynasty. It was the trend of this era to invoke the knowledge of Western medicine for interpretation. From the historical view of warm diseases, the evolution of warm diseases also took a long time. Under the comprehensive influence of a wide range of medical knowledge, social culture, the spread of medical books in the south of the Yangtze River and the discussion of local circumstances, the warm disease school gained a solid foothold. Experts who were well versed in warm diseases during this era were more engaged in analyzing classical medical books and discussion with Western medicine, than creating new "general theories". The mission of TCM at that time was to create an overall discussion similar to Western infectious diseases from the classic works of the Qing Dynasty and reflect on the disease interpretation in its own academic system according to the disease names of Western medicine.

During the Republic of China period, the most popular medical books on warm diseases were Wu Tang's *Analysis on Febrile Diseases*. The book had been published with 22 editions, followed by Wang Mengying's *Perspectives on Febrile Diseases*, with 20 editions. These two medical books on warm diseases were published once every two years on average, and their influence was obvious. In addition, *On Seasonal Diseases* by Lei Feng (1833–1888) in the late Qing Dynasty was also published with 13 editions. There were as many as 7 editions of the *Syndrome Table of Seasonal Diseases* annotated by Peng Guangqing, and 2 editions of *Annotations of On Seasonal Diseases* by Chen Lianfang. It can be seen that *On Seasonal Diseases* was also a very

[19] Cao Yingfu, *Cao's Golden Collection of Exploring Typhoid Fever*. Preface of the reprint, pp. 2–3.

[20] Fan Xingzhun, *A Brief History of Chinese Medicine*, p. 240.

important document of warm diseases during the Republic of China period. As for the works on warm diseases in the Ming Dynasty, the only book was *Updated Complete Book on Heatstroke* written by Zhang Heteng (llll) and further updated by Ye Li, which was published more than 3 times. The works of the Qing Dynasty include Liu Baoyi's *Finding the Source of Febrile Diseases* and Zhang Ruzhen's *3 character Formula of Febrile Diseases*, all of which have 5 versions; there are 4 versions of Liu Hengrui's *New Book of Exorcism,* Ji Piaozi's *Words on Febrile Diseases*, Lou Jie's *Guide to Febrile Diseases*, and Cao Huafeng's *Summary of Febrile Disease Treatment*; there are 3 versions of Ye Lin's *Therapies to Febrile Diseases*. To my surprise, compared with typhology, doctors during the Republic of China period did not pay special attention to the annotations of the classic original texts in the early stages of the development of warm diseases, such as Ye Tianshi's *On Febrile Diseases* and Xue Shengbai's *On Damp Heat*, which were not specially published as a single book, nor annotated or interpreted according to the original.[21] On the other hand, *Analysis on Febrile Diseases, Perspectives on Febrile Diseases* and *On Seasonal Diseases*, which caught more attention from doctors during the Republic of China period, are actually medical books after the eighteenth century, drawing close to modern times and belonging to the later generation. Perhaps this is related to the fact that the works of Wu Tang or Wang Mengying also contain part of *On Febrile Diseases*. The publishing market of medical books during the Republic of China period seemed to prefer these "later classics" with more complete prescriptions and comprehensiveness.[22]

The doctors of the Republic of China period who made the effort to interpret *On Febrile Diseases* are Chen Guangsong's *Annotations of On Febrile Diseases* (1915), which was meant to "annotate Ye's intention and correct the loss of all schools".[23] However, the annotations made by Chen are only to explain the chapter of "warm diseases" in the *Perspectives on Febrile Diseases* and there were only 3 editions during the whole Republic of China period. There is no evidence to prove that his contribution exceeds that of Wang Mengying and others. As for the *Syndrome Table*

[21] In fact, neither *On Febrile Diseases* nor *On Damp Heat*, which is scattered in the works of doctors in the Qing Dynasty and being included in the introduction of medical books, has its separate edition. See Li Shunbao, *Complete Book of Warm Diseases, Vol. I,* Beijing: Xueyuan Publishing House, 2002, pp. 2, 118. However, during the Republic of China period, no one collected them for identification and annotation. In fact, doctors only read *Perspectives on Febrile Diseases*, which includes both but the problem is that it is Wang Mengying's interpretation and tailoring, rather than that of the original. On the contrary, the original version of *Treatise on Febrile Diseases* was highly valued by doctors, and was duly published in various versions.

[22] Another possibility is that the texts of *On Febrile Diseases* and *On Damp Heat* are quite short, and sometimes they are included in other medical books for interpretation. For example, *On Febrile Diseases* was included in *Perspectives on Febrile Diseases*, under the title of "Exogenous Febrile Diseases". It is also found in *Doctor Wu's Medical Talk, Vol. 1*, under the title of "On the Treatment of Febrile Diseases". Zhang Xugu included it in his book *Warnings in Medicine*, with the title of "Ye Tianshi's Theory of Febrile Diseases". Zhao Faxin, Hu Yongxin, Lei Xinqiang & Ding Hongzhan et al. (eds.), *Dictionary of TCM Philology*, Beijing: TCM Classics Publishing House, 2000, p. 418.

[23] Chen Guangsong, Annotations of On Febrile Diseases, included in *Three Books of Advancing Febrile Disease Studies*, Beijing: Xueyuan Publishing House, 2007, pp. 330–332.

of Seasonal Diseases compiled by Peng Guangqing, even with the "supplementary notes to the syndrome table of time and disease" at the end of the book, the content of the supplementary notes is only tailoring to various discussions, with no involvement of bacteria and offered few novel ideas.[24] Another phenomenon is that at this time, there were many handouts or scattered transcripts of epidemic warm diseases, or their own privately printed and manuscripts, which were not widely circulated and had limited influence; or they were just mnemonic rhyme or charts made out of previous works.[25] All this shows the lack of creativity in the study of warm diseases at the time.

Another example is Shen Lin (Hanqing)'s *Interpretations of Febrile Diseases*, which had 4 editions during the Republic of China period. At that time, Yan Xishan (1883–1960), the warlord in Shanxi, advocated medical studies and set up a "Research Association for TCM Improvement", which solicited contributions in newspapers. Shen had his book completed, printed by the Association and distributed to Shanxi TCM agency. Later, due to insufficient supply and the poor printing quality, it was subsidized and reprinted after revision. The book emphasizes that "Qi" was the gist in the long-term TCM accumulation. Although it is the work of febrile diseases, it strongly emphasizes the principle of Qi in *Treatise on Febrile Diseases*, and even criticizes that modern doctors only paid attention to the works of febrile diseases but ignored the principle of personal Qi established in classical medical books. Shen believed that Chinese and western customs are different due to different races. Western people are prone to internal diseases, while Chinese people concerned themselves with more external diseases, which indicates they must be treated in different ways. Moreover, as Western medicine does not understand Qi, it naturally does not know how to treat epidemics.[26]

As for the publication of epidemic medical books during the Republic of China period, they were influenced by Western medicine mostly, and had a tendency of focusing on infectious diseases. Meanwhile, such medical books were also the major forum of discussing "antibacterial". The most noted were: *On Warm Epidemics* known to medical historians. It had 4 versions then. If taking into account of *Supplemented Annotations on Warm Epidemics* annotated by the Zheng Chongguang in the Qing Dynasty, and *Supplemented Annotations of on Epidemics*, which was written by Hong Tianxi in the Qing Dynasty, there are a total of 14 versions. Another important

---

[24] Peng Guangqing (ed.), Supplement to Syndrome Table of Seasonal Diseases, *Syndrome Table of Seasonal Diseases*, Shanghai: Shanghai Book Company, 1955, p. 1.

[25] For example, during the Republic of China period, there were 9 versions of medical books with formulas or directions put into rhyme on the basis of warm diseases such as *Systematic Differentiation of Warm Diseases*. They were written by Zhong Shaotao, Yan Zhixin, Liu Benchang, Jiang Zifang, Zhao Zhuyan, Li Houkun, Wu Zaojiang, Wang Xinmin and Anonymous. Jiang Zifang's *Fu on Warm Diseases* even published 4 editions; there were *Prescription Songs of Warm Disease* published in 1921 and *3 Character Classic of Febrile Disease,* similar to Zhou Yunzhang's work, published in 1932. They were all mnemonic books of primary introductions. He Zhonggao's *Syndrome Table of Warm Diseases* in 1921 belongs to the chart type.

[26] Shen Lin, Interpretations of Febrile Diseases, included in Cao Bingzhang (ed.), *Great Achievements in Chinese Medicine*, Vol. 18, Shen Lin's original preface, pp. 1–2.

medical book is *Analysis on Typhoid Fever and Warm Diseases* (also known as *Analysis on Typhoid and Warm Diseases*—with Appendix of Warm Disease Syndrome) written by Yang Xuan (Lishan) in the Qing Dynasty, which had 8 versions. The original book was published in 1784. Later, Lv Tian (Xinzhai) excerpted it, together with his excerpts of Chen Liangzuo's *Febrile Diseases of Spring and Autumn*, he compiled *Excerpts of Analysis on Epidemics* (also known as *Excerpts of Analysis on Typhoid and Warm Diseases*) in 1811, which also had 5 editions. Dai Tianzhang of the Qing Dynasty, published the *Generalizations on Epidemics* in 1722. In 1750, the book was published by Zheng Dianyi as *Analysis on Epidemics*. The two books were exactly the same, which had 7 versions during the Republic of China period. Later, Lu Maoxiu (Jiuzhi) changed the title of the book into *Generalizations on Febrile Diseases* and published it in 1866 with omissions and supplements. After all, Dai had the most, as many as 10, revised versions during the Republic of China period.[27]

The epidemic medical books summarized above are mostly general, but they are different from the above generalized medical books. In the epidemic medical books of the Republic of China period, there are many books on certain particular infectious diseases. These medical books mostly aim at a specific disease, borrowing some new definitions of Western medical theory, and then applying them to the relevant theories of classicism, trying to inherit and give play to traditional medicine when expounding a single infectious disease. For example, Yan Cangshan wrote *Collection of Self-Treatment of Epidemic Spasm (Meningitis)* in 1932 and Liu Caiwu's *The Complete Book of Spasm and Meningitis* in 1935 is a book on meningitis. In ancient times, there was no such Western disease name, so TCM found the classical disease name of "spasm" as reference.[28] In fact, TCM also used the names of "convulsion" and "epilepsy" then. However, in 1931, Liu Yanong, a TCM doctor, believed that his diagnosis and treatment of many cases were effective by using the treatment of "spasm" or febrile diseases. Therefore, the "spasm" named by Zhang Zhongjing

---

[27] In this regard, the statistics in the *Catalogue* are wrong. According to Lu, the updated version should be called *Generalizations on Febrile Diseases* instead of *(Revised) Generalizations on Febrile Diseases* in *Catalogue. Catalogue* mistakenly attributed the *Revised Generalizations on Febrile Diseases* (or *Re-supplemented Generalizations on Febrile Diseases*) revised by He Lianchen (1861–1929) to Lu, without indicating He Lianchen's role of revising. Moreover, according to the statistics of *Catalogue*, it is his revised edition, not Lu's, that was published by Shaoxing Zhedong Book Company in 1914. See Library of the Chinese Academy of TCM (ed.),*National Joint Catalogue of TCM Books*, p. 391. For the above textual research, see Li Shunbao (ed.), *Dictionary of Warm Diseases*, Beijing: Xueyuan Publishing House, 2007, pp. 20, 184. However, it also had mistakes. It claimed that He Lianchen's work were published in 1909. According to the current edition, He Lianchen said at the end of the preface that it was written in "October, 469th year of the Yellow Emperor era". The preface should be written in November 1911, so the later version of the book is the 1914 version. See (Qing) Dai Tianzhang (Linjiao), revised by He Lianchen, *Revised General Febrile Diseases*, Fuzhou: Fujian Science and Technology Press, 2006, Introduction, pp. 3–4.

[28] The name of the disease (convulsion disease) originally came from *Synopsis of the Golden Treatise.* Now it mostly refers to febrile spasm and tetanus. It can be seen that a disease name of TCM can be compatible with several diseases of Western medicine. During the Republic of China period, what doctors cared about was the unification of the names of Chinese and Western medicine. See He Dongcan, *Research on Internal Diseases in Synopsis of the Golden Treatise*, Taipei: Zhengzhong Publishing House, 1995, pp. 21–32.

was the most proper.[29] In addition, from the publication of some medical books, it can be found that the most serious or concerned disease during the Republic of China period was cholera. The more published medical book during the Republic of China period was Wang Mengying's *On Cholera*, which had as many as 15 versions. In establishing a new treatise on infectious diseases, TCM theory was still very important, although it is influenced by Western medicine, including bacteriology. *On Cholera* is the first book to publish cholera in the form of a special book from the perspective of exogenous fever. The status of the book was even more distinguished with the emergence of the general theory of febrile diseases and infectious disease specialty during the Republic of China period.

Liu Minshu's *Interpretations on Cholera in Treatise on Typhoid Fever* (with Zhang Taiyan's *Treatise on Cholera*) is the only contemporary work with 3 versions. In addition, a large number of medical books have also been published on the treatment and discussion of "Sha" diseases.[30] Some have more than three versions, including the *Complete Book of Sha Diseases* compiled by Wang Kai in the Qing Dynasty, with a total of six editions, followed by Guo Zhishen's *Sha Treatment*, with 5 editions. Other books are the *First Aid to Sha Diseases* (also known as *Therapies on Sha Diseases*) compiled by Taoist Jueyin in the Qing Dynasty and Xu Zimo's *Diaojiao Sha Disease*, each has 4 editions. "Sha" disease during the Republic of China period mainly referred to gastrointestinal infectious diseases, but such "Sha" books mostly discuss cholera.[31] As for the causes of its occurrence, the "Sha" books of the Republic of China period rarely use bacteriology to explain it, but mainly use the traditional discussion of epidemic Qi. For example, "Sha, the epidemic Qi between heaven and earth".[32] This may be related to too many types of diseases contained in "Sha", but the details remain to be discussed.[33] The medical books of doctors in the Qing Dynasty were still very important during the Republic of China period. On the contrary, the

---

[29] Liu Yanong, Discussion on the Names of Meningitis in TCM, *Medical Adviser*, 19th Annual of the Republic of China Period (1931), pp. 32–34.

[30] Ji Zhenghan, Systematic Examination of Medical Records of Sha Disease in the Qing Dynasty, *Journal of TCM Literature*, 2009 (4), pp. 1–4.

[31] Although "Sha syndrome" finally developed into a general term containing many diseases, it is believed to be an infectious warm disease caused by feeling the wind, cold, heat and dampness between summer and autumn, or by feeling the pathogenic factor of epidemic Qi and filth. See *Dictionary of Warm Diseases* compiled by Li Shunbao, p. 268. Zhang Gang explained: "Since the Ming and Qing Dynasties, the term 'Sha' had been used to refer to cholera, 'lethargy', or the cases of throat rash and measles. However, the name of Sha should be derived from 'sand'. In the Wei and Jin Dynasties, the so-called 'Sha' was the sick ear of the sand lice entering the muscle. The skin rash was caused by the rotation of the sand lice into the muscle, so the ancients took the leaves from Maoming to pick and scrape. The disease was originally called Sha, which is the origin of the expressions of picking Sha and scraping Sha. Without knowing its meaning, later generations used the term extensively, so there was no definite meaning for it, or it was defined in different ways ".Refer to his book, *On the Source of Disease Names in TCM*, pp. 98–99.

[32] Chen Jingqi, *Treatment of 72 Kinds of Sha*, Taichung: Ruicheng Publishing House, 1972, p. 31.

[33] For the interpretation and social history, see Zhu Pingyi, Sha in the Qing Dynasty: the Birth of A Disease Category, *Sinological Research* 31.3 (2013), pp. 193–238; Pi Kuoli, Discourse of Chinese and Western Medicine and Modern Business Discussion: from the Example of "Sha Potion" in Shen Bao, *Shanghai Academic Monthly*, 2013 (1), pp. 149–164.

new publications did not receive much attention. In contrast, Western medicine in the early Republic of China period, when comparing with Chinese medicine, would also study Chinese medical books and explore the disease theory of China along with Western medicine. For example, when Yu Fengbin vigorously promoted the benefits of cholera bacterial slurry, he also discussed the "seizure" of possible cholera in his book. In terms of the position of Western medicine, it was better to abolish this common name, but this kind of discussion offered many references in the comparison of disease names between Chinese and Western medicine, which has its own literary value.[34] Other important diseases or medical books are worth noting: (1) malaria: Both *Guide to Malaria* written by Zheng Quanwang in the Ming Dynasty and *On Malaria* written by Han Shanzheng in the Qing Dynasty (also known as *Self-therapy for Malaria and Dysentery*) had 4 editions, and Cai Luxian's *Malaria Q & A* had 3 editions. At that time, old works were republished and sometimes they were re-entitled by adding "*self-therapy*" to highlight the needs of daily life. (2) Dysentery: Both *On Dysentery* (also known as the *Complete Collection of Dysentery* compiled by Kong Yuli in the Qing Dynasty, attached with the theory of infantile acute convulsion syndrome and the theory of diphtheria) and *Updated Essentials of Quick Therapy for Dysentery* by Ding Guorui had 3 editions. At that time, some medical books were also attached with the treatment of some other infectious diseases in order to enhance its practical and reference value. (3) Pestis: *Compilations of Pestis* by Wu Xuanchong and revised by Zheng Fenyang in the Qing Dynasty had 4 editions. There were also 3 editions of *Pestis Selections* written by Yu Dexun. It is worth noting that Yu's writings, in the lead printed edition by the capital police headquarters, the section of "Plague Syndrome Differentiation and Treatment" was attached at the back. It may have been printed by the police, as effective prescriptions for the treatment of plague, for the public to use as reference in the second plague in 1918.[35] However, the former was no longer published after 1928 and the latter after 1918. They were only included in medical books.[36] At the beginning of the Republic of China period, medical books on fever were mostly published as charity books when the epidemic broke out, and even directly announced by the police. This is not only an important function of traditional medicine in epidemic prevention, but also an important channel for the production and transmission of medical knowledge. For example, in 1915, when diphtheria and throat scraping were prevalent in the capital city, Yang Xiling, a TCM doctor, wrote to the police department to recommend the TCM epidemic treatment methods, and

[34] Yu Fengbin, *Series on Cholera*, Publisher unknown, 1922, pp. 20–24.

[35] Cao Shuji, Public Health of the Nation and the Regions—A Case Study of 1918 Shanxi Epidemic, *Chinese Social Science,* 2006 (1), pp. 178–190. Zhang Zhaoqing, 1917–1918 Epidemic and the Reaction of the Republic of China Period, *History Teaching,* 2006 (1), pp. 19–23.

[36] The former was included in the *Collection of Rare Medical Books* (1936), while the latter was included in the *Great Achievements in Chinese Medicine* (1936). The two books are very representative in pestis studies, though neither addresses the theory of bacteria. Instead, they integrate the western health discourse since modern times. See (Qing) Yu Dexun (Botao), Pestis Selections, included in Cao Bingzhang's *Great Achievements in Chinese Medicine, Vol. 17*, pp. 6–7.

printed them as epidemic treatment booklets for distribution.[37] In addition, there were more than 3 editions of epidemic medical books, as well as Liu Fu's *Dispelling Doubts about the Current Epidemic* (4 editions), Xu Xiangren's *Therapies to Acute Epidemic* and Cao Bingzhang's *Essentials of Autumn Epidemic Treatment* (3 editions for each).

3.3 The Influence of Western Medicine and the Gradual Formation of "TCM Infectious Diseases"

In view of the publication of epidemic medical books, special books on individual infectious disease came out. From all TCM medical books on warm diseases, the discussion of "infectious diseases" of modern TCM had gradually taken shape. There were infectious diseases in ancient China, and the ancients also knew about "infections". However, before modern times, they were commonly referred to by their ancient disease names, which did not have the significance in health modernity and bacterial pathology, and was essentially different from the infectious diseases in Western medicine. Yu Yunxiu, an opponent of TCM, pointed out that China's "epidemic" could not be defined as an "infectious disease" on the basis of bacterial pathogens. It goes with the saying "no infectious disease is possible without pathogenic microorganisms". The TCM interpretation of epidemic was not to be equated with infectious diseases.[38] Fu Sinian, another opponent of TCM, said: "The examination of micro bacteria is the most important diagnosis of all infectious diseases". But Chinese medicine has no diagnostic device nor any diagnostic techniques except pulsing.[39] Although the ancient "seasonal diseases" can be compared with infectious diseases of Western medicine, there was obviously no discussion of microorganisms. The TCM opponents would never admit that there is "epidemiology" in TCM.

However, the transformation of medical knowledge still took place. After the Republic of China period, TCM gradually used the term "infectious disease" as the title of books and gave them the Western medical definitions and knowledge of microbiology. The earliest medical books listed as "infectious diseases" in the early Republic of China period were the *Summary of Warm Diseases* compiled in 1915, which were included in the series of "4 Kinds of Huang's Infectious Diseases". Other representative TCM books under the name of "infectious diseases" include: *8 Kinds of Infectious Diseases Syndrome and Their Treatment* by Cao Xunxuan (Yuansen) et al. in 1918, *Chinese Acute Infectious Diseases* by Shi Yiren in 1933, *Infectious Diseases of Four Seasons* by Yang Zhiyi Ji, *Infectious Diseases by* Ru

[37] Yang Xiling, Q & A on Throat Rash, Medical Talk in Zhu Garden, included in Lu Zheng (ed.), *Collection of Rare Modern TCM. Medical Talk*, pp. 587–588.

[38] Yu Yunxiu, *Microbiology*, Shanghai: Commercial Press, 1929, Preface, p. 1.

[39] Fu Sinian, On the So-called National Medicine, Vol. 6, *Fu Sinian's Complete Works*, Taipei: Lianjing Publishing House, 1980, pp. 309–310.

Shimei, *Commentaries and Annotations on Typhoid Fever* (also known as *General Theory of Acute Infectious Diseases*) by Tan Cizhong (style name Xingyuan, 1893–1955) in 1935, and *Three Parts of the Convergence of Chinese and Western Infectious Diseases* by Wang Zhizhou in 1947. The name of "infectious disease" had been gradually established in the TCM during the Republic of China period. The names of seasonal diseases and seasonal Qis were related to infectious diseases. Of course, typhoid and warm diseases were also the synonyms for infectious diseases. Doctors may have different views,[40] but no one would deny that a doctor knowledgeable about exogenous fevers was incapable of treating infectious diseases. The status of TCM based on treatment of infectious diseases was gradually established. Shi Yiren was an insightful doctor among them. He said:

> In 1922, I advocated that infectious diseases should be an independent specialty, the writings of which should be edited and compiled into a special book that can be used as reference materials for Chinese medicine in epidemic prevention and diagnosis, as well as for the treatment of infectious diseases. Considerable attention and investigation should be given to the experiences and methods of diagnosis and treatment of infectious diseases contained in the writings of doctors of the past. The heritage of ancient history should be clarified with modern scientific theories and combined with modern science, so as to achieve the goal of "scientization of TCM".[41]

Shi held that the establishment of infectious diseases is the basis for TCM in its future task of public health, and we must lose no time in the development of it. Hong Guanzhi stated: "While it is not determined if warm diseases and typhoid fever in TCM belong to infectious diseases, and there are no accurate definitions yet, how can we set it as a special department?"[42] TCM can not clearly define its epidemiology unless it can classify its own disciplines. In this circumstance, there were still many possibly unknown problems to be solved. The name of the infectious disease was officially used in *8 Kinds of Infectious Diseases Syndrome and Their Treatment*. The book clearly aimed at the pestis and cholera epidemics from 1918 to 1919.

Xu Shichang said in the preface of his book: the book is aimed at the so-called "8 kinds of acute infectious diseases" in Western medicine according to separate syndromes. Cao Xunxuan said: "There are cures for such infections, which are the specialty of TCM. They are overpowered and can't be put into practice".[43] It can be seen that at that time, TCM had the pressure from Western medicine in the treatment of

---

[40] Shi Yiren advocated that the epidemics in TCM should be set apart and referred to as "acute infectious diseases" (similar to Western Medicine); and it seems more appropriate to discuss typhoid fever and warm diseases in the "seasonal diseases" category. See Shi Yiren, *Chinese Acute Infectious Diseases*, Shanxi: Council of Research for TCM Improvement, 1933, pp. 1–5. However, some people mainly wrote on infectious diseases based on typhoid fever. See details below.

[41] Shi Yiren, *Chinese Epidemiology*, Hong Kong: Qianqing Hall Publishing House, 1952, Preface, p. 1.

[42] Hong Guanzhi, Proposals to the Educational Authorities and Those Who Are Passionate in TCM Education for the Prerequisite Problems of TCM Education", *New TCM*, 1947, New Issue (1), p. 1.

[43] Kong Bohua's Classic Study Office (ed.), *Answers to the Queries on the Treatment of Eight Infectious Diseases*, Beijing: Chemical Industry Press, 2010, Xu Shichang's preface. Sean Hsiang-Lin Lei had made a special research on the 8 major infectious diseases. See Sean Hsiang-Lin Lei, Microscope and Sovereignty: Constituting Notifiable Infectious Diseases and Containing the

infectious diseases. It was wished that books be written as soon as possible to explain the treatment methods and discipline norms. However, it still focused on Qi and had no place for bacteria theory. The book starts with "heaven and earth, both are out of Qi". The Qi of heaven and earth has a natural law, so "the research of disease in China focuses on Qi, while those in Japan and Europe focus on natural science". It holds that we must include the Qi of heaven and earth in the study of infectious diseases.[44] Tan Cizhong (Xinyuan)'s *Commentaries and Annotations on Typhoid Fever* emphasizes that typhoid and warm diseases are acute infectious diseases. Although the book recognizes the authenticity of bacterial discussion, it does not particularly talk about it. Instead, attention was paid to the concept of "syndrome group". Tan believed that it is not necessary to keep on emphasizing the six meridians, but that they should be classified as a concept of 'syndrome group' of infectious diseases of Western medicine, which is in line with the scientific discussion of infectious diseases.[45]

On the other hand, even with the title of "epidemic diseases" or ancient diseases, many TCM doctors also borrowed the definitions and discussion of Western medicine in the process of actual diagnosis and treatment, and then responded with traditional medicine. For example, *On the Damp Warm Seasonal Epidemic Treatment* compiled by Shaoxing Medical Association and He Lianchen in 1913, which had 3 editions, takes the name of infectious disease in Western medicine "infection" as the subject of discussion, and discusses the position of "infectious bacillus"—microorganisms in pathology.[46]

Another example is Xu Xiangren (1881–1959), a native of Wu County, Jiangsu Province. He studied medicine with his father-in-law Fei Shengfu. He was one of the heirs of Menghe medical school and later practiced in Shanghai. In the summer and autumn of 1908, an epidemic, mostly cholera, was prevalent in Shanghai. Influenced by traditional medicine, he was employed as a doctor and consultant by the epidemic hospital attached to Shanghai Red Cross Society of China, and served in the Standing Committee of Shenzhou Medical Association.[47] At that time, the Red Cross Society of China in Shanghai was actually a Western-style organization, including many Western doctors. They even established an epidemic hospital together. The Red Cross Society was good at using local medical resources, including the power

Manchurian Plague, included in Angela Ki Che Leung and Charlotte Furth (ed.), *Health and Hygiene in Modern Chinese Eastern Asia: Politics in the Long Twentieth Century*, Durham: Duke University Press, pp 73–108.

44 Kong Bohua's Classic Study Office (ed.), *Answers to the Queries on the Treatment of Eight Infectious Diseases*, p. 2.

45 Tan Cizhong, *Commentaries and Annotations on Typhoid Fever*, Taichung: Jingning Science and Technology Bookstore, 2003, p. 69.

46 Shaoxing Medical Association, Treatment of Damp and Warm Epidemics, included in Li Shunbao (ed.) *Complete Book of Warm Diseases*, pp. 2090–2091.

47 Yang Xinglin, Learn from the Past and Follow the Good—Thoughts of Xu Xiangren, the Successor of Fei's Medicine, *Journal of TCM Literature* (2009) 27.1, pp. 36–38. For the social network of Menghe medical school, see Volker Scheid, Wujin Medicine Remembered: Memory, Identity and Social Networks in Chinese Medicine 1800–2000, *Taiwanese Journal of Studies for Science, Technology, and Medicine,* 2002 (2), pp. 121–184.

of TCM or local gentry.[48] When the epidemic occurred, Western medicine often determined the name of a disease and even published the information to the public, which gave TCM access to the infectious disease framework defined by the West, and TCM also intervened in treatment. Basically, an epidemic hospital was a treatment laboratory integrating Chinese and Western medicine.[49] At that time, although the epidemic was mostly cholera, there were many other infectious diseases, including influenza, smallpox, diphtheria and even Sha.[50] In 1920, Xu wrote *Therapies to Acute Epidemics*, which mainly expounds the treatment of acute infectious diseases such as laryngeal Sha, cholera and meningitis. He wrote a general prescription, which may be related to his treatment.[51] Moreover, Volker Scheid's research also shows that Ding Ganren took advantage of this charitable medical opportunity to accumulate contacts and obtain various resources provided to him by the social network, including funds or patients.[52] The author believes that many doctors might have accumulated their own views and experiences on the treatment of diseases in this process. The nature of the epidemic hospital allows us to reasonably speculate that a large part of the diseases handled by TCM at that time were infectious diseases.

Zhang Juren, a TCM doctor, described his experience in treating the epidemic diseases in Beijing in 1919, so that we can understand the history of Chinese medicine doctors visiting the epidemic areas at that time. He said that even though there was an epidemic prevention hospital then, it was just the prevention without treatment. The epidemic was becoming more and more serious. The hospital sent Yang Haoru, Chen Boya and some acupuncture doctors to the epidemic area for treatment. At first, there were few patients due to the fact it was not widely known. They decided to use the method of touring, going door to door for treatment. In each village, they had one person in charge of publicity and one person giving treatment. Due to the immediate effect of drug administration, more and more patients were treated, and the diseases were generally eliminated in just ten days. Zhang said: "Most of the sources of cholera this time are farmers working in the fields who were thirsty and picked the hot melons being exposed to the sun. The heat-against-heat contact was the cause of the epidemic". It can be seen that the occurrence of diseases was still explained based on the characteristics of "Qi"—touching heat with heat. Moreover, Zhang admitted

---

48 Chi Zihua, *The Red Cross and Modern China*, Hefei: Anhui People's Publishing House, 2004, p. 71; Chi Zihua & Hao Ruyi, *Modern Jiangsu Red Cross Movement*, Hefei: Anhui People's Publishing House, 2007, pp. 132–133.

49 For other information on the status of hospital and medical education and personnel training of the Red Cross Society, see Zhang Yufa (ed.), *Centennial History of the Red Cross Society of the Republic of China period*, Taipei: Federation of the Red Cross Society of the Republic of China period, 2004, pp. 108–117. For charity medical undertakings in Shanghai, see Zhou QiuGuang & Zeng Guilin, *A Brief History of Charity in China*, Beijing: People's Publishing House, 2006, p. 303.

50 Shanghai Shen Bao (ed.), The Opening of Epidemic Hospital, Compliments from the Medical Officer of the Ministry of Industry for the Epidemic Hospital", *Shen Bao*, July 2, 1918, p. 3, and July 6, 1918, p. 3.

51 Li Shunbao (ed.), *Dictionary of Warm Diseases*, pp. 189–190.

52 Volker Scheid, *Currents of Tradition in Chinese Medicine 1626–2006*, Seattle: Eastland Press, 2007, pp. 228, 229, 240, 242.

that the treatment back then was still "imitating the treatment of Wang Mengying". Obviously, the theory of doctors in the Qing Dynasty had a great influence on it, but there was no discussion on microorganisms.[53] Another example is from Cao Bingzhang (1878–1956). When the worldwide influenza spread to China in 1918, he set a disease name of "autumn plague" according to the standard of "season-based" naming in TCM, with the reference of the news in newspapers, including the world epidemic situation and the diagnosis of Western medicine, along with his understanding of the epidemic situation of influenza. He wrote a medical book *Essentials of Syndrome and Treatment of Autumn Plague* which clarifies its treatment. This style of writing in response to infectious diseases had inevitably integrated the factors of Western medicine. Moreover, Cao also admitted: "The diagnosis of TCM is only to examine phlegm, saliva and discharges. Due to the lack of microscope, there is no way for further examination, which is truly a missing part".[54] As TCM has no "microscope" for the test, the book does not discuss bacteria, but the understanding of "autumn plague" in TCM has taken into account the interpretation of Western medicine. After all, it is different from the ancient "plagues".

If Western medicine or bacteriology began to have an impact on TCM, we should review the important fever literature as the basis for further discussion. *Spring and Autumn of Medical World* published an article in 1937, pointing out that "the theory of acute infectious diseases in China is the same as that of typhoid fever. It is applicable to use a typhoid prescription. The prescription collection of TCM in internal medicine completely adopts the disease names of Western medicine and typhoid prescriptions were used the most".[55] It can be seen that typhology had become an important connotation of infectious diseases during the Republic of China period. Under the influence of Western medicine, among the typhoid medical books that discussed the concept of new bacteriology or infectious diseases, the more popular publication was Zhu Fu's *On the Compromised Essence of Typhoid and Miscellaneous Diseases*, which had a total of 6 editions. Yun Tieqiao's *Research on Typhoid Fever* and Huang Zhuzhai's *Collected Annotations on Typhoid Miscellaneous Diseases* had 5 editions; Lu Yuanlei's (1894–1955) *Current Interpretation of Treatise on Febrile Diseases* and Pan Chenglian's *New Interpretation of Treatise on Febrile Diseases* had 4 editions; Yu Wuyan's *Chart Notes on New Meanings of Typhoid Fever* and Zhu Weiju's *New Meanings of Typhoid Fever* had 3 editions.

Zhu Hushan once taught at North China Medical College and Peking Medical College. In the name of "compromising", his book was deeply influenced by Zhang

---

[53] Zhang Juren, *Ju Ren's Mecical Talk*, Beijing: People's Health Publishing House, 2006, pp. 28–29. For the treatment history at this stage, see Yang Haoru, Langfang Epidemic Prevention Record, Kong Bohua's Classic Study Office (ed.), *Answers to the Queries on the Treatment of Eight Infectious Diseases*, pp. 106–142.

[54] Cao Bingzhang, Chapter IV: Diagnosis of Autumn Plague, *On the Essence of Typhoid and Miscellaneous Diseases, Collection of Rare Modern TCM*. Warm Diseases, pp. 749–752.

[55] Xie Zeren, Answers to Mr. Zhang Xinyi's Questions about Typhoid Fever, *Spring and Autumn of Medical World*, 1937 (122), p. 32.

Xichun and Tang Zonghai. He called Tang a "teacher" and Zhang a "friend".[56] According to Zhu's theory of three energizers, all the routes of Qi transmission in the human body are based on the essence of the Tang Dynasty.[57] Both of them held that the actual route of Qi flow in the human body.[58] In his book, he reviewed the academic history of typhoid fever before the Republic of China period, affirmed the historical position of Zhang Zhongjing in the Eastern Han Dynasty to carry forward the past and forge ahead into the future, refuted all typhoid fever work from Wang Shuhe and those after in the Jin Dynasty, and considered the development of typhoid fever as having gone through "five misfortunes". In short, it was "chaotic in the Jin Dynasty, different from the Tang and Song Dynasties, and wrong in the Yuan and Ming Dynasties". This theory is the legacy of Tang Zonghai's view that "after the Jin and Tang Dynasties, the truth had been gradually lost, and many mistakes were passed down to the Song and Yuan Dynasties".[59] Tang believed that doctors after the Jin Dynasty failed to carry forward classical medicine, which led to the questioning of the anatomical form and quality of Western medicine. This argument was based on the fact that ancient China (before the Jin Dynasty) had a good knowledge of anatomy and viscera essence, which indicates the intention to restore and respect ancient times. Most modern doctors believe that if classical learning can be restored, TCM will be able to compete with the newly developed Western medications. The last of the five misfortunes was "using Western medicine to improve national medicine, but destroying national medicine instead".

Zhu published *Complete Annotations of Treatise on Febrile Diseases* in 1940, which obviously absorbed more Western medicine theories than previous medical books. Of course, he still took "Qi" as the focus of medical theory, without believing that Western medicine anatomy could prove the truth of the human body, but Chinese and Western medicine could still be connected, "the treatment of TCM is detoxification, and the treatment of Western medicine is sterilization". He held that the West attached importance to "the science of human organs without studying the principle of Qi", which resulted in many questionable cases. Knowing that some doctors in the world had noticed the theory of Qi, he held the optimistic view that Qi medicine would be demonstrated in the medical field in the future.[60] Though not knowing when that era would come, some TCM doctors were still filled with confidence in the basic medical theory of Qi during the Republic of China period.

Pan Chenglian's *A New Interpretation to Typhoid Fever* is another important work. Pan graduated from Shanghai Special School of TCM in 1929 and learned

---

[56] Zhu Fu, *The Latest Compromised Essence of Typhoid Fever Theory*, Vol. 1, Peking: North China Medical College, 1936, Introduction, p. 1b.

[57] Zhu Fu, *The Latest Compromised Essence of Miscellaneous Diseases*, Vol. 1, pp. 2a-3a. For the discussion of Tang Zonghai's three energizers, see Pi Kuoli, Image, Shape, Quality and Viscera Knowledge—the Enlightenment of Tang Zonghai's Triple-Energizer Theory, *Discourse in Ancient and Modern Times,* No. 15 (2006.10), pp. 71–98.

[58] Zhu Fu, *The Latest Compromised Essence of Miscellaneous Diseases*, Vol. 1, pp. 1a-3a.

[59] (Qing) Tang Zonghai, *Essence of Medical Classics*, Taipei: Lixing Publishing House, 1998, p. 1.

[60] Zhu Fu, *Complete Annotations of Treatise on Febrile Diseases*, Beijing: Zhuhu Mountain Medical Hut, 1940, pp. 7b–8b.

from famous doctors such as Cao Yingfu and Ding Ganren. After graduation, he started his practice in Wenzhou and helped in a Western medicine clinic. In 1937, he moved to Shanghai and taught at Shanghai College of TCM and Shanghai Chinese Medical College.[61] He recalled that the most important aspect at school was to systematically study books such as *Internal Canon of Medicine*, *Treatise on Typhoid Fever*, *Synopsis of the Golden Treatise*, *Perspectives on Febrile Diseases* and *Classic Materia Medica.* The deficiency of other subjects was supplemented by the *Gold Mirror of Medical Forbears.* It can be seen that with all the medical schools then, they still focused on some classics, and there was no disagreement between typhoid fever and warm disease schools.[62] Pan could read freely at the school, attended other medical schools, taught by correspondence, and conducted anatomical experiments of physiology and pathology. He also read the works of Japanese scholars, such as the *Iron Vertebrae of the Medical World* by Wada Keijuro, *Royal Han Medicine* by Yumoto Kyushin and the *Japanese Han Medicine* by Matsuzono Yasuhiro. These works of Japanese Han Medicine were born at the moment when they wanted to bolster Han medicine and try their best to fight against the pressure of Western medicine, which moved many Chinese doctors. Pan Zengyan said that in the 1930s, he had the desire and attempt of "filling the gap between classic and modern schools, and integrating TCM and Western medicine", and eventually wrote the book *A New Interpretation to Typhoid Fever,* which shows the influence of Western medicine and Japanese Han Medicine.[63] The study of Huang Zhuzhai is similar to that of Cao Yingfu, with the remnants of "revising the classics" and "retaining the old theory" in the Qing Dynasty. Huang Zhi's *Collected Annotations on Typhoid Miscellaneous Diseases* had a great influence in several provinces in Northwest China. As for the theory of treating typhoid by Yun Tieqiao and Lu Yuanlei, it was most influenced by Japanese typhologists.[64]

Another famous scholar of warm diseases, He Lianchen, was also knowledgeable of both the typhoid fever and warm disease systems. One of his main achievements is to annotate the important books of doctors in the Qing Dynasty, and to publish typhoid rhymes.[65] In addition to the previously mentioned *(Revised) Generalizations on Febrile Diseases*, he also reprinted and annotated the works of Yu Genchu and

[61] Sheng Zengxiu et al. (eds.), *Biographies of Doctors, Chronology, 100 Chinese Medicine Clinicians in a Century.* Pan Chenglian, Beijing: China Chinese Medicine Press, 2001, pp. 1–10, 357–360.

[62] Zhu Shipei (ed.), *Pan Chenglian's Views on Warm Diseases*, Shanghai: Shanghai University of TCM Press, 2009, Preface, p. 1. However, it was impossible for all doctors to share one idea. Honestly, this was a response influenced by the revival of classical medicine then. At that time, there were indeed many voices against febrile disease, but few voices against typhoid fever.

[63] Zhu Shipei (ed.), Pan Chenglian's Views on Warm Diseases, pp. 1–2.

[64] Ren Yingqiu, Schools in the Research on Typhoid Fever, included in Liu Shien and Mao Shaofang (ed.), *Commentaries of Contemporary Famous Doctors on Zhongjing's Typhoid Fever,* Beijing: Xueyuan Publishing House, 2008, pp. 114–127.

[65] He Lianchen (ed.), *Updated Annotations on the Song of 100 Typhoid Fever Syndromes*, Fuzhou: Fujian Science and Technology Press, 2008, Introduction, pp. 5–6. In addition, for the historical significance of the medical rhymes of the Ming and Qing Dynasties, see Angela Ki Che Leung, Introduction and Popularization of Medicine in China in the Ming and Qing Dynasties, *French*

Wu Zhen (Kun'an), doctors in the Qing Dynasty. The former book was compiled into *Popular Treatise on Typhoid Fever.* The latter was originally entitled *A Survey of Febrile Diseases.* He Lianchen said that he couldn't find the book after a 10-year search in the late Qing Dynasty. Eventually he found the manuscript. As he couldn't bear to see it being obliterated, he managed to have it published, renaming it as *Treasure Raft of Influenza.* The categorization of diseases also contribute to the integration of typhoid fever and warm disease schools by naming it "influenza". In fact, it also discusses typhoid fever and warm disease symptoms. The two books have 4 or 5 editions each.[66]

As for the warm disease medical books influenced by Western medicine, there were relatively few. Among them, the works on warm diseases relating to infectious diseases and even bacteria were *Chinese Seasonal Diseases* compiled by Shi Yiren in 1931, which was published in 5 editions according to *Catalogue.* However, the book had been revised repeatedly. Shi Yiren's first statement in 1953 edition indicates that he had updated the book 9 times, and compiled it into typhoid and warm diseases *of TCM* in 1956. The book advocates the integration of typhoid fever and warm diseases, but highlights some of their respective characteristics, with the expectation of subsiding the dispute between the two as well as resolving the contradictory views of ancient and modern schools. It's probably not the individual opinion of Shi Yiren himself, but a trend of the time in the academic field of TCM then.[67] Moreover, Shi put forward a very insightful view that there were some problems in editing medical books in ancient times: "First, due to the limitations of the environment and customs, they treated patients within a hundred miles and thought that everything in the world followed the same rule as what they could see and hear. This speculation is wrong. Second, due to inconvenient transportation, it was difficult to mail books. With limited reference materials, this self-reliance and blind obedience was inevitable. Third, personal knowledge is limited but rational research is infinite. Making one's own knowledge as worldly knowledge is not only fallacious but also impossible".[68] During the Republic of China period, the changes brought about by the technology of book printing and convenient transportation made the circulation of books easier and the publication of medical books more prosperous. Intellectuals were more eager to explore new knowledge than holding on to their own views and attack the opposing party as they had done in the past. Medical education was no longer the teaching–learning mode between doctors and their apprentices. In the modern public TCM schools, medical knowledge could be openly exchanged and discussed, which was the reason for the prosperity of medical integration. This was the popular academic

---

Sinology, Vol. 8 (Special Issue of Education History), Beijing: Zhonghua Book Company, 2003, pp. 155–179.

66 (Qing) Wu Zhen, updated by He Lianchen, *Treasure Raft of Influenca,* Fuzhou: Fujian Science and Technology Press, 2004, Introduction, pp. 1–2.

67 Shi Yiren, *Typhoid and Warm Diseases in TCM,* Shanghai: Shanghai Health Publishing House, 1956, Preface and Introduction.

68 Shi Zhensheng, *Medical Talk of Modern School,* Beijing: TCM Ancient Books Publishing House, 1994, p. 680.

trend, whether for Western medicine, or typhoid fever and warm disease school in TCM.

In addition, Yun Tieqiao's *Understandings of Febrile Diseases* also has 5 editions. Although the book is classified as a work of febrile diseases, it spared no effort to attack the theory of febrile diseases. The book harshly criticizes the epidemic warm disease school that "its fallacies spread and killed thousands of people, a crime past forgiving. It has the fundamental fallacies without reasoning, and its medication makes no sense. House hygienism, fluid enhancement, various components of breathing-controlling pills are nothing but nourishing or moist ingredients, telling of fantastic tales. These fallacies are found in *Analysis on Febrile Diseases, On Febrile Disease,* as well as *Perspectives on Febrile Diseases.* In the note added in his book *On Febrile Disease,* Wang Mengying was demonstratively outspoken. Today it's no more than a posturing, the sayings of a swindler".[69] At this time, the warm disease science was weak, and no doctors came out to defend it against Yun's attack. Yun tried to attack the theory of warm diseases to expound on its correctness and orthodox position of the theory of typhology, which is a case to show the conflict of the two schools.

The most insightful work on febrile diseases during the Republic of China period, with the integration of TCM and Western medicine, is the *Interpretations of Chinese and Western Febrile Diseases* by Wu Xihuang (Ruifu) in 1920. At present, there are 7 editions of the manuscript. The book mainly introduces the treatise on febrile diseases in TCM. Some articles are annotated with the names of Western medicine and infectious bacteria as the explanations. For example, "there are eight febrile diseases in Western medicine. In addition to gangrene, rash and smallpox, they are divided into enteritis, infectious fever diseases, recurrent fever diseases and mild fever diseases. The last four are classified in TCM as febrile diseases. Enteritis is recently taken as China's typhoid fever, which as we now know is a big mistake".[70] He took warm disease to respond to Western infectious diseases, rather than typhoid fever. As for the warm diseases of pregnant women, Wu also introduced the Western puerperal fever. This disease is caused by the midwife's "not being sanitized properly, and the toxic mold is brought into the birth gate by the hands of the midwife or the woman in labor, as well as utensils, cloth and other items", "in the case of sepsis, the virus is absorbed by the lymphatic vessels, first invades the genitals, then the peritoneum, and finally damages the whole body".[71] Wu's theory is more avant-garde among doctors of the same generation in explaining TCM diseases with the theory of bacteria in Western medicine. In addition, Wu wrote a book entitled *Lecture Notes on Diseases of Four Seasons*, which is not included in the febrile disease category of *Catalogue*, and may have been published in 1936. As the lecture notes of Xiamen

[69] Yun Tieqiao, Understandings of Febrile Diseases, included *in Four Kinds of Medical Books, Vol. 4,* Fuzhou: Fujian Science and Technology Press, 2007, p. 123.

[70] Wu Xihuang, *On Febrile Diseases, Plagues and Warm Toxin—the Light and Severe Syndromes of Febrile Diseases, Vol. I, Interpretations of Chinese and Western Febrile Diseases*, Fuzhou: Fujian Science and Technology Press, 2003, p. 21.

[71] Wu Xihuang, *Interpretations of Chinese and Western Fever*, pp. 21, 114.

National Medical College, the book was jointly written by teachers and students, including Ye Zhencheng, a student living in Tainan, Taiwan.[72] The book mostly deals with bacteria of Western medicine, physiology and febrile diseases of TCM, but rarely expounds the *Treatise on Typhoid Fever. I*t should be classified as a work of febrile diseases. The author believes that Wu was the most neglected scholar of warm diseases during the Republic of China period. In addition, it can not be ignored that Wu also wrote a pamphlet, *An Outline of Treatise on Typhoid Fever*. It is said in the preface: "*Treatise on Typhoid Fever* is also a book for regulating six Qis".[73] He thought that the attack from Western medicine to the six Qis of TCM by using the theory of pathogenic bacteria was due to the fact that it didn't understand that the growth of bacteria depended on the "climate", as the epidemics were related to seasons, instead of bacteria.[74]

As for the publisher who collected the essence of various books during the Republic of China period, there was also the book *Orthodox School of Warm Diseases*. The book was a handout for Wang Dexuan to teach warm diseases at the Hunan National Medical College. Another designated textbook of the school was Shen Xiaogu's *Complete Book of Warm Diseases* adapted from Shi Yiren's work. As Wang felt that "there never have been orthodox books on warm diseases", he particularly hunted for the ancient and modern medical books and compiled them into one book, including the excerpts of Wu Xihuang and He Lianchen's works.[75] He believed that it was wrong for doctors in the Qing Dynasty to say that there was no method to treat febrile diseases in the *Treatise on Typhoid Fever.* However, it would be too much to completely disregard the science of febrile diseases like Yun Tieqiao's attitude toward warm diseases. He stated that as long as it can be consistent with the classical theory, even the study of warm diseases should be preserved. This is the "real implementation to Zhongsheng's theory", which fully demonstrates the compromising concept febrile disease study.[76] The book was written in the form of lecture notes. Although it has not been reprinted, it can be seen that the development of the warm disease school was the acme of that time. But it just collected old theories and compiled them into lecture notes, with less involvement of bacteriology. For example, "The pathogen of plagues is pathogenic factors from heaven and earth, that is, turbid Qis, filthiness and bacteria. As it is a sticky substance, it can not enter from the pores of the skin, but only from mouth and nose. As for pestis, it is also infected by skin stabbing or flea bite of dead rats. When the skin is injured, the toxins got into

---

[72] Wu Xihuang, *Lecture Notes on Diseases of Four Seasons*, Taipei: Xinwenfeng Publishing Company, 1991, Preface by Li Lichen, p. 2 and "Name List of the Proofreaders" at the end of the book.

[73] Wu Xihuang, *Handout of Typhoid Outline*, Taipei: Xinwenfeng Publishing Company, 1985, Preface by Yang Tingshu, p. 9.

[74] Wu Xihuang, *Interpretations of Six Qis, Handout of Typhoid Outline*, pp. 9, 20.

[75] Wang Deshuan, Orthodox School of Warm Diseases, included in Lu Zheng (ed.), *Collection of Rare Modern TCM· Medical Talks Warm Diseases*, p. 195.

[76] Wang Deshuan, Orthodox School of Warm Diseases, included in Lu Zheng (ed.), *Collection of Rare Modern TCM Medical Talks Warm Diseases*, p. 200.

the blood, which allows the entry of toxins, rather than the pores of the skin."[77] This statement generally acknowledges the correctness of the theory of bacteria, nothing different from the views of contemporary doctors. According to the medical books on warm diseases in the statistical table, the theory of infectious diseases in Western medicine was not favored by the doctors then. Instead, the focus was on typhoid and epidemics.

3.4 The Influence of Japanese Medical Books

In the late Qing Dynasty and the early Republic of China period, various books on medicine and health were translated from Japanese into Chinese. Many people made their contributions during this process. According to Zhang Zhongmin's research, the translation of medical books in the late Qing Dynasty was mostly written by missionaries. However, at the beginning of the twentieth century, many Chinese, especially students studying in Japan, began to translate Western medicine books by themselves. They mostly learned Western medicine with the help of Eastern medical books. Kang Youwei first put forward the method of using Japanese books to introduce western learning. Cai Yuanpei said: "The translation of Japanese books were prevalent and promoted at schools, turning into a type of fashion in the academic world".[78] According to the author's statistics, the most important publications of Japanese medical books are ranked in the following order: *A Survey of Typhoid Fever* and *Interpretations of Typhoid Fever* by a Japanese named Tanba Motoken (style name Yirou, pseudonym Luoting) with 6 editions for each, of which the former was updated by He Lianchen and then became a book entitled *Updated Survey of Typhoid Fever* with 4 editions, but actually it had more than 10 editions. In fact, these two books were published more times than many medical books in China during the Republic of China period. As for the famous Yumoto Kyushin, his *Royal Han Medicine* had 4 editions; other Japanese Han medical classics published in more than 3 editions, including the *Treatise on Typhoid Fever in 1060* which was annotated by Otsuka Keisuke, *Views on Typhoid Fever* by Asada Tadatsune (style name Zongbo, pseudonym Liyuan) and *Compilation of Typhoid Fever* compiled and annotated by Tanba Motojane (style name Lianfu).

After the Meiji Restoration, the fate of Japanese Han medicine was quite similar to that of Chinese medicine. Both being faced with the fate of being abolished, which gave Chinese medicine a feeling of solidarity with Japanese Han medicine. Japanese traditional Han medicine was faced with the pressure of Western medicine earlier. When TCM wanted to seek the anti-West experience and comfort from Japanese traditional Han medicine, they saw the glory of the TCM ancient prescription school.

---

[77] Wang Dexuan, Orthodox School of Warm Diseases, included in Lu Zheng (ed.), *Collection of Rare Modern TCM Medical Talks Warm Diseases*, pp. 195–200.

[78] Zhang Zhongmin, Publication and Cultural Politics: A Study of "Health" Books in the Late Qing Dynasty, pp. 114–120, 184–188, 193.

Liao Yuqun believed that the admiration for the Chinese ancient school from modern Japanese, such as Yoshimasu Todo, reached its peak. Liao held that this was rooted in national self-esteem and the need to build academic idols, like Wu Xiusan, a Doctor of Medicine, said: "The status of Han medicine in our country is equal to the status of the Chinese ancient prescription school". The impact of Western medicine turned to be an enhancement of the ancient prescription school, because the scholars who studied Chinese prescriptions automatically used the empirical method of modern science as the evaluation standard. The ancient school took the *Treatise on Typhoid Fever* as the golden rule. It did not pay attention to the syndrome differentiation of the six meridians, nor the mysterious theories of Yin and Yang, five elements and viscera in the *Internal Canon of Medicine*. What it advocated was "where there is a syndrome, there should be the medicine". Scholars promoting Han medicine in modern times believed that the *Treatise on Typhoid Fever* itself did not attach importance to the philosophical medical theory and admired the ancient prescription school for "having long been devoted to experiments and personal trials by abandoning all empty discussions"[79] before the flourishing of Western medicine. Modern Chinese medicine also noticed such a research model. For example, Lu Yuanlei said: "200 years ago, a famous Japanese doctor, Yoshimasu Todo, emerged. He marked each of Zhongjing's prescription with the dosage standard. Now, the revival of TCM in Japan owes its credit to Yoshimasu Todo. The medication standard of Yoshimasu Todo has very clear regulations, which is different from the Chinese vague expressions like cold, heat, warm, invigorating blood and regulating Qi. Now the Japanese who turned from the new school into the old one carried it further with some experimental modifications."[80] In addition to the above information, many Chinese doctors, including Lu, held that the research methods of the Japanese Han medicine were so desirable that it was enough to prove the deficiency of Chinese medicine. Another example is Huang Zhuzhai's *Treatise on Typhoid and Miscellaneous Diseases*, which also uses many explanations of Japanese Han medicine, and it is all based on the attention paid to Chinese medicine from ancient Japanese Han medicine.[81] History is like a mirror. Under the dual pressure of national self-esteem and modern science, Japanese Han medicine confronted the difficulties instead of withdrawing, showing TCM doctors the light for the "revival of Royal Han medicine". TCM was greatly concerned with the interpretations and the development of the movement. Lu Shige (1879–1944) said in his *Shige's Medical Talk*:

> "Royal" means Japanese native herbal therapy, while "Han" means Chinese medicine that has been handed down from China. Since tens of thousands of people jointly supported the revival of Han medicine, which had been officially practiced in Japan ever since. It was more and more popular among the people, who preferred folk therapy to Western medicine. The so-called folk therapy is to treat diseases with herbal medicine. In reality, Han Medicine have

---

[79] Liao Yuqun, Overlooking *Royal Han Medicine—Understanding Japanese Traditional Medicine*, Taipei: Dongda Book Company, 2007, pp. 130–131.

[80] Lu Yuanlei, Medication Standards, Lu's Collection of Medical Theories, included in Zhang Yuping (ed.), *Two Kinds of Lu Yuanlei's Medical Books*, Fuzhou: Fujian Science and Technology Press, 2008, p. 331.

[81] Huang Zhuzhai, *Treatise on Typhoid and Miscellaneous Diseases*, pp. 492–497.

> always been popular ever since the reform, in a relatively open way. Once the ban was lifted, Chinese medicine stood out, springing up like mushrooms. The practitioners of Japanese Royal Han Medicine had prosperous careers.[82]

The success of this movement was a boost for TCM during the Republic of China period. Japan has a long history of absorbing TCM knowledge, and has also preserved many precious TCM books. In the *Annals of Visiting Japan* at the end of the Qing Dynasty, it was pointed out that "climate in Japan, though not as damp as that of the southern Yangtze River in China, is no less erosive as that of Hebei in China. Why can much of the heritage of the Tang dynasty survive till today? It's due to the fact that it has been planted in the homes of the powerful so that they could be protected from the repeated housefires. As for the manuscripts, they were made of cocoon paper from other countries, which are more durable than cloth and silk, and they have lasted for thousands of years without breaking apart."[83] The well-preserved classical medical books in Japan were in line with the Han medicine revival movement dominated by ancient prescription schools at the time, which led to the reflection from the TCM doctors on the importance of classical medicine. Guo Ziguang maintained that the characteristic of Japanese Han medicine was to adopt the methods of *Treatise on Typhoid Fever* and *Synopsis of the Golden Treatise*, which is different from the treatment of warm diseases in modern Chinese medicine.[84] This tendency is also consistent with the new trend of TCM at that time.

The following is the discussion for a few important medical books. The first is Yumoto Kyushin's *Royal Han Medicine*. Chen Cunren had been to Japan when preparing another set of famous *Royal Han Medicine Series*. Like many TCM doctors, he bought some Japanese Han medicine works and brought them back for reference. Cao Bingzhang also said that he had more than 350 kinds of typhoid medical books in his possession. He commented on some typhoid works, among which "only Asada Weichang's *Compilation of Typhoid Fever* of 6 volumes can be called the perfect compilation with innovative essence". As for Chen's teacher, He Lianchen, according to Cao Bingzhang: "(He) enjoys reading typhoid fever books, and had his particular views. There had been other typhoid fever publication series, such as Tanba Motoken's *A Survey of Typhoid Fever*, *Interpretations of Typhoid Fever*, Xu Shuwei's *Annotations on the Song of 100 Typhoid Fever Syndromes* and Asada's unpublished *Views on Typhoid Fever* that is in my collection. Mr. He had supplemented or annotated the theories, which later was put into publication".[85] It can be seen that TCM

---

[82] Lu Shige, The Revival of Chinese Medicine in Japan, Shige's Medical Talk, included in Shen Hongrui and Liang Xiuqing (eds.), *General Views Medical on Chinese Medicine in China*, p. 2046. Lu had a profound observation and explanation on the revival of Japanese Royal Han Medicine.

[83] (Qing) Yang Shoujing, Annals of Visiting Japan, included in *Updated Complete Library in the Four Branches of Literature History Catalogue, Vol. 930*, Shanghai: Shanghai Ancient Books Publishing House, 1997, p. 472.

[84] Guo Ziguang, *Essence of Japanese Han Prescription Medicine,* Chengdu: Sichuan Science and Technology Press, 1989, p. 363.

[85] He Lianchen (ed.),revised by Wang Zhipu et al., *Updated Popular Treatise on Typhoid Fever*, Cao Bingzhang's preface, p. 19.

doctors were very interested in reading and annotating Japanese medical books. Lu Yuanlei even made a lot commentaries on the study of typhoid fever. He said:

> Of the authors in the modern medical world, no one is as knowledgeable as Xu Lingtai, as smart as Ke Yunbo and as moderate as You Zaijing. They are all assets of today's world. In the Sui and Tang Dynasties, this eastern neighbor stole from China the thoughts and took them as the civilization of their three islands, including the study of medicine. After generations of endeavor, it tends to excel its master. The medical books of that country, like ones by Yoshimasu father and son, are as incisive as those by Ke and You, but only more profound. The Tanba father and son are as profound as Lingtai, but only more incisive and moderate. Others, such as Odaiyodo, Masahiro Yamada and Nakanishi Koretada, were all vigorous writers with their own established schools. During my teaching of the classes "Generals" and "Synopsis" at Shanghai National Medical College, I have been searching and collecting old books, and browsed many of the schools of thought, on which basis the above is by no means just flattery. Recently, Yumoto Kyushin wrote *Royal Han Medicine* with three volumes by taking Yoshimasu's *Collection of Prescriptions*, attached with the notes of previous sages, along with his own ideas that are incisive to some extent. It is from Zhang Zhongjing's theory, rather than the study of Ye Tianshi and Wu Jutong, that Chinese doctors learned the revival of Han Medicine in the East.[86]

Lu believed that the study of typhoid fever in Japan even surpassed that in China. At that time, he taught classical medicine and took the theory of the ancient Japanese prescription school in his teaching. In his search for more Chinese medical works, Chen Cunren traveled to Japan and met Yumoto Kyushin, who entertained him with a tea ceremony and presented him two out-of-print Han medical works. Returning to China, Chen spent a year sorting out all his Chinese medical works. Together with the medical books successively purchased in Japan, there were more than 400 volumes, which were all published after the procedure of compilation and revision. He said: "Most of the Han medical books are the fluent writings in Chinese characters as they were written in the styles of the Han and Tang Dynasties, and the only revision needed is to add punctuation." It can be seen that it was quite popular for the publishing houses to consign people the work of editing and collecting Japanese medical books then.[87] In 1928, Zhou Zixu stated that, when he was translating *Royal Han Medicine*, the value of translating the book lies in its integration of the Qi of TCM and the experiments of Western medicine. His pioneering spirit lies in "being based on scientific experiments without adhering to any mysterious explanations", "what Yumoto said is exactly what I wanted to say but failed to express. The declining TCM can thus be revived".[88] This book had a great influence on doctors. Pan Chenglian said in his *A New Interpretation to Typhoid Fever*: "The dosages of all prescriptions in this book are based on *Royal Han Medicine* written by Yumoto Kyushin".[89] In regard to the form, conception and feasibility in the scientization of TCM, Japanese

---

86 Lu Yuanlei, Preface to 'Clinical Application of Han Medicine', Lu's Collection on Medicine, included in Zhang Yuping (ed.), *Two Kinds of Lu Yuanlei's Medical Books*, pp. 105–106.

87 Chen Cunren, *Life History of the Silver Dollar Era*, pp. 309–310.

88 Yumoto Kyushin, translated by Zhou Zixu, *Royal Han Medicine*, Beijing: People's Health Publishing House, 2007, Translator's introduction, p. 2.

89 Pan Chenglian, *A New Interpretation to Typhoid Fever*, Taipei: Xinwenfeng Publishing Company, 1976, Introduction, p. 1.

Han medicine provides a guideline for Chinese doctors to start dialogues. Even the pathological changes caused by infections or microorganisms, as well as the understandings and treatment of infectious diseases, are all related to Japanese Han medicine.

Yumoto studied Western medicine at first. Later, he found that something was missing in Western medicine. He turned to learn TCM and became a believer of it. In his book, he did not completely exclude science and experimentation, but pointed out the weaknesses in Western scientific methods, and used its valuable part to prove the theory of TCM. With his experience of turning from "a Western medicine learner" to "a follower of TCM", he "criticized science" without rejecting scientific demonstrations. These positions were consistent with the TCM development, and became an example that TCM often cited during the Republic of China period.[90] This also annoyed some intellectuals opposing TCM, such as Yu Yunxiu who hated TCM and wanted to have it abolished. He hated Yumoto and the Han medicine revival movement, took Yumoto's *Royal Han Medicine* as a book written by a Western medicine doctor with mixed thoughts of new and old, and particularly wrote the book *Criticism to Royal Han Medicine* to attack the cooperation between China and Japan in Chinese medicine (see Fig. 3.1),[91] Yu said:

> What is said in the book is to overstate the benefits of China's old medicine and Japanese Han medicine to attack modern medicine. The TCM doctors in the past generally thought that Yumoto, who started learning new medicine then the old medicine, then turned to attack the new medicine, happened to be the opposite of Yu Yunxiu (who turned from studying old medicine to the learning of new medicine, and then attacked the old medicine). This *Royal Han Medicine* is the life-saving talisman of China's old medicine. It can greatly promote the momentum of resisting new medicine, be used as a sharp weapon against the enemy's medical revolutionary army, misleading the tycoons and dignitaries by using it as an anesthetic to reduce their innovative ideas and restore the soul of their retro ideas. For this purpose, a lot of time was spent in translating his works, a lot of money was spent on its publication, advertisement and promotion. Sure enough, it was admired by quite a few having hazy notions of science.[92]

From this, we can see the status of Yumoto, the admiration for him from TCM and the hatred for him from Western medicine. In China, there is a saying that "ancient prescriptions can't cure current diseases".[93] Many people even attacked the

[90] Lu Shige, The Revival of Chinese Medicine in Japan, Shige's Medical Talk, included in Shen Hongrui and Liang Xiuqing (eds.), *General Medical Views on Chinese Medicine in China*, pp. 2048–2049.

[91] Shanghai Social Medicine Newspaper Office, *Social Medicine Paper*, Vol. 1, 1934 (6), Back Cover Advertisement.

[92] Yu Yunxiu, *Criticism on Royal Han Medicine,* Shanghai: Shanghai Social Medical Mewspaper Office, 1931, p. 1.

[93] Jia Dedao, *A Brief History of Chinese Medicine*, Taiyuan: Shanxi Science and Technology Press, 2002, pp. 231–247. The doctor who first put forward this view may be Zhang Yuanyuan (style name Jiegu) of the Jin Dynasty. It is originally from what Zhang Jifu said: "Jiegu cures diseases without ancient prescriptions. It is said that ancient prescriptions are not suitable for new diseases. Instead, they are harmful". Quoted from (Jin) Zhang Yuanyuan, *Medical Enlightenment*, Beijing: people People's Health Publishing House, 1978, Zhang's preface, p. 1.

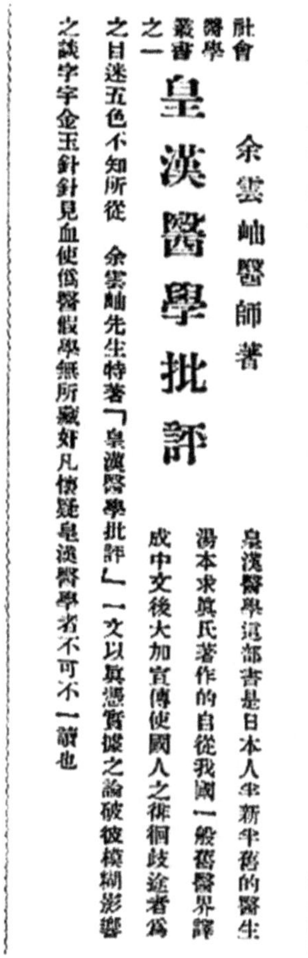

社會醫學叢書之一

余雲岫醫師著

皇漢醫學批評

皇漢醫學這部書是日本人半新半舊的醫生湯本求眞氏著作的自從我國一般舊醫界譯成中文後大加宣傳使國人之徘徊歧途者爲之目迷五色不知所從　余雲岫先生特著「皇漢醫學批評」一文以其憑實據之論破彼模糊影響之談字字金玉針針見血使僞醫假學無所藏奸凡懷疑皇漢醫學者不可不一讀也

Fig. 3.1 Criticism to Royal Han Medicine by Dr. Yu Yunxiu

ancient prescriptions for typhoid fever for not being able to treat new warm diseases. However, Yumoto believed that Zhongjing prescriptions were the most basic foundation. They can be used flexibly by adding flavors or other ingredients, but "Zhongjing prescriptions must be taken as the criterion". Using the ancient prescription rigidly without increasing or decreasing the dose, it would definitely fail in the treatment of today's disease. Yumoto's affirmation of the value of ancient prescriptions for typhoid fever had influenced Chinese doctors. In the academic development of TCM during the Republic of China period, typhoid fever gradually gained the upper hand. Affected by this, doctors began to advocate Zhongjing's medicine and belittle the warm disease school of Ye and Wu.[94] Lu Yuanlei said: "Western medicine has been practiced in Japan for 50 years, and TCM has almost lost its footprint. Currently, TCM in Japan has been revitalized, and the Oriental Medical Association and Royal

94 Yumoto Kyushin, translated by Zhou Zixu, On the Relationship between Ancient Prescriptions and Later Prescriptions, *Royal Han Medicine*, pp. 163.

Han Medical Community have been established, where gongs and drums are trumpeted. Now from their books and newspapers being available, I knew that all TCM in Japan is Zhongjing school. Many of their Western medicine doctors changed to TCM, admiring Zhang Zhongjing. They said that Zhongjing's prescriptions have more efficacy than" foreign prescriptions. "Moreover, many diseases that cannot be cured by "foreign doctors" can be cured quickly by Zhongjing methods. However, there has never been a word of compliment to Ye Tianshi. It can be seen that a fast-talking fellow like Ye Tianshi can only coax the Suzhou people, but not the Japanese."[95] Lu's criticism is harsh enough to confirm the desire of TCM to resist Western medicine by restoring the glory of classical medicine, which has been enhanced by the research of Japanese Han Medicine.

Focusing on the interpretation of microorganisms, Yumoto quoted the Chinese medical book "typhoid fever is taken as a toxin and is the most fatal Qi" in *Royal Han Medicine.* He explained: "This pathology is due to the lack of knowledge in bacteriology, but it can not be blamed as it did no harm to the actual treatment".[96] Yumoto believed that the treatment method in *Treatise on Typhoid Fever* still had its value, and the ignorance of bacteriology did not hinder its therapeutic efficacy. Yumoto once used the physiological view of Western medicine to explain the context of infectious diseases in classical medicine. He said: "The delirium and mumbles of intestinal typhoid patients can be explained by the invasion of bacteria into the brain, which is what Zhongjing meant".[97] He annotated the provisions of classical medicine with new Western medicine theory and put scientific makeup on traditional classics. What's more, he also compared the influence of bacteria in the body with the "toxin" in the literature. He said: "If the blood and the Qi are not stagnant, there are no toxins in the body. No harm can be done even though there are toxic pathogenic factors or having thousands of bacteria".[98] He emphasized the "stagnancy" of Qi and blood, indicating that as long as the Qi and blood in the human body are smooth, neither "toxins" nor "bacteria" can harm the human body. This statement shares the common ground with the views of Chinese doctors back then, especially "detoxification", which became one of the important ideology of many TCM doctors in the early Republic of China period that TCM could treat bacterial infectious diseases.[99]

The discussion of new warm diseases in Chinese medicine is more than what was written above. The most important theory in Yumoto Kyushin is probably the "sweating method" of TCM, a way to release the toxins from the body. For example,

---

[95] Lu Yuanlei, Medication Standard, Lu's Collection of Medical Theories, included in Zhang Yuping (ed.), *Two Kinds of Lu Yuanlei's Medical Books,* p. 331.

[96] Yumoto Kyushin, translated by Zhou Zixu, Notes on Muskmelon Pedicel Powder, *Royal Han Medicine,* p. 224.

[97] Yumoto Kyushin, translated by Zhou Zixu, Notes on Yangming Disease, *Royal Han Medicine,* p. 296.

[98] Yumoto Kyushin, translated by Zhou Zixu, On the View of Infectious Diseases Not Being Established if No Toxin is Found in One's Body, *Royal Han Medicine,* p. 21.

[99] Nie Yuntai, Typhoid Detoxification Therapy, included in Liu Bingfan and Zhou Shaoming et al. (eds.), *Essence of Famous Hunan Medical Classics. Internal Medicine,* Changsha: Hunan Science and Technology Press, 1999, pp. 823–863.

the article *Scientific Basis for the Application of Sweating Agents* explains the theoretical basis of sweating and detoxification: "According to the test of Aluroa, sweat is toxic. Injecting 10–15 cubic centimeters of it into the blood vessels of a dog of one kilo, it will cause gastrointestinal symptoms and death within 15 to 84 h". It is also said that the sweating method is limited. In the field of warm diseases, "sweating drugs can be used in the early stages of febrile infectious diseases, or acute catarrh and cold in the airway".[100] He tried to construct a reasonable scientific explanation of TCM therapies, as how Chinese and Japanese doctors connected with the knowledge of bacteriology through the explanation of sweating. In addition, he did not think that the disease names of Western medicine are absolutely important, because TCM is the treatment of "syndromes" (the symptoms of patients), rather than the treatment of "causes" (such as bacteria and parasites). The so-called "cause" of Western medicine is not the root of the disease, but the syndrome treatment of TCM seemed to be "particularly effective".[101] As for the specific methods and the responses of TCM, further details will be given in the following chapters. Now let's take a look at the impact of other Japanese medical books.

Let's examine the influence of Tanba on Chinese medicine. As early as the end of the Qing Dynasty, in *Annals of Visiting Japan*, it has been discussed that "Japanese doctors are more knowledgeable, and there are more collections of books among doctors, such as Kitamura, Taki, Shibue, Kojima and Mori. So there has been a wide collection of medical classics".[102] The book mentions the contribution and erudition of Tanba (Taki), a famous family in the history of Japanese medicine. Among the modern TCM researchers, Motojane should be ranked at the top. In the several editions of *Compilation of Typhoid Fever* published in the early Republic of China period, it is explained: *Treatise on Typhoid Fever* takes "cold Qi" as the theme of the book, because cold is the most serious external pathogen among the six Qis, which exists in all seasons. Unlike heat, dampness and dryness only occur in certain seasons. So "all harmful external pathogenic factors are called typhoid fever". However, Zhongjing's book is not all about "typhoid fever".[103] It can be seen from the discussion that Motojane mainly focused on typhology, rather than the discussion of warm diseases during the Qing Dynasty. This argument also affected his son and extended to some doctors in Japan and China. He Lianchen quoted from Asada: "Zhang Zhongjing's *Treatise on Typhoid Fever* has been admired by great doctors

[100] Yumoto Kyushin, translated by Zhou Zixu, Scientific Basis for the Application of Sweating Agents, *Royal Han Medicine*, pp. 140–141.

[101] Yumoto said: "As mentioned above, we must choose the three methods of sweating, vomiting and excreting according to the symptoms, which is what Zhongjing meant in "giving treatment according to the symptoms". The right cure can only be prescribed after discovering the constitution of the patient and the location of the virus, regardless of the pathogens or the names of the diseases." Quoted from Yumoto Kyushin, translated by Zhou Zixu, On the Treatment of the Most Infectious Diseases Based on Their Symptoms Instead of Pathogens, *Royal Han Medicine*, p. 22.

[102] (Qing) Yang Shoujing, *Annals of Visiting Japan, included in Updated Complete Library in the Four Branches of Literature History Catalogue*, Vol. 930, p. 472.

[103] Tanba Motojane, *Selected Medical Books of Yu Xiu Hall Compilation of Typhoid Fever*, Beijing: People's Health Publishing House, 1983, pp. 8–9.

of all times. It is the divine book of medical Tao for all ages, and the secret code of saving people's lives". He was highly valued by Japanese Han doctors.[104]

Motojane's son Motoken wrote *A Survey of Typhoid Fever,* for which he selected 148 kinds of TCM works in the past. Unlike Chinese doctors in the Qing Dynasty who only repeatedly annotated the classics, he explored various diagnostic and treatment methods of various typhoid fever diseases, which expanded the research scope of typhoid fever.[105] On the other hand, it was said that Tanba Motoken's *A Survey of Typhoid Fever* "takes the strength of the past and eliminates their weaknesses, especially brings the epidemic warm disease into the three Yang Syndromes of typhoid fever, initiating the unity of typhoid fever and warm diseases".[106] In short, warm diseases were taken into account of the discussion of the typhoid fever system, rather than being regarded as the two opposing sides. Motojane discussed it in another book:

> Pathogenic Qi changes according to individuals. It is not proper to distinguish the syndromes from the cold or warm seasons. Therefore, what Zhongjing called apoplexy, typhoid fever, and warm disease are only names given to describe their pathogenesis, rather than their nature. Typhoid fever is not named for wind, cold, seasonal Qi or epidemic diseases.

This statement explicates the general and comprehensive status of "typhoid fever". Motoken also believed that people have different symptoms due to different "Qis", and it was not needed to seek particularly the names of the diseases, because the "Qi" of each era or season was different. He said: "Zhongjing didn't classify the disease by pathogenic causes but used typhoid fever as a general name instead". Motoken held that there was no need to stick to the "distinction between climate or epidemic reasons". It was due to the fact that "disease differs in each individual", so a good doctor could take the "Qi" in each "individual" as the standard of syndrome differentiation.[107] He was not led by the discussion of disease names like some Chinese doctors. Finally, Motoken attached great importance to reading medical classics. When his disciple Ye Yuanxi recalled the teacher's words in *Selected Medical Books of Yu Xiu Hall Interpretations of Typhoid Fever*, he recorded:

> My teacher (Motoken) often told his disciples that reading medical classics is different from reading other books. In reading medical classics, we should be open-minded, humble with a peaceful mind. To study the principles of life, it is to seek the compatibility of textual meanings and clinical experiences. Even if it is grounded, it still needs to be proved from classics and tested with various cases. Only by summarizing all the classics, exploring its essence with periodical accumulations, could one come up with the proper treatment for various cases. This is what we call a good reader.[108]

---

[104] He Lianchen (ed.), *Updated Annotations on the Song of 100 Typhoid Fever Syndromes,* Introduction, pp. 4–5.

[105] Tanba Motojane, A Survey of Typhoid Fever, included in Chen Cunren(ed.), *Royal Han Medicine Series, Vol. 5,* Shanghai: World Book Company, 1936, pp. 1–4, 263–279.

[106] Tanba Motojane, collated by Xu Changqing, *A Survey of Typhoid Fever,* Xu Changqing's preface.

[107] Tanba Motojane, *Selected Medical Books of Yu Xiu Hall Treatise of Typhoid Fever*, pp. 61–69.

[108] Tanba Motojane, *Selected Medical Books of Yu Xiu Hall Treatise of Typhoid Fever, Postscript of Ye Yuanxi*, pp. 74–75.

On the whole, the inspiration the Chinese doctors received from Motojane's study of typhoid fever can be briefly summarized as respecting the classics and restoring the ancient. To put it in a simple way, syndrome differentiation is based on the "Qi" of the human body rather than the "names of the diseases", and practicality is the key. The characteristics of other important medical books and academic thought found from literature statistics also tend to be respecting classics and restoring antiquity of the ancient school. For example, Koretada's *Research on Typhoid Fever* takes the opportunity of correcting the name of "cold pathogen (typhoid)" to endorse the position of Zhongjing's *Treatise on Typhoid Fever* as the general theory of fever. He said that "typhoid fever" was the ancient meaning of pathogenic Qi, and the names of warm diseases, spring epidemic and epidemic virus in later generations were developed by Wang Shuhe, which was not being deceitful on purpose, but they are not what Zhongjing meant.[109] Akiyoshi also put forward the similar view in his *Personal Review on the Theory of Warm Epidemics*: "In his *Cases of Typhoid Fever*, wang Shuhe was not aware of the fact that typhoid fever was the general categorization of warm diseases. He stuck to the name on the basis of the Qis of the four seasons, taking the cold in winter as typhoid fever, and the incompatible climate in the four seasons as the cause of epidemic diseases".[110] Yuan Yuankai, the author of another book entitled "Warm Diseases", criticized Wu Youke's theory of "miscellaneous Qi" and "epidemic Qi" as nonsense, which are still within the scope of classical "six Qis".[111] He also denounced Wu Youke's theory that "typhoid fever is different from epidemic disease", and strongly defended the general position of "typhoid fever, the general name of epidemic disease".[112] Another example is Akiyoshi's *Personal Review on the Theory of Warm Epidemics*, which believes that "typhoid fever" and "epidemic disease" are basically two names associated with one disease, and their starting point is very different from Wu Youke's view that "epidemic disease is not typhoid fever". He even said: "Wu's so-called epidemic warm disease is the so-called Yangming disease in Changsha (Zhongjing's theory-translator's note); Wu's epidemic Qi is the so-called pathogenic wind in Changsha".[113] Although it does not completely deny

[109] Nakanishi Koretada, Research on Typhoid Fever, included in Chen Cunren(ed.), *Royal Han Medicine Series, Vol. 5*, pp. 10–11, 15–16. From the literature of the Republic of China period, it seems that Japanese Han doctors generally disagreed with Wang Shuhe's theory. As Wang Shuhe said in the *Treatment of Cold*, "it's all the empty talk about the transformation of pathogenic cold into febrile disease". All kinds of modern epidemics and febrile diseases were just caused by "pathogenic wind", so "cold" could be used to summarize their symptoms. The treatment principle was still based on the six meridians. It can be seen that the theory of fever in Japanese Han Medicine has a feature of reducing complexity to simplicity. See Goto Satoru, *Treatment of Cold*, included in Chen Cunren (ed.), *Royal Han Medicine Series, Vol. 5*, pp. 3–4.

[110] Wu Youke, reviewed by Akiyoshi, Personal Review on the Theory of Warm Epidemics, included in Chen Cunren (ed.), *Royal Han Medicine Series, Vol. 8*, p. 4.

[111] Yuan Yuankai, Miscellaneous Qi Theory, Research on Warm Diseases, included in Chen Cunren (ed.), *Royal Han Medicine Series, Vol. 8*, p. 35.

[112] Yuan Kai, Identification of Typhoid Epidemic, Research on Warm Diseases, included in Chen Cunren (ed.), *Royal Han Medicine Series, Vol. 8*, p. 14.

[113] Wu Youke, reviewed by Akiyoshi, Personal Review on the Theory of Warm Epidemics, included in Chen Cunren (ed.), *Royal Han Medicine Series, Vol. 8*, pp. 3–4.

Wu Youke's view, it is used to restore the essence of Zhongjing theory. At that time, the Chinese medicine research in Japan was widely known. Japanese Han doctors were skeptical of the "mistaken" inference that Zhongjing's *Treatise on Typhoid Fever* "lost" the treatment methods of warm diseases, and disagreed with the view that the supplementary theories or prescriptions of later generations were more effective than those of *Treatise on Typhoid Fever*. With regard to the research and discussions in the field of TCM warm diseases, Japanese Han medicine obviously strengthened the position of TCM typhology at that time.

3.5 The Revival of Classical Medicine During the Republic of China Period

On the resurgence of the study of *Treatise on Typhoid Fever* during the Republic of China period, Chen Wujiu (1884–1948) once said: "From the Ming and Qing Dynasties to the present, it have been an era of typhoid fever. Medical scholars have firmly taken the study of typhoid fever as the only task, and deemed it a shame for not reading *Treatise on Typhoid Fever*". He believed that since Western medicine was extensively introduced into China, the only missing part in Western medicine that could be made up by TCM was "to start with typhoid fever and it's doubtlessly an area of exploration".[114] It presents the optimistic attitude toward the development of typhology. Many TCM doctors believed that the revival of TCM must start from the subject of "typhoid fever". Many journals also had columns like "National Medicine Typhoid Lessons", "Typhoid Q & A" or "Typhoid Essentials… to explain some problems of typhology.[115] However, it was impossible to see the developmental characteristics of the whole history of warm diseases by completely abandoning the medical books of the febrile school. No matter how much attention had been paid to *Treatise on Typhoid Fever*, I'm afraid we can't ignore the fact that many doctors were of warm disease school, and there were still some warm disease medical books in the Qing Dynasty. Furthermore, the formation of epidemiology and bacteriology posed the challenge for both systems of typhoid fever and warm diseases.

In the minds of many TCM practitioners during the Republic of China period, there might be a developmental history of warm diseases in TCM. There is no doubt that the Qing Dynasty was almost dominated by the epidemic warm disease school. Yang Zemin (1893–1948) believed that "typhoid fever and warm diseases are the general names of acute warm diseases, which were arbitrarily called by the ancients. After the Qianlong and Jiaqing reigns, they set up the banner of warm diseases to confront typhoid fever. Logically speaking, it was only the argument at the verbal

---

[114] Chen Wujiu, On the Transformation of Typhoid Fever, included in Jiang Hongjun, et al. (eds), *Eight Books of Chen Wujiu Medicine*, Beijing: China TCM Press, 2010, p. 254.

[115] Tianjin Institute of TCM (ed.), *Authentic National Medicine,* 1934 (3), pp. 9–22.

level. In terms of treatment, it was the practical view, which was more important".[116] "Verbal argument" and "practical treatment is more important" can represent the opinions on the developmental of warm diseases, which was a linear and progressive approach. However, more doctors believed that this developmental was gradually regressive. Until the Qing Dynasty in the development of medical history, the ancient prescriptions had been overthrown and evolved to the so-called "light-dose school". For example, Te Tianshi founded the theory of "upward movement of febrile pathogens, first attacking the lung and transmitting the pericardium inversely", and "played down" (used light doses) all his life. Later, Wu Jutong worshiped Ye Tianshi and wrote the *Analysis on Febrile Diseases*, changing the "six classics theory" to the "treatment of three energizers", which "was practiced all over China, such as Jiangsu, Zhejiang, Anhui, Fujian and even some remote provinces. These prescriptions were quoted, taught by doctors to their disciples and from fathers to their sons, making 'a world of mint and burdock!'".

In addition, Yao Shichen thought that as Ye and Wu practiced in the south, their patients were mostly princes, nobles or rich merchants. These people lived in luxury, indulging themselves in fine food and lust, with occasional physical discomfort. Their sickness were no more than the minor cold or physical fatigue. Therefore, their prescription of "no need of hemp and cinnamon, just schizonepeta, divaricate saposhniovia root, burdock and downy moonwort would be enough for their cold cases". Their prescriptions were made according to the particular circumstances and constitution of their patients.[117] The prosperity of warm diseases was probably related to the ease of studying warm diseases and the ease of using warm disease prescriptions. Lu Jinsheng, who practiced medicine in Shanghai in 1913, explained in *Reviews of Medical Essence*: "It is not difficult to study the family of warm diseases. If you are well versed in the books of Ye, Wu, Xue Shengbai, Wang Mengying, Zhang Xugu and Lei Shaoyi, you would have a good grasp of the wisdom; if you can further distinguish the concurrent symptoms from the bad symptoms (symptoms not to be cured by sweating or discretion–translator's notes) and give them separate prescriptions, the cure rate will be nine out of ten".[118] Although there were many medical books on warm diseases during the Qing Dynasty, read a few most important books would be enough to practice. Patients also preferred doctors using lighter prescriptions, rather than the heavy ones from classics. Jiang Zuojing once commented on the crisis and the tricks of practicing in Shanghai:

> How easy can it be to practice medicine in Shanghai? People here were shallow and ignorant. Fearing dizziness, they preferred light dose for their treatment. When the doctors were seen living in grand houses, wearing fur coats, driving cars, they seemed to show themselves in high status, possessing high credentials. Their business was so good that they wouldn't bother to make house calls, even without adequate skills. It was said: 'this is what the famous doctors are'. Patients scrambled to them despite their high fees. Upon seeing a doctor, they

[116] Yang Zemin, Reviews on Systematic Differentiation of Warm Diseases, *Medical Talk in Seclusion*, Beijing: People's Health Publishing House, 1986, p. 37.

[117] Cao Yingfu, *A Record of Classical Prescription Experiments*, Yao Shichen's preface, pp. 17–18.

[118] Lu Jinsheng et al. (eds.), On Northern Febrile Diseases, Medical Talk on Preserving the Essence, included in Lu Zheng (ed.), *Collection of Rare Modern TCM. Medical Talk*, p. 973.

> would say: I'm weak and can't take the strong dose, tonics would be fine. The doctor would have to give the light prescription. He was then known for being good at keeping safe but the development of the disease was unknown.[119]

If the patient died later, the two sides would confront each other in court. The relevant medical association in charge of identification would also think that the medicine prescribed by the doctor was too light to cause death, leading to the abandoning of the effective TCM prescriptions, and finally it was the patients who suffer. Particularly when some patients also knew a little about medicine, they could make a whole list of the harm of the classic prescriptions, which even intimidated the doctors more. It is mentioned in the *Treatment of Damp and Warm Epidemics*:

> The worst pain is the person who knows a little about medicine. A patient who makes less and breaks more is the doctors biggest headache for whom no strong agent is to be used, with the excuse: to avoid the wrong treatment; neither the most effective prescription is to be used, with the excuse: it's too overbearing. The patient then gets the light prescription, and takes it at their own chosen time. Being ineffectively treated, he would blame it on the doctor, saying there are no good doctors nowadays. Like patients, like so-called famous doctors who cater to their needs. Therefore, a good doctor is not to comply with the patients, but to give them enlightenment instead.[120]

The situation of typhoid-fever-oriented in the North and febrile-disease-oriented in the South began to change in the late Qing Dynasty. Lu Jinsheng commented that Zhongjing had always been enshrined in the North, as well as in the Royal Hospital, in the Qing Dynasty. It is for this reason that there came a saying "doctors in Beijing don't know how to treat warm diseases". Among the medical books sold in the capital bookstores, the books of Chen Xiuyuan were very popular, while the books of Ye Gui and Wu Jutong were rarely purchased. Since when had this situation changed? Lu said in his *Medical Talk on Preserving the Essence*: "After the hospitals were set up with the funds from Emperor Xiaoqin, many southern doctors came to Beijing, and books by Ye and Wu were popular. Now those who are practising in Beijing have also switched to the Southern school".[121]

It can be seen that when the warm disease school began to decline in modern times, it was still influential. However, the medical authorities were mainly engaged in classical school practices. Xu Dingchao from Yongjia said that the Emperor tried to established schools in 1902, including medical schools. He was asked to teach in one of the universities. While teaching *Internal Canon of Medicine*, he also compiled the *Handouts on Typhoid Fever*, elucidating that in terms of the disputes between the two schools of typhoid fever and warm diseases, all the laws governing the treatment had been recorded in the classical medical books. He said: "Those who never read Zhongjing's book are incapable of understanding the theory of typhoid fever, nor the

---

[119] Jiang Zuojing, Biography of Mr. Cao Yingfu; Cao Yingfu, *A Record of Classical Prescription Experiments*, pp. 25–26.

[120] Shaoxing Medical Association, Treatment of Damp and Warm Epidemics, included in Li Shunbao (ed.), *Complete Book of Warm Diseases,Vol. II*. p. 2099.

[121] Lu Jinsheng et al. (eds), On Northern Febrile Diseases, Medical Talk on Preserving the Essence, included in Lu Zheng (ed.), *Collection of Rare Modern TCM. Medical Talk*, pp. 972–973.

principles of warm diseases".[122] However, the school of warm diseases was often valued based on some external factors. Yao Shichen said in the preface of *A Record of Classical Prescription Experiments* by Cao Yingfu that by neglecting the theory of typhoid fever and taking the theory of warm diseases as the golden rule was not the original intention of Ye and Wu. This tendency was probably enhanced by the following few factors stated later:

> (1)Teachers and disciples learn from each other, which turns out to be a rule. (2) *Treatise on Typhoid Fever* belongs to the classic Chinese, its words being simple but its meaning being abstruse. It is not as easy to read as *Guide* and *Analysis,* which stops the less learned from reading. (3) Misunderstanding Ye and Wu's theories and insisting on their own ways, ending up with being more and more confused. (4) Stubbornly holding *Treatise on Typhoid Fever* as ancient theory, which is out -of -date and should be prevented. (5) Most of the patients prefer light to strong doses, and the cunning doctors would take the opportunity to please them. One or two righteous doctors might try to give full play to the effectiveness of *Treatise on Typhoid Fever*, but they held themselves back for fear of accusations. In addition, coupled with the boasting of the so-called "modern prescription school", the social psychological pressure increased day by day. Even the classic book of the saint Zhongjing was thus ridiculed! I think this should not be blamed on Ye and Wu. It seems that we misunderstood it![123]

Since modern times, with the surge of medical innovation, the restoration of ancient classics has also been upgraded to another level. The development of ancient medicine can always be equated with national self-esteem and cultural foundation. Zhu Hushan believed that the revival of classical medicine had been around since modern times. The essence of classical medicine is "Qi", which can compete with Western medicine once it's restored. He further pointed out:

> For this purpose, one should first study the theories of *Internal Canon of Medicine, Materia Medica* and *Typhoid and Miscellaneous Diseases*, acquiring the profound knowledge before exploring Western medicine in understanding the structure of the human body, the movement of blood and Qi. The magic functions of circulation naturally merge and complement each other. Why do people hold on to one view and oppose another? It is truly self destructive, a laughing stock for the knowledgeable.[124]

In other words, before communicating and competing with Western medicine, we must first understand TCM classics. The content of ancient medical books is the noumenon and trunk of Chinese medicine, while the theories and medical books of warm disease school later are not. This is why Zhang Taiyan taught Zhang Cigong the way of learning medicine is "to take Changsha (Zhongjing-translator's note) prescriptions as the master without following *Lingsu Medicine*, *Internal Canon of Medicine* and *Classic on Medical Problems* in the past, nor Xue and Ye's theory at present", and "integrating the theory of the West so as to identify errors".[125]

---

[122] Xu Dingchao (ed.), Mr. Yongjia's Handouts on Typhoid Fever, included in Liu Shijue: (ed.), *Wenzhou Literature Series Collection of Wenzhou Modern Medical Books, Vol. I,* Shanghai: Shanghai Academy of Social Sciences Press, 2005, p. 268.

[123] Cao Yingfu, *A Record of Classical Prescription Experiments,*Yao Shichen's preface, pp. 17–18.

[124] Zhu Fu, *The Compromised Essence of the Principles for the Latest Miscellaneous Diseases*, Vol. II, pp. 116b–117a.

[125] Zhang Nianchi, *My Grandfather Zhang Taiyan*, Shanghai: Shanghai People's Publishing House, 2011, p. 107.

From the discipline structure of some new TCM schools during the Republic of China period, we can also find that in addition to the influence of Western medicine, classical medicine is the most important. Lu Yuanlei recorded in "II. Internal Medicine. Applied Medicine" in his *Course Description of Shanghai National Medical College*: "After Ye Gui gave his explanations on warm diseases, his disciples Wu Tang and Wang Shixiong followed, promoting and admiring them, sometimes to the extent of using them to competing with those of Zhongjing classics. Of their views, there are more mistakenly missing points than merits. It is a sign that TCM is declining. This class is intended to clarify the confusion on typhoid fever and warm diseases, which is attached to internal medicine, so that scholars won't be misled. The weekly schedule is: 6 h on *Treatise on Typhoid Fever*, 6 h on *Golden Treatise*, 5 h on modern prescriptions, 2 h on the clarifications on typhoid fever and warm diseases, which totals the classes of a year."[126] It shows the proportion of the curriculum formulated by the medical schools at that time. *Treatise on Typhoid Fever* accounted for the most, and warm disease was actually an auxiliary subject, though not being completely ignored. Lu Yuanlei said: "For a medical student, reading medical classics is like mining in the mountains and making salt by the ocean. They are abundant and inexhaustible". It would be too narrow to compile the teaching materials by adapting from one or two sources of the later medical scholars. It is stated: "The standard for the teaching materials is to limit the character to Zhang Zhongjing, books to *Treatise on Typhoid Fever*, *Golden Treatise*, *Zhouhou Prescriptions*, *Qianjin Prescriptions*, *The Secret Therapies of the Censors*, *Materia Medica* and *Supplementary Records of Famous Prescriptions*, with scientific methods."[127] It can be seen that the curriculum design and arrangement of the school focused on the interpretation of classical medicine, which was consistent with the spirit of adhering to classics, especially the medical books before the Tang Dynasty. This is a very special trend, that is, when the theory of TCM was questioned by Western medicine, it urged TCM to reflect the following: the strengths of ancient Chinese doctors were metaphorically referred to as lost technologies or the lost past, the situation which was caused by doctors not reading classics. But now they must be restored and developed. The evolution of the time tended to see the past as being better than the present, and even the wise were not knowledgeable about it. This may be called the degradation of medical development. Influenced by the comments of Japanese Han Medicine, it was said that TCM had declined since the Song Dynasty, and the real academic essence was all in the classical medical books. Lu Yuanlei even suggested that strict inspections should be made to the modern medical books, rather than the classical medical books. He said:

> Before the Jin and Tang Dynasties, the records of the facts were relatively faithful, and the facts were deduced into theories which were not too far from the truth. The facts were more

[126] Lu Yuanlei,Course Descriptions of Shanghai National Medical College, Lu's Collection of Medical Theories, included in Zhang Yuping (ed.), *Two Kinds of Lu Yuanlei's Medical Books,* pp. 96–97.

[127] Lu Yuanlei, On Sorting Out the Academic Works of TCM, Lu's Collection of Medical Theories, included in Zhang Yuping (ed.), *Two Kinds of Lu Yuanlei's Medical Books,* p. 104.

> reliable and the theories could also trigger ingenious thinkings, though they were not entirely correct. This is a treasure house for research and reference, for which no urgent inspection is needed. After the Song and Yuan Dynasties, there were many records being involved with exaggerations, and the books were not totally reliable as they were likely to be made up by the author on the basis of inadequate facts. For the books in modern times, it's been more available due to the progress of printing, and it was also easier to have them copied and resold, among which there was more misinformation than good points. The misinformation will spread widely if inspections doesn't follow quickly, then more people will be misled.[128]

Probably at this time, doctors thought that the publication of medical books of later generations was excessive and the academic degradation was too deplorable to be evaluated. Only the classic medical books could stand the test of time. Moreover, the purpose of medical development must focus on clinical efficacy. Under the challenge of Western medicine, TCM seemed to need stronger and more effective drugs and treatments, and classical medicine had become the source area to fulfil a wish list. Lu Yuanlei believed that with in-depth study of the description of disease types in *Treatise on Typhoid Fever*, one can discover that many treatments for acute warm diseases are included, such as malaria, measles and scarlet fever. Although their names are not found in *Treatise on Typhoid Fever,* they can be treated according to the syndrome differentiation of the six meridians in the book. What's more, many drugs having heavy agents that the warm disease school were afraid to use, including cinnamon twig, ephedra, bupleurum, plaster, aconite, would "shorten the course of the disease by half, comparing with drugs used by warm disease school". Just because "it's generally taken as warm disease", they would stop themselves from using the most effective and correct prescriptions. Lu sighed: "I believe that *Treatise on Typhoid Fever* is practical and that the modern theory of warm disease school is a medical degradation."[129] "Heavy agent" is more effective than "light agent". The trend behind this discussion is worth noting. The typhoid prescription, which was not popular with doctors, slowly regained its orthodox status.

Yu Yunxiu, who also shared great views on the theory of warm diseases in TCM, believed that the warm disease prescriptions were used by many doctors during the debate between the two schools in the Qing Dynasty. He analyzed the reasons: "No doctor trusted the prescriptions of Zhongjing in curing warm diseases, nor believed there was even typhoid fever in the south. Everyone was intrigued and trying to make some differences, among whom Ye's school was the most popular. Why? It's due to his high reputation and numbers of disciples, but his methods were mediocre. A weak medication can do no harm. If the disease is cured, it can get the credits of heavenly treatment; if it gets worse, there is not too much to be blamed for. This is what Gu Tinglin said as "a quack doctor who neither kills nor cures", and Xunzi's "a corrupt scholar who has no fault nor credits".[130] There were many criticisms

---

[128] Lu Yuanlei, Outline on Sorting Out the Academic Works of TCM, Lu's Collection of Medical Theories, included in Zhang Yuping (ed.), *Two Kinds of Lu Yuanlei's Medical Books,* p. 149.

[129] Lu Yuanlei, Principles of Medication for Acute Febrile Disease, A Survey of Treatise on Typhoid Fever,included in *Two Kinds of Lu Yuanlei's Medical Books,* pp. 48–49.

[130] Yu Yunxiu, On the Syndromes of Febrile Diseases, *Selected Works on Medical Revolution,* Taipei: Art and Culture Press, 1976, p. 190.

to the warm disease school, and "modern mild dosage prescriptions" were often questioned. Cao Yingfu said: "Aha, the modern prescriptions got such popularity when they are far from being tested. How can TCM be revived and compete with Western medicine?"[131] This was the change took place when many people began to pay attention to the effectiveness of classical prescriptions.

Although the overall development of the warm disease study in TCM during the Republic of China period was the revival of typhology, it does not mean that warm diseases are not important, or that they will not be developed in the future. In fact, with the convenience of circulation and printing of medical books, and the mode of medical practitioners' learning from ancient teachers to apprentices, self-study, and gradually to academic learning,[132] and even practicing in TCM hospitals,[133] most of the TCM training since the Republic of China period got the spirit of "syndrome differentiation and treatment". As Lu Yuanlei said, "any new academic invention of Western medicine, once recognized, were implemented by all. Although there are different schools of Western medicine in Germany, Japan, Britain and the United States, it is still consistent in theory. TCM had been divided into many branches after the Jin and Yuan Dynasties. Each successor had his own master to follow and there had been no unity. To achieve the unity, there should be medical academic research societies organized so as to preserve the right and eliminate the wrong".[134] Lu believed that it is not necessarily to prove which school is more prevailing, nor to view medical development from the perspectives of typhology or warm diseases. It was needed to have the medical integration within the academic system by eliminating the coarse and retaining the fine.

3.6 "Renewed Canonization" of TCM Classics

To sum up, this chapter discusses two academic perspectives based on TCM warm disease studies: externally, the dialogue with Western medicine on bacteriology or infectious diseases, and internally, the development of typology and warm disease schools. Yun Tieqiao, a modern Chinese doctor, believed that it was not easy for

---

131 Cao Yingfu, A *Record of Classical Prescription Experiments*,Yang Zhiyi's preface, p. 12.

132 From ancient times to the present, there have been several approaches in studying medicine.For the examples of ancient doctors' teaching (medicine) books through exclusive tutoring and case-based instructions, see Li Jianmin, *A New Vision for the Study of Chinese Medical History, Life history—Viewing Chinese History from Medical Treatment*, pp. 1–16. For the history of TCM education and the debate between TCM and Western medicine, see Deng Tietao, *Modern History of TCM*, pp. 277–307. For thoughts and ideas on the course from ancient medical texts to medical practice and clinical experiences, see Nathan Siven, Text and Experience in Classic Chinese Medicine, included in Don Bates (ed.), *Knowledge and the Scholarly Medical Traditions*. Cambridge: Cambridge University Press, 1995.

133 Volker Scheid, *Currents of Tradition in Chinese Medicine 1626–2006*, pp. 239–242

134 Lu Yuanlei, Declaration upon Abolishing Classic Medicine in the Central Health Conference, Lu's Collection of Medical Theories, included in Zhang Yuping (ed.), *Two Kinds of Lu Yuanlei's Medical Books*, p. 90.

Zhang Zhongjing to write *Treatises of Typhoid Fever* in his era. Most insightful people were modest and introvert with brief writing style, so that it was difficult to understand their meanings. Without oral instructions, most doctors could not understand the classics. The same is true for the ancient medical books.[135] The recognition and reinterpretation of classical medical books by the doctors of the Republic of China period and the new meaning of infectious diseases may be regarded as the process of "renewed canonization".[136] For example, Zhu Chenghan, a TCM doctor, investigated the so-called "epidemic dysentery", "red and white dysentery", "intestinal distension" and "retention" in ancient Chinese medical books. Zhu also talked about bacteria when discussing dysentery. He believed that the cause of the diseases in the ancient books was based on the intuition of doctors, but it was insightful and effective in clinical treatment.[137] This kind of treatment norms and confidence was developed through clinical verification, and the exploration of ancient books have unparalleled influence on the development of TCM then and in the future.

As for the publication of ancient books, medical books after the Tang Dynasty on warm diseases were published and printed repeatedly during the Republic of China period to strengthen the internal recognition and reflection of the knowledge system of TCM on warm diseases, to establish a position similar to that of ancient medical books. But in view of the overall situation of academic development, the books specializing on warm diseases were a lot less. We can't say that the problem between typology and warm disease debates have been solved. We can only say that when facing the challenge of Western medicine, the scholars of the two schools basically shared the common ground: theoretical dispute is one thing, facing the challenge of the outside world is another. In this context, the value of TCM classics had not been diminished by the new bacteriological theory, instead, a limited integration emerged. To this day, we still see that TCM continues to emphasize the importance of reading classics, which is self-evident.[138] During that period of time, confidence and optimism for TCM prevailed in the process of continuously publishing and interpreting classic medical books. Zhang Shanlei said in the *Collection of Medical Talk—An Official Letter to the Directors of the Central National Medical Museum*:

> In recent years, with the progress of printing and the great enlightenment of civilization, the medical profession in China has become a speculative enterprise in response to the

---

[135] Yun Tieqiao, *Understandings of Febrile Diseases,* Taipei: Huading Publishing House, 1988, Vol. 1, p. 6.

[136] For the history of "canonization" of ancient medical books, see Li Jianmin, *A New Vision for the Study of Chinese Medical History, Life History—Viewing Chinese History from Medical Treatment*, pp. 1–16.

[137] Zhu Chenghan, Dysentery—An Introduction to Diseases, *Wuxing Medical Monthly*, 1947 (13), pp. 15–16.

[138] When commenting and interpreting *Treatise on Typhoid Fever*, *Synopsis of the Golden Treatise, On Febrile Diseases* and so on, Liu Gongwang said that these three works are the basis of TCM. Among the numerous medical books, the classic medical books are no more than *Systematic Differentiation of Warm Diseases, A Survey of Febrile Diseases, Exogenous Febrile Diseases of Ye Xiangyan, Interpretation of Xue Shengbai's Treatise on Damp and Heat* and the recent *Revision of Popular Typhoid Fever,* besides *Treatise on Typhoid Fever.*

> current trend, just like the spring blossoms after the rain. In Japan, there is a series of *Royal Han Chinese Medicine*, which has been re-translated in Shanghai. With admiration for its great name, I bought a copy and read it. It turned out to be quite naive. It was hard for me to compliment. Nothing but a waste of money, a total disaster. It was more misleading than helpful for beginners. Domestic talents are good at writing. They are ambitious and innovative. In contributing their writings, they have their annotations on *Typhoid Fever* and *Golden Treatise* published widely in the past three to five years, and more of them are coming out continuously.[139]

Zhang believed that this trend was a sign of the creativity of Chinese medicine. He did not think much of *Royal Han Medicine*, but expected Chinese medicine to "eliminate the old pedantry" and "seek truth from facts, learn about each other and respect experience", rather than copying from old works. This seems to be a bright prospect. Time flied to 1959. Pu Fuzhou delivered a report at the "National Academic Conference on Acute Infectious Diseases" held at the Beijing Institute of TCM, which incorporated the ideas of the three systems of typhoid fever, warm disease and epidemics into acute infectious diseases. This process had gradually taken shape during the Republic of China period. These classical "warm disease" theories have become important national medical weapons, which are good enough to combat pathogenic infectious diseases. Nobody would insist on the proposition that "there is no acute infectious disease in the TCM theory". TCM only dealt with "eliminating pathogens and strengthening health", "adjusting the unity of contradictions in the body" and "internal contradictions". It was not necessary to have overdue research on "external pathogens" or "bacteria", and a patient's physical condition was the real "source". The "acute infectious diseases" of TCM began to be more related to public health and people's lives, which was quite different from the thought of "no knowledge of bacteriology, no qualification for health work" during the Republic of China period.[140]

More and more comments show that in this era, being educated with the understandings of both typhoid fever and warm diseases, ancient and modern, was often the highest level that doctors aspired to. At this time, the debate between typhoid fever and warm disease school was no longer the focus, and the comment of their being integrated might be too teleological. But the medical practitioners could clearly understand this phenomenon. Facing the challenge of pathogen theory brought by Western medicine bacteriology, the scientific transformation of TCM became imperative. Zhang Shanlei believed that the collation of TCM learning must start with practicality, focusing on the collation of classical medical books,[141] and then expanding

[139] See Liu Gongwang (ed.), *A Survey of Classics of Typhoid, Golden Treatise and Warm Diseases*, Beijing: Huaxia Publishing House, 2003, Preface, pp. 1–2, 358. Zhang Shanlei, An Official Letter to the Directors of the Central Chinese Medical Center, Collection of Medical Talk, included in the Editorial Board of Zhejiang Provincial TCM Administration (ed.), *Medical Collection of Zhang Shanlei Vol. II*, Beijing: People's Health Publishing House, 1995, p. 423.

[140] Pu Fuzhou, *Research Report on Acute Infectious Diseases in TCM, Syndrome Differentiation and Treatment of Several Acute Infectious Diseases*, Beijing: People's Health Publishing House, 2006, pp. 1–19.

[141] Zhang Shanlei, An Official Letter to the Directors of the Central Chinese Medical Center, Collection of Medical Talk, included in *Medical Collection of Zhang Shanlei Vol. II*, p. 422.

to warm diseases. Warm disease study is still an important asset in comparison with Western medicine. The confluence of Chinese and Western medical systems and the academic study of the typhoid fever and warm disease schools is the general development of the times, but the inconsistency of disease names due to the academic debate of TCM itself was still a source of pain. When the National Medical Center released the "Proposal for Unifying Disease Names", Yun Tieqiao held that the problem of fever disease names should be dealt with first. Otherwise "unifying disease names" would be a fantasy, and the punishment based on it would be meaningless.[142] When there was no consensus within the TCM academic circles, it would be inevitably one-sided by using the pathogen of Western bacteriology to define the names of the diseases. When a Western medicine disease name was adopted, the problem was not as simple as what could be used as reference nor if it should be based on the prevailing school as typhoid fever or warm disease. This trend must include some problems neglected in the past controversies between TCM and Western medicine: how were the reflections in TCM academic circles and the responses of TCM to the definition of Western medicine bacteriology presented at that time?

---

[142] Yun Tieqiao, *Treatise on Medicine,* p. 11.

Chapter 4
The Interpretation of Diseases in the Chinese and Western Medical History: The Emergence and Regeneration of "Typhoid Fever"

In old Shanghai, most adults suffered from typhoid fever, while most children suffered from sore throat or the diseases caused by bad food. From Ding, I learned a set of prescription medication procedures for the treatment of typhoid fever. At this time, I had the opportunity to "apply what I learned". Shanghainese used the water from the Huangpu River, which easily led to typhoid fever, a disease that is fatal. Once it was cured, the patients were not only grateful, but would also publicize it widely.[1]

4.1 Preface

This chapter follows the development of "typhoid (theory)" and discusses the problem of "typhoid (disease)". Although scholars had noticed the innovation of working procedures and theories when discussing the history of fever in modern Chinese medicine, they still played the old tune of "integration of TCM and Western medicine" and "integration of typhoid and warm disease schools".[2] If we do not discuss the difficult transformation of Chinese and Western disease concepts with specific examples, it is easy to fall into the "natural process" inference and ignore the complexity of the whole historical development.

The data cited at the beginning of this paper shows the prevalence of typhoid during the time of the early Republic of China period. "Typhoid fever", the infectious diseases defined by Western medicine, shares the same name as in the modern "re canonized" *Treatise on Typhoid Fever*, which is really thought-provoking. What is typhoid fever? This chapter will focus on how Chinese medicine responded to the Western definition of a disease. It involves the response to the definition of diseases incidental to Western bacteriology, and the reflection and reconstruction of the TCM

[1] Chen Cunren, *My Medical Career,* Guilin: Guangxi Normal University Press, 2007, pp. 7–11.

[2] Zhu Jianping (ed.), *A Hundred Years' History of TCM*, Vol. I, Shanghai: Shanghai Science and Technology Press, 2016, pp. 195–208.

© Zhonghua Book Company 2026

K. Pi, *The Contest of Modern Chinese and Western Medicine*,
https://doi.org/10.1007/978-981-95-2832-5_4

study itself. Typhoid fever is a disease name in modern Western medicine.[3] The book *Renewing the Treatment of Infectious Diseases* has the following descriptions: "Typhoid is an acute infectious disease caused by typhoid bacilli. The most significant lesion is the proliferation and necrosis of intestinal wall lymphoid tissue. The clinical features include the lasting high fever, relatively slow pulse, roseola, splenomegaly and leucopenia. Severe cases can have complications such as intestinal bleeding and perforation. The disease can occur all year round, but mostly in summer and autumn".[4] Modern medicine has the thorough study and definition of it. There is a standard and consensus on the knowledge of etiology, prevention and treatment. However, during the Republic of China period, the discussion of "typhoid fever" in TCM was not so simple. Try to think: why does "typhoid", an English name coined from the disease name of Chinese medicine, is also accepted by Chinese medicine? The classical term "typhoid fever" in TCM could be the generalization of several major exogenous warm diseases. It was recorded in several chapters[5] in the *Inner Canon of the Yellow Emperor· Basic Inquiries*[6] and the statement in the *Classics on Medical Problems· No.58* that "there are five kinds of typhoid: stroke, cold, dampness and warmth, fever and warm disease, and their symptoms are different". It was generally explained in *Interpretations to the Basic Inquiries* by Zhang Qi (1763–1832) of Qing Dynasty that the so-called "typhoid fever" refers to classical "typhoid" of all types, including warm diseases.[7] There were definitely still many disputes between the two schools before modern times. In such discussions and debates, how can TCM further reflect on its own academic problems and integrate

[3] Typhoid had caused great disasters and numerous discussions in western history. For a discussion on the history of typhoid (including typhus) in Britain, see William Budd, On the Causes of Fevers (1839), included in Dale C. Smith (ed.), *The Henry E. Sigerist Supplements to the Bulletin of the History of Medicine, No.9.* Baltimore: Johns Hopkins University Press, c1984. Another interesting narrative writing is about the social attention and reports caused by typhoid in the United States. The perspective of Medical Science reported by the media often shapes people's understanding of the disease itself. For example, "Diphtheria is related to children, typhoid is related to uncleanness, and syphilis is a sexual disease". See Terra Ziperyn, *Disease in the Popular American Press:the Case of Diphtheria, Typhoid Fever, and Syphilis, 1870–1920.* New York: Greenwood Press, 1988, esp. Chapter 3. Typhoid in Britain in the middle of the eighteenth century was often referred to as the general name of several febrile diseases. Compared with the definition of bacteriology, it is broad and vague. Moreover, its definition and clinical practices also focus on the personal opinions of a few doctors, such as Cullen (1710–1790)'s concept of typhus or Cullen' s textbook. See Dale C. Smith, Medical Science, Medical Practice and the Emerging Concept of Typhus in Mid-18th Century Britain, included in W.F. Bynum and V. Nuttoned (ed.), *Theories of Fever from Antiquity to the Enlightenment, Medical History, Supplement No.1.* London: Wellcome Instutution for the History of Medicine, 1981, pp. 121–134.

[4] Li Zhaohua, *A New Approach to the Treatment of Infectious Diseases,* Shijiazhuang: Hebei People's Publishing House, 1981, p. 191.

[5] For more information, see Guo Aichun (ed.), *Interpretations to the Basic Inquiries of the Inner Canon of the Yellow Emperor*, Beijing: People's Health Publishing House, 1996, pp. 192–205.

[6] (Warring States) Qin Yueren, annotated by Zhang Dengben, *A General Explanation to Classics on Medical Problems,* Xi'an: Sanqin Publishing House, 2001, p. 335.

[7] (Qing) Zhang Qi, *Notes on Basic Inquiries,* Beijing: Science and Technology Literature Press, 1998, p. 108.

the different views on the names of diseases from different schools? What are the connotations of Western medicine that were adopted by TCM?

Behind a disease name, there must be a series of definitions or explanatory factors related to society, history and even science and technology. In the Chinese language-based medical environment, the introduction of western scientific terms is bound to go through a process of translation, recognition and definition.[8] For example, Bridie Andrews discussed the definition of "malaria" in TCM since the late Qing Dynasty. She first analyzed that TCM would seek the explanation of "malaria" in the classics. When bacteriology was introduced into China, the definition began to change slowly, and people began to recognize that there was a set of stereotyped pathogenesis factors and bacteria behind the disease. There was a set of concepts to protect health and seek sanitation to prevent diseases in this knowledge system. The history of "malaria" is relatively simple, because no matter whether doctors believed in the bacterial theory or not, except for some common names (such as malaria ghost, miasma), there was only one disease name that everyone agreed on—malaria, which was not involved in the internal debate in TCM itself.[9] Another interesting example is that both Sean Hsiang-Lin Lei and Bridie Andrews interpreted the history of "tuberculosis" during the Republic of China period. In the comparison between "bacteria" and "tuberculosis", whether TCM accepted the bacterial theory or not, we can at least see that the naming of diseases tended to be simple. Namely, to correspond roughly to the dualistic disease discussion on the basis of the two systems of China and the West: the Western medicine attached importance to tubercle bacillus, while TCM attached importance to the concept of "tuberculosis". Although they disagreed with the physical sense and disease explanations,[10] the definitions and interpretations of disease names have become more and more clear and specific since the Republic of China period, unlike ancient times when the only word "plague" was used to summarize many febrile infectious diseases, which confused medical historians.[11]

Does the term "typhoid", a Chinese translation from Western disease, involve the reorganization, reinterpretation and integration of the internal system of Chinese medicine? Or does TCM present a new kind of knowledge after absorbing many interpretations of Western disease treatment and diagnosis? In the past, those who studied the history of modern Chinese medicine only paid attention to how the *Treatise on Typhoid Fever* developed,[12] without exploring the changes of disease discussions in

---

[8] Ruth Rogaski, *Hygienic Modernity: Meanings of Health and Disease in Treaty-port China*, Berkeley, London: University of California Press, c2004), especially Chapter 5.

[9] Bridie Andrews, *The Making of Modern Chinese Medicine, 1895–1937*, PhD. Dissertation, included in *History and Philosophy,* University of Cambridge, London, 1996, pp. 232–225.

[10] Sean Hsiang-Lin Lei, Why Health Is Not Protecting Life—Alternative Health, Self and Disease during the Republic of China period, *New Historiography,*2003 (14.1), pp. 45–96. Bridie Andrews, "Tuberculosis and the Assimilation of German Theory in China, 1895–1937, *Journal of the History of Medicine and Allied Sciences,* 1007(52), p. 1141.

[11] Yu Xinzhong, *Plague and Society in the South of the Yangtze River in the Qing Dynasty—A Study of Medical Social History*, pp. 79–82.

[12] Zhao Hongjun, *The History of Modern Debates between TCM and Western Medicine*, pp. 231–235.

the field of TCM under the influenced of Western medicine theory. This chapter will elaborate on the story of the new "typhoid" under the influence of Western medicine during the Republic of China period.

4.2 The Origin of the "Chinese Translation for Typhoid Fever" from the West

In the part of "Modern Disease Names" in his *History of Chinese Medicine* (1936), Chen Bangxian introduced the comparison of several Western diseases, including "typhoid fever", between ancient and modern times. Under the item of "infectious diseases", the term "typhoid fever" classified by Chen is mainly a new disease name of Western medicine, with reference to the classical TCM disease name. As a matter of fact, Chen just listed the names of various warm diseases in TCM as a comparison. If Chen's textual research skills and opinions are acceptable, it means that this book highlights a very important problem: after the introduction of Western medicine disease names, it was difficult for TCM to match them on one-to-one basis with ancient disease names.

Chen Bangxian believed that the typhoid[13] of Western medicine could correspond to the disease names of Yin syndrome typhoid, damp warmth, warmth, summer warmth and winter warmth used in ancient Chinese medicine, including a variety of disease names of the two systems of typhoid and warm diseases in TCM. As they have different connotations, Chen's discussion can only reflect a hodgepodge of disease names. The later "stomach intestinal fever", "small intestinal fever" and "typhus fever" are the old translated names, which should refer to the disease names from the introduction of Western medicine to the early Republic of China period.[14] "Syndrome" and "intestinal fever" are the terms translated by China Medical Missionary Association. "Enteromorphus" is a Japanese translation.[15] It can be roughly clarified with the textual research. In the late Qing Dynasty, typhoid had various translated names. The China Medical Missionary Association took "intestinal fever" as its translated name, which should have been introduced earlier than the Japanese translation. However, the term "intestinal fever" was obviously not favored by TCM. Many new medical terms originally translated by Westerners were later replaced by new Japanese terms.[16] Subsequently, Japanese medical and health books translated

[13] To avoid confusion with the "typhoid fever" in TCM, if there is a modern definition of typhoid fever in the following text, "typhoid" will be used.

[14] There are also "enteritis" in TCM. See Wu Xihuang, *On Febrile Diseases, Epidemics and Warm Toxin—the Light and Severe Syndromes of Febrile Diseases, Vol. I, Interpretations of Chinese and Western Febrile Diseases*, p. 23.

[15] Chen Bangxian, *History of Chinese Medicine*, Taipei: Taiwan Commercial Press, 1992, p. 233.

[16] Benjamin Schwartz, *In Search of Wealth and Power: Yen Fu and the West,* Cambridge: Belknap Press of Harvard University Press, 1964, pp. 9596. For the Japanese translation of names in the late Qing Dynasty, see Douglas R.Reynolds, translated by Li Zhongxian, *The New Deal Revolution and Japan: China, 1898–1912*, Nanjing: Jiangsu People's Publishing House, 2006, pp. 116–125.

the terms of Western medicine from Japanese into Chinese in a more extensive and continuous manner. The term "intestinal Mifusi" (肠チフス-the Japanese translation of typhoid) was known to the Chinese medical community.

According to the research of Fujikawa, the formal establishment of the name of Mifusi in Japan should be in the *Updated Epidemic Treatment* published by Ogata in 1855. It has replaced the previous names of nerve fever and rotten fever, as well as the explanations of many fever diseases in the *Treatise on Typhoid Fever* from China.[17] However, an interesting point must be made: Typhoid bacteria were officially isolated by George Gaffky in 1884. Long before that, Westerners could not distinguish between "typhus" and "typhoid". It was not until the 1930s that the French Pierre Louis (1787–1872) and the American William W. Gerhard (1809–1872) gradually discovered that they were different diseases.[18]

I can't see the *Updated Epidemic Treatment* by Ogata, but I am sure that the original "mifus" should be a transliteration[19] from German typhus. This is very confusing, as typhus means "scrub typhus" today, instead of "typhoid". Why did Japanese translators use the transliteration of "mifus" from typhus, rather than typhoid that is acknowledged today to represent typhoid fever? To this end, the author explored the transformation of the modern translation of typhoid in Japan, and made a chart as follows:

Table of evolutionary Japanese translation of typhoid fever

No	Translated disease names	Sources of translation data
1	Taifeitu syndrome[a]	Health Bureau of the Ministry of Internal Affairs (ed.), a *Chronicle of the Epidemic of Trigonella Disease,* Tokyo: Collected copy in the Health Bureau, 1877, p. 4
2	Zhifus	Written byエステルレン, *General Theory of Medical Statistics* (German original edition), Tokyo: Wenchang Hall, 1889, p. 35
3	Intestinal fus disease; rash fus disease	Health Department II of Fukushima Prefecture (ed.): *The Ninth Annual Health Report (January—December in the 21st year of Meiji,* published by the editor,1890, p. 41
4	Intestinal fus	Hirosaki Matsui, Study on the Feces of intestinal Fus Patients, *Journal of the Army Medical Association* (1890). Quoted from Army Medical School (ed.), *The 50-year History of the Army Medical School*, Tokyo: Buer Publishing, 1988, p. 391

(continued)

[17] Fujikawa, *History of Japanese Diseases*, Tokyo: Ordinary Society, 1994, pp. 276–277.

[18] K.F. Kiple (ed.), translated by Zhang Daqing: *Cambridge World History of Human Diseases*, Shanghai: Shanghai Science and Technology Education Press, 2007, p. 963.

[19] Liu Yuanxiao (ed.), *Yongda Contemporary Japanese Chinese Dictionary*, Taipei: Yongda Publishing House, 1989, p. 1730.

(continued)

No	Translated disease names	Sources of translation data
5	Intestinal zhifus; rash zhifus	Cabinet Record Bureau (ed.), T*he Complete Classification of Laws and Regulations, Part I,* published by the editor, 1891, pp. 13–14
6	Zhifus "バチルレン" (typhus bacillen)	Translated by Shinhei Goto, *Atlas of Mold* (original German Edition), Tokyo: Tokyo Tsukiji Letterpress, 1893, p. 8 and Table 8
7	Intestinal zhifus (typhus abdominalis)	Meiji Life Insurance Co., Ltd. (ed.), *Table of Death Statistics,* Tokyo: published by the editor, 1899, p. 9. (According to the statistics of the insured of an insurance company in 1881 from to 1898, the mortality rate of typhus abdominal is ranked at the third place in the death list, only second to tuberculosis and cerebral hemorrhage, higher than trigonella disease and dysentery.)
8	Intestinal zhifus	Bureau of Statistics of the Cabinet (ed.), *Drawings and Statistical Tables of Health Statistics,* Tokyo: Publishing Department of the Tokyo Statistical Association, 1911, 11th edition
9	Intestinal zhifus	Health Survey Association of the Ministry of Internal Affairs (ed.), *Report II of the Health Survey Association,* Tokyo: Health Survey Association, 1917, p. 58
10	Intestinal "チフス"or intestinal zhifus	Health Bureau of the Ministry of Internal Affairs, *References for the Prevention of Intestinal "チフス",*Tokyo: Prince Printing Co., Ltd., 1923, p. 1
11	Intestinal "チフス"(typhoid fever)	Health Bureau of the Ministry of Internal Affairs, *Statistics of Notifiable Infectious Diseases,* Tokyo: Administration Institute of Printing, 1937, p. 16

[a]"土Tu" should be "士Shi", but the original text is indeed marked as "土"

From the context of this table, various Japanese translated nouns of typhus, including "taifeishi", "zhifus", "intestinal fus" and "intestinal zhifus", all indicate the changes caused by translators' use of different translated nouns in different periods. The most interesting translation of the German *Atlas of Mold* by Shinhei Goto is the term "窒扶斯バチルレン" which means that this typhus is named after the name of the bacteria. In addition, the fact that intestinal "チフス" and "intestinal zhifus" have been used together was after the 1920s. Upon the textual research, the author found that Japanese public health documents in this period used "肠 'チフス" to express typhoid, and the frequency of "intestinal zhifus" came up less frequently. The last column (Item 11) is also very important. The author found from a lot of data that Japanese public publications on disease statistics don't have the format of attaching Western disease names. It was not until 1937 that the book *Statistics of*

Notifiable Infectious Diseases had a comparison as "typhoid fever", which is consistent with the modern English translation of typhoid. Thus we can see that the word "typhoid" was used relatively late in Japan. In addition, according to the records in *Suxuan Medical Talk* by Shao Canzhi in 1935, "there are still rash cases of infectious diseases similar to intestinal zhifus. According to Li's *Modern Typhology*, the original name of intestinal zhifus was regarded as a typhoid fever, and the name typhus fever referred to rash zhifus".[20]

By scanning the data without in-depth exploring, it is easy to fall into the thinking that Japan has been "misusing" translated terms. In fact, in modern Japan, "typhus" was translated into the so-called "typhoid" in its present meaning, which was different from the definition of names understood later. In addition, according to Yu Wuyan (1900–1963, style name Zeming), "typhus" is a German term, while "typhoid" is an English term.[21] In the early days of Japan, the German word "typhus" was quoted, which was consistent with the development background of Japanese medical circles with German medicine as the mainstream. If we do not make an investigation and comparison of the evolution history of such a disease name, we can easily be misled in the understanding of history by the modern definition (typhus).

What is more interesting is that the books in the above table have never used the term "typhoid" as the Japanese translation of the name of typhoid, and "typhoid" was obviously not accepted by orthodox Western medicine circles in Japan. In the document edited by the Health Bureau of the Ministry of Internal Affairs of Japan, it was pointed out that "in ancient times, Japan had the name of the so-called typhoid disease (harmed by cold), which was a kind of warm disease. This word was spread from China, and its interpretation was also a warm disease and infectious, which was consistent with the intestinal 'チフス (fever)'. However, this is doubtful, because the ancient name of "typhoid" may include various diseases with fever and infectious characteristics. It was not until modern times that the widely-ranged scope of disease definition was narrowed down."[22] It can be seen from this that although "typhoid" is an ancient term, it is too extensive to meet the domestic demand for accurate translation of disease terms in Modern Japan. On the contrary, it is Japanese Chinese medicine that put forward the translation of "typhoid": in 1911, the book *Iron Vertebra in Medicine* by Wada Keijuro (1872–1916), which protects Japanese Han medicine, was translated into Chinese and published in China. Many TCM doctors have read it. The chapter on "Treatment of Typhoid" is explained by "intestinal zhifus disease".[23] This is the symbol that the relationship between "intestinal zhifus" and "typhoid fever" was established, which was soon known by Chinese doctors. In other words,

---

[20] Shao Canzhi, 47. The Functions of the Six Classics of Zhongjing, *Suxuan Medical Talk*, included in Lu Zheng (ed.), *Collection of Rare Modern TCM. Medical Talk*, p. 645.

[21] Yu Wuyan, *New Treatise on Infectious Diseases, Vol. 1. Damp and Warm Typhoid Fever*, Shanghai: Yu Zeming Clinic, 1954, p. 3.

[22] Health Bureau of the Ministry of Internal Affairs (ed.), *Reference Materials for the Exchange and Inspection Meeting of Health Experts of the International Alliance*, Tokyo: Xiufanshe Printing, 1926, p. 171.

[23] Wada Keijuro, *Iron Vertebrae in Medicine,* Tokyo: Association of Chinese Han Prescription Medical Books and Periodicals, 1971, p. 103.

the modern meaning of the term "typhoid" was first given to Japanese Han medicine, but its Chinese translation benchmark was Chinese medicine instead of bacteriology.

Although various disease names have been translated into Japanese, these terms must have undergone a process of being reinterpreted and accepted after being introduced in China. For example, based on the research of Chen Jianhua, Huang Yuhe on the revolutionary course of Sun Yat Sen, it can be seen that when Sun was about to overthrow the Qing Dynasty, he was regarded as a bandit (pirate) and a danger. However, when *London Disaster* written by his mentor Cantline was translated into Japanese by Miyazaki Torazou, Sun was immediately shaped into an ideal and an admirable revolutionary leader. The reason is that the Japanese word "revolution" had become a modern term endowed with the meaning of ideal and justice, a confrontation with power, like the Western revolution.[24] Later, Zhang Shizhao (1881–1973) translated Miyazaki's works into Chinese and published them in Shanghai in 1903. At this time, Sun had become a new hope for the weak China.[25]

It was probably common that the new meanings were endowed during the process of a noun translation in the late Qing Dynasty and the early Republic of China period. In terms of medical exchange, the background can be traced back to the 10 years from the late Qing Dynasty to the founding of the Republic of China. Chinese students studying in Japan, who were the intellectuals acting as an intermediary between Western new learning and Chinese traditional learning, founded many academic groups and journals, and compiled or published popular medical books. With the translation and publication of Japanese medical books,[26] many medical and health terms have been used since then. For example, according to Liu Shiyong's research, the word "hygiene" was translated into "health" by Sensai (1838–1902) in 1870, which reinterprets the old word "health" that originally used in the Chinese world, and provides it with a new meaning of "being a special administrative organization responsible for the general health protection of the people", which is a "brand-new cause".[27]

The grammar and word formation of Chinese characters in Japanese are mostly similar to that of Chinese, and Chinese scholars mostly copy them when translating Japanese books. This trend began in the late Qing Dynasty.[28] During the Republic

---

[24] Chen Jjianhua, Textual Research on Sun Yat Sen's "Revolutionary" Discourse and Eastern-Western Political Cultures—on the Historization of "Revolution" and the Interpretation of "Post-establishment", *Chinese Academy of Sciences,* 2001 (3.2), pp. 67–109.

[25] Huang Yuhe, *The Truth of Sun Yat Sen's London Disaster: Undisclosed Historical Facts*, Taipei: Lianjing Publishing House, 1998, pp. 201–203.

[26] Niu Yahua, Medical Students Studying in Japan in the Late Qing Dynasty and Their Contributions to Modern Chinese Medicine, *Historical Materials of Chinese Science and Technology*, 2003(24.3), pp. 228–243.

[27] For the translation and practice of the word "health" in East Asian society, we can refer to Liu Shiyong: "Cleanliness", "Hygiene" and "Health Care"—the Change of the Concept of Public Health in Taiwan During the Japanese Rule, *Research on the History of Taiwan*, 2001 (8.1), pp. 41–88.

[28] Zhen Liucheng, Modern Chinese Traditional Medicine, Japan—the Influence of Japanese Medical Books during the Republic of China period, *Clinic of Han Medicine*, 1999 (46.12), 1928–1944.

of China period, Jiang Yong wrote in his *Casual Notes*: "In the reign of Guangxu, Japanese nouns prevailed. Zhang Xiaoda came to Hunan from Hubei and the Board of Education was also under his charge. Whenever seeing new terms in the official documents, he would wiped them out with a pen, and mark them as 'Japanese terms'. Later, the terms were taken as new terms, which were renamed as Japanese' vernacular'". It can be seen that Japanese new terms had been unconsciously integrated into the Chinese language system in the late Qing Dynasty. There are many terms in modern Chinese that were not created and translated by Chinese, but by Japanese.[29] The influence of Japanese translation is evident.[30] After the Republic of China period, Tang Erhe, an intellectual studying in Japan, and others established a "Medical Terminology Unification Committee" (later renamed "Scientific Terminology Association") to work on terminology unification in histology and anatomy.[31] In terms of disease discussion, there must be a large number of Chinese intellectuals who had made efforts to make ripples in comparing Chinese and Western disease names. The most important person among them is Ding Fubao.

Although Ding Fubao was not a medical student studying in Japan, his contribution to the translation of Japanese medical books was greater than that of medical students studying in Japan. In his youth, Ding studied Chinese traditional culture. Later, he came into contact with many pioneers who translated Western books and spread Western knowledge, such as Hua Hengfang (1833–1902), Zhao Yuanyi (1840–1902). However, upon realizing that it was easier to learn Western medicine through Japanese medical books than to translate Western medical books, he turned to study Japanese and medicine in 1901.[32] In 1908, he translated and published the *New Treatise on Typhoid Fever* by Miyamoto, Kanesada Hashimoto and Terao Kunihei.

In the book, "zhifus bacillus" is introduced, and the symptoms of the patients are attributed to the toxins of the bacteria.[33] The name of this bacterium was derived from the Japanese translation. Ding said: "What eastern and Western countries referred to as typhoid is also called intestinal zhifus in Japan, which means that the small intestine festering febrile. Therefore, it was translated from the church hospital as

---

[29] Xiong Yuezhi, *Western Learning Spreading to the East and the Society of the Late Qing Dynasty*, Shanghai: Shanghai People's Publishing House, 1995, pp. 673–674.

[30] Chen Cunren, Zhu Weiju and Ding Fubao have all experienced traveling in Japan and even copying Japanese Chinese medicine books. Younger modern physicians, such as Cheng Menxue (1902–1972), claimed to have found the "correct academic track", which was also inspired by the annotated medical books of Japanese Chinese medicine. See Zhu Shizeng (ed.),*Cheng Menxue's Study on Exogenous Diseases*, Shanghai: Shanghai University of TCM Press, 2008, p. 2.

[31] Li Jingwei (ed.), *History of Sino-foreign Medical Exchanges*, Changsha: Hunan Education Press, 1998, p. 275.

[32] Niu Yahua, Ding Fubao and Modern Sino Japanese Medical Exchanges, *Historical Data of Chinese Science and Technology*, 2004 (25.4), pp. 315–329. For Ding Fubao's life and his contribution to the translation of Japanese medical books, see Gao Yuqiu & Zhen Liucheng, *Ding Fubao and the Exchange of TCM between China and Japan, Journal of Chinese Medical History,* 1992 (22.3), pp. 175–180. Gao Yuqiu, Ding Fubao's Chronology, *Journal of Chinese Medical History,* 2003 (33.3), pp. 184–188.

[33] Miyamoto, translated by Ding Fubao, Chapter 1. Preliminary Typhoid Fever, *New Treatise on Typhoid Fever*, Shanghai: Medical Publishing House, 1908, p. 3.

small intestinal fever".[34] Compared with "typhoid fever", a term that Chinese people can understand better, "intestinal zhifus" is a completely Japanese translation term. These two terms had been given new and bacteriological meanings. It can also be said that Ding introduced the Western meaning of "typhoid fever" to the Chinese earlier than Wada Keijuro. According to Zhang Taiyan, it was the Han doctors who first translated the current typhoid into "typhoid fever" directly in Japan, because:

> Western people often failed to cure diseases in China, especially typhoid and warm diseases. Their skills were clumsy. Intestinal zhifus syndrome could last for 4/ 7 days. The fever is not high on the first 7 days, the highest fever is on the second 7 days, and it lasts till the third 7 days. The fever on the fourth 7 days gradually decreases, and eventually disappears. On the second and third 7 days, patients with extreme fever often go crazy. If the fever invades the heart, they will die. It is said that if fever occurs in the intestines, it would cause ulcers and purulence. The fever is high if there is no purulence, it will decline once there is purulence. The Eastern translator read from *Treatise on Typhoid Fever* that it can be cured in 6 or 7 days, along with the term "typhoid fever" in the text, intestinal zhifus is thus being called typhoid.[35]

That is to say, the eventually established Chinese name for the western disease typhoid in Chinese medical circles was translated by the Japanese Han medicine doctor after reading *Treatise on Typhoid Fever*, comparing the onset process of typhoid with similar provisions in the TCM classics and putting "intestinal zhifus" into "typhoid". Yun Tieqiao (1878–1935), a TCM doctor, also said: "The fluctuation of (this disease) fever seems to be typhoid. The Japanese translated it as typhoid fever, which is used by Chinese in the translation of western books".[36] Therefore, in the early Republic of China period, typhoid had the name of "typhoid fever", and "intestinal zhifus" continued to be used by some Chinese doctors, presenting two Chinese translations of a single disease.

"Typhoid fever" in Japan was not officially adopted as the name of "typhoid" by the dominating Western medicine. On the contrary, it was adopted by the Beiyang Government of China. As one of the exclusive Chinese names of infectious diseases, it was juxtaposed with "intestinal zhifus". As early as 1913, the name of Typhus Abdominalis was found in *The Table of the Current Deaths and Their Age in X County* attached with the *Comparison of Terms of 8 Infectious Diseases*, which was standardized by the Ministry of Internal Affairs of China.[37] Of course, this refers to the infectious diseases of Western medicine, which had been officially recognized. By 1916, the government promulgated the *Regulations on the Prevention of Infectious Diseases*, with intestinal zhifus (typhus abdominales)[38] included, which was a clear example. Although the regulations on the prevention of infectious diseases in the early

---

[34] Miyamoto, translated by Ding Fubao, *New Treatise on Typhoid Fever*, Preface, p. 1.

[35] Zhang Taiyan, Chapter 11. On Intestinal Zhifus, *Zhang Taiyan's Medical Theory*, Beijing: People's Health Publishing House, 2006, p. 31.

[36] Yun Tieqiao, Conclusion, Febrile Diseases, included in *The Wisdom of Experts*, p. 34.

[37] Cai Hongyuan (ed.), *Collection of Laws and Regulations of the Republic of China Period,* Vol. 16, Hefei: Huangshan Publishing House, 1999, p. 243.

[38] Cai Hongyuan (ed.), *Collection of Laws and Regulations of the Republic of China Period,* Vol. 16, Hefei: Huangshan Publishing House, 1999, p. 243. Vol. 26, p. 23.

Republic of China period were completely copied from Japan,[39] the terms favored by the two countries were obviously different. This is related to Ding Fubao's active translation of Han medical works. According to Yu Wuyan's textual research, both Chinese and Western medicine recognize "typhoid fever" as the Chinese name of typhoid, which owes entirely to some works like Ding Fubao's translation of *New Treatise on Typhoid Fever.* "Typhoid" was then used as often as "intestinal zhifus", and even more later. Finally, it was officially adopted by Chinese-Western medicine.[40]

Although Japanese and Chinese governments, both attaching importance to Western medicine, had adopted different names for the disease, their official interpretations of the disease were backed by bacteriology, just like Western medicine. No matter how the terms were translated, the definition was standardized as: typhoid is introduced by "bacillus typhosus", the test had standard procedures and methods, and even the test time had strict regulations (to complete the test in the first week of the disease) to avoid misdiagnosis.[41] Although the translation of disease names was still seeking unity, bacteriology had been a factor that must be considered when Western medicine pursued the definition of a disease name, which was very different from the TCM definition, a topic to be discussed later. The complexity of classical medical books can not be ignored, because in the modern Chinese medical system, the term "typhoid fever" itself also needs to be reinterpreted, and the situation is more complicated than "the comparison of disease names".

4.3 "Typhoid Fever" in the Chinese Medical Context

According to Ding Fubao's view, Zhang Zhongjing's *Treatise on Typhoid Fever* has "as much accuracy... As doubts". After the great chaos in the last years of the Western Jin Dynasty, its original copy had long been lost. Therefore, Ding said in the preface of the *New Treatise on Typhoid Fever*: "Today, *Treatise on Typhoid Fever* can not be perfect unless it is annotated with the interpretations from the East and the West".[42] That is, "typhoid fever" in Chinese classical medicine can be defined with either Eastern or Western interpretations to clarify some disputes in classical theory, which means that the era of convergence of typhoid theory would come into focus. Just a few years after Ding translated the concept of "new typhoid", Chinese medicine quickly absorbed the new ideas, and accepted the explanation of diseases

---

39 Huang Shengbai, *Commentaries on the Regulations on the Prevention of Infectious Diseases* (published in the official gazette on March 20, the Republic of China period), Tongji,1918 (01),External, p. 4.

40 Yu Wuyan, *New Treatise on Infectious Diseases, Vol. 1. Damp and Warm Typhoid,* pp. 1–2. For reference, see Hua Fuxi, *Outline of Microbiology, Vol. II,* Shanghai: Zhonghua Book Company, 1935, pp. 220–225.

41 Zheng Ziying, *Bacteriology*, Taipei: Taiwan Commercial Press, Original, 1945, Taiwan 1st Edition 1968, pp. 123–125.

42 Miyamoto, translated by Ding Fubao, *New Treatise on Typhoid Fever*, Preface, p. 2.

from Western medicine. Such prompt acceptance was different from the stereotype of "conflicts between TCM and Western medicine (concepts)".

As for the etiology of typhoid, He Lianchen and members of Shaoxing Medical Association noticed the "mycobacterium zhifus precisely studied by Herbert Griffith Institute" in 1880, and introduced its characteristics and microscopic examination methods. He said, "there were no microscopes in China and there was no accurate description for the state of bacteria. However, the ancients knew that all kinds of infectious diseases were the filthy toxins of mildew, and they had found the signs of bacteria. From this point of view, it had generally been recognized that there was a pathogenic factor, even though theories between China and foreign countries are different".[43] At this time, as there were no microscopes to verify bacteria, TCM could only passively compare their findings with the theory of Western medicine. However, it can be seen that TCM was also positive, rather than completely negative, to the theory of bacterial pathogenesis.

Generally speaking, since TCM had the traditional theory of warm diseases, and the medical books translated from Western medicine then often referred to infectious diseases such as warm diseases, some knowledge could be easily converged at the beginning. This includes similar theories in both Chinese and Western medicine: for example, judging the disease by observing the body after the body temperature rises. Ding Fubao observed that Western medicine used science to explain the body temperature and fever of the human body: "When we are alive, our bodies are often warm, which is similar to the warm phenomenon when a steam engine is running".[44] Therefore, Ding's translation of "the principle of fever" introduces in detail the body feeling of "fever" caused by severe infectious diseases in Western medicine, as well as the symptoms of headache, palpitation or general fatigue, which "is generally called warm disease".[45] However, the "fever" is only a general term. To distinguish which kind of fever it is, we must use other methods to identify it. At that time, the instruments and techniques for diagnosing typhoid were not as sophisticated as today. Apart from simple observation, such as observing rosette rash, splenomegaly, and the fever types, the most accurate diagnostic method was to use the patient's blood for bacterial cultures, but the process was complicated. Moreover, it was not very popular to select a special "bacteriology classroom or hospital" for testing. It is possible that the naked eyes were used, while the culture medium was needed. The so-called incubator should be able to control the constant temperature between 37 °C and 38 °C, and the clues could be seen in 24 h, which was time-consuming and laborious. It was even more dangerous at that time to take a blood test by puncturing the spleen.[46]

43 Shaoxing Medical Association, Treatment of Damp and Warm Epidemics, included in Li Shunbao (ed.), *Complete Book of Warm Diseases*, Vol. II, p. 2090.

44 Ding Fubao, The Principle of Heat, *The Principle of Heat*, Shanghai: Wenming Book Company, 1910, p. 1.

45 Ding Fubao, The Name of Febrile Disease, *The Principle of Heat*, p. 6.

46 Miyamoto, translated by Ding Fubao, Chapter II: The Essence of Typhoid, *New Treatise on Typhoid Fever*, pp. 44–45.

As many practical testing techniques could not be widely applied in daily medical treatment, the feeling of "heat" in Western medicine had become the basic method for diagnosing most fever diseases. In other words, it is to observe the pattern of fever in patients. *The Principle of Fever* introduces the observation of Western Medicine on the process of body fever, so as to diagnose a disease: "A certain infectious disease has its own fever syndrome, and the reproduction of the virus spreading in the body. This condition can be inferred from the fever syndrome".[47] For example, the definition of "continued fever" in Western medicine is that there is very little difference between the rise and fall between day and night, which is the case for general infectious diseases. The "remittent fever" refers to the fever with great difference between day and night, such as tuberculosis. Typhoid is classified as "heat dissipation", also known as "ladder type", which is gradually ascending or descending. Since typhoid is no different from the common cold at the beginning, it included headaches, chills and other symptoms. Doctors hoped that patients could also record their own fever pattern and provide it to doctors as an important reference for clinical diagnosis. The daily operation of this technology was actually beyond the TCM discussion.[48]

Japanese and Chinese share "a common writing system", and a large number of modern Japanese words use Chinese idioms, which expand the original meaning in usage.[49] It should be noted that Ding, after learning from Japanese Chinese medicine, re-recognized or redefined the names of the diseases according to the traditional knowledge of TCM. In terms of typhoid, from the perspective of the feelings and patterns of "fever" in Chinese and Western medicine, western medicine referred to it as "heat type" at that time, while Ding compared it with the changes of "six meridians" in the traditional *Treatise on Typhoid Fever*. In view of the observation of the fever state of the patient, Ding expressed, in the preface of the *New Treatise on Typhoid Fever*, that it was quite in line with the ancient Chinese medicine books: the light stage intestinal zhifus was the so-called "taiyang disease" in Chinese medicine. The disease with stagnant or intermittent fever was called "shaoyang disease". If the patient was seriously ill and continued to have fever, it was called "yangming disease".[50] This is completely put in reference of the six meridians syndrome differentiation theory in the classical typhoid theory of TCM. In this way, Ding classified the Western typhoid as the Chinese "fever".

Zhang Taiyan had a broader definition. In addition to treating typhoid and fever in China with the same heat type, he believed that the typhoid system of TCM includes all warm diseases[51] and it covered more than the "intestinal zhifus disease".

---

[47] Ding Fubao, Types of Febrile Diseases, *The Principles of Febrile Diseases*, p. 11.

[48] Miyamoto, translated by Ding Fubao, Chapter 1. Preliminary Typhoid Fever, *New Treatise on Typhoid Fever*, p. 9.

[49] Douglas R. Reynolds, translated by Li Zhongxian, *The New Deal Revolution and Japan: China, 1898–1912*, p. 119.

[50] Miyamoto, translated by Ding Fubao, *New Treatise on Typhoid Fever*, Preface, p. 3.

[51] Zhang Taiyan, Chapter 5. On Yangming Disease Being Warm Disease, *Zhang Taiyan's Medical Theory*, pp. 15–18.

Typhoid is the "counter decoction syndrome" in *Treatise on Typhoid Fever*.[52] There is a problem in translating "intestinal zhifus" into "typhoid", which will lead doctors to misuse the laws mentioned in *Treatise on Typhoid Fever* in dealing with all the clinical symptoms of typhoid. Intestinal zhifus is just a proof in *Treatise on Typhoid Fever*, rather than an accurate translation. That is to say, the "six meridians" of TCM is the syndrome differentiation method for various warm diseases. Of course, it can cover typhoid, but typhoid can not be the equivalent to the TCM "typhoid" and "fever".[53] Wang Shenxuan praised Zhang's views when he sorted out the *Compilation of New Theories of TCM*.[54] The article "Intestinal Zhifus and Typhoid Fever" in *Spring and Autumn of the Medical World* also shows that typhoid in China represents a broad classification of febrile diseases, while typhoid is only one part, and can not be taken as an equivalent. The common ground between them is that both of them are "caused by cold".[55] Yun Tieqiao thought that typhoid in the West was named after bacteria, while typhoid in China was not, which indicates the difference of the two. The term shares the common ground with the Western name should be the so-called typhoid in the narrow sense in *Classics on Medical Problems* (one of the "five typhoid fevers").[56] Although these statements are different from each other, they all take the typhoid theory of TCM as the starting point to understand Western disease names; "typhoid fever" in China was a broader meaning than typhoid. In fact, it just shows the difficulty of translating the names of TCM under the definition of Western medicine.

Once it was confirmed that western typhoid could be found in Chinese medicine, it can also be found that TCM was full of confidence in the treatment of this disease, because it was not supposed to be "a new disease". From the name of a disease, its symptoms to its treatment, TCM could draw up the knowledge they needed from ancient classics. However, TCM did not stop the dialogue with Western medicine. Based on the various pressures and public opinions in the comparisons and debates between TCM and Western medicine in the early Republic of China period, sometimes it was necessary for TCM to take the initiative to communicate or discuss with Western medicine. For example, when translating medical books, Ding Fubao once said, "Untalented as I am, it is my wish to converge Chinese and Western medicine from medical books. The ancient prescriptions that can be used will be kept to protect the quintessence of China. Chinese medications should be used if it can replace Western medication". In cases that "Western medicine is the only option, one or two kinds of them will have to be used to make up for the deficiency of

---

[52] Nie Huimin (ed.), *The Collected Explanations of the Treatise on Typhoid Fever*, Beijing: Xueyuan Publishing House, 2001, pp. 466–470.

[53] Zhang Taiyan, Chapter 11. On Intestinal Zhifus Being Taiyang Stagnation with Meridian and Its Treatment, *Zhang Taiyan's Medical Theory*, pp. 32–34.

[54] Wang Shenxuan (ed.), *Compilation of New Theories of TCM*, Shanghai: Shanghai Bookstore Press, 1991, Part 8: Internal Medicine (I), p. 4.

[55] He Peiyu, On Intestinal Zhifus and Typhoid Fever, *Spring and Autumn of the Medical World* 95,1934 (11), p. 4.

[56] Yun Tieqiao, Narration, Febrile Diseases, included in *The Wisdom of Experts*, p. 34.

TCM".[57] It can be seen that the original intention of convergence is to preserve TCM as much as possible, so as to prove the value of TCM and the difference between TCM and Western medicine, and to prove the advantages and strengths of TCM.

In the discussion of typhoid in his *Treatment of Damp and Warm Epidemics*, Zhang Zanchen believed that Western medicine attached importance to anatomical pathology, which is difficult for TCM to match. However, the treatment of Western medicine at that time was quite simple and ineffective. He believed that Western medicine not only recognized that bacteria propagated in the intestines, but also used "calomel" to release intestinal toxins and reduce fever syndrome, or use "folia digitalis leaf" for diuresis, "sulfuric acid" for antipyretic, "natrium acid" for injection to sterilize and prevent corrosion, which can still be called "the magic method". However, the new serum therapy was "questionable and cannot be fully implemented". Zhang believed that the internal medicine therapy of Western medicine was too simple and rigid, which is the best annotation of "Western medicine is good at treating external diseases and TCM is good at treating internal diseases".[58] In spite of this, Chinese and Western medicine still shared many common methods to treat fever. Ding Fubao said: "Only ancient books have extremely effective prescriptions, which are often in line with the West. Relaxing decoction for excretion goes with calomel as the agent; sweating decoction goes with antipyrinum as the antipyretic agent".[59] It can be seen that in the treatment of fever, both Chinese and Western pharmacology have the technology of utilizing sweating and purgation (defecation) methods to treat fever.

Xu Renfu's *Practical Medicine Handout* (1929) affirmed the benefits and necessity of comparing the names and connotations of Chinese and Western medicine. He said that typhoid "is actually an infectious bacterium when examined under a microscope", but the ancients often named it "evil". He also said: "Today's medicine is changing with each passing day. It is a progress noted by comparing the names of diseases in the past and present of China and the West. Zhongjing would agree if he were reborn. It is not to follow the beaten track and degenerate TCM".[60] Xu was not against learning from Western medicine, as innovation was what TCM could not avoid at that time. However, the contradictory point was that TCM believed that the diagnosis and treatment techniques of new Western medicine were not as good as the old and TCM. For example, Li Jianyi pointed out that the so-called "typhoid" in TCM means that "there are five typhoid diseases" in the *Classics on Medical Problems*, including "exogenous syndromes of wind, cold, warm, heat and dampness", which almost covers all exogenous febrile diseases. He considered that there were various treatments in this system, which were enough to cope with all exogenous fevers.

---

[57] Miyamoto, translated by Ding Fubao, *New Treatise on Typhoid Fever*, Preface, pp. 3–4.

[58] Shaoxing Medical Association, Diagnosis and Treatment of Western Medicine, Treatment of Damp and Warm Epidemics, included in Li Shunbao (ed.), *Complete Book of Warm Diseases, Vol. II*. p. 2090.

[59] Miyamoto, translated by Ding Fubao, *New Treatise on Typhoid Fever*, Preface, p. 3.

[60] Xu Renfu, *Handouts on Practical Medicine*, Taipei: Xinwenfeng Publishing Company, 1997, p. 179.

On the contrary, Western medicine does not know TCM therapy for typhoid except for the "expectant therapy", such as "a person suffering from typhoid would heal himself after three weeks. For the mild cases, expectant therapy will do no harm; for the severe cases, it will lead to catastrophe". He further pointed out that the use of medication was quite complicated regarding the "stages" of typhoid. According to the experience of TCM, if drugs are not used according to the order of "stages", "hundreds of diseases" will be caused. Western medicine's passive waiting for recovery is a helpless move.[61]

After the 1930s, this situation did not change much. In addition to TCM therapies, it seemed that the quiet rest and waiting for the recovery of Western medicine were also a choice in the passive treatment of typhoid fever. The Western medication occasionally used did not take much effect. He Peiyu elucidated:

> According to the *Complete Book of Internal Medicine,* which was translated from Western medicine and recently published by Shanghai Commercial Press, it is said of acute infectious diseases (typhoid fever) that "as for its treatment, honestly there has been no invention of effective drugs, except for the serum therapy which has achieved better results. Since ancient times, the commonly used drugs, such as calomel, vodol, etc., are not safe. So far, not much to be done except for prevention and symptomatic treatment". From this, we can see that no effective method had been found for the outbreak period and the recovery period was often disappointing.[62]

What He said shows that at that time, TCM held that its therapy had its advantages. In addition, many prescriptions were cited by the TCM doctors, specifically confirming that their curative effect was remarkable. Xu Renfu said: "Typhoid bacilli can spread throughout the body, causing inflammation of various organs, pneumonia and swelling of throat mucosa. A lectin occurs in the patient's blood, such as macula. The sweat of the newly infected person will have it dissolved immediately. If it lasts for many days, the only treatment will be cleaning up".[63] According to Xu Lie's prescriptions, most of them are based on the prescriptions in *Treatise on Typhoid Fever*. Sweating and purgation are still the two main treatments. He believed that TCM could change medication according to symptoms. There are several prescriptions that can be used, such as cassia twig decoction, ephedra decoction and other well-known prescriptions, whether in the incubation period or the outbreak period.[64] Generally speaking, TCM believes that the disease theory of Western medicine has some merits, but the treatment methods are not very innovative, because the treatment methods in *Treatise on Typhoid Fever* not only cover the "sweating" and "purgation" of Western medicine, but also are more flexible. The real problem in TCM is that there was no consistent point of view to explain typhoid at that time. However, another group of doctors responded to typhoid from the viewpoint of epidemic warm diseases, which can not be ignored in interpreting the modern disease history of TCM.

---

[61] Li Jianyi, On the No Cure for Typhoid Fever in the West, *Spring and Autumn of the Medical World,* 23,1928 (05), pp. 3–4.

[62] He Peiyu, *Intestinal Zhifus and Typhoid Fever*, p. 4.

[63] Xu Renfu, *Handouts on Practical Medicine*, pp. 188–189.

[64] He Peiyu, *Intestinal Zhifus and Typhoid Fever*, pp. 4–5.

4.4 Another Voice—Context of Warm Diseases

At the turn of spring and summer in 1912, the epidemic broke out in Shaoxing, China, and spread to all villages and towns. Shaoxing Medical Association in Zhejiang made a collective study and explains in its investigation report: "Western medicine names it as intestinal bad fever, while Eastern medicine names it as intestinal zhifus (inflammation and ulceration of small intestine). TCM gave it the name of damp and warm epidemics".[65] Later, this report was compiled into the *Treatment of Damp and Warm Epidemics* (hereinafter referred to as damp and warm diseases) by He Lianchen, Chen Yueqiao, et al., which was printed and distributed to the members of the Association.[66] From the order of the data, the interpretations of the authors were different from that of Ding Fubao, and it was several years later than that of Ding's translation work. Although the translation of "Eastern medicine" still had a profound impact on the interpretation of diseases, these Chinese doctors chose "damp and warm diseases", a disease name in the warm disease system, rather than "typhoid fever" on the basis of what they learned from the real epidemic situation and went back to think about the newly translated names of diseases.

The book *Damp and Warm Diseases* classifies the treatment of typhoid into two parts: acute epidemic and chronic epidemic. The former starts from "warm toxin" and the latter from "dampness and filth". Most of the discussions were based on the theory of warm diseases. The book quoted Yu Botao as saying: "Mouth and nose are most directly connected with the brain meridian. The Qi of the nose passes through the brain, the Qi of the mouth passes through the stomach, and also through the brain. People caught in the pathogens of epidemic disease instantly would have the whole brain shaken, leading to the burst of brain blood vessels and the loss of physical feeling. It is featured with easy infection and quick death".[67] This theory is roughly related to the theory of warm diseases, which discusses the process of pathogenic Qi entering the human body from the mouth and nose. In addition to infection, this is the same as the statement in *On Febrile Diseases*, the classic theory of febrile diseases of TCM, that "when the pathogenic Qi is absorbed, it first invades the lung and reversely transmits to the pericardium".[68] All the diseases invade the human body from the mouth and nose. However, the most serious situation is that the pathogenic factors invade the "pericardium" instead of the "brain", which should be modified due to the influence of Western medicine theory, but the theoretical prototype of its convergence is the theory of febrile diseases. If the disease is explained according

[65] Shaoxing Medical Association, Disease Names, Treatment of Damp and Warm Epidemics, included in Li Shunbao (ed.), *Complete Book of Warm Diseases*, p. 2089.

[66] Shaoxing Medical Association, Treatment of Damp and Warm Epidemics, included in Li Shunbao (ed.), *Complete Book of Warm Diseases*, Vol. II, Notes on Annotation, p. 2086.

[67] Shaoxing Medical Association, Diagnosis and Treatment of TCM, Treatment of Damp and Warm Epidemics, included in Li Shunbao (ed.),*Complete Book of Warm Diseases*, Vol. II, pp. 2091–2093.

[68] (Qing) Ye Gui, Ye Xiangyan's Exogenous Febrile Diseases, included in Shen Fengge et al. (eds), *Interpretations of Ye Xiangyan's Exogenous Febrile Diseases and Xue Shengbai's Damp Febrile Disease*, Nanjing: Jiangsu Science and Technology Press, 1983, p. 1.

to the "six meridians" system in the *Treatise on Typhoid Fever*, the pathogen should invade from the muscle surface of the human body, not from the mouth and nose.

Why do these doctors think that typhoid is "damp heat"? The understanding of the pathogenic "dampness" of febrile diseases in Chinese medicine can be traced back to the chapter of "Differentiation of Spasm, Dampness and Heatstroke Syndrome" in *Treatise on Typhoid Fever*. Although the original book has emphasized that the "damp" disease must be distinguished from typhoid fever,[69] there was no obvious disease classification boundaries in Zhang Zhongjing's era. Zhu Qiong, a doctor in the Northern Song Dynasty, was from the south of the Yangtze River. When he was living in Hangzhou, he thought about the system of *Treatise on Typhoid Fever* and wrote *Book of Syndromes of Living People*. The book introduces "damp warmth", an external disease ignored in the past: "The patient was harmed by dampness, which results in heatstroke. When dampness goes with heat, it is damp warmth". Zhu also explained that perspiration is not proper to treat damp warmth, which is different from the thinking of the typhoid school in treating exogenous diseases with perspiration. Until the emergence of warm disease school in the Qing Dynasty, "dampness" not only became the main cause of the "damp warmth" disease, but was also more systematic in its treatise than the previous generations. Xue Shengbai's *On Damp Heat* in the Qing Dynasty can be the representative in the discussion of this warm disease. After the Republic of China period, some scholars as He Lianchen also believed that damp warm disease could not be mixed as "typhoid fever". He strongly objected the Western and Japanese translated versions of "typhoid fever" for both small intestinal bad fever and intestinal zhifus: "It is obvious that those practicing new medicine had never studied our medical books".[70] He held that according to the context of Chinese medicine, typhoid should be translated as "damp warm disease" rather than "typhoid fever".

Another example is that TCM tended to compare the theory of Western medicine with the Chinese inherent theory at that time. For example, Yang Zemin put "dampness" and "bacteria" of Western medicine together in his discussion. He wrote in *Medical Talk in Seclusion*:

> Western medicine prefers discussing bacteria, while TCM prefers discussing dampness. There are similarities between dampness and bacteria. The ulceration of skin diseases in TCM is called dampness toxin, which causes bad swelling. The large swollen area is called dampness fire, the brain fever is called dampness warmth, and the malaria is called dampness malaria. Erysipelas are attributed to dampness fire, and dysentery is attributed to dampness heat. All these diseases are caused by bacteria. TCM generally treats them with agents that promote dampness, clear away heat and can detoxify. Bacteria in Western medicine are known by using a microscope, and dampness in TCM is distinguished by symptoms. Bacteria and dampness are significantly related.

---

[69] (Han) Zhang Zhongjing, annotated by (Song) Cheng Wuji, Differentiation of Spasm, Dampness and Heatstroke Syndrome. No.4, *Annotations of Treatise on Typhoid Fever, Vol. 2,* Beijing: People's Health Publishing House, 1997, p. 49.

[70] Shaoxing Medical Association, Definitions, Treatment of Damp and Warm Epidemics, included in Li Shunbao (ed.), *Complete Book of Warm Diseases*, Vol. II, p. 2089.

This seems reasonable, but the concept and statement of "dampness" is still too broad, and this is just the tip of the iceberg in comparing the names of Chinese and Western diseases. On the whole, the "damp warmth" is only one link in the epidemic warm disease system. The "epidemic warm disease" actually includes many infectious diseases. However, isn't it true for the "damp warm disease"? From the context of "damp warm disease", "typhoid" is by no means an accurate translation, even though they correspond to each other, because "damp warm disease" can also correspond to other diseases with "damp warm disease" characteristics. Zhang Zanchen said: "Shaoxin is along the seaside and is damp. There is actually an endemic disease all year round. With the right treatment, 8 or 9 out of 10 can be cured."[71] Although it is the theory of damp warm disease that is under discussion, it can be inferred that "the diseases in summer and autumn are included by half, which can be the clinical help for the doctors".[72] It can be seen that "damp warm disease" is a comprehensive system of all specific warm diseases at one time and one place. This does not accurately refer to a single disease. It can be said that typhoid is a "damp warm disease", but the meaning of "damp warm disease" is not just about typhoid.

From the prescriptions selected by Shaoxing Medical Association to deal with damp and warm diseases, it can also be seen that there was a tendency of "multiple packages for one disease" in the discussion of TCM treatment. In the section of "Detoxification Pills" in the book, the explanation made by TCM is very interesting:

> Mr. Hui Xi said: the first part of this secret medicine is amazing. It is specially used to treat all kinds of toxins, such as medical toxin, wild rice seed, rat mangrove, pathogenic bacteria, cattle and horse toxin, fugu, and it attacks plague, malaria, acute laryngeal infection, jaundice, red eye, sore boil fever, or self hanging, drowning, beating and flapping injury, carbuncle and gangrene on the back, fish umbilical ulcer, and injury caused by insects, snakes and dogs. It is to be taken by men and women who are haunted by pathogens with crazy walking or have ghost foetus and ghost spirit. From this point of view, this pill is indeed the first important agent for sterilization. In the prescription, it is noted that it is the killer for the pathogenic bacteria. Whatever disease caused by bad bacteria, it is highly recommended for the doctors to use. However, it is referred by TCM generally as pathogenic bacteria, while in Western medicine it is generally called toxic bacteria. Bacteria is translated into Xi Jun (fine bacteria) in Chinese because of its extreme fineness. It is also called mould because it can corrupt substances. Those who have learned new medicine often slander TCM for being ignorant of toxic bacteria. It is due to the fact that they are not well-read in Chinese medical books. It is the way to put TCM down in general by picking one or two of its weakness and to ignore all its strengths. New scholars who learned about it tend to think of TCM as nothing of value. As a result, the old and new ideas are irreconcilably opposed to each other.[73]

This paragraph describes the curative effect of "detoxification pills", which shows that this drug is not specific to a single disease, but to treat a series of "toxic"

---

[71] Shaoxing Medical Association, Introduction, Treatment of Damp and Warm Epidemics, included in Li Shunbao (ed.), *Complete Book of Warm Diseases*, Vol. II, p. 2089.

[72] Shaoxing Medical Association: Introduction, Treatment of Damp and Warm Epidemics, included in Li Shunbao (ed.), *Complete Book of Warm Diseases*, Vol. II, p. 2089.

[73] Shaoxing Medical Association, Treatment of Damp and Warm Epidemicss, included in Li Shunbao (ed.), *Complete Book of Warm Diseases*, Vol. II, pp. 2102–2103.

diseases.[74] In addition, it is explained under the item "Taiyi Purple Golden Pill": "This pill is similar to the two prescriptions of detoxification pills mentioned above. It is a true TCM elixir for sterilization and detoxification. It produces immediate effects regardless of a current epidemic, major epidemic and pandemics, whatever listed in the notes of prescriptions for each disease".[75] It can be seen that many ancient prescriptions were not made specifically for one disease, but most of them had the effect of treating several diseases with the same symptoms. The above prescription can "sterilize and detoxify" without specifying what disease it is aimed at, but it can be "commonly used" for several "toxic" diseases. Does this also mean that ancient Chinese medicine only needed to bring up the name of a disease when diagnosing febrile disease, instead of defining a disease name? Problems surfaced when people began to review the names of TCM diseases from the perspective of Western medical standardization.

4.5 Reinterpret Disease Names or Vanish in the Debate Between China and the West

The process of Sinicization of a Western disease name is actually diverse and complex. After being translated from Japanese to Chinese, typhoid had become a disease that can be explained by both typhoid system as well as warm disease system (damp warmth). In this way, modern Chinese medicine still had to face the old problem of "typhoid verses warm disease debate" which led to different names for the same disease. This difference may be understood by TCM doctors who are familiar with the history of warm diseases, but it is absolutely unable to convince Western medicine doctors who believe that "each disease has its own origin".

Yu Yunxiu, the opponent of TCM, also noticed "typhoid" and its interpretation by TCM. He said: "I have been practicing medicine in Shanghai for more than ten years. Patients diagnosed of having warm pathogens in the old medical cases were tested by blood, and most were proved to be infected intestinal zhifus". It can be seen that in Shanghai, typhoid was often regarded as "warm pathogens" by TCM. This interpretation is biased toward the theory of warm diseases. Yu also cited the item in the theory of warm diseases in TCM to compare the symptoms of typhoid in Western medicine: "Item 13 of Xue's *Damp and Warm Diseases* says: "the root of the tongue is white, and the tip of the tongue is red, which is the triangle tongue of the intestine zhifu". It is said in Item 23: "when a warm disease lasts for over 10 days, stomach ache and hematochezia would occur. This is the intestine bleeding of intestinal zhifus."[76] From the observation and diagnosis of symptoms, Yu believed

[74] For "toxin" and "bacteria", see the detailed discussion in Chapter 4.

[75] Shaoxing Medical Association, Definitions, Treatment of Damp and Warm Epidemics, included in Li Shunbao (ed.), *Complete Book of Warm Diseases*, Vol. II, p. 2103.

[76] Yu Yunxiu, On the Syndromes of Febrile Diseases, *Selected Works on Medical Revolution*, pp. 194, 197.

that typhoid should be doubtlessly the damp warmth in the TCM theory of warm diseases. If so, it seems that the integration and comparison of the names and theories of Chinese and Western medicine has had a good start.

Later, in 1936, Yang Zhiyi mentioned that Zhongjing's classical prescriptions had a good therapeutic effect on infectious diseases. At that time, there were some tacit agreements between Chinese and Western disease names, such as "Hu Lyra" for "cholera", "acute pneumonia" for "lung wind", "scarlet fever" for "laryngitis". What corresponds to "intestinal zhifus" is "damp warm diseases".[77] This assumption is too simplistic, because there was no nation-wide consensus in the field of TCM as the name of "typhoid" should be put into "damp and warm diseases" or "typhoid fever", or the treatment mode represented by it. Yu Yunxiu criticized in his *Medical Revolution* that "warm diseases are caused by wind warmth as well as heat, known as damp and warm diseases. The symptoms are complex and related to a variety of diseases, which can not be covered by a single disease name. Based on today's knowledge of syndromes, most of the descriptions are about intestinal zhifus".[78] That is to say, even though it is reasonable for damp and warm diseases to correspond to typhoid, the name "damp and warm diseases" includes many diseases and is not suitable to have an one-to-one translation.

Yu Yunxiu's many criticisms of TCM are not groundless. He was knowledgeable about the TCM theory, and even had a very accurate grasp of the theoretical conflicts within the TCM warm disease circle. He believed that in ancient Chinese medicine, no matter "typhoid fever", "warm disease" or "epidemics", none of them was a single disease, but a "kind" of disease, which should be classified into the category of acute warm diseases. Just like intestinal zhifus has intestinal zhifus bacteria, all the so-called warm diseases have their own characteristics of "infection", and each disease has a pathogen to be tested. He said:

> The civilization of China had stopped its development, and there is no microscope for the study, so the pathogenic bacteria of fever infectious diseases is beyond our knowledge. All human knowledge is nothing but changes in nature. Therefore, it is speculated that the origin of the disease is from the six Qis of wind, cold, heat, dampness, dryness and fire. It's understandable when they were from the pre-civilized age. How can they be applied to today's world of advanced science?[79]

As for the definition of infectious diseases, TCM used to discuss diseases within the six elements of wind, cold, heat, dampness, dryness and fire, which were not accurate enough. Yu said: "What old medicine called damp warmth and damp heat, obviously including epidemic cerebrospinal meningitis, intestinal zhifus, dysentery and so on". New medicine has explained convincingly in detail the pathogenic bacteria, pathological changes and the location of the diseases. These diseases are generally referred to as warm pathogens or heat toxin which is the first to invade the lungs and the upper-energizer. Some tend to stick to the old rules without being able to tell

---

77 Cao Yingfu, Experimental Records of Classical Prescriptions, Yang Zhiyi's preface, p. 12.

78 Yu Yunxiu, On the Syndromes of Febrile Diseases, *Selected Works on Medical Revolution,* p. 196.

79 Yu Yunxiu, On the Syndromes of Febrile Diseases, *Selected Works on Medical Revolution,* pp. 190–191.

the difference between good or bad. It is a society where ignorance is admired and believed by the knowledgeable and be accepted as a Tao to the general public. Alas!" I believe that the definition of medical treatment and disease during the Republic of China period should completely adopt the new and western defined methods", rather than the thinking of "multiple dimensions for one disease" in the TCM warm disease system in the past. What's more interesting is that I saw many doctors at that time following the twelve words of Ye Tianshi's "warm pathogens move up, attacking the lung first, infecting the pericardium next" as the holy Bible. They looked up to him as a God and dared not innovate. This statement was extremely absurd, because intestinal zhufus was not a respiratory disease, but a disease of the gastrointestinal system. It would never "attack the lung first", and it was completely wrong.[80]

A so-called unified and scientific disease name can not be illustrated by these two ancient disease names. Based on this idea, I think the typhoid verses warm disease debate should come to an end. For example, modern Chinese medicine was known for its view that typhoid fever school gives more attention to "incubating Qi" (typhoid incubative pathogen), while warm disease school gives more attention to "new sensation" (warm pathogenic exogenous sensation). The most consistent discussion with these two concepts were the viewpoints of Western medicine. Yu used to explain the situation of virus "incubating" on the human body, which is called "incubation period" in Western medicine. Scientific experiments have proved that the incubation period of intestinal zhifus lasts for only one to two weeks, and it is impossible, as some TCM doctors said, that "the severe cold in winter would cause typhoid in winter, warm disease in spring, and heatstroke in summer", which takes it as a "seasonal" disease. In this case, the theory of "incubation" is not tenable at all. As for the theory of "new sensation", TCM scholars could only find "pathogenic Qi" outside the six Qis to discuss it as they had no microscopes in the past and could not see bacteria. Although it was more understandable than "incubating warmth", when bacteriology was prosperous, typhoid and warm diseases could be justified by various "infectious diseases". Yu Yunxiu said: "The distinction between typhoid and warm disease, as well as the dispute between incubating Qi and external sensation can be stopped".[81] Whether it is "typhoid" or "warm disease", it is a very general statement. If the name is not proper, it is not compatible with the medical study of the new era. To name diseases and understand pathogens more accurately had gradually become an unavoidable topic for TCM.

---

[80] Yu Yunxiu, On the Syndromes of Febrile Diseases, *Selected Works on Medical Revolution*, pp. 196–198.

[81] Yu Yunxiu, On the Syndromes of Febrile Diseases, *Selected Works on Medical Revolution*, pp. 192–195.

4.6 Discussion on the New Typhoid in TCM

From the example of typhoid, the definition of it in the field of TCM was not unified, but when there was a dominant party, that is, the Western medicine, the naming and discussion of fever diseases in TCM became a big problem. Yun Tieqiao once said, "The most inconsistent names of diseases in TCM are fever diseases. In the Ming and Qing Dynasties, there were many disputes, causing a lot of confusions. This is the crux of name unification".[82] Yun believed that the divergent views on fever diseases in TCM was the biggest weakness when being faced with Western medicine theory, which coincided with Yu Yunxiu's above-mentioned views. After such a comparison between China and the West, seeking a unified explanation of the disease names had gradually become the primary goal of the survival of the TCM theory during the Republic of China period. However, as for the principle of reform, Yun specified the premise that the TCM community should adhere to. In the *Discussion on the Proposal for Unified Disease Names*, he said:

> *Treatise on Typhoid Fever* includes bronchitis, pleurisy, peritonitis, pleural effusion, ascites, and even epidemic cerebrospinal meningitis, heatstroke, cholera, etc. If these names were used, the book itself will no longer be studied in the first place. Next, no one would use its prescriptions, and furthermore, injection sterilization would be widely used. In this way, TCM and its study will be gone. It is compulsory that the Chinese disease names are to be used as the unified names, and it is more than a matter of name ownership.[83]

Yun thought that the work of unifying the names of diseases should be explained mainly by the names of diseases in TCM, because they were connected with ancient classics. Once the standard of Western medicine was adopted, the knowledge of TCM would also turn to "sterilization". At that time, the TCM classics would automatically be eliminated. This is the most critical part, and it was also the worry of most TCM doctors during the Republic of China period. However, such persistence brought about setbacks for the TCM movement, which was facing reform or scientization. After the establishment of the National Medical College in 1931, a series of works related to "academic collation" was carried out. In 1933, important documents, including The *Proposal for Unified Disease Names by the Academic Collation Committee of the Central National Medical Museum*, were issued, with the aim of achieving a unified statement between Chinese and Western disease names and reaching a national consensus. After this document was distributed to all parts of the country, it immediately triggered a lot of controversies, and TCM doctors with different views made their voices heard. TCM warm diseases became a major focus of the controversies in this debate, and the movement ended hastily because it could not get the consensus of most doctors.[84] As for the translated term "typhoid", the official statement of TCM was that "typhoid fever" overwhelmed the "damp warm diseases" of the warm disease school. The study of warm diseases produced no new

---

[82] Yun Tieqiao, Discussion on the Proposal for Unified Disease Names, *Treatise on Medicine*, p. 7.
[83] Yun Tieqiao, Discussion on the Proposal for Unified Disease Names, *Treatise on Medicine*, p. 4.
[84] Deng Tietao, *Modern History of TCM*, pp. 93–100.

ideas during the Republic of China period. In addition to the repeated publication of medical books in the Qing Dynasty, doctors gradually turned to the study of individual infectious diseases, such as diphtheria, pestis, cholera, dysentery. However, typhology, which was once surpassed by warm disease school and reduced to the status of "tiller and vassal", had a great potential of revival during the Republic of China period.[85] Xie Guan regarded *Treatise on Febrile Diseases* as a classic example for medical learners to make inference. Whether it is about warm diseases or epidemics in general, typhology actually had been occupying the position of the "general theory" at the top level. It is thus said that "by following this pattern, its effect will multiply".[86]

In its *List of Disease Names Approved by the Central National Medical College*, the Central National Medical College confirmed that "typhoid fever (伤寒)" is the name of "typhoid", which is the "original name of all national medicine" and is suitable for a unified disease name. This consideration is also based on the fact that the word "typhoid" has been used in Western medicine, and "typhoid bacteria" has been used to name bacteria. The term "typhoid" has converged the meaning of China and the West. It is closely connected with classical medicine, and conforms to the prosperity of the typhoid study during the Republic of China period, as well as to the name of Western bacteriology.[87]

The new term of typhoid can lead us to examine the development of TCM infectious history during the Republic of China period. In the definition of most doctors in the Qing Dynasty, "typhoid" itself was not contagious.[88] However, after comparing with Western medicine, the new term "typhoid" was given the feature of infectious disease, and TCM turned to define ancient typhoid as an infectious disease. For example, Ding Fubao said that typhoid "was generally recognized as fever, a major infectious disease, even though there were different theories in ancient and modern times, at home and abroad". He added: "According to Zhongjing, typhoid was known as an infectious disease, with both fever and infection that fulfill the conditions of typhoid."[89] Compared with Western medicine, "typhoid" had become a synonym for infectious diseases. In the Qing Dynasty, the fact that *Treatise on Typhoid Fever* became a classic of TCM was not due to its being a guidance for doctors in treating infectious diseases. However, since the Republic of China period, the new treatise on typhoid has indeed extended to the field of infectious diseases. The *Commentaries and Annotations on Typhoid Fever* by Tan Cizhong in 1935 affirms that typhoid is an

---

[85] Fan Xingzhun, *A Brief History of Chinese Medicine*, p. 240. For the development of turning febrile diseases into a separate infectious disease during the Republic of China period, see Deng Tietao, *Modern History of TCM*, pp. 407–411.

[86] Xie Liheng, You Zaijing, *Febrile Diseases, On the Origin and Development of Chinese Medicine· Notes of Corrective Medicine*, p. 83.

[87] Central National Medical College (ed.), *List of Disease Names Approved by the Central National Medical College, Vol. 1, Documents between the National Medical College and Yun Tieqiao*, Nanjing: Central National Medical College, 1933, pp. 32–33.

[88] (Qing) Lu Jiuzhi, Fu Qingzhu & Dai Tianzhang, *On Febrile Diseases* II, Complete Collection of Medical Books in Shibu Room, p. 82.

[89] Miyamoto, translated by Ding Fubao, *New Treatise on Typhoid Fever*, Preface, p. 1.

acute infectious disease, and the "Six Classics" represent the concept of syndrome in Western medicine.[90] Moreover, the book was also called *General Theory of Acute Infectious Diseases,* which indicates that its significance is self-evident.

This is an interesting change, but it also means that we must respond positively to the Western theory of infectious diseases. The status of other individual infectious diseases can only be clarified with further studies. After the movement of unifying disease names in the 1930s, several TCM doctors wrote important books specializing on "typhoid". Let's first look at the example of Zhu Weiju (1884–1951). Zhu grew up in Sichuan and was proficient in Western and Chinese medicine. As for the attitude toward Western medicine, he was not in line with the Sino-west convergent school, such as Tang Zonghai or Zhu Peiwen, who had only read some Western medicine books in the late Qing Dynasty. More similar to Ding Fubao's experiences, he graduated from a Western medicine school and then went to Japan to study medicine. All this was completed before he was 30 years old.

When he came to Shanghai, he saw that the local TCM doctors mostly used the cold prescriptions of the warm disease school to treat patients. As many of them were wrongly treated, he turned to advocate the use of warm prescriptions to treat typhoid, and gradually integrated this method into the TCM circle in Shanghai.[91] In 1932, he published *New Meaning of Typhoid Fever* and *Modern Interpretations of Treatise on Febrile Diseases.* He used the physiology of Western medicine, such as new concepts of nerve and body temperature, to explain the *Treatise on Typhoid Fever*. For example: "Fever means that the terminal nerve is stimulated and reflected in the warming center, resulting in hyperthermia of exothermic function and the rise of body temperature on the surface".[92] He believed that "typhoid fever" was not just "typhoid", but it actually included most fever diseases in Western medicine, and the "typhoid fever" he referred to was "generalized typhoid fever". This "broad sense" is like putting the *Treatise on Typhoid Fever* in Fan Xingzhun's so-called "general theory" of warm diseases, so as to further explore the inducements of various exogenous febrile diseases. Its theoretical origin is still attached to the "generalized typhoid fever" (including apoplexy, specified typhoid, damp and warm diseases, febrile disease, etc.) under the context of "five typhoid fevers" in the *Classics on Medical Problems,* rather than the "typhoid in the narrow sense" defined by western bacteriology under "generalized typhoid fever".[93]

At that time, TCM was satisfied with this explanation. In addition to respecting the status and contributions of classics and the saint (Zhang Zhongjing), it was also able to bring the diseases of the warm disease school into the broad system of typhoid to reorganize the names of the diseases. Wang Shenxuan commented: "*Treatise on*

---

[90] Tan Cizhong, Commentaries and Annotations on Typhoid Fever, pp. 1–2.

[91] Zhao Haihua (ed.), *Biography of Zhu Weiju, Collection of Zhu Weiju's Medical Cases,* Shanghai: Shanghai Technology Press, 2007, pp. 1–10.

[92] Zhu Weiju, Distinguishing the Pulse Syndrome of Taiyang Disease and Its Treatment, New Meanings of Typhoid Fever, included in Xing Bin and Huang Li (ed.), *Reviews of Zhu Weiju's Five Medical Books*, Beijing: China TCM Press, 2008, p. 302.

[93] Zhu Weiju, Introduction, New Meanings of Typhoid Fever, included in *Reviews of Zhu Weiju's Five Medical Books,* p. 302.

Typhoid Fever written by Zhang Zhongjing covers typhoid in both broad and narrow senses. All the so-called acute infectious diseases in Western medicine and various fever diseases undiscovered by science have been included".[94] This became the definition of the disease scope recognized by TCM at that time.[95] It defined typhoid and warm diseases as being in a subordinate relationship, rather than an antagonistic and contradictory relationship.

Zhu Shengping's representative work, *Inquiries for Typhoid Fever*, was completed in 1945 (published in 1950). He almost completely adopted the disease staging method of Western medicine, that all febrile diseases were divided into incubation period, prodrome period, progressive period, polar period, regression period and recovery period. He believed that these discussions were the ways of "controlling the complexity by targeting on the cause of the disease", which was the characteristic of TCM. He had the wish to sum up a set of effective treatment methods, rather than arguing about the cause of disease (bacteria).[96] Many Chinese doctors maintained that it was more important to understand the treatment methods and rules than to determine the name of a disease. Of course, this may also reflect the problem that TCM was still too broad in determining the names of diseases, and it could only selectively adopt the disease staging method of Western medicine, without discussing or paying much attention to bacteriology and the naming mechanism behind it. This is the contradictory part.

At the same time when Zhu Weiju's works came out, an important writing of defining typhoid also came into being after the failure of the disease name unification movement. It was the work of Chen Cunren, a famous doctor in Shanghai. Chen was the disciple of Ding Ganren, who was a famous doctor in Shanghai with enormous prestige and numerous disciples. Many famous modern Chinese doctors, such as Ding Jiwan, Qin Bowei, Xu Banlong, Zhang Cigong, Wang Shenxuan, Cheng Menxue took him as their teacher. Chen belonged to the younger generation. Ding was good at treating many diseases, especially fever. He mainly believed in *Treatise on Typhoid Fever*, especially the *Annotated Treatise on Typhoid Fever* by Shu Chiyuan of the Qing Dynasty. Ding agreed with the *Basic Inquiries. Heat Theory* that "warm disease today are all typhoid". Therefore, in clinical practices, *Treatise on Typhoid Fever* was a medical book that must be read. However, due to the different weather conditions from the ancient till modern times, diseases have spread, new diseases have emerged one after another, and doctors should duly learn the traditional theory of warm diseases at different periods. In line with the purpose of "melting the school of typhoid and warm diseases into one furnace", he had made great efforts in the clinical treatment of exogenous febrile diseases, emphasizing that we should focus on the combination of classical and modern prescriptions without neglecting either

---

94 Wang Shenxuan (ed.), Part 8: Internal Medicine (I), *Compilation of New Theories of TCM*, p. 4.

95 Cao Yingfu, *A Record of Classical Prescription Experiments*, p. 56; Zhu Weiju, *Inquiries for Typhoid Fever*, Fuzhou: Fujian Science and Technology Publishing House, 2005, Zhou Zongqi's preface, p. 3.

96 Zhu Weiju, Introduction I, Inquiries for Typhoid Fever, included in *Notes to Reviews of Zhu Weiju's Five Medical Books*, pp. 23–28.

of them.[97] It is obvious that there was few "typhoid verses warm disease debates" among his disciples. Instead, they tended to find out various methods in the theory of warm diseases and take the treatment as the priority.

Chen Cunren followed Ding Ganren in the 1920s. At that time, the situation in TCM clinics was as follows: "At 6 o'clock in the morning, the room was filled with patients of typhoid fever, all of whom were carried by their families with rattan chairs and planks". It can be seen that typhoid was very serious in Shanghai, which coincided with Yu Yunxiu's statement that typhoid was often prevalent in Shanghai. In 1926, when the Shanghai epidemic broke out, Chen recalled the situation: "Many doctors fell ill, and the number of patients seeking treatment in various charity halls increased two or three times. Mr. Ding Ganren also caught damp and warm typhoid rapidly. He was ill for a month and died at the age of 55".[98] What was the "damp and warm typhoid" that led to Ding's unfortunate death? The other scene was in 1933, when Chen was referred to treat Yu Youren (1879–1964) who was a well-known figure in support of TCM. He once declared: "I have been seeing TCM doctors and taking traditional Chinese medications all my life".[99] The first thing Yu asked the referrer was "is it TCM or Western medicine?" The man replied, "It's TCM." Upon hearing this, Yu nodded and replied, "yes, I have to see TCM doctors". Then he reached out to let Chen feel his pulse. What disease must be treated by TCM? After diagnosis and treatment, Chen concluded that it was "damp and warm typhoid", which was the same disease that took his teacher's life, and he advised him to have a blood test to confirm it. Yu immediately responded that he had gone to the hospital for blood tests (white blood cell) three days ago, and it was confirmed to be the earliest stage of typhoid. Yu said, "As soon as I heard the term 'typhoid', I knew I needed to see a TCM doctor".[100] Then, after about 15 days of diagnosis and treatment, Yu's fever slowly decreased and he finally completely recovered.

The above story is from *Life History of the Silver Dollar Era.* They are some fragments of Chen Cunren's memories of his medical and daily life before the Sino Japanese War. The term "typhoid fever" heard by Yu Youren when he went to have a blood test had become the Chinese name of typhoid, but with some TCM elements. It was a very popular mode to use Western medicine to confirm the name of a disease before seeing a TCM doctor for treatment. It is surprising for Chen to name it "damp and warm typhoid ", a name surprisingly consistent with Western medicine diagnose without any modern testing equipment. "Damp and warm typhoid" is just another name of typhoid disease. It is a new compound noun that combines the two disease names of warm disease and typhoid systems, with the combination of both "damp febrile" and "typhoid". From Chen's diagnosis of "damp and warm typhoid", we can see a new direction of reforming the names of fever in TCM, that is, "generalized

[97] Shen Zhongli(ed.), Biography of Ding Ganren, *Collection of Ding Ganren's Clinical Cases,* Shanghai: Shanghai University of TCM Press, 2000, p. 2.

[98] Chen Cunren, Life History of the Silver Dollar Era, pp. 32–38.

[99] Wen Xiang, Chiang Kai Shek and the Administration of TCM, *Journal of Huaiyin Normal University* (Philosophy and Social Sciences), 29.4, 2007 (07), p. 504.

[100] Chen Cunren, Life History of the Silver Dollar Era, p. 185.

typhoid fever" that includes all fever diseases. However, to refer to all warm diseases as "typhoid fever" is not adequate to explain all infectious diseases including typhoid. So doctors tended to choose terms other than typhoid fever, such as names of warm diseases, to make a detailed analysis so as to find out the terms that can correspond to the disease names of Western medicine.

Since 1937, Chen Cunren had gradually summarized his experience in treating "damp and warm typhoid", and spent about 10 years writing a book. After the book was completed, it was submitted to his predecessors and fellow friends for review. A total of 13 people wrote prefaces for him. These prefaces were summarized and completed in 1949. However, due to the war, this book was not published until 1955 in Hong Kong under the title of *A Manual of Typhoid Fever.* A year after that, *A Manual of Damp Febrile Typhoid* was published in Shanghai, with almost the same content as the previous book. It can be described as a compilation of his experiences in seeing and treating typhoid during the Republic of China period. This book is featured with the complete TCM academic development in the debate between typhoid fever and warm disease schools in the Qing Dynasty. Xie Guan praised the book for "combining the theory of the West for confirmation, regardless of the six meridians and the triple energizers, classifying the four stages of symptoms, being adaptive and practical, defining standards, identifying gains and losses without any vague discussions", so "the dispute between typhoid and warm diseases is dissipated".[101] Xie referred to the fact that the typhoid manual does not take the six meridians of the typhoid system nor the triple energizer of the warm disease system as the proof for examination, but absorbs the stage theory for diseases in Western medicine, divides the onset of typhoid into four weeks, with each week having various changes in symptoms, which are listed in the chart below for comparison by doctors,[102] and shelves the dispute between the six meridians and the triple energizer. This is quite consistent with the above-mentioned way of distinguishing diseases by the "heat types" of fever in the medical books translated by Ding Fubao, which is equivalent to rethinking the syndrome differentiation method of TCM for specific infectious diseases. It is also similar to Zhu Weiju's theory of stages. These classifications were obviously influenced by Western medicine.

Chen believed that "typhoid fever" has three meanings: "The first is the collective noun of all warm diseases, which generally refers to all kinds of warm diseases; next is the narrower sense which may refer to the syndrome of ephedra decoction in *Treatise on Typhoid Fever*; the last one is new, specifically referring to damp and warm typhoid, which is the most confusing".[103] The first two are in the TCM context, and the last new definition refers to the typhoid of Western medicine. Chen sorted out around 10 items relating to typhoid in the classic *Treatise on Typhoid Fever,* thinking that they account for only one twentieth of the whole *Treatise on Typhoid Fever*.

---

[101] Chen Cunren, *A Manual of Typhoid Fever*, Hong Kong: China Medical Press, 1955, Mr. Xie Liheng's preface, p. 3.

[102] Chen Cunren, *A Manual of Typhoid Fever*, pp. 2–3.

[103] Chen Cunren, Table of Comparisons between Ancient and Modern Unified Disease Names (I), *Handbook of TCM Practitioners,* Taipei: Hongye Book Company, 1991, p. 160.

Treatise on Typhoid Fever only focuses on "syndrome", that is, a syndrome of large-scale fever, without a single, unified definition of the disease name, so the "six meridians" are no longer supposed to serve as the facade of TCM fever theory in modern times. A more accurate and detailed definition of the disease is to be explored.[104] As mentioned above, "damp and warm diseases" and "typhoid fever" are often mixed up. Yun Tieqiao once said, "Dampness (usually called damp and warm diseases)... is often indiscriminate with typhoid fever... In the early stage of clinical diagnosis, it is often impossible to distinguish. What is the reason for their indiscernibility and how slightly different their symptoms are, should be explained so that there is a detailed definition. The book is specialized, and is read by people all over the country."[105] In the 1930s when Yun was troubled by the names of the diseases, and it seemed that there was no solution. So Chen's thinking may be a breakthrough in the entanglement of disease names.

Chen Cunren further explained the reason for defining typhoid as "damp febrile typhoid". It is written in *A Manual of Typhoid Fever*: "In TCM, the blood test results of those who got damp and warm typhoid are mostly typhoid of infectious diseases in Western medicine. Those who had serious damp and febrile symptoms generally belong to positive typhoid fever, and the light symptoms belong to paratyphoid fever".[106] This is a conclusion based on the scientific demonstration of Western medicine as well as TCM experiences. In addition, he also pointed out: "Blood tests in Western medicine are divided into typhoid and paratyphoid fever according to their pathogen classifications. If the symptoms are similar, the treatment is the same. TCM doesn't have a bacteria test and there is no difference between positive and negative."[107] It can be seen that he did not define the disease according to the bacteriology of Western medicine, but summarized the experience and came to the conclusion that the typhoid referred to by Western medicine was "damp febrile ". It is worth mentioning that Chen did not have the ability to conduct Western medicine experiments nor to test bacterial methods. Western medicine knowledge was only a tool to confirm his experience, which can only be regarded as an "indirect" scientific demonstration.

In addition, Lu Yuanlei once said, "There is no need to take typhoid as being so different from warm disease. It is more caused by bacteria than by environment or Qi".[108] This shows the contradictory feelings of TCM for Western medicine bacteriology: on the one hand, Lu believed that the bacteria theory could dissolve some disputes of typhoid verse warm disease debate in order to establish the name of a disease, which was a theory that TCM had to respond to positively. On the other hand, as the examples of Yun Tieqiao and Chen Cunren mentioned above, they were not

---

104 Chen Cunren, Lecture on Typhoid Fever, II—Methods of Reading Ancient Medical Books, *Handbook of TCM Practitioners*, pp. 181, 186–187.

105 Yun Tieqiao, Discussion on the Proposal for Unified Disease Names, *Treatise on Medicine*, p. 7.

106 Chen Cunren, A Manual of Typhoid Fever, p. 1.

107 Chen Cunren, Table of Comparisons between Ancient and Modern Unified Disease Names (I), *Handbook of TCM Practitioners*, p. 161.

108 Chen Cunren, *A Manual of Typhoid Fever*, Mr. Lu Yuanlei's preface, p. 4.

willing to completely adopt bacteriology, for fear that classical medicine would be replaced by bacteriology, or for reasons such as "TCM does not test bacteria". This means that TCM can only indirectly and passively use the knowledge of Western medicine. TCM was "vague and aloof", and its passive and partial learning of Western medicine bacteriology was criticized. For example, Fu Sinian criticized that TCM was quite ignorant of bacteriology and just "plagiarized things they didn't understand", in a way like "asking someone knowing nothing about electricity to come home and install a power grid on the wall, and the danger is indescribable". For Fu, to accept Western science, one must accept it "completely". It is impossible for TCM to achieve "scientization" by starting from the "classical" thinking and adopting the theory of Western medicine in fragments.[109]

For what reason did Chen Cunren use the combination of "damp febrile" and "typhoid"? Chen explained: "Nowadays, it is generally recognized that the word 'typhoid' is the name of a legally acknowledged infectious disease, which has been widely used and does not need to be changed. However, if colleagues in the TCM circle use the word 'typhoid' alone in their writing, it is still easy to cause misunderstandings. Only the term 'damp and warm typhoid' is more common and obvious".[110] The reason is that "typhoid" not only has the broad sense (generally refers to all warm diseases) and narrow sense (specifically refers to ephedra decoction syndrome) definitions of TCM, but also represents the typhoid of Western medicine. In order to avoid confusion, the term "damp febrile" was added as a more detailed identification. Of course, "damp febrile typhoid" was not originally created by Chen. A disease name may involve new theories, new interpretations, and even a commonly known name. Ding Zhongying (1886–1978) said, "The term 'damp febrile typhoid' in Shanghai has become a medical idiom".[111] Chen was born in Shanghai. He named typhoid as damp febrile typhoid, which may also be due to conventional reasons. In the early 1950s, on the basis of *A Manual of Typhoid Fever,* Chen reorganized his comparative analysis on Chinese and Western disease names that he had continuously been interested in, and wrote *Table of Comparisons between Ancient and Modern Unified Disease Names* and *Table of Various Febrile Diseases,* so as to compare the disease names between Chinese and Western medicine in retrospect. Chen Yudai explained the naming of "typhoid" in a refrained way: "There must be many opinions on the naming of this disease. 'Damp febrile typhoid' will be used for the time being before it is determined after public discussion."[112] The term "damp febrile typhoid" represents the temporarily consistent name of some diseases in TCM identity, which was a transferring name from the late Qing Dynasty to the Republic of China period rather than a the definition of the disease agreed upon. Later, in 1954, Yu Wuyan published a special book, *New Treatise on Infectious Diseases, Vol. 1. Damp and Warm Typhoid,*

[109] Fu Sinian, On the So-called National Medicine, *Complete Works of Fu Sinian*, Vol. 6, pp. 323–324.

[110] Chen Cunren, A Manual of Typhoid Fever, pp. 1–2.

[111] Chen Cunren, *A Manual of Typhoid Fever*, Ding Zhongying's preface, p. 2.

[112] Chen Cunren, Table Comparison of Ancient and Modern Unified Disease Names (I), *Handbook of TCM Practitioners,* p. 161.

which holds that "typhoid fever" was "generalized" in classical Chinese medicine and was not suitable for an individual disease name, "Damp febrile" was included in the generalized typhoid fever, which was more suitable for the comparison with the disease names of Western medicine.[113] At this time, the definition of "damp febrile typhoid" was quite different from the idea of "typhoid and damp febrile are completely different" among some TCM doctors in the Qing Dynasty. The boundary of its name and definition had been redrawn.

The meanings of new disease names are different from those of classical medicine due to communication and re-translation. All this process can only be called "slow change"—TCM did not completely adopt western disease names, but still looked for the possible position of each disease in ancient classics. Of course, for people like Zhu or Chen, the definition of Western medicine was still the basis of their "experience". In this regard, Sean Hsiang-Lin Lei had noticed the discussion of the valuable "experience" of TCM during the Republic of China period, which is extremely important but easy to be ignored. Classical Chinese medicine did not particularly emphasize "experience", but after the impact of the TCM abolition movement in 1929, it also began to discuss the unique "experience" accumulated by classical medicine, trying to compete with the scientific "experiment" of Western medicine.[114] This chapter combs the theory of typhoid and warm diseases in TCM, and proves that without accurate bacteriological and scientific experimental evidence, the TCM "experience" could only remain at the level of defining diseases based on classical medical training and doctors' personal identification (typhoid or damp febrile). The one-way diagnosis of diseases based on "experience" without scientific "experiment" confirmation might only become the forum of doctors' individual statements. Due to the consistent definition of disease names in Western medicine for comparison, TCM during the Republic of China period began to narrow the scope of its discussion, and strive to find new connotations that were not only in line with classical discussions, but also comparable to the disease names of Western medicine.

4.7 Translation, Interpretation and Regeneration of Chinese Medical History

Xie Guan once analyzed the general trend of the development of TCM history in his book *On the Origin and Development of Chinese Medicine*: "The convergence of Chinese and Western medicine will be the great cause of doctors in the future". However, they might need two qualifications, that is, to be well versed in Chinese and Western medical books, and also be able to "match the disease names in TCM

[113] Yu Wuyan, *New Treatise on Infectious Diseases, Vol. 1. Damp and Warm Typhoid*, p. 1.

[114] Sean Hsiang-Lin Lei, How Did Chinese Medicine Become Experiential? The Political Epistemology of Jinyan, *Positions: East Asian Culture Critique*, 2002 (10.02), pp. 333–364.

with that in the west, as well as the common ground they share".[115] It can be seen that understanding the theory of Western medicine and comparing the names of diseases was the most basic skill of TCM during the Republic of China period, and it was also the biggest problem faced by febrile diseases. TCM knew they needed to match the disease names with those of Western medicine, but it was unwilling or unable to adopt the whole meaning of scientific knowledge behind the definition of Western medicine names, or even to give up some conflicting traditions. For example, Lu Yuanlei said that even though TCM must be scientific, science is only a supplement, and it is not acceptable to "sacrifice itself and assimilate into Western medicine".[116] With the expectation to maintain its autonomy in some degree, TCM was unwilling to assimilate into Western medicine. Yun Tieqiao said: "Adopting the Western disease names in today's disease name unification is in conflict with its original intention of collation and improvement".[117] Instead of seeking the unified disease names of Western medicine and assimilating or eliminating TCM, it is better to continue to adopt the interpretations and definitions of some diseases in Chinese medicine. If so, TCM doctors might have their individual set of views, which will certainly increase the difficulty of internal integration of TCM febrile disease study. To look at Chen Cunren's medical theory discussed in this chapter, some names are still "tentatively" used. Whether "typhoid fever" or "damp febrile" is used as the name for "typhoid", TCM is still having a dialogue with Western medicine. It will be a long and unfinished undertaking for the whole TCM to retranslate and reinterpret ancient classics and unify the disease names of Chinese and Western medicine.[118]

At the beginning of this chapter, we see the whole process of a noun being introduced from Japan, later incorporated into the regulations on infectious diseases by the Chinese authorities, and finally integrated and reinterpreted with the ancient classic *Treatise on Typhoid Fever*. Then it went through the "slow change" of the definition of Chinese medical diseases. Its significance lies in that even TCM adopted some Western medicine theories to explain diseases, the valuable parts of classical medicine considered by TCM were still preserved, and TCM had not completely overturned the disease name of classical medicine. The impact of Western medicine made TCM reflect on the original definition of disease. While combing the internal integration and unification of febrile diseases, they redefined the attributes and names

115 Xie Liheng & You Zaijing, The Convergence of Chinese and Western Medicine, *On the Origin and Development of Chinese Medicine· Notes of Corrective Medicine*, p. 137.

116 Yun Tieqiao, compiled by Zhang Yuping, Mr. Yun Tieqiao's Life and Academic Thoughts, *Four Kinds of Yun Tieqiao's Medical Books*, p. 10.

117 Yun Tieqiao, Discussion on the Proposal for Unified Disease Names, *Treatise on Medicine*, pp. 4–5.

118 "The movement of unifying the names of diseases" has constantly appeared in the history of the debate between Chinese and Western medicine. See Gan Zuwang, The Lawsuit of the Names of Diseases, *Gan Zuwang's Medical Remarks*, Beijing: People's Health Publishing House, 1996, p. 64.

of new diseases with classics, "in order to rebuild the order and authority of the discipline".[119] TCM more or less reinterpreted infectious diseases with bacteriology, with a distance, trying to weaken the major influence of "bacteria" on diseases, for fear that the complete adoption of bacteria will lead to the demise of TCM. This part of the history can be the insistence of TCM on its right to explain the diseases, and it also shows the endless discussion of Chinese doctors on Western medicine and classical medicine.

Attention needs to be paid to a few aspects of the topic "facing Western medicine": First, the theory of a bacterial incubation period in Western medicine has changed some concepts of "febrile incubation" in TCM. Second, the interpretation of "infection" changed the theory of classical medicine. For example, "typhoid fever" was a "non infectious" fever in the typhoid fever verses warm disease debate in the Qing Dynasty. But after the Republic of China period, it became a very important infectious disease under the influence of Western medicine. And *Treatise on Typhoid Fever,* instead of being criticized that it could not treat infectious diseases in the debate in the Qing Dynasty, became an important theoretical book discussing the treatment of infectious diseases, occupying the position of "general theory". Third, certain corresponding relationships between some Chinese abstract nouns and western concepts, like the "dampness", "toxins" and "bacteria", have been determined. We still don't know what TCM thought about the bacterial discourse of Western medicine. Although the preliminary comparison of some disease names can not be accurately named one-to-one, it seems that TCM was very confident to find terms in classical medicine comparable with Western medicine theories, and many definitions are still kept, remaining the important knowledge in TCM febrile disease until today.[120]

From the perspective of the history of science, Fu Dawei had a very simple and concise metaphor: China has its own tradition of alternative science and technology, and to directly absorb the latest western scientific theories would be as unlikely as to expect the westerners to give up Newtonian mechanics. The true scientific revolution must accumulate scientific knowledge in the new system,[121] rather than taking classical medicine as the benchmark before taking into account the bacteriology of Western Medicine, like what the TCM doctors during the Republic of China period did. This can not be a sign that TCM had created a kind of scientific knowledge by integrating Chinese and Western medicine. From the perspective of laboratory studies, TCM had no experimental instruments and had not developed a set of scientific methods to examine and study bacteria even though bacteriology was one of the pressures facing TCM reform. Moreover, it was not enough just to "see" bacteria. In

---

[119] Li Jianmin, *The History of Life—Viewing Chinese History from Medical Treatment*, Taipei: Sanmin Book Company, 2005, p. 18. For example, there is still a saying in modern TCM infectious diseases that "typhoid and paratyphoid belong to the category of 'damp febrile' in TCM febrile diseases". The source of this certification was in the early years of the Republic of China period.

[120] Zhang Xiuhui, *Modern Chinese Medicine Epidemiology*, Tianjin: Tianjin Science and Technology Press, 1999, p. 208.

[121] Fu Dawei, *Three Answers to What Science Is: STS, Gender and Philosophy of Science*, Taipei: Qunxue Press, 2009, pp. 45–53, 249.

addition to establishing a one-to-one correspondence between bacteria and diseases, Western medicine should also be able to prove that bacterial infection will be affected by environmental conditions, and tell the world that scientific medicine can control these conditions, so that people outside the laboratory can find the possibility to have a dialogue with such scientific research and apply its results.[122] At that time, TCM had no laboratory for practice and production of knowledge, meaning it had no power in either controlling infectious diseases nor leading health work brought by bacteriology to Western medicine.

It can be seen that the so-called "new" bacteriological knowledge absorbed by TCM was still second-hand. When TCM decided to go back to the world of classical medicine, they chose to continue to interpret classical literature. Since "there is little to learn from today", they could only "retreat to the ancient",[123] rather than choose to enter the laboratory and show results.[124] So why didn't TCM try to go into the laboratory to study bacteria and testing methods? This may be answered from various angles, but the author believes that the attitude of TCM toward bacteriology may be the key. This problem will be sorted out in the next chapter of the book.

Chinese medicine did not go into the laboratory to find the positive stimulation and influence brought by bacteriology, which may disappoint those who were concerned with the development of Chinese medicine. However, through this "indirect" science, TCM had carried out a lot of academic introspection. These changes might not be good, but after all, there have been "changes" concerned by historians, such as the innovation of disease names. During the Republic of China period, compared with the Qing Dynasty, the demand for disease names had a relatively fixed range though it did not achieve the accuracy of "one disease, one cause". Yin syndrome, typhoid fever, warm heat, summer warmth, winter warmth, metabolizing decoction syndrome, etc., were actually no longer the disease names that can represent typhoid. Lei Feng criticized the confusion of "typhoid fever" as the main disease name in the *On Seasonal Diseases* written in the late Qing Dynasty, based on his "learning from the typhoid experts that typhoid are classified as febrile, heat, cholera and sore syndromes". What is more surprising is that there were more names[125] as sputum typhoid, food typhoid, air typhoid, blood typhoid, dirty typhoid, bottom leakage

---

[122] Bruno Latour, translated by Lin Zongde, Give Me A Laboratory and I Will Lift Up the World, included in Wu Jialing, Fu Dawei and Sean Hsiang-Lin Lei (ed.), *Science and Technology Yearn for Society*, Taipei: Qunxue Press, 2004, pp. 219–263.

[123] This is what Zhang Taiyan said in his preface in the *Dictionary of Chinese Pharmacy* in 1934. From Chen Cunren, *Life History in the Silver Era*, p. 263.

[124] At the beginning of the Republic of China period, even TCM integrated Western physiology and pathology into the modern school education and laboratory working, it was not enough to master the skills by just reading the operational manuals or bacterial atlas. It can only be acquired by learning the correct experimental methods with the repeated failures in operation and the guidance from the highly experienced. For the characteristics of laboratory research, see Sergio Sismondo, translated by Lin Zongde, *Introduction to Scientific and Technological Research,* Taipei: Qunxue Press, 2007, pp. 152–167.

[125] (Qing) Lei Feng, *On Seasonal Diseases*, Beijing: People's Health Publishing House, 1964, p. 138.

typhoid, stabbing typhoid, fatigue typhoid, chaos typhoid and even doctors at that time felt it to be confusing and irrational.

However, by the Republic of China period, the disease name "damp febrile typhoid", which was interpreted and regenerated from classical medicine, had specifically referred to typhoid, which was a major change and agreed by most doctors. It was still the scientific verification of Western medicine that contributed to this change. Bacteriological tests made the diagnosis of diseases more accurate, just like the story of Chen Cunren's diagnosis recorded in Yu Youren's writing. Can "damp febrile typhoid", which was diagnosed by Chen, be diagnosed by another TCM doctor with a different disease name? However, the "accuracy" of this diagnosis was confirmed by scientific blood tests. In other words, the process of using Western medicine to confirm the name of a disease before seeking the treatment of TCM won TCM the patients. Although it lost some dominance in defining diseases, after all, TCM during the Republic of China period successfully achieved its original intention of preserving classical medicine and did not come to an impasse of abolishing classical medicine. In addition to blending into the background and situation of the whole medical development and adapting to the environment, we should not lose our academic identity, which was an important topic faced by TCM during the Republic of China period. All of the above turned to be the epitome of the achievements and limitations of the development and transformation of TCM during the Republic of China period.

Chapter 5
Bacteria and Qi: The Absorption, Elimination and Rejection of the Western Bacteria Theory by TCM During the Republic of China Period

> Of the most effective technologies in modern medicine, the first is surgery, the second is sterilization, and the third is the treatment of infectious diseases. There have not been perfect treatments for the interior disorder of the human body even if it is clearly diagnosed. Modern medicine is not deceptive. It doesn't boast of being able to cure all diseases in the world. Nothing like the absurd books as the *Demonstrations of Typhoid Fever and The Secret Therapies of the Censors*, maintaining that nothing is incurable, which is comforting for the foolish but not true in reality.[1]
>
> —Fu Sinian

> The Chinese believe in the five elements and six Qis, while westerners believe in the performance of bacteria, flagella or amoeba action. Each follows its own concept and theory, which are very different from each other. The theory of the five elements and six Qis may not necessarily be true and, by the same token, the theory of immunology is not entirely perfect.[2]
>
> —Ye Guhong

[1] Fu Sinian, On the So-called Chinese Medicine, *The Complete Works of Fu Sinian,* Vol. 6, Taipei: Lianjing Publishing House, 1980, p. 322.

[2] The author commented that "amoeba action" should refer to the concept of amoeba protozoa moving in the body by extending the meaning of "Qi" in the body of TCM, which is significantly different from the body view of "bacteria" in Western medicine. The methods TCM used in treating bacterial diseases can be found in the publication of Ye Guhong, *Chinese Therapies for Infectious Diseases*, National Medical News, No. 1 (1939), pp. 70–72.

© Zhonghua Book Company 2026

K. Pi, *The Contest of Modern Chinese and Western Medicine*,
https://doi.org/10.1007/978-981-95-2832-5_5

5.1 Preface

Since the end of the nineteenth century, Western bacteriology has developed vigorously, taking infectious diseases as quite important disciplines.[3] Influenced by the Japanese media in the late Qing Dynasty, this theory was gradually introduced into China. Since the beginning of the Republic of China period, the Beiyang government began to adopt the standard of "eight infectious diseases"[4] of Western medicine, which enhanced the development of Western medicine in health work and its status on behalf of progress and modernity.[5] The most important work of modern health is the prevention of infectious disease. Undoubtedly the essential theory in the early twentieth century is the knowledge system of bacteriology. At present, the research on health history has been carried out in all aspects,[6] but the role of TCM is still "undetermined" or "aphasia". So, how did TCM use its knowledge system to respond to Western bacteriology at that time? This is the key issue of this book.

This book also attempts to record the process of integration, dialogue and transformation of pathology between traditional Chinese fever and Western infectious diseases.[7] How does TCM make use of "Qi" in traditional classics to have a dialogue with Western bacteriology? Did Chinese medicine ever try or how did they try to change traditional interpretation of some treatments? We will even see the surprising

---

[3] For general works, see William Bulloch, *The History of Biology* (New York: Dover Publications, 1979, c1938). On the impact of bacteriology on history, for example, David S. Barnes used the development of bacteriology in France at the end of the 19th century to discuss the new public health cause and its impact on social life. See *The Great Stink of Paris and the 19th Century Struggle against Filth and Germs.* (Baltimore: Johns Hopkins University Press, 2006.) For the daily life and medicine in the United States at the beginning of the 20th century, see Nancy Tomes, *The Gospel of Germs: Men, Women, and the Microbe in American Life* (Cambridge, Mass.: Harvard University Press, 1998).

[4] For the records and comments on these eight diseases, see Huang Shengbai, *Commentaries on the Regulations on the Prevention of Infectious Diseases*, Official Gazette (Announcement) in March 20, the Republic of China period 5th year and *Commentaries on the Regulations on the Prevention of Infectious Diseases*, (continued No. 1), Tongji, No. 1 and 2, 1918, pp. 4–6 and 169–170.

[5] Angelic Ki Che Leung & Charlotte Furth (eds.), *Health and Hygiene in Modern Chinese East Asia: Policies and Publics in the Long Twenties Century* (Durham: Duke University Press,2011).For the study of the eight major infectious diseases, see the article by Sean Hsiang Lin Lei in the book, pp. 73–108.

[6] In addition to western scholars, many researchers, such as Wataru Iijima from Japan, Hu Cheng, Yang Nianqun, Cao Shuji, Zhang Daqing and Zhang Zhongmin from the mainland, have also made achievements in all disease and health aspects in modern China. Yu Xinzhong shared some particular insights. See Yu Xinzhong, What Is Health—Research on the History of Health in Modern China, *Theoretical Studies on History*, No. 3, 2011, pp. 132–141. For the latest summary of results and research review, see Yu Xinzhong, *Health and Epidemic Prevention Mechanism in the Qing Dynasty and Its Modern Evolution*, Beijing: Beijing Normal University Press, 2016, pp. 1–35. For the works from Taiwan, see Chen Xiufen, Medical History Research in Taiwan (1990–2010) and Its Relationship with "New Historiography", *Sinology Research Newsletter*, Vol. 29, No. 3, 2010, pp. 19–28; Jiang Zhushan *Trends, Methods and Practice of Contemporary Historical Research: from New Cultural History to Global History,* Taipei: Wunan Publishing House, 2012, Chapter 4.

[7] Fan Xingzhun, *A Brief History of Chinese Medicine*, Beijing: TCM Classics Publishing House, 1986, pp. 240–241.

invention of "sterilization" of TCM. Generally, the acceptance of bacteriology in TCM should also be divided into different historical stages. In the late Qing Dynasty when bacterial theory was not quite introduced, Qi theory of TCM was able to hold the dialogue with Western medicine, without being repulsed by the ideas of Western medicine. The subsequent situation during the Republic of China period still needs to be continuously clarified. This chapter focuses on the phase analysis of "Qi" and "bacteria". The author has the hope of making up for the blank of bacterial discussion in the modern history of TCM.

5.2 The Track of Western Bacteriology

After 1880, Western medicine made a leap forward in the development of "microorganisms". The theory of pathogen" was firmly established.[8] This suspicion dates back to the sixteenth century. Unfortunately, there were no microscopes to help scientists further verify this fact.[9] At the end of the eighteenth century when the Chinese School of warm diseases was getting more mature, "fever" was a common diagnostic term. But it is often confusing, because many diagnoses of diseases did not mark the exact disease names. The differences of opinions among doctors were similar to TCM. From the eighteenth century to the early nineteenth century, doctors continued to make "correct" classifications of diseases, but all were based on the symptoms of patients, not on the disease protoplasm. For example, according to the famous *Cambridge Medical History* translated by Zhang Daqing, "Cullen" (William Cullen, 1710–1790) took the order of symptoms occurring in a patient as the main reference indicator.[10] He summarized the common characteristics of several warm diseases, such as fever, anger, rash and fluid flow. It has the characteristics of loss and dissolution, and fever was connected with the nervous system,[11] which is applicable to descriptions and definitions of several fever diseases at the same time. The diagnosis of fever in China and the West were both inaccurate and subjective. The

---

[8] William Bulloch, *The History of Bacteriology*. (New York: Dover Publications, 1979, c1938). The practice of moving from theory and laboratory to daily life can be referred to Christoph Gradmann, translated by ELborg Forster, *Laboratory Disease: Robert Kochs Medical Bacteriology* (Baltimore: John hopkins University Press, 2009), pp. 105–170.

[9] P.E. Baldry, translated by Chen Yinian, *The Battle of Antibiosis*, Taipei: Great China Book Company, 1972, p. 14.

[10] Ruth Rogaski also mentioned case of a doctor. For details, see Ruth Rogaski, translated by Xiang Lei, *The Modernity of Health: the Meaning of Health and Disease at China's Commercial Ports*. Nanjing: Jiangsu People's Publishing House, 2007, pp. 94–98.

[11] For the history of Colleen's fever taxonomy, see W.F. Bynum, *Culle and the Study of Fevers in Britain, 1760–1820,* W.F. Bynum & V. Nutton (ed.), *Theories of Fever from Antiquity to the Enlightenment*, Medical History, Supplement No. 1 (London: Wellcome Institute for the History of Medicine, 1981), pp. 137. Cullen is also good at explaining madness by the nervous system disorder of the human body, and integrate psychosis into the medical discourse on madness. See Roy Porter, *A Brief History of Madness*, Taipei: Zuo'an Culture Press, 2004, pp. 133–134.

occurrence of diseases were even explained according to their own beliefs.[12] After the mid-nineteenth century, Western medicine began to look for the damage caused by specific causes of diseases, then gradually moved toward the thinking of one disease with one cause.[13]

When Europeans were hit by waves of infectious diseases in the nineteenth century, medical scientists tried to solve the mystery of "cause of disease". At that time, many people supported the "miasmatic theory". This school believed that the original cause of the disease was the foul gas emitted by dirt and rotting materials, which enabled the infectious diseases to occur. The other school supported "contagionism", which was a school believing that diseases were caused by the transmission of certain substances. Some people may have thought of micro life being the cause, but there was no direct proofs.[14] However, malaria and bacteria are not mutually exclusive. Dirty air and an unsanitary environment would lead to disease according to both views.[15] In the late nineteenth century, Pasteur discovered yeast by studying the process of wine fermentation. British surgeon Joseph Lister published a paper on surgery, affirming the view that trauma infection was caused by microorganisms.[16] However, many people still held the malaria theory, or used chemical and other factors to explain the causes of thermal infectious diseases, and even openly challenged Pasteur. It was not until Koho in Germany successively isolated tuberculosis and cholera bacteria from the blood since 1880, that the "malaria pathogenic theory" withdrew from the stage of disease history. At the beginning of the twentieth century, the theory of bacterial pathogenicity was completely accepted by western society.[17] An excellent physician must be an excellent bacterial pathologist.[18] Unfortunately, bacterial theory was not much of a help in treatment except for diphtheria serum. The cure rate was often low when the antitoxin of epidemics and other diseases, such as tuberculosis, tetanus and cholera, was injected into the patient's body at the time of onset.[19] At the beginning, the "bacteria" summarized by Bridie Andrews in modern China had quite an extensive coverage, including not only many "virus" invisible

---

[12] W.F. Bynum, *Science and the Practice of Medicine in the Nineteenth Century* (Cambridge; New York; Cambridge University Press, c1994), Chapter 1.

[13] Margaret Pelling, *Cholera, Fever and English Medicine,* Oxford, New York: Oxford University Press,1978.pp. 1825, 1865.

[14] Li Shangren, *Healthy Moral Economy: Dezhen's View on Chinese People's Living Habits and Health,* Collection of Institute of History and Language, Academia Sinica, 2005, Vol. 76 (3), pp. 473–474.

[15] Kenneth F. Kiple (ed.), translated by Zhang Daqing, *Cambridge World History of Human Disease,* Shanghai: Shanghai Science and Technology Education Press, 2007, p. 15.

[16] Micheal Worboys, *Spreading Germs: Disease Theories and Medical Practice in Britain,* 1865–1900 (Cambridge, UK; New York, NY; USA: Cambridge University Press, 2000), pp. 34–39.

[17] In fact, since the middle of the 19th century, microorganisms have been discovered continuously. See Castilloni, translated by Cheng Zhifan, *The History of Medicine,* Vol. 2, Guilin: Guangxi Normal University Press, 2003, pp. 731–741.

[18] Castilloni, translated by Cheng Zhifan, *The History of Medicine,* Vol. 2, p. 750.

[19] Roy Porter, The Greatest Benefit to Mankind: A Medical History of Humanity (New York: W.W. Norton, c1997), pp. 442–443.

under the microscope, but also parasitic diseases.[20] For example, Chen Qiu explained in 1902 that the epidemic of Hong Kong in 1894 was an "internal worm", which was then called "epidemic worm".[21] When several epidemics broke out in the late Qing Dynasty, "the micro worm" was almost ubiquitous, and the discussion it caused was significant and diverse. In TCM Classics, epidemic worms, corpses worms and toxic worms seemed to be common for Chinese people before "bacteria" were incorporated into the fever disease interpretation system.[22] At that time, the term "microorganisms" still included parasitic diseases, but after several deliberations on the terms, the Japanese translation of "bacteria" was used. Jiang baimin said: "The common reference varies from country to country. It is called Bakterien in Germany, bactereis in France, bacteria in Britain and America, and Xijun in Japan, which was used by most scholars in China."[23] As infectious diseases based on bacterial pathogenicity was gradually established in China, the importance of bacteriology and the process of theoretical innovation were eventually recognized by the Chinese people.

With the introduction of Chinese doctors, the intellectual community learned the origin of fever. For example, in 1910, Ding Fubao commented on bacteria: "The old translation is microorganism, which is the vector of various infectious diseases. Bacteria being divided are seen under a microscope as broken hairs or spirals. The origins of the diseases such as pneumonia, tuberculosis and nose gangrene, splenic gangrene, tiger spur, tetanus, black death, returning fever, intestinal zhifus and diphtheria, all belong to this subdivision.[24] The process of understanding bacteria started from the late Qing Dynasty, but it was not until the Republic of China period that bacteriology became a specialized discipline to be studied in the laboratory".[25]

In 1919, Beijing set up the "Central Epidemic Prevention Office", which became the major agency of microbial research in China. Subsequently, western medical colleges and universities successively set up bacteriology courses or bacteriology research departments. Most of the text books included English and American materials. For the needs of teaching, local Western medicine also compiled or translated

[20] Bridie Andrews, "Blood Disease" and the History of Chinese Medicine, Diseases, Medical Treatment and Health since the Qing Dynasty, p. 180.

[21] Chen Qiu, et al. (eds.), Collection of Liji Medicine Questions and Answer Epidemics and Cholera, included in Liu Shijue (ed.), *Wenzhou Literature Series Integration of Wenzhou Modern Medical Books*, p. 66.

[22] Lu Caixia, Research on the Evolution of Public Health Mechanism in Beijing and Tianjin in the Late Qing Dynasty (1900–1911), Wuhan: Hubei People's Publishing House, 2010, pp. 145–149.

[23] Jiang Baimin, *Practical Bacteriology*, Shanghai: Commercial Press, 1922, p. 1.

[24] Ding Fubao, Proper Names in Pathology, The Collection of Medical Reviews, included in Shen Hongrui and Liang Xiuqing (eds.), Medical Reviews in the Past Dynasties in China, p. 1520.

[25] Dong Mei & Li Zhiping, The Spread of Western Bacteriology in China: 1894–1949, *Medicine and Philosophy* (Humanities and Social Medicine Edition), 2010, (2), pp. 72–74. The first generation of Japanese bacteriologist Ogata returned Japan from his study in Germany in 1884.He brought new bacteriological knowledge to Japan and strongly led the medical development of the country. See Liu Shi Yong, *Samurai Sword and Lancet: the Formation and Diffusion of Western Medicine in Japan*, Taipei: Publishing Center of Taiwan University, 2012, pp. 83–123.

some microbiology books.[26] Li Zhenpian, who once served in the Serum Research Institute of the military medical school, once made the comments that the test and application of bacteria were "still in need of special books for reference".[27] Special books on bacteriology can provide necessary theories, but they must rely on laboratory practice in order to obtain clinical practical knowledge. For Western medicine, medical books are a practical and basic operation manual, which provides basic knowledge and experimental steps for doctors. However, in the late nineteenth century, medical textbooks were based on experimental results and new knowledge. Compared with the respect for medical classics of TCM, there have been no medical books with classical significance for repeated reading in modern Western medicine.[28] For modern Western medicine, medical books are just a collection of practical basic knowledge at different times, similar to operation manuals that are not to be read repeatedly and annotated.

When it comes to the application of bacterial science, it can be seen from both inside and outside the laboratory. In the laboratory, doctors must be familiar with the technology of bacterial testing and the basic knowledge of serum production. In 1943, Hu Ding'an said, "Bacteriology is the mirror for the discovery of infectious diseases, and it is also the essence of preventive medicine".[29] The knowledge of bacteriology is essential in bacterial research and the operation of health work.

Chen Shaobo, who was teaching at the national Jiangsu Medical College at that time, accused the Chinese-Western medicine doctors practicing in China of not being knowledgeable about the operation technology of bacterial experiment, so he was eager to provide a good bacteriology textbook to solve the problem in Chinese people's poor implementation and experimental procedures.[30] Outside the laboratory, bacteriology also served the daily life of the public. Westerners had a saying that the fact that people were accidentally killed by microorganisms was the "proof of inadequate medical skills", and that the deceased was a "fool".[31] There were many problems related to public health. Books, even popular science books,[32] sprang up, and the ignorance of bacteriology became a danger. Ding Fubao once published a medical case:

Proficient in English, he worked as a teacher at a school in Shanghai in 1908. In April, he got an urgent telegram that his wife was suffering from scarlet fever and was in danger. He sent for his wife to come to Shanghai for medical treatment, but

---

[26] Deng Tietao & Cheng Zhifan, *General History of Chinese Medicine Modern History*, Beijing: People's Health Publishing House, 1999, pp. 374–375.

[27] Chen Shaobo, *Test Methods of Experimental Bacteriology*, Li Zhenpia's preface, Beijing: Longmen United Press, 1943, p. 1.

[28] Li Jianmin, *Knowledge Form of Classical Medicine, included in Zhu Pingyi, New Theory of Chinese History, Science and Technology and Chinese Society*, pp. 153–177.

[29] Chen Shaobo, *Test Methods of Experimental Bacteriology*, Prefaced of Hu Dingan, p. 1.

[30] Chen Shaobo, *Test Methods of Experimental Bacteriology*, p. 1.

[31] Bayne Joness, translated by Chen Zhaoxi, *Microorganisms and Human Life,* Taipei: Taiwan Commercial Press, 1970, pp. 102–103.

[32] Gao Shiqi, *Complete Works of Gao Shiqi*, Beijing: Aviation Industry Press, 2005, Vols. 1, 4 and 5.

before his wife was cured, he was infected. They were treated with the old medicine, which was ineffective. So they went to Zixin Hospital. The hospital turned them down, for this hospital did not have an infectious disease department, and referred him to the hospital of the Ministry of Work. He died in the carriage. His wife killed herself the next morning by taking opium, as she felt her husband's death was due to her infection. With even a little general medical knowledge, his wife would have had a serum injection, with strict disinfection and isolation methods to prevent infection. Early injection of serum would leave the disease a very slim chance to develop. This is known by everybody today. How miserable for the young couple to have lost their lives in this way![33]

The vigilance of this story is quite strong. Without knowing the harm of "infection" and the necessity of isolation, disinfection and serum injections, it became quite dangerous. It also directly pointed to the ignorance of the "old-fashioned" treatment. This is just the beginning of the challenges that the Chinese medicine profession must be faced with.

5.3 Origin of the Acceptance of Bacteria Theory in TCM

How does TCM treat bacteriology? During the entire period of the Republic of China period, TCM did not share "one attitude" toward bacteriology. The attitude of acceptance was generally adopted at the beginning. He Lianchen said: "The patients tend to take it as the doctor's responsibility to cure a disease, without taking into account the condition of a patient's home. When they live in a improper place with an uncleaned body, unsuitable temperature, disordered time schedule, it would be only promoting the breeding of bacteria, rather than helping the medical treatment."[34] Mr. He's words show that TCM had paid attention to daily hygiene and the harm of bacteria. In addition, Lu Yuanlei explained in the item "Basic Medicine Pathogenic Bacteriology" in his *Course Description of Shanghai National Medical College* in 1929, "this is the most updated and advanced science ever since the invention of the microscope", "it would be deemed as being ignorant of commonly known infectious diseases if there is no such subject in medical schools. The subject includes bacterial protozoa and immunology, which is to be completed two hours per week within one year".[35] Here, the number of teaching hours is no more than other subjects, but as time went by, other TCM bacteriology courses in schools were often added.[36] However, understanding a certain area of knowledge does not mean accepting a

[33] Ding Fubao, *Collection of Medical Reviews, Medical Reviews in the Past Dynasties in China*, p. 1513.

[34] He Lianchen (ed.), *Updated Popular Treatise on Typhoid Fever*, p. 502.

[35] Lu Yuanlei, Course Descriptions of Shanghai National Medical College, Lu's Collection of Medical Theories, included in Zhang Yuping (ed.), *Two Kinds of Lu Yuanlei's Medical Books*, p. 94.

[36] Zhu Jianping (ed.), *Research on Major Innovations in Modern Chinese Medicine*, Beijing: Ancient Books of TCM Press, 2009, No. 98, p. 118.

set of values and research methods behind it. The fact may be that most of the study of TCM was to understand the knowledge of public health. There was no relevant experimental course design for the method of serum manufacturing and bacteria testing. Therefore, Fu Sinian once commented: "The examination of micro bacteria is the most important diagnosis of all infectious diseases. This diagnostic instrument is not found in the National Medical University, and these diagnostic processes, except for the pulse, are unknown or barely known to National Medical University".[37] This became the accusation for TCM's lacking the knowledge of new medicine. How to gain the bacteriological knowledge was also a big problem. We can't just rely on school education. In 1934, Jian Pao (pseudonym) mentioned, in an article published in a magazine, that Yu Yunxiu would compile supplementary teaching handouts for young TCM doctors and set up TCM supplementary research classes, which would be completely based on science and take into account the old theory, in order to explain medical theory for the purpose of laying the foundation for the scientization of TCM. He cited the example that "diagnosis of infectious diseases" and "disinfection methods" were also in the regulations of TCM, calling on doctors to learn this new knowledge.[38] This bacteriology course offered by the anti-Chinese medicine camp was probably not bought by Chinese medicine, and it was only offered sporadically. It was a flash in the pan and had little impact. On the contrary, if Yu's move was true, it is quite thought-provoking. Yu's "anti TCM" may not be intended for what it claimed, which is worth pondering.[39]

TCM often used the traditional knowledge of exogenous fever, including typhoid and warm diseases to communicate with the bacteriology of Western medicine. Tan Cizhong believed that traditional medical books should be explained with the thinking of "scientific sorting", equating infectious diseases with typhoid fever.[40] Lu Yuanlei noticed the omission of bacteriology in traditional medicine. He said, "As this study is missing in TCM, it is more difficult to establish an outline. The prevention of epidemic diseases is closely related to bacteriology and it should be placed under the category of bacteriology."[41] Bacteriology and the measures under its guidance became the key of "scientific standards". Tan said frankly that the shortcoming of TCM is that there were no microscopes, so that bacteriology was unknown.[42] Tan was a TCM doctor that can accept bacteriology, as opposed to those who denied bacteria being the "cause of the disease". In addition, Yun Tieqiao held that TCM could not give the logical

---

[37] Fu Sinian, On the So-called National Medicine, *Complete Works of Fu Sinian*, Vol. 6, pp. 309–310.

[38] Jian Bao, *Supplementary Education Young Chinese Medicine Doctors Need*, Social Medical Journal, 1934 (207), pp. 4618–4619.

[39] Pi Kuoli, Medical Revolution and Medical History Research during the Republic of China Period—Yu Yan (1879–1954) "Modern Medical History" and Its Practice, *Journal of TCM*, 2013 (24), pp. 159–185.

[40] Tan Chuang's theory of "five treatments of typhoid fever" is the categorization of *Treatise on Typhoid Fever* according to the interpretation of infectious diseases by Western medicine.

[41] Lu Yuanlei, Proposal to the Central National Medical Institute,
Lu's Collection of Medical Theories, included in Zhang Yuping (ed.), *Two Kinds of Lu Yuanlei's Medical Books*, p. 161.

[42] Tan Cizhong, *Commentary on Typhoid Fever*, p. 1.

explanation to its excellent curative effect. "It's always difficult for the contemporary intellectuals to be convinced".[43] How to give "the logical explanation"? Bacteriology turned to be an opening for a good frame of reference for TCM to explain the "Qi" theory Ever since the 1930s, it had been an important scientific procedure to find out the "material" basis involved in the theory of Western medicine, including the interpretation of pathology in TCM with bacteriology. For example, when explaining the "wind" of TCM, Zhang Ninan commented on the "infectious effect": "It is air infection that carry diseased bacteria and spread it into the air".[44] TCM compared the Chinese and western theories in order to clarify the material basis of "Qi".

In the TCM warm disease system, doctors began to use the perspective of bacteria to explain various theories. Generally speaking, it can be seen from two aspects: basic theory and prescriptions. In the theoretical part, TCM first affirmed that many epidemics were caused by "bacteria". He Lianchen explained in his medical book revised and published in 1914:

The air is the most turbid in summer and autumn, with the stagnant steam of water and soil evaporating in sunlight. What comes up in summer is called steaming with mildew and rain. What comes up in mid-autumn is called osmanthus steaming. It is also a disease, which is a mixture of water, soil and foul gas. However, people take the interior heat and dampness, rather than having cold drinks, as the cause of their diseases, without knowing the fact that in summer and autumn, the water and soil are stagnant and steamy, with heat in dampness, dampness in hot heat, being turbid, hot, sticky and moldy, which is called damp warmth or damp heat. In Western medicine, mold toxin gas is the most harmful and causes various diseases, which is more difficult to be treated than the diseases caused by wind, cold and summer heat.[45]

He stated:

> The British doctor Hobson said: Dry heat in the air does not hurt people, but damp heat hurts people the most. Due to the fact that low-lying land contains latent heat of stagnant water, or rotten vegetation (that is, soil and water are polluted, gassed and moldy), the mildew gas would explode after being exposed to 60 degrees of sunlight. Therefore, in the southeast hot land, toxins are especially severe at the turn of summer and autumn. It can be seen that wet temperature and damp heat are tangible and greasy, but it is invisible in Western medicine. Alas! A man is in the midst of filthy air all day long, fighting against gas, namely against microorganism, living unknowingly in the midst of danger. How scary it is![46]

Here, He Lianchen had noticed the influence of bacteria. Please note that Benjamin Hobson's (1816–1873) theory of miasma was still influential, and it did carry the idea of "bacteria". Based on the concept of hidden pathogenic Qi and the discussion of seasonal Qi in TCM, what was actually more consistent with TCM was the discussion

[43] Yun Tieqiao, *On Medical Collection*, p. 1.

[44] Zhang Ninan, *Material Principles of Chinese Medicine*, National Medical Bulletin, (2), 1932, p. 47.

[45] (Qing) Dai Tianzhang, revised by He Lianchen, *On Febrile Diseases of Four Seasons, Revised Generalizations on Febrile Diseases*, p. 7.

[46] (Qing) Dai Tianzhang, revised by He Lianchen: *On Febrile Diseases of Four Seasons, Revised Generalizations on Febrile Diseases*, p. 8.

of the "toxic gas" in the miasma theory. Yu Xinzhong had a summary of various pathogenic effects on the epidemics in the Qing Dynasty. It was found that Chinese doctors were aware of the fact that unclean environment, rotten and smelly gas could cause plagues.[47] When they saw the west medicine theory transferred from miasma theory to bacteria theory, it naturally returned to the original knowledge system to find the various possible explanations, and the concept of "bacteria" caused by bad Qi was rationalized. Actually in the west, the two were slightly conflicting concepts. Another example is that Angela Ki Che Leung had also studied various diseases caused by environmental factors and put forward the concept of "depressed steam".[48] The above citation also mentioned the theory of water and soil miscellaneous gas evaporation, together with "mold toxic gas" and "mold" of Western medicine, which is a justified new exposition.

In addition, the most important thing is that TCM also discussed the relationship between "toxic gas" and bacteria, as Zhang Xichun said: "Those who suffer from epidemic diseases are caught by bad luck. This discord contains toxic gas, causing disease to whoever comes into contact with it."[49] It is common to use "toxic gas" to explain the epidemic. Moreover, it shares the same concept of "toxin" with "bacterial toxin", which became a new discussion of TCM, and there was even a mixing up of "detoxification therapy" and "sterilization".[50] In fact, there was also the concept of "bacterial toxin" in ancient times, but this visible bacteria could be referring to fungi. For example, there was "Taiyi golden pill" in the *Authentic Surgery* of the Ming Dynasty that could treat "all dietary drugs, toxins, miasma, pathogenic bacteria", etc. It can be seen that "bacteria" and "toxins" were extremely related in the Chinese medical system. As for the image of "toxins", it is also highly related to the bad "Qi" in nature. For example, toxins are often associated with "mountain miasma" and "epidemic smog". As for the description of "bacteria", it had also been widely used in surgery or laryngology where "visual inspection" was more needed. There was an example in surgery: "the node in the genitals have large heads but small pedicle, the small ones were the size of beans, and the large ones were like bacteria, causing no pain".[51] There was a description of a woman's vaginal ulcer: "the protrusion in the middle is like fungus, as chicken crowns, the swelling and pain on the four sides

[47] Yu Xinzhong, A Preliminary Study of the Qing People's Understanding of the Plague—with the Focus on the Jiangnan Area, *China Social and Historical Review,* Vol. 3, Beijing: Zhonghua Book Company, 2001, pp. 238–258.

[48] Angela Ki Che Leung, The Relationship between Disease and Locality: the Medical Views from the Yuan to the Qing Dynasty, included in his *Facing Diseases: Medical Concept and Organization in Traditional Chinese Society*, pp. 231–242.

[49] Zhang Xichun, Prescriptions for the Plague and Pestilence, *Chinese Medicine with Reference to the West*, Shijiazhuang: Hebei Science and Technology Press, 2001, p. 174.

[50] Fudan University, A Survey of the Theories in the Treatment of Acute Infectious Diseases, *Chinese Medical Journal,* Vol. 1 (10), pp. 1–2, 1941.

[51] (Ming) Chen Shigong, Section 49 Carcinoma of the Skin, *On Surgery*, Tianjin: Tianjin Science and Technology Press, 2000, p. 247.

are caused by liver depression and spleen deficiency".[52] This is based on the shape. Others include "oral bacteria"[53] "born in the mouth or on the gum". There were also the "tooth fungus" "born in the root of teeth". They look purple and black, like "fungus",[54] or as described in *On Laryngology*: "a disease of white rot in the throat, commonly known as white fungus, that is, white entanglement on the throat".[55] It refers to the pathogenic factors with sore throat and ulceration, coated with white fungus like membrane. Also, the disease of "bacteria growing on the tongue…starts like beans and grows like fungus. It is red, rotten and painful, which is caused by the heat toxin of the heart and spleen".[56] There are also "throat bacteria… which look like duckweed, purple in color… soft as a pig's lung", which is infarcted in the throat and hinders normal diet.[57] "Lip fungus" means "the abrupt turn of the lips, like a pig's mouth".[58] All of the references are based on the shape of the lesion, rather than seeing the "bacteria". The birth of "bacterial toxin" may be related to the damp and heat inside the body.[59] Of course, the allegation of "toxins" is very extensive. Even in visual based surgery, the source of "toxins" may be attributed to the bad Qi of the outside world, such as "the toxins of the time, the disease of the prevailing Qi of the day", which is related to the fever study of internal medicine.[60]

The term "virus" in early modern times is slightly different from what it means today. At that time, the meaning of "virus" was vague. Originally, it might refer to microorganisms, which is our understanding today. Another meaning of it was that the "toxins" caused by bacteria stems from the fact that some bacteria can "release secrete toxins and make people sick".[61] *Imperial Chinese Medicine,* written by Yumoto Kyushin from Japan (1876–1941), was translated into Chinese and published in 1928. He vigorously promoted the Chinese medicine, respected Zhang Zhongjing and was trusted by Chinese doctors. He believed that some of the symptoms of patients suffering from fever were due to "virus accumulation". Sweating, vomiting

[52] (Ming) Chen Shigong, Sect. 39 Erosion of Vulva, *On Surgery*, Tianjin: Tianjin Science and Technology Press, 2000, p. 234.

[53] (Ming) Zhu Di, *Updated Prescriptions for the Diseases of Mouth and Throat*, Beijing: Xueyuan Publishing House, 2009, p. 302.

[54] (Ming) Zhu Di. *Updated Prescriptions for the Diseases of Mouth and Throat*, Beijing: Xueyuan Publishing House, 2009, p. 308.

[55] (Ming) Zhu Di, *Updated Prescriptions for the Diseases of Mouth and Throat*, Beijing: Xueyuan Publishing House, 2009, p. 315.

[56] (Ming) Zhu Di, *Updated Prescriptions for the Diseases of Mouth and Throat*, Beijing: Xueyuan Publishing House, 2009, p. 319.

[57] (Ming) Zhu Di, *Updated Prescriptions for the Diseases of Mouth and Throat*, Beijing: Xueyuan Publishing House, 2009, p. 354.

[58] (Ming) Zhu Di, *Updated Prescriptions for the Diseases of Mouth and Throat*, Beijing: Xueyuan Publishing House, 2009, p. 345.

[59] As the saying goes: "Bacteria toxin is caused by the condensation of heat accumulated in the spleen," quoted from ((Ming) Chen Shigong, Section 120 Ophthalmomonas Toxin, *On Surgery*, p. 296.

[60] (Ming) Chen Shigong, Section 22 Seasonal Toxin, *On Surgery*, p. 130.

[61] Hu Hongji, *Introduction to Public Health*, Shanghai: Commercial Press, 1933, p. 16.

and other methods of TCM can have the effect of "detoxification".[62] This may have strengthened the "solution" of TCM. The "detoxification" method was interpreted as "detoxifying bacteria" and affected later TCM. If Ye Guhong believed that the Chinese medicine had used Qi to explain efficacy on the human body, now it integrates the bacterial theory and identifies the three methods, such as sweating, vomiting and excretion commonly used in the treatment of infectious diseases in the past, are to "eliminate toxins". So TCM was good enough to treat infectious diseases.[63] In fact, as early as 1921, Wu Xihuang pointed out the influence of "bacterial toxin" or "virus" on the body in many parts of his book, which might have been enhanced by the theory of Chinese medicine. For example:

> Neurosis is often found in the conditions of spring warmth, winter warmth, dampness or summer heat, without being caused by improper sweat. It is all introduced into the medulla by viruses. After being infected, the mental state is not clear.[64]

In the early stage of a critical infectious disease, some may die from fever. This is due to the obstruction of infectious toxic bacteria, but death is not caused by fever.[65]

When fever lasts for one or two days, the tongue is covered with thick white coating. This is the sign of weak digestion actually due to digestive organ damage caused by pathogenic bacteria.[66]

TCM also integrated bacteriology into the traditional body view. For example, the typhoid school held that the wind and cold enter the body (invading the human body from the surface), while the warm disease school held that pathogenic Qi invades the human body from the mouth and nose. Combined with the omnipresence of bacteria, this gave TCM a feasible interpretation. Wu Xihuang said: "The invasion of bacteria can be from the mouth and nose, from the hairy orifices. Tuberculosis, pneumonia and epidemic diseases are transmitted through the mouth and nose; malaria is caused by the stings of mosquito, and the parasite enters the blood from the pores. Most infectious diseases belong to the above two, and there are many new theories in modern times."[67] After reading books related to bacteriology, the doctors during the Republic of China period started their more convincing new interpretations with their knowledge of classical medicine.

Another example is from Pan Chenglian. He recalled his work experience in a western hospital during 1932 when he treated many infected patients: "Even though

---

62 Yumoto Kyushin, translated by Zhou Zixu, Introduction, On the Ineffectiveness of Western Cardiotonic, *Royal Han Medicine,* pp. 6,13.

63 Ye Guhong, Medical Treatments in the Country of Infectious Diseases, *National Medical Bulletin,* Vol. 1 (5), 1933, p. 71.

64 Wu Xihuang, *Interpretations of Chinese and Western Febrile Diseases*, p. 164.

65 Wu Xihuang, *Interpretations of Chinese and Western Febrile Diseases*. p. 53.

66 Wu Xihuang, *Interpretations of Chinese and Western Febrile Diseases*. p. 57.

67 Wu Xihuang, Notes on Ye Xiangyan's Theory of Tepidity, *Interpretations of Chinese and Western Febrile Diseases*. p. 89.

it was a Western medicine hospital, TCM was used in most cases except for emergencies. In six years, the systematic observation of many cases was obtained".[68] It can be seen that hospitals had carried out treatment similar to integrated TCM and Western medicine,[69] and there was no evidence showing that doctors like Pan had ever received any training in Western medicine. His treatment and observations of modern infectious diseases were entirely like a bystander. As for the practical treatment, we still have to rely on the knowledge system supported by TCM. Pan believed that though the treatment of TCM was more general than disease-specific, "cinnamon twig decoction" could have good therapeutic effects in cases of influenza, intestinal zhifuz and malaria. This was not dominated by bacteria-based "cause therapy", but a unique "case specific therapy" of TCM.[70] Pan advocated the method of "scientific sorting" of ancient medical books and the new treatment by taking into account Western medicine theory or the essential medical theory, so as to do the textual research of medical classics and treatment methods.

Various explanations of TCM treatment based on bacteriology came into being. Mr. He Lianchen explained the pulse condition of bacteria absorption with pulse science: "Epidemics are mostly caused by the absorption of various molds, which leads to infectious diseases. A disease is due to either Yang or Yin toxin. Yang toxin results in thick and hot blood with many visible veins on the right hand and irregular pulse on the left hand; Yin toxin results in cold deficiency in Qi and a weakening pulse".[71] More interestingly, archaeologist Shi Zhangru (1902–2004) recalled the medical procedure that a doctor in his hometown (Dongcai Village, Yanshi County, Henan Province) used. He said that there was a surgeon named Li Le who knew acupuncture. There was a very bad epidemic in his hometown village, and many people died. Li Le said that needles could be inserted into the human body to prevent infection, saying "bacteria can flow out through acupuncture and bloodletting." According to Shi, he didn't know whether if what the doctor said was true, but the village where he lived at that time was not infected.[72] It can be seen that during the Republic of China period, many TCM doctors tended to use bacteriology to prove the effect of TCM treatments.

In addition to adopting this kind of argument, TCM also raised some questions about the theory of bacterial pathogenicity. Although Lu Yuanlei believed that knowledge such as pathogenic bacteria must be learned, he said: "Bacterial protozoa are not absolutely the pathogen of infectious diseases,"[73] which was contradictory with his own argument. Why is bacteriology not the main cause of infectious diseases?

---

[68] Zhu Shipei(ed.), *Pan Chenglian's Views on Warm Diseases*, Shanghai: Shanghai University of Chinese Traditional Medicine Press, 2009, p. 4.

[69] Volker Scheid, *Currents of Tradition in Chinese Medicine* 1626–2006,Seattle: East Land Press,2007. pp. 228, 229, 239, 242.

[70] Pan Chenglian, *A New Interpretation to Typhoid Fever*, pp. 5–6.

[71] He Lianchen (ed.), *Updated Treatise on Popular Typhoid Fever*, p. 38.

[72] Chen Cungong, et al., *Interview Records of Mr. Shi Zhangru*, Taipei: Institute of Modern History Academia Sinica, 2002, p. 27.

[73] Lu Yuanlei, Lu's Collection on Medicine, *Two Kinds of Lu Yuanlei's Medical Books*, p. 266.

Pan Cheng put forward an explanation: all kinds of infectious diseases may have the same symptoms at the beginning, but different bacteria and protozoa inhabit the human body, and the symptoms they cause vary from person to person, so the theory of bacterial pathogenicity has the characteristics that cannot be accurately predicted.[74] Tomoto also pointed out that bacteria were not the only cause of infectious diseases, and bacteria were also organisms. "If there are no suitable nutrients, water and temperature, it can not maintain its lifeline".[75] This is the reason why an infectious disease can not occur unless there is a "retention of food, water and blood" in the body, which leads to the weakening of resistance and illness. This means that bacteria are a kind of organism, and must have a suitable environment to survive. TCM can change the internal environment, which is not conducive to the survival of bacteria, and the disease will be cured naturally.[76] Huang Guocai, a TCM doctor, pointed out that as the superstitious age of believing in the Shinto and the pestilence ghost had passed, it's been known that the cause of the epidemic is bacteria. But no matter how different the way of infection is, it is always for the "physical loss" and "insufficient resistance" that the bacteria can take advantage, though bacteria are not the only pathogenic factor.[77] As early as 1910, TCM used Chinese medicine to enhance Qi and blood to enhance the "resistance" of the body.[78]

TCM also brought up the possible difficulties in the academic development of integrated bacteriology. Lu Shige said, "All studies must be grounded with their foothold, which is an absolute rule". Now TCM takes six Qis as the external cause, "if there is an accommodation for the theory of Western medicine, all the cases would be filled with inflammatory bacteria, and the ground would be totally lost".[79] Lu's worry was that many using TCM had doubts about the use of bacteriology, but comparing with Japanese medicine and Chinese medicine, the latter was much bolder in explaining the relationship between bacteria and traditional medicine. In addition to those conservatives who stuck to traditional medicine and refused to adopt bacteriology at all, most TCM doctors swung between these two kinds of thinking.

In the discussion of Chinese and Western medicine during the Republic of China period, people had seen the differences between the epistemology and technical operation of the two. TCM expressed their doubts. For example, Yun Tieqiao held the view that to adopt the terms and the names of Western medicine, it is necessary to accept the whole set of technology and cognitive systems behind western bacteriology, including the use of Western textbooks and experimental instruments, which

---

74 He Lianchen (ed.), *Updated Popular Treatise on Typhoid Fever*, pp. 6–7.

75 Yumoto Kyushin, translated by Zhou Zixu, On the Untenability of Infectious Diseases without Self Poisoning, *Royal Han Medicine,* pp. 20–22.

76 Lin Qingping, *On the Traditional Chinese Therapies for Infectious Diseases*, Vol. 1 (1), 1947. p. 23.

77 Huang Guocai, Methods and Agents of TCM in Preventing Infectious Diseases, *Medical Journal*, (86), 1935. p. 22.

78 He Xichen, On the Pathogenic Qi in TCM and Microorganism in Western Medicine, *Journal of TCM and Western Medicine* (2), 1910. pp. 26–29.

79 Lu Shige, Shige's Medical Talk on Chinese and Western Medicine, *General Views on Chinese Medicine in China*, p. 2062.

was truly frustrating.[80] The biggest worry for Chinese medicine then was how much classical medical theory could be preserved.[81] When the two problems of bacteria being pathogenic and how to overcome it came up, TCM showed its persistence while agreeing with some western views. More observations and objections to bacteriology from Chinese medical circle may be another perspective of TCM.

5.4 Zhang Taiyan's "Views on Bacteria Based on the Ancients"

When Japanese and Chinese doctors opposed a theory, they either accused it simply for the purpose of opposing it, or just ignoring it. In academic discussions, the response of TCM was quite similar to the views of modern intellectuals that "western learning originated from China".[82] Joseph Levinson once made the comment that the returning to the traditions of modern Chinese intellectuals did not stem from their rational belief, but from their wish of catching up with the west, the emotional appeal of reducing and alleviating the suffering from the impact of western culture.[83]

The so-called "ancient" here includes not only the classics of TCM, but also the ancient Chinese culture and thought, such as philosophy, even Confucian classics and Buddhism. Zhang Hao maintained that the "internal dialogues" of Chinese intellectuals could gather together the problems and thoughts that would arouse the interest of intellectuals of all generations. Tradition is not a dead heritage, but should be regarded as the common thought community of knowledge and concern of any period.[84] Perhaps the focus of this book, which is on the discussion of fever disease in TCM, is also in line with this trend. Likewise Yu Yingshi believed that textual research in the Qing Dynasty advocated "returning to classics" through "exegesis" to clarify the six classics and the traditions of Confucianism. Their basic point of view was to "believe in the ancient" rather than "doubt the ancient", to have "exclusive

---

[80] Yun Tieqiao, *Collection on Medicine*, p. 5.

[81] Pi Kuoli, *The Connotation of "National Medicine"—on the Modern Transformation and Reconstruction of Chinese Medicine*, Journal of Zhongshan University (Social Science Edition), 2009, Vol. 49 (1), pp. 64–77.

[82] See my book *Body View and Ideological Transformation of Modern TCM—Tang Zonghai and the Era of Convergence of TCM and Western Medicine*, Chapter 2.Wang Ermin said that the "ancient support" of intellectuals in the late Qing Dynasty was needed for "reform". See Wang Ermin, *On the History of Political Thought in the Late Qing Dynasty,* Taipei: Taiwan Commercial Press, 1995, pp. 33–35. And Wang Ermin, *On the History of Modern Chinese Thought,* Beijing: Social Science Literature Press, 2003, pp. 39–43.

[83] Joseph R. Levenson, *Confucian China and Its Modern Fate.* Berkeley: University of California Press, 1958. p. 1319. However, at the beginning of the Republic of China period, the pursuit of "shared cultural identity" from TCM could not only assort to emotional factors, but also to the curative effect and clinical experience. From the perspective of Joseph R. Levenson's "shared cultural identity" in the context of Chinese medical history, the example of Zhang Taiyan's "ancient bacteria interpretation" may be more representative.

[84] Zhang Hao, *Chinese Intellectuals in Crisis*, Beijing: Xinxing Publishing House, 2006, p. 12.

respect for Confucianism", rather than the equal respect for all schools of thoughts.[85] The development of TCM during the Republic of China period may be similar to the development of Confucianism. "Respecting the ancient" and "deriving from the ancient" in the exploration of the original medical classics and taking the ancient knowledge as the database for the creation in the new era are quite similar to the development of academic thought in the Qing Dynasty.

It is necessary to bring up Zhang's observation when exploring the thought of TCM during the Republic of China period in explaining bacteria "according to ancient sayings". In 1899, he examined the existing bacteria on the basis of the article "On the Battle of Man and Microorganism" published in the *Journal of Science*, a popular science magazine introduced into China earlier. He said, "It is said in the book *Zhuang Zi. The Common Nature of Material Beings*: 'Joy comes out of emptiness, which is turned into fungi in steam', without explaining why. The joy of the heart comes from emptiness and can be turned into tangible fungi in steam".[86] If Zhang represents some intellectuals or doctors, it can be said that at the beginning, the perspective of Chinese people's understanding of bacteria was not the "observation of bacteria", but to observe the negative behavior of people leading to the breeding of bacteria. This is particularly important because different research objects will lead to differences in the whole knowledge system. In addition, he compared the observation of "worms" in China with the bacteriology of Western medicine. He said:

The infected (by bacteria), though having nothing to do with joy, must start from joy. Doctors agreed: "when the female private part turns dark, the disease of internal heat and noxious agents induced by worms will occur if she has sex", though it's not particularly lust that can produce bacteria or noxious agents. When fungi and noxious agents have been produced, they can be seductive, leading to sexual indulgence.[87]

Zhang's discussion does not involve exogenous harmful air or environment, which indicates that his explanation of bacteria tends to be from the influence of human behavior and human feelings, by leaving out "Qi" completely and just taking "worms" as the reference in his observation of physical objects.

Between 1921 and 1927, Zhang had more and more publications in medical journals. Later, he also served as the president of Shanghai Chinese Medical College and continued to work on the theory of TCM ever after.[88] Since the 1920's, he

---

[85] Yu Yingshi, *Hu Shi in the History of Modern Chinese Thought*, Taipei: Lianjing Publishing House, 1984, p. 79.

[86] Shanghai People's Publishing House (ed.), *Bacteria Theory, Complete Works of Zhang Taiyan*, Vol. 8, p. 2. It is quoted from *Zhuang Zi*, "They are moody with joy, worry, sigh, and fear. They are restless, frivolous and pretentious. Joy comes out of emptiness, which is turned into fungi in steam. This process recycles all the time with no revelation of how its started". It refers to all kinds of repeated modalities, and from the view of All-in-One, changes are indistinguishable. Wang Shumin interpreted this sentence as "steaming produces fungi", which means that damp and hot gas leads to the formation of fungi (bacteria).Wang Shumin, *Annotation of Zhuang Zi*, Taipei:: Institute of Modern History Academia Sinica, 1988, Vol. 1, p. 13.

[87] Shanghai People's Publishing House (ed.), On the Non Typhoid Fever Etiology of Micro Bacteria, *Complete Works of Zhang Taiyan*, Vol. 8, pp. 2–3.

[88] For the medical discussion of Zhang, see the preface by Zhang Nianchi and Pan Wenkui, *Complete Works of Zhang Taiyan*, Vol. 8, pp. 1–49; Zhao Yongjin, Zhang Taiyan and His Medical Views,

gradually separated himself from the theory of the *Internal Canon of Medicine* and began to devote himself to the research of *Treatise on Typhoid Fever.* His focus began to turn to the clinical treatment of exogenous fever, and brought the role of "bacteria" into its discussion.[89] In the late 1920s, when the debate between TCM and Western medicine became increasingly fierce, he believed that TCM did not need to defend itself totally against Western medicine. It is true that TCM had a weakness of "ignoring anatomy, lacking proficiency in physiology", but in typhoid fever, the key issue is not about human organs, but Qi—the "floating Qi". TCM should keep its effective treatment, rather than "taking Western medicine as the better", a view prevalent in TCM circles.[90] Exploring Zhang Zhongjing's treatment study and interpreting the mystery of Qi theory, the effective treatment should always be the highest criterion, which can compete with Western medicine. During this period, he completed the famous book *A New Theory of Acute Diseases*,[91] which focuses on infectious diseases and bacteria in TCM. The discussion on the comparison between TCM and Western medicine covers a wide range of topics such as typhoid fever and warm diseases.

Zhang's understanding of bacteria may sound irrational today. He said: "Micro bacteria were invented in the Far West in modern times. Previously, only micro worms were mentioned, and they were also found in the central plain area. The term 'five corpses' is recorded in ancient books, "corpses" here refer to worms."[92] This is to regard bacteria and worms as the same. Zhang also gave play to his ability of historical research, investigated "worms" from literature and traced the possible routes of bacteria. In addition, as bacteria produce "toxins", Zhang also explained "bacteria" with "toxic air".[93] TCM had long been using "toxins" to explain the occurrence of infectious diseases. For example, Zhu Fu quoted Zhang Yanshan, "The infected in epidemics feel the noxious rotten Qi, which contains toxins and pathogenic factors, spreading in the air that is unavoidable. As it spreads door to door and village to village, just like the taxation, so there came the name. (the epidemic disease in Chinese "疫Yi" is taken after the term "taxation役Yi"—note from the translator)".[94] The fact that TCM had noticed the factor of "air" indicates the obvious influence of Western medicine.

History Studies, 1998, (1), pp. 127–134; Zhang Nianchi, *My Grandfather Zhang Taiyan*, Shanghai: Shanghai People's Publishing House, 2011, pp. 101–114, 292–298.

[89] Duan Xiaohua (ed.), *On Zhang Taiyan's Medical Thoughts*, Beijing: Doctoral Dissertation of Beijing University of TCM, 2006. p. 1.

[90] Tang Zhijun (ed.), *Zhang Taiyan's Chronicle*, Vol. 2, Beijing: Zhonghua Book Company, 1979, p. 890.

[91] The book was first named *A New Theory of Acute Diseases, and was revised after 1957 as Zhang Taiyan's Theory of Medicine.* See *Complete Works of Zhang Taiyan*, Vol. 8, p. 9.

[92] Shanghai People's Publishing House (ed.), On the Micro Bacteria Being Not the Cause of Typhoid Fever, *Complete Works of Zhang Taiyan*, Vol. 8, p. 245.

[93] Shanghai People's Publishing House (ed.), On the Pathogenesis of Micro Bacteria, *Complete Works of Zhang Taiyan,* Vol. 8, p. 449.

[94] Zhu Fu, *Compromise of the Essence of the Latest Miscellaneous Diseases*, Vol. I, p. 29B.

Zhang also used his accomplishment in ancient Chinese literature and TCM to prove "Ke toxin" (Ke, a small plant) and all kinds of "harsh air", "pathogenic air" and "miasma" are related to "micro bacteria".[95] Shi Yiren thought it makes sense, that "Ke toxin" is connected with "strong wind", which means that it is only harmful when bacteria spread through the air.[96] Zhang noted that the biggest challenge of bacteriology to TCM was that there was a definition of pathogen behind the theory of Western medicine, rather than "six indulgence" or "six Qis (air)". However, Zhang challenged it by specifying that it is the "(heat) air" of nature that causes diseases, not bacteria. He said, "I think bacteria is generated by heat, rather than the other way round. Bacteria is originally based on damp and heat. It is caused by plum rain and heated with Qi. At this point, both bamboo and wood can produce bacteria".[97] To the fact of "infection", Zhang did not believe it to be caused by bacteria, but by a kind of "electrical" induction. He said: "Human bodies are similar, which makes it easy to infect one another. The revived corpses are led by the electrical connections from animals. The same is true for diseases. The volatilization of Qi causes infection".[98] Zhang only recognized that some diseases are caused by bacteria, such as Yin-Yang toxins,[99] warm toxin, tuberculosis, ulcer, phthisis, sores. However, typhoid and warm diseases in the category of exogenous fever should be "caused mainly by wind, cold and heat, supported by bacteria".[100] He also cited many examples of diseases to show that bacteria are not the fatal cause of disease but only the "side cause" at most. He did not deny the existence of bacteria but took it only as a rise and fall phenomenon of life in nature,[101] which does not necessarily lead to infection.[102]

Zhang's examples are not isolated ones. Luo Xieyuan, a doctor in Sichuan, in his *On the Invention of Microbiology in Chinese Medicine,* commented that bacteriology had actually been recorded in Chinese medical history even though it is supposed to be the "unprecedented invention" of Western medicine:

> Micro bacteria has been examined in Chinese medical books. Although there had been no significant names given, it is not uncommon to find it from the Chinese medical books with intensive studies. For example, in *Internal* and *Difficulties,* it is said that pathogenic wind,

95 Shanghai People's Publishing House (ed.), On the Pathogenesis of Micro Bacteria, *Complete Works of Zhang Taiyan,* Vol. 8, pp. 449–450.

96 Shi Yiren, *Shi's Internal Canon of Medicine,* Taipei: Tailian Guofeng Publishing House, 1969, p. 30.

97 Shanghai People's Publishing House (ed.), On Infectious Diseases in China, *Complete Works of Zhang Taiyan,* Vol. 8, pp. 321–322.

98 Shanghai People's Publishing House (ed.), On infectious Diseases in China, *Complete Works of Zhang Taiyan,* Vol. 8, p. 322.

99 Shanghai People's Publishing House (ed.), On Bacteria and Toxins, *Complete Works of Zhang Taiyan,* Vol. 8, p. 447.

100 Shanghai People's Publishing House (ed.), On the Pathogenesis of Micro Bacteria, *Complete Works of Zhang Taiyan,* Vol. 8, p. 453.

101 Shanghai People's Publishing House (ed.), On the Non Typhoid Fever Etiology of Micro Bacteria, *Complete Works of Zhang Taiyan,* Vol. 8, p. 248.

102 Shanghai People's Publishing House (ed.), On Bacteria and Toxins, *Complete Works of Zhang Taiyan,* Vol. 8, p. 446.

> devious emptiness or mixed toxins, the five epidemic diseases in the chapter *Supplement*, the five pathogenic factors in chapter *True Pathogens*, and worm toxin and ghost abscess to be eliminated in *Shennong's Herbal Classic,* are all the implications of micro bacteria. However, the descriptions are ambiguous without too much credibility. In *Source of Diseases*, there are worms in leprosy and ringworm; in *Golden Cabinet,* there are worm-induced ulcers and roundworm parasites; Yin-Yang toxins are similar to the sepsis of pestis; cachexia is similar to the adenoma of pestis. Pests are categorized into nine kinds, while burying beetles were categorized into three types. Gonorrhea has worms; sores start from typhoid fever and dysentery brings out pinworms. Countless examples are recorded in the books, which can be the proof based on precise observations.[103]

Luo believed that TCM in its development "had focused on Qi but ignored the physical beings", and now "the learning of Asia is studied in the west", which proves the contribution of TCM. He sighed that the Chinese people did not cheer up and did not cherish the treasure of their own, calling on people's attention to its values. Although this kind of research was not helpful to the real research of bacteriology, it promoted the review of TCM books. Zhang's vision was "to study traditional Chinese literature, as well as western literature, and return to the study of medicine",[104] mainly ancient medical books, alongside other ancient books, searching for materials that can respond to bacteriology. The concepts of "Qi", "toxins" and "worms" in the discussion help us understand the major ideological context of TCM at that time.

5.5 The First Focus in the Debate on Bacteriology Between TCM and Western Medicine—Adherence to the Theory of Qi

When Hu Ding'an wrote the preface to *Practical Bacteriology* in 1922, he praised the progress of science and doubted the theory of "six Qis" in traditional medicine. He believed that the traditional views that diseases are led by "pathogenic Qi" and "demons" is out of date.[105] But in the knowledge of TCM, "Qi" is a part of nature and the basis of material growth, in which human survival and diseases are inseparable parts. Lu Jinsheng said that "(heaven and earth) have human beings, first as Qi and then the form, with the father's sperm and mother's blood, making it possible for the reproduction of generations", "both plants and animals are transformed by the Qi of Yin and Yang in heaven and earth". He clearly stated that "Qi" is the foundation of

[103] Luo Xieyuan, *On the Invention of Microbiology in Chinese Medicine,* Modern TCM, Vol. 2 (1), 1941, pp. 19–24.

[104] Zhang said, "Primary school, classics by the saints and medical science can be called three wonders. Among the three wonders, medical study is my favourite topic, which is the pleasure of my life". See Zhang Nianchi, *My Grandfather Zhang Taiyan,* p. 113.

[105] Jiang Baimin, *Practical Bacteriology,* Preface, pp. 1–2.

life. Here "Qi" can be a verb, representing the basic material on which all substances grow.[106]

Lu Jinsheng, a native of Jiangsu Province, went to Shanghai in 1913 to practice medicine by using TCM and Western medicine. He had quite a lot of detailed observations on treatment methods, and he was also a productive writer. *Collection of Medical Manuscripts in Jingjing* was published in 1920 by his son, and another book with a similar name, *Jing Jing Medical Talk*, co-edited by his son and nephew, was also published.[107] In his *Significance of Qi in the Application of TCM*, Lu maintained that Qi is the fundamental reference in diagnosis and treatment in medical practice.

Since the birth (of a person), one absorbs the five Qis to maintain peace and preserve health, and can be sick when the absorption is not proper, such as suffering from cold and heat, or when dryness and dampness are not balanced. Gold, stone, grass, birds, animals, fish and insects in heaven and earth also get the Qi of Yin and Yang in the four seasons to survive. As they are not proportional nor pure enough, they are taken as the medicine to cure diseases caused by this imbalance. The reason is that medicine is based on the principle of Yin and Yang in the four seasons, which indicates the unity of heaven and humans. If the treatment is detached from the Qi of Yin and Yang, and human beings are treated as objects, how can it be effective, even with sophisticated anatomy?[108]

Lu criticized that Western medicine regarded people as "objects", which is probably consistent with the thinking "a microscope can examine, but it can not make any changes; a dissection can be done, but the organs may no longer be the same," a view held by some Chinese doctors since modern times.[109] Both are the reflections on the material culture of Western medicine. There were many discussions on the ineffectiveness of Western medicine in the treatment of epidemic diseases, for being "not knowledgeable of the Qi theory".[110] The debate between Chinese and Western medicine then can be regarded as the debate between the view of natural history and the view of material and cultural history. Modern science, based on the progress of material culture and the progress of technology such as a microscope, laboratory and dyeing methods, had the dominant role in the medical discussion. However, bacteria made its presence in both. It was not only a part of natural history, but also a part of material and cultural history. However, TCM didn't have much to argue at this point but only emphasized that "bacteria" belong to the characteristics of natural organisms

---

[106] Lu Jinsheng, Collection of Medical Manuscripts in Jingjing Theory of Qi, *General Views on Chinese Medicine in China*. p. 1730.

[107] Li Jingwei (ed.), *Dictionary of TCM Characters*, Shanghai: Shanghai Dictionary Publishing House, 1988, pp. 305–306. Lu Jinsheng, Collection of Medical Manuscripts in Jingjing, *General Views on Chinese Medicine in China*. p. 1726.

[108] Lu Jinsheng, Collection of Medical Manuscripts in Jingjing Significance of Qi in the Application of TCM, *General Views on Chinese Medicine in China*. p. 1730.

[109] Xu Runzhi (ed.), *Songling's Medical Bell, Wenzhou Literature Series Collection of Modern Wenzhou Medical Books*, Vol. II, p. 449.

[110] Chen Zedong, On Fu Mengzhen's Insult to Chinese Medicine—A Letter from the Chinese Medicine Association, *Complete Works of Fu Sinian*, Vol. 6, p. 315.

first so as to devalue bacterial pathogenesis. Zhang Taiyan shared the same view as mentioned above.[111]

Yu Yunxiu, who held the opposite position, believed that less educated people could only pray to God and worship Buddha, while the more educated could only talk about the "six Qis" without any effective measures for infectious diseases. Yu criticized the experience and theories of traditional doctors and average people on infectious diseases. "It's ridiculous that there had been no progress in the past 2000 years."[112] Zhang Taiyan believed that bacteria is not the only factor to cause infection. Human blood and Qi are similar, so they can sense each other, because "Qi" is transmittable.[113] Shen Lin of the warm disease school said, "In Western medicine, Qi is ignored and infectious diseases are regarded as plagues, without knowing that Qi can also be transmitted. When a cough is caused by hot wind, its Qi enters the lungs from the nose and the disease is infected, which is mistaken by the westerners as lung disease, namely pestis. They don't know that wind produces worms, which is a common sense of Qi. The wind removes the worms and destroys them. If the wind doesn't go away, the long term cough will turn into tuberculosis. This is not the fatal local Qi."[114] This is to enhance the status of wind and Qi to the highest. The discussion of worms and bacteria is only the "side cause" of disease. In line with the concept of "Qi" (climate and season) producing "bacteria", Wu Xihuang explained the mechanism behind the theory of microbial pathogenicity with the theory that "pathogenic worms can only be produced seasonally".[115] In fact, it is still a climate matter.[116] Shi Yiren believed that the system of typhoid and warm diseases defined and explained by TCM according to the Qi of climate can make up for the deficiency of pathological discussion of Western medicine.[117] The treatment of TCM is still effective in the treatment of epidemics, so the "Qi Theory" still has its value.[118] Yun Tieqiao also took "season" as the basis for naming the disease when competing with Western medicine. He said: "Now the nouns and idiomatic terms in *Treatise on Typhoid Fever* are to be used to describe its symptoms. According to the example of naming on the basis of seasons in *Internal Canon of Medicine*, they are called typhoid fever in winter, warm disease in spring, summer warmth after the summer solstice, and summer heat after the beginning of autumn".[119] Yun did not use the

[111] Shanghai People's Publishing House (ed.), On the Micro Bacteria Being Not the Cause of Typhoid Fever, *Complete Works of Zhang Taiyan*, Vol. 8, p. 245.

[112] Yu Yunxiu, *Criticism on Royal Han Medicine*, pp. 24–25.

[113] Shanghai People's Publishing House (ed.), On the Micro Bacteria Being Not the Cause of Typhoid Fever, *Complete Works of Zhang Taiyan*, Vol. 8, pp. 245–246.

[114] Shen Lin, Interpretations of Febrile Diseases, included in Cao Bingzhang (ed.), *Great Achievements in Chinese Medicine*, Vol. 18, p. 2.

[115] Wu Xihuang, *Interpretations of Chinese and Western Febrile Diseases*, p. 172.

[116] Wu Xihuang, *Lecture Notes on Diseases of Four Seasons*, Chen Yinghe's preface, p. 1.

[117] Shi Yiren, *Typhoid and Warm Diseases in TCM*, Shanghai: Shanghai Health Publishing House, 1956, Notes of the editor, p. 1.

[118] Shi Yiren, *Seasonal Diseases of TCM*, Tainan: Donghai Publishing House, 1977, Xue Yizhai's preface, p. 11.

[119] Yun Tieqiao, *Collection on Medical Study*, p. 7.

definition of bacteriology to redefine the names of the diseases, which indicates that he did not trust bacteriology. He said:

> In short, just like Confucianism can not be appropriately used to be mixed up with Mohism, western theories can only be more appropriately applied to physiology, anatomy, pathology and histology, than to micro bacteriology. In my book *Annotations of Typhoid Fever*, I oppose microbiology, stating that bacteria comes after disease, rather than the other way round. The theory that bacteria are pathogens is just to take the result as the cause.[120]

In terms of disease names, the benchmark of bacteriology is less adoptable. The reason is: "Chinese and Western medicine name the diseases on different basis. In foreign countries, the name is given by focus and bacteria, while in China, the name is given by viscera and climate, which is due to different cultures of China and the West."[121] He also said, "I believe that science is progressive". Today's science will be overthrown in the future. What's the rush to adopt "bacterial" standard as the only one?[122] Wu Xihuang said, "To use six Qis for disease diagnosis is the most sophisticated science of TCM."[123] The theory of Qi was not only aimed at typhoid or warm diseases in a narrow sense, but was actually the basic discussion of infectious diseases in TCM. A notable example is *Answers to the Queries on the Treatment of Eight Infectious Diseases* which sorts out the infectious diseases of Western medicine on the basis of Western disease classification with reference to TCM theory. Among them, the cause of the epidemic disease (pestis) is mainly from Qi, as is stated in the book:

> Epidemic is probably caused by the presence of a different Qi in the air, also known as impure Qi, or the excretion of an filthy gas from people or other objects, which becomes epidemic after being absorbed. This does not specifically refer to rats, but rats are used as objects. They are ambushed in the day and out at night, hiding from sunlight, and lurking in dirty places. They easily catch the epidemic Qi. They travel through walls of many houses, infecting more than anything else. Nowadays, there are wars all over the world. Troops in the country have being engaged in the war for a while, with heavy casualties and injuries. In addition, the flood last autumn was disastrous and the earth was blocked from air in winter. Once the early sun rises, the pathogenic Qi is evoked anytime.[124]

At that time, China was in a period of warlord scuffles around the country. TCM used "human affairs" and "time of Heaven" to speculate on the possibility of "Qi" being the cause of diseases, which was the law used by TCM to explain diseases in the early Republic of China period.[125]

TCM used Qi to summarize the principles of biology and bacteriology, which seems to be rational. However, the Qi theory of TCM had no achievements in the

---

[120] Yun Tieqiao, *Collection on Medical Study*, p. 2.

[121] Deng Tietao, *Modern History of TCM*, pp. 93–100.

[122] Yun Tieqiao, *Collection on Medical Study*, p. 4.

[123] Wu Xihuang, *Interpretations of Chinese and Western Febrile Diseases*, p. 148.

[124] Kong Bohua's Experts' Research Office (ed.), *Answers to the Queries on the Treatment of Eight Infectious Diseases*, p. 10.

[125] For the new theory of individual infectious diseases, see Zhu Jianping (ed.), *Research on Major Innovations in Modern Chinese Medicine*, esp. Chapter 3.

construction of practical public health. Yu Yunxiu criticized: "Taking that 'epidemic (Qi)' is as irresistible as natural disasters such as earthquakes, floods and droughts, the only way is to attributed it to fate and luck. Therefore, what else can they do for the public epidemic prevention methods, except praying for heaven and earth, hanging runes and performing sacrificial rites?".[126]

However, the "Qi Theory" of TCM did not remain the same. In terms of fever disease, doctors during the Republic of China period seldom explored the relationship between Qi and "fortune", but focused on the observation of nature by Western science and proposed the comparison among the components of the air and associations based on it. For example, Yun Tieqiao said, "At the turn of June and July, the air in the mountains and forests is clear and contains less acid; the air in cities is turbid and contains more acid. The disease of dampness often occurs in densely populated areas in the city, because the air is the source of the disease."[127] In fact, the discussion of this epidemic Qi is similar to the western "miasma theory". More disputes between Chinese and Western medicine on Qi and bacteria, will be sorted out later.

5.6 Observations, Experimental Methods and Therapeutics—the Second Focus in the Debate on Bacteriology Between TCM and Western Medicine

This section continues to talk about the controversy between TCM and Western medicine on the theory of bacterial pathogenicity. Firstly, it starts from the perspective of scientific experiment, the cornerstone of bacterial research in Western medicine. As TCM has no laboratory to observe the relationship between bacteria and pathology, it was dwarfed in this regard. Yumoto Kyushin, a Japanese doctor who specialized in Chinese medicine, criticized Western medicine in view of the essence of scientific experiment. His remarks are quite similar to those of TCM at the time. He said that medicine is to be applied to human beings, namely the spirits of all living beings. But Western medicine, by holding the "scientific omnipotence", "treats test tubes as human bodies and takes the animal test as the golden rule". The theory derived from scientific experiments is not be applied to the most wonderful and unpredictable human body. Yu Yunxiu retorted in his book: "The old-fashioned doctors denied the "experiment" process. In fact, the reason behind it was that they were afraid that the traditional doctors would lose all their status once they were scientifically tested, so they had to push their views with their eyes closed.[128] Yu also refuted Yumoto Kyushin's argument: "To take a step back, even taking 'test tubes as human body' is a progress to the doctors who think out of thin air or of their own limited experiences

---

[126] Yu Yunxiu, *Criticism on Royal Han Medicine*, pp. 23–24.

[127] Yun Tieqiao, *Understandings of Febrile Diseases, Four Kinds of Medical Books by Yun Tieqiao*, pp. 117–125.

[128] Yu Yunxiu, *Criticism on Royal Han Medicine*, pp. 11–12.

and knowledge of the human body…. Those who know neither the strength nor the weakness of laboratory test tubes are not entitled to criticize these laboratory test tubes."[129] That is to say, TCM was not in the status of commenting on Western medicine nor science unless it had the same equipment and observations.

The inspection and research of bacteria had to rely on microscopes, test methods, test tubes, petri dishes and other instruments. We can use more critical remarks of TCM on the material science of Western medicine to see the debate between TCM and Western medicine at that time. Lu Shige reflected on the development of TCM through the example of the revival of Chinese medicine in Japan. He talked about the problems of "bacteria" and "inflammation", and believed that only by "recognizing the evidence"—this evidence does not refer to the data and results of the laboratory, but the growth and decline of various Qis, the occurrence of symptoms and the body information revealed by clinical observations—could we grasp the detailed differences among regions and of human bodies, rather than only trust one result or one treatment of bacterial testing.[130] However, Yu Yunxiu ignored the Qi or seasonal factors except bacteria. He affirmed that bacteria are an observable organism, which also conforms to the biological rule of "survival of the fittest". If the environment of the infected body is suitable for the survival of bacteria, the bacteria can give play to their "virulence", and people will get sick. However, if "conditions are not suitable for its survival" in the human body, bacteria will definitely not be able to move, nor give play to their "virulence" and can only live in the body as a parasite. Yu Yunxiu criticized that such facts could not overturn the argument that "bacteria are the main cause of infectious diseases".[131]

Lu Shige quoted *Yao Mingda's Inquiries on Diseases* that TCM does not exclude bacteria, nor deny the existence of bacteria, nor its "annoying" characteristics. It is an act of bartering the trunk for the branches for the Western medicine to pay attention to bacteria only and ignore the significance of meridian thought, Qi, blood and other knowledge related to the body in diagnosis.[132] At that time, TCM still believed that the relevant discussion of Qi could better explain the occurrence of diseases. For example, Wu Xihuang explained: "The so-called bacteria of Western medicine is the so-called performance of Qi in China." The seasons are mostly related to summer and autumn. As long as one can read books on warm diseases and understand them thoroughly, one can deal with them. In contrast, West medicine had no special effect on treating fever disease then, except for cinchona that could "sterilize" for malaria. However, many people had diarrhea and new symptoms after using this medicine. So the method of "sterilization" is questionable.[133] Wu believed that even if Western medicine really sees microorganisms through a microscope, the lesions are

---

[129] Yu Yunxiu, *Criticism on Royal Han Medicine*, pp. 28–29.

[130] Lu Shige, Shige's Medical Talk the Revival of Chinese Medicine in Japan, *General Views on Chinese Medicine in China*. pp. 2047–2048.

[131] Yu Yunxiu, *Criticism on Royal Han Medicine*, pp. 26–27.

[132] Lu Shige, *Shige's Medical Talk Yao Mingda's Inquiries on Diseases, General Views on Chinese Medicine in China*. pp. 2050.

[133] Wu Xihuang, *Interpretations of Chinese and Western Febrile Diseases*, p. 96.

infinite. Killing one bacterium brings up another disease, which has no substantive significance. It is not necessary to stick to the law of pathogen inspection.[134] Yu Yunxiu criticized that TCM "could only" see and observe the superficial part but had no ability to conduct experiments for further analysis. It's just "knowing the symptoms without the knowledge or technology for the truth of the disease". It is thus a waste to discuss the disease, and can't but be ridicules for making "spontaneous prescriptions". Yu held that what TCM could do was only "discussing medicine but not diseases" without knowing the true nature of the "diseases". The claim that TCM is the real "cure" is actually the real "nonsense".[135]

There was also a debate between Chinese and Western medicine on a medical case, which had a great impact on the bacteriology, inspection and diagnosis of Western medicine. Many doubts had been raised. The complete record comes from *Shige's Medical Talk*. The author is Lu Shier of Shanghai. He had written more than 100 novels in his life, which can be described as the best in both medical and literary world.[136] Between 1919 and 1924, Lu had written more than ten medical books at his Songjiang residence. It was the time of his early attention paid to TCM and his intensive writing of medical books. Ge Gongzhen (1890–1935) was the victim in the story. He was the important founder of "Journalism" during the Republic of China period. It is said that "there are people in Europe and America who don't read books, but all of them read newspapers". He vigorously advocated the social function and academic research of newspapers, and wrote the *History of Chinese Journalism.*[137] On October 22, 1935, he died from the wrong treatment of Western medicine at the age of 45. Lu said the results of the autopsy of Ge's body by doctors of the Red Cross Society were published in *The News*, revealing it was a body "with a lot of diseases". In that case, why couldn't the diseases be diagnosed before he died? Lu questioned:

> Mr. Ge had a lot of diseases. In addition to sepsis and peritonitis, there are also diseases all over his body including his lungs, stomach, waist, heart and brain. However, when Ge went to the hospital for treatment, Western medicine doctors should have had him carefully examined but they never found out any of these diseases. This is enough to show the make-believe science and technology of Western medicine.[138]

Lu criticized that the cause of Gore's death was discovered after the autopsy, but he was "disorderly treated" for a while before his death, as a multitude of his diseases were not discovered until after his death. This is to prove that the scientific inspection technology of Western medicine can not be trusted. After that, Western medicine doctor Cheng Hanzhang's defense of it was published. For this reason,

---

[134] Wu Xihuang, Volume II: Dai Linjiao's Demonstrations, *Interpretations of Chinese and Western Febrile Diseases*, pp. 40–41.

[135] Yu Yunxiu, *Criticism on Royal Han Medicine*, pp. 90–91.

[136] Tian Ruohong, Chronology of Lu Shige, *Research on Novels of the Ming and Qing Dynasties*, (3), 2002, pp. 119–138. *A Textual Research on Lu Shige's Novels*, Shanghai: Shanghai Sanlian Bookstore, 2005, pp. 285–333.

[137] Ge Gongzhen, *History of Chinese Journalism*, Taipei: Students' Publishing House, 1964, p. 1.

[138] Lu Shige, Shige's Medical Talk·Western Medicine Academic, *General Views on Chinese Medicine in China*. pp. 2084–2085.

Lu You said sarcastically: Cheng Hanzhang listed 7 kinds of septic bacteria and 18 kinds of complications, which is as far-fetched as "catching the moon in the clouds and seeing flowers in the fog". According to Cheng, the reason why there are great differences in pathological tests before and after death is that there are too many kinds of "bacteria", which are unpredictable and difficult to test. Cheng believed that the bacterial infections found in the postmortem pathological examination can not be used to question the patient's pre-mortem diagnosis.[139] It can be understood that the fact that TCM attacked Western medicine, or distrusted Western medicine were mainly due to the two kinds of technologies: diagnosis and testing. As for Ge's death, there was a sequel. Lu said:

> Today, I read a Western medicine doctor's paper about Ge Gongzhen's death in the *News*, saying he just died of an insignificant cold. The so-called cold syndrome in Western medicine is just the rough feeling of wind cold and wind heat in our TCM. How can this disease be fatal? It would be cured by having a few afternoon teas even if there is a delay in taking medicine. Thanks to the Western medicine doctor, he was injected and operated on, which caused his immediate death. The Western medicine doctor knew neither wind cold nor wind heat, let alone how to cure them. I'm really shocked and feel ashamed of it.[140]

Lu believed that many Western doctors in charge of diagnosis and subsequent comments didn't know the exact cause of the diseases with all their talk about "bacteria". Yun Tieqiao also questioned the clinical value of bacteriology. According to him, it is impossible for Western medicine to analyze every disease in clinical treatment with all its efforts to distinguish the types of bacteria. Though not being able to distinguish bacteria, TCM can control the disease symptoms caused by the changes of traditional "Qi" and come up with the antidote against the disease. This is the biggest difference between modern Chinese and Western medicine in the efficacy of bacteria clinical treatment.

5.7 Thoughts on the Treatment of Bacterial Infectious Diseases

With so many remarks against the discussion of bacteria in the field of TCM, it should be noted that oppositions did not stop the communication. Readers may feel that TCM might just study the theory of Qi and ignore the development of bacteriology. On the contrary, the TCM circles tried their best to make repeated comments on this topic, which represents their keen interest. Moreover, the story ended up in TCM combining the treatment rules of Western medicine and "found" many "bactericidal" drugs, which is worth pondering.

---

[139] Lu Shige, Shige's Medical Talk· the Explicitness of Western Medicine Diagnosis, *General Views on Chinese Medicine in China,* pp. 2085–2086.

[140] Lu Shige, Shige's Medical Talk·the Death of Ge Gongzhen, *General Views on Chinese Medicine in China*. P. 2090.

Before 1949, many drugs used in Western medicine for fever diseases were not aimed at "sterilization". Even in the middle and late 1940s, antibiotics were still very rare and even only used during wars. In the early Republic of China period, the drugs of Western medicine for fever were mainly aimed at "antipyretic", but there was little thinking of "sterilization" (the treatment of syphilis in early Republic of China period was an exception). For example, in the *Dictionary of Western Medicine* published in 1936, except that the classification of "antipyretic" was related to the treatment of exogenous febrile diseases,[141] other so-called "fungicide" substances, which had the effect of "preventing the fermentation of substances and instant killing of all molds", were mainly used for surgical disinfection, traumatic ulcer, mouthwash and environmental sanitation for disinfection products, but were rarely taken orally for sterilization. Probably the exceptions were "creosotum or, creosot" and "thiocol", which were mainly used to kill bacteria in tuberculosis, bronchitis and laryngitis. In addition, myrtolum had the function of "disinfection and antisepsis", and could also be used in the early stages of acute and chronic bronchitis, as well as lung disease.[142] These were probably the only oral bactericides used before the war of resistance against Japan.

During the early Republic of China period, the therapeutic drugs of Western medicine for bacterial diseases were serum slurry vaccines made of special pathogenic bacteria or dead bacteria, also known as "biological products (agents)". The "bacterial serum" (see Fig. 5.1)[143] specially developed for specific infectious bacteria was used as a preventive injection and treatment. The 1938 special pharmacology books also introduced the new mixed vaccine, such as the "Beiling flu bacteria vaccine" that could be added to the "pneumonia vaccine" or "streptococcus vaccine", which was said to be more effective. However, the efficacy of these drugs was to enhance the resistance of the human body to the "virulence" produced by bacteria, and they were not direct sterilization.[144] Drugs that really focus on "sterilization" were not introduced to China until the late 1930s and early 1940s (see Fig. 5.1).[145] For example, prontosil album, which had been famous in the history of medicine, was one of them,[146] though the research report at the time also indicates that the effect of the drug on "staphylococcus" was not ideal.[147] Another drug called "uleron" has the characteristics that can just make up for the deficiency of previous

[141] Li Longgong (ed.), *Dictionary of Western Medicine*, Shanghai: Dazhong Publishing House, 1936, pp. 38–47.

[142] Li Longgong (ed.), *Dictionary of Western Medicine*, pp. 121–132.

[143] Shanghai National Medicine Guide Press, *National Medicine Guide,* Vol. 1 (3), 1939, p. 7.

[144] Bayer Pharmaceutical Company, *Supplement to A Collection of Bayer's New Drugs,* Shanghai: Bayer Pharmaceutical Company, 1938, pp. 42–47.

[145] Shanghai National Medicine Guide Press, *National Medicine Guide,* Vol. 1 (3), 1939, p. 17.

[146] Magne, translated by Liu Xueli, *Medical History*, Shanghai: Shanghai People's Publishing House, 2009, pp. 492–494.

[147] Bayer Pharmaceutical Company, *Supplement to A Collection of Bayer's New Drugs*, pp. 14–18.

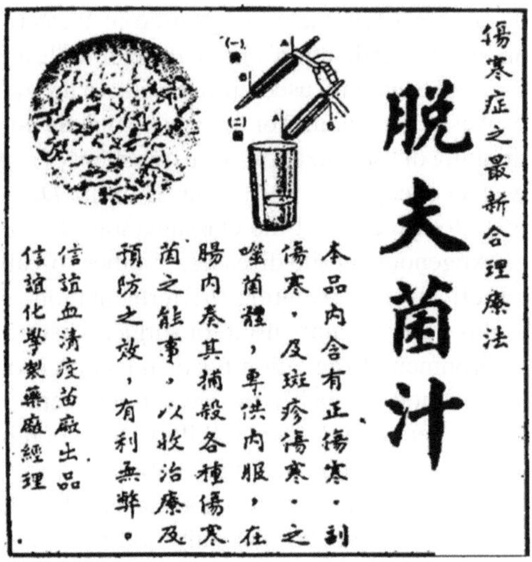

Fig. 5.1 The latest reasonable treatment of typhoid fever—bacterial serum

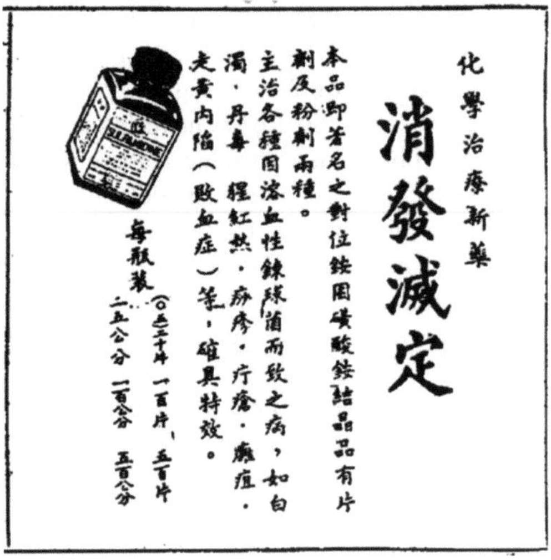

Fig. 5.2 A new chemical drug—disinfection

drugs.[148] However, these two drugs were regarded as new drugs, and their utilization rate and popularity were very doubtful.

Before the 1940s, the overall display of "sterilization" thinking was mostly seen in the "hygiene" measures of daily life. For example, the famous disinfectant "Lowesol" at that time emphasized that "disinfection and sterilization" could be achieved

---

[148] Bayer Pharmaceutical Company, *Supplement to A Collection of Bayer's New Drugs*, Shanghai: Bayer Pharmaceutical Company, 1938, pp. 28–32.

through flushing.[149] It was the favorite consumption of the social "health movement" in the early Republic of China period. Today we often call it "disinfection", but its function should be "sterilization".[150] As for the material culture of Western medicine, the operation of instruments and the identification and use of solvents were taken as common knowledge. For example, experimental glassware "should be washed or boiled with a soap solution, followed by another solution composing of 46 percent sulfuric acid, 6 percent potassium chromate and 46 percent of water. After washing it with the solution, rinse it with distilled water, and then wrap it with a fresh paper. Never disinfect with high-pressure steam sterilizer or dry sterilizer". There are also several physical disinfection methods, all of which involve precautions for instruments, physical laws and chemical reactions.[151] Potassium chromate (K_2CrO_4) is a toxic solvent. I'm afraid the acquisition of these chemicals is another problem. Its operation steps can only be understood through laboratory implementation. Therefore, the difficulty and complexity of studying bacteriology may far exceed the imagination of TCM. For example, Yun Tieqiao also said that these procedures were "specialized knowledge, which can not be imitated by laymen easily".[152] It was in the late 1930s that Western medicine was widely used for sterilization. There were "immune agents" that claimed to be able to treat infectious diseases and various warm diseases, but the composition was unknown (see Fig. 5.3).[153]

To my surprise, Chinese medicine had the idea of "bactericide" for a long time. Although TCM emphasized Qi, it had gradually lost the trust of the "Nation" by using "Qi" or "Yin and Yang" to discuss pharmacology. Though the thinking of the TCM community was multifarious, it was known that TCM had its strength in practice[154] and could make up for the missing part in Western medicine. So it simply cut in from the bacterial discussion to define and explain the composition and characteristics of TCM, which gradually became a scientific discourse of a new TCM.

As for the treatment of "bacteria" drugs, TCM during the Republic of China period mostly got inspiration from the traditional thinking of body view and treatment, rather than from the drug classification of Western medicine. Ding Fubao's *A Brief Introduction to Chinese Medicine* published in 1933 divides TCM into 10 categories according to the classification of Western medicine. "Antipyretic drugs" are more related to febrile diseases. Most of these drugs have the effect of "sweating and antipyretic".[155] In addition, drugs commonly used in TCM to treat fever, such

---

[149] Sino French Pharmacy, *Health Essentials*, Shanghai: Shanghai Sino French Pharmacy, 1919, pp. 34–36.

[150] Cheng Hanzhang, *A Brief Introduction to Western Medicine,* Shanghai: Commercial Press, 1934, pp. 28, 33.

[151] Xie Enzheng (ed.), *New Drug Materia Medica*, Peking: Hua'an Pharmacy, 1943, pp. 2364–2366.

[152] Yun Tieqiao, *Collection on Medicine,* pp. 8–9.

[153] Shanghai National Medicine Guide Press, *National Medicine Guide,* Vol. 1 (3), 1939, p. 28.

[154] Yang Xiling, Medical Talk in the Garden. TCM Is Not Useless, *Collection of Rare Modern TCM.Medical Talk*, p. 515.

[155] Ding Fubao, *A Brief Introduction to Chinese Medicine*, Fuzhou: Fujian Science and Technology Press, 2008, pp. 20–29.

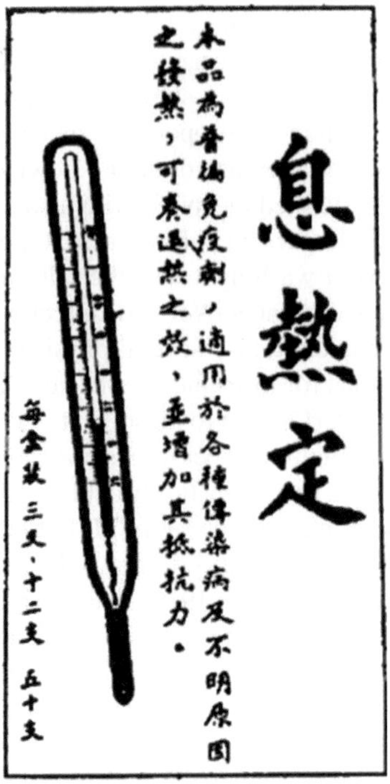

Fig. 5.3 The immune agent heat pacifier

as "ephedra", were classified as "analgesic, sedative and antispasmodic drugs".[156] The classification method determines their attributes. Since Western medicine had no bactericidal medicine for oral administration, no matter how it was subdivided according to the classification method of Western medicine, the thinking of "sterilization" did not come up. Another famous work on TCM was Chen Bangxian's *Preparation of New Materia Medica.* It may have been completed in a small tea house in Sichuan later bombed by artillery during Anti-Japanese War.[157] Although Chen used the classification method of traditional pharmacology to distinguish the types of TCM, the drug of "coptis chinensis" was marked with "antibacterial effect",[158] which is different from Ding's book. The "coptis chinensis" in Ding's book can only "strengthen the stomach and stop diarrhea" or treat enteritis and jaundice, but

[156] Ding Fubao, *A Brief Introduction to Chinese Medicine*, p. 51.

[157] For Chen Bangxian's life and contributions, see Zheng Jinsheng & Li Jianmin, The Origin of Modern Chinese Medical History Research, *Mainland Journal*, Vol. 95 (6), 1997, pp. 26–35; Li Jingwei, Chen Bangxian, The Famous Chinese Medical Historian, *Journal of Chinese Medical History*, Vol. 16 (4), 1986, pp. 193–198; Cai Jingfeng, *Mr. Chen Bangxian's Contribution to the History of Chinese Diseases*; Wang Zhipu, *Mr. Chen Bangxian's Research on Early Medical History;* Chen Dinghong, The Personality and Academic Cultivation of Professor Chen Bangxian—A Medical Historian, published separately in *Journal of Chinese Medical History,* Vol. 20 (1),1990, pp. 11–13, 14–16 and 17–19.

[158] Chen Bangxian, *Essentials of New Materia Medica,* Taichung: Ruicheng Publishing House, 1983, pp. 20–21.

can not "sterilize".[159] Unfortunately, this is the only item with "antibacterial" function discovered by Chen. Chen adopted the analysis of western pharmacology in the drug compositions, such as the commonly used drug "cinnamon twig" for the treatment of fever, which contains volatile cinnamon oil (cinnamon oil) and other components, "ephedra" has "ephedrine of plant base",[160] and his conclusion did not go beyond the experimental results of Western medicine. Therefore, I believe that Chen's "antibacterial" discovery may be just a coincidence.

The discussion of "sterilization" in TCM during the Republic of China period could come from two kinds of thoughts. The first thought was that TCM did not treat bacteria, but it could eliminate bacterial toxicity. Bacteria was not the main cause of fever. Those who held this view did not think that it was necessary to think about the treatment of TCM from the perspective of "sterilization". Zhang Taiyan believed "sweating is also an inflammatory agent." "Although typhoid fever contains bacteria, it must take cold as the main cause and bacteria as the auxiliary cause. Although warm disease contains bacteria, it must take heat as the main cause and bacteria as the auxiliary cause."[161] Zhang believed that the main cause of fever was not bacteria, but "external Qi" such as heat and cold. Further, Zhang concluded that the efficacy of TCM was not "sterilization", but it could expel the "toxin" of bacteria.[162] However, Zhang did not specify which TCM might have the function of sterilization or expelling toxins. The second thought is to further demonstrate the thinking that "TCM can eliminate toxins, so it can also kill bacteria", an idea that probably originated from Yumoto Kyushin's *Royal Han Medicine*.[163] However, Zhang Xichun, in his *Chinese Medicine with Reference to the West* published in 1924, stated "camphor is good at invigorating the heart, activating the blood vessels of the whole body, especially eliminating toxic bacteria."[164] It seems that Zhang had not read Chinese medicine books.[165] Probably, a lot of comments on "sterilization" in later Chinese medicine works and its modern history questioned by Western medicine could quite arouse the resonance and sympathy of TCM circles at that time. Yang Xiling believed that if TCM was not reformed, it would have been wiped out within

[159] Ding Fubao, *A Brief Introduction to Chinese Medicine*, p. 13.

[160] Chen Bangxian, *Essentials of New Materia Medica*, pp. 65, 126–127.

[161] Shanghai People's Publishing House (ed.), On the Pathogenesis of Micro Bacteria, *Complete Works of Zhang Taiyan,* Vol. 8, pp. 451–452.

[162] Shanghai People's Publishing House (ed.),On the Pathogenesis of Micro Bacteria, *Complete Works of Zhang Taiyan,* Vol. 8, pp. 453–454.

[163] Zhang Taiyan, Lu Yuanlei, Wu Xihuang, Yun Tieqiao, Yu Wuyan and Pan Chenglian were greatly influenced by Japanese Han Medicine. Their discussions were indeed in line with Tang Ben's discussion. As for Cao Yingfu and Zhu Fu, there was no proof that they had been affected.

[164] Zhang Xichun, Prescription for Cholera First Aid Reviving Pill, *Chinese Medicine with Reference to the West*, Vol. I, p. 182.

[165] Zhao Hongjun, Chronicle of Zhang Xichun, *Journal of Chinese Medical History*, (21.4), 1991, pp. 214–218.

ten years like Japanese Han Medicine. But where to start the reform? The example of Chinese medicine in Japan can be reversely taken as the reference for TCM.[166]

A Japanese doctor in Chinese Medicine Yumoto Kyushin once studied Western medicine. His discussion on "sterilization" often expressed the integration of Chinese and Western medicine. In addition to his inspiration from ancient Chinese medical classics, I'm afraid the study of Chinese pharmaceutical study in Japan had also inspired him a lot. He once pointed out that the main component of "almond" in *Hehan Pharmacology* was fatty oil (almond oil), which took up more than 50%. Supported by some proofs, the drug was said to "have the function of making rot and fermentation, making it possible to treat animal and bacterial diseases".[167] Here, he held that almond has the function of "making rot and fermentation" due to the fact that the substance is affected by bacteria, and it has the characteristics of acid rot and odor. Its function of "decreasing the acidification of cells" is an important pharmacological support for the treatment of bacterial diseases. In fact, TCM often speculates on the basis of western pharmacology that some Chinese medicine can also be disinfecting and sterilizing. For example, Zhang Xichun said: "(Cinnabar) is composed of sulfur and mercury, which can eliminate toxic bacteria, so it can treat fulminant disease infection, cholera, vomiting and diarrhea."[168] In addition, other bactericidal thoughts were extended discussions based on the fever disease treatment of classical medicine, that is, they first affirmed the treatment of classical medicine, then explained the relationship between bacteria and drugs, and especially emphasized the concept of expelling "toxins". Yumoto said:

When being invaded by the same pathogen, the patients may have different symptoms due to the patients' different constitution and the different locations of the virus... It is necessary to use the three methods of sweating, vomiting and excreting according to the symptoms, which is Zhongjing's "treating the disease according to its symptoms".[169]

Regardless the pathogens and the name of a disease, Yumoto maintained that sweating, vomiting and excretion are the methods for the "toxins" of the patient's constitution and body, and the "toxins" are extended into "bacterial toxins". On the contrary, Yu Yunxiu criticized Yumoto's theory and attacked his most respected book *Treatise on Typhoid Fever* that the way he annotated the classics is the most mediocre writing method of modern Chinese medicine. By putting some Western medicine or scientific statements in the framework of classic texts, it is simply "a groundless lie with no support by any studies nor proofs".[170]

---

166 Yang Xiling, Medical Talk in the Garden. TCM Is Not Useless, *Collection of Rare Modern TCM.Medical Talk*, p. 516.

167 Yumoto Kyushin, translated by Zhou Zixu: The Therapeutic Effect of Almonds, *Royal Han Medicine*, p. 115.

168 Zhang Xichun, Interpretation of Cinnabar,*Chinese Medicine with Reference to the West*, Vol. 2, p. 281.

169 Yumoto Kyushin, translated by Zhou Zixu, *Royal Han Medicine*, pp. 36–37.

170 Yu Yunxiu, *Criticism on Royal Han Medicine*, pp. 36–37.

Going through the medical books of Yumoto in detail, there are indeed many "bactericidal" drugs "found". The provisions of the book on sterilization thinking were sorted out as follows: one is the malaria drug "Changshan".[171] According to the ancient herbal books, Yumoto explained that the drug "has insecticidal and bactericidal properties, but it is toxic and can not be freely used". Perhaps the "strong medicine" and "toxins" that can treat fever have the function of sterilization. The expressions of "removing blood stasis" and "killing worms" came up at the same time as "sterilization". For example, in his book *Shengsheng Hall Treatments,* he recorded the case of a woman curing typhoid fever by menstrual blood: "It is clear that the toxin of intestinal typhoid fever can be eliminated by menstrual blood."[172] It can be seen that "menstrual blood" is also a way of detoxification, and Yumoto explained that this treatment was to expel bacteria and toxins. The second drug was "lead pill": Tang Ben cited the main prescriptions from the medical books such as *Compendium of Materia Medica* to explain that lead pill "is a compound of lead, so it has the functions of convergence, sedation, antispasmodic, insecticidal and bactericidal".[173]

By analyzing his exposition, it seems like as long as the drugs conformed with the "antipyretic and detoxification" as well as "insecticidal" functions recorded in classical medical books, they could be proved as having "sterilization" function. The third is the example of "sophora flavescens". Yumoto said: "According to *Preparation of Materia Medica*: 'sophora flavescens... heat generates wind and dampness generates worms. It can also dispel wind, expel water, kill worms and sterilize.' From this point of view, this medicine is a powerful antipyretic medicine with insecticidal and bactericidal effects".[174] It is obvious that the drugs he believed having insecticidal and antipyretic effects could be sterilizing. During the Republic of China period, the relationship between "worms" and "bacteria" was close, which was not necessarily the influence of Japanese Han Medicine. As mentioned above,[175] the theory of Yumoto did add the best footnote to the relationship between sterilization and insecticidal.

Except for the insecticidal effect which is mainly for exogenous use, the idea of sterilization may also involve TCM for surgical sore disease and detoxification. For example, when speculating on the efficacy of "peach nucleolus", Yumoto said: "This medicine is an anti-inflammatory anticoagulant for expelling blood stasis, which has

[171] Yumoto Kyushin, translated by Zhou Zixu, The Therapeutic Effect of Shu Chi, *Royal Han Medicine,* pp. 62.

[172] Yumoto Kyushin, translated by Zhou Zixu, Abdominal Syndrome of Xiaochaihu Decoction, *Royal Han Medicine,* p. 160.

[173] Yumoto Kyushin, translated by Zhou Zixu, The Therapeutic Effect of Lead Pills, *Royal Han Medicine,* pp. 179–180.

[174] Yumoto Kyushin, translated by Zhou Zixu, The Therapeutic Effect of Sophora Flavescens, *Royal Han Medicine,* pp. pp. 258–259.

[175] "Although the ancient Chinese medicine book writers did not know bacteria, they believed that there were insects, so every insecticide used to treat sores and scabies can also kill bacteria." It shows that TCM believed that the concepts of insecticidal and bactericidal were similar. From Pan Shuren, Random Talk on Bacteria and Insects, *China Medical Monthly*, 1941 (8–9), p. 21.

the functions of antitussive, analgesic, defecation, insecticide and sterilization."[176] "Scallion", a convenient prescription commonly used in the treatment of exogenous diseases, can also be sterilizing. Yumoto quoted the *Preparation of Materia Medica* as follows: "(Scallion) ventilation can detoxify the toxins of medicine, fish, earthworm and smear dog injury." And onion is a warm excitatory drug, which can kill insects and bacteria.[177] There are also "realgar"[178] and "Dry Paint",[179] which were also considered to have bactericidal effect because they can kill insects or have slight toxicity, or can treat surgical and trauma injuries. However, there are still many "insecticidal" drugs in TCM that had not been listed.[180]

The "sterilization" thinking of TCM had been influenced by Japanese Chinese medicine, but it is not exactly the same. For example, Wu Xihuang said, "Since micro bacteria come from the climate and change with the change of climate, they are taking the essence of heaven and earth as the source of treatment. They prescribe them according to the six Qis, which is why they can cure the disease and eliminate micro bacteria."[181] The thinking of "sterilization" discussed in TCM was very extensive. Drug sterilization was just a method, and it was also a method to adjust the influence of external "Qi" on the body. Here is an example: Cao Yingfu, who might not have been influenced by Han medicine, commented that sweating can expel bacteria from the body, on the basis of the explanation of the debate context of Chinese medical fever, so as to criticize the febrile school for blocking bacteria from going out of the body with Yin nourishing products.[182] Sweating methods were badly stigmatized in the Ming and Qing Dynasties, especially those with drugs like cassia twig and ephedra. Many patients regarded them as severe as tiger and wolf medicine. In contrast, during the Republic of China period, many doctors gave "sweating method" a new status, which may be used as a side observation of the revival of classical prescriptions.

In addition, Zhang Taiyan once mentioned that TCM began to pay attention to the problems of "resistance": "The treatment for the five fever diseases and five infectious diseases is to promote the spleen Yang to produce white blood, producing

---

[176] Yumoto Kyushin, translated by Zhou Zixu: The Therapeutic Effect of Peach Kernel, *Royal Han Medicine,* pp. 347–348.

[177] Yumoto Kyushin, translated by Zhou Zixu: The Therapeutic Effect of Scallion, *Royal Han Medicine,* p. 417.

[178] Yumoto Kyushin, translated by Zhou Zixu: The Therapeutic Effect of Realgar, *Royal Han Medicine,* p. 456.

[179] Yumoto Kyushin, translated by Zhou Zixu: The Therapeutic Effect of Resina Toxicodendri, *Royal Han Medicine,* p. 365.

[180] For example, rehmannia, glutinosa and flax can also kill insects, but Yumoto did not explain it. From (Qing) Wang Ang, Essentials of Materia Medica, included in Xian Changshen (ed.), *Wang Ang's Complete Book of Medicine,* Beijing: China TCM Press, 1999, p. 375.

[181] Wu Xihuang, *Lecture Notes on Diseases of Four Seasons,* Chen Yinghe's preface, p. 1; Watanabe Hee, *The Oriental Beacon of Modern Medical Transformation and the Collection of Experimental Chinese Medicine,* Osaka: Oriental and Chinese Medical Research Association, 1927–1932.

[182] Cao Yingfu, *Typhoid Fever Development, Combined Issue of Typhoid Fever from Cao's Golden Cabinet*, p. 124.

the effect of sterilization."[183] This also shows that Chinese doctors had perceived the cultivation and recovery of the patient's own antibacterial ability rather than focusing on "sterilization". TCM also held that we should not stick to the view of "sterilization", because bacteria could be good or bad. "Pathogenic bacteria" can be called "evil", and TCM can attack it with drug toxin. For the bacteria beneficial to the body, tonics can be used.[184] As Yang Zhiyi expressed, some infectious diseases often occurred during cold spring, such as meningitis; some are more likely to occur in summer, such as cholera, because the seasons dominated by six Qis or climate are conducive to the growth of certain bacteria. TCM is used to treat diseases caused by six Qis ("six Yin"), rather than focusing on sterilization. Western medicine uses saline injections to treat cholera, food recuperation to treat tuberculosis, and expectant therapy to treat typhoid fever. They don't focus on sterilization. How did it come that TCM can not be bactericidal?[185] Yang aimed to treat infectious diseases by adjusting the deviation of six Qis in the body, and did not take sterilization as the key issue.

TCM is more based on the contents of classic medical books than on the impact of chemical components of drugs on bacteria. In particular, the *Treatise on Typhoid Fever* begins with the discussion of "taiyang disease", by laying out the importance of the sweating method in the treatment of febrile diseases. Many TCM doctors started from this thinking and discussed the problem of treating "bacteria". For example, Cao Yingfu used the sweating method to sort out the physical pathology and meanings of "bacteria" and "blood stasis". He had the view that "dampness" disease is that water dampness (Qi) condenses in the muscle, and the blood is blocked, resulting in pain; similarly, carbuncle and gangrene are also a kind of "blood stasis", which must be alleviated. At this time, moxibustion, ironing or charcoal are used for fumigation, so that the hot air can force out the "bacterial sweat", the blood will circulate and the disease will be cured.[186] Cao was very confident in the treatment of sweating to eliminate the virus. He once said: "All toxins (including foreign pathogens and blocked excreta) would be gone with this smooth sweating. This is the so-called 'sweat solution'."[187] Cao believed that this was derived from daily "experiments". In fact, it is just the practical experience of putting the writings of classical medical books into clinical practice.

Zhang Taiyan also said, "If the wind, cold, heat and dampness do not invade, the constructive and defensive Qì won't be competing with them. How can there be bacteria?" Although ancient people didn't have the term "sterilization", the prescribed drugs had the sterilization effects. Cinnamon twig decoction was used for apoplexy, ephedra decoction was used for typhoid, and ephedra decoction

183 Shanghai People's Publishing House (ed.), On Infectious Diseases in China, *Complete Works of Zhang Taiyan,* Vol. 8, p. 322.

184 Tan Linbo, TCM on Bacteria, *Jiading TCM Weekly*, Vol. 1–20,1947, p. 16.

185 Yang Zhiyi, My Views on "Epidemic Treatment" of TCM and Western Medicine, *Spring and Autumn of the Medical World,* 1930 (49), pp. 3–4.

186 Cao Yingfu, *Typhoid Fever Development, Combined Issue of Typhoid Fever from Cao's Golden Cabinet*, p. 23.

187 Cao Yingfu, *Experimental Records of Classical Prescriptions*, p. 40.

also contains cinnamon. *Supplementary Records of Famous Prescriptions* says that cinnamon can be harmlessly used with different drugs. It is stated in *On Medical Properties*: "As cinnamon can kill the toxins in plants, how can it not be the bactericide!"[188] Probably the fact that sweating can treat fever was taken, by the same token, as the possibility that TCM can treat bacterial diseases. Zhang did not quite agree with the bacterial pathogenic theory. On the contrary, he held that TCM can detoxify or sterilize, which is an interesting idea.[189] As for the discussion of "purgation", in fact, there had been many discussions in the chapter of "Yangming Disease" of *Treatise on Typhoid Fever*. From the discussion of some doctors, we can see the convergence of Qi and bacterial theory. Pan Chenglian said, "Yangming disease can be called the second step of acute fever." It is also said that the high fever in its symptoms is due to "bacterial invasion and dysfunction of thermoregulation". The use of Qi Activating Decoction and other purgative agents for treatment can "expel the virus from the body".[190]

For individual infectious diseases, the description of "sterilization" is more clear. The drugs in individual prescriptions for the treatment of epidemic diseases are directly classified as "sterilization" without involving sweating, vomiting, purgation, bleeding and blood stasis removing. We can't examine every infectious disease in detail,[191] but we can see its outline by looking at the major discussions on the treatment of "epidemics" and several examples of cholera. Zhu Fu said: "For severe epidemic cases, TCM attributed it to toxin and heat in blood fever, while Western medicine to bacterial infection. In fact, they are the same. However, TCM had no test equipment and could not clearly define it as bacteria, but generalized it as toxin… The function of clearing heat and detoxification of TCM is not different from the treatment of clearing blood and sterilization of Western medicine."[192] Zhu discussed the "heat clearing and detoxification" of TCM and the "blood clearing and sterilization" of Western medicine, believing that they have the common ground to share. The prescriptions discussed in "heat (fire) clearing and detoxification" were all said to have the function of sterilization, which shows that Zhu admitted the theory of bacterial pathogenicity. The concepts of sterilization and detoxification of TCM came up repeatedly in the discussion of TCM during the Republic of China period, and became the assets of establishing the new views in the discussion of infectious diseases.

---

[188] Shanghai People's Publishing House (ed.), On Worms and Bacteria, *Complete Works of Zhang Taiyan*, Vol. 8, pp. 444–445.

[189] Shanghai People's Publishing House (ed.), On Bacteria and Toxins, *Complete Works of Zhang Taiyan*, Vol. 8, p. 447.

[190] Pan Chenglian, *A New Interpretation to Typhoid Fever*, pp. 87, 89.

[191] Cao Hongxin (ed.), "The Prevention and Control of Modern Infectious Disease (1840–2006)", *Summary of Warm Diseases*, Fuzhou: Fujian Science and Technology Press, 2008, Vol. VI.

[192] Zhu Fu, *The Compromised Essence of the Principles for the Latest Miscellaneous Diseases*, Vol. I, pp. 28b–29b.

5.8 "Western Knowledge Learned from Asia"—The Discussion of Bacteriology in TCM

There is no doubt that TCM could treat epidemics. However, there was no consensus on whether it could treat infectious diseases in the modern sense in the era of bacteriology. Since the Republic of China period, through continuous dialogue between TCM and western bacteriology, efforts have been made to reinterpret and affirm the experience and treatment methods in classical medical books, establish the confidence in treatment, give a new definition of exogenous fever, and urge TCM to construct a more complete analytical framework.

Since the introduction of Western medicine bacteriology into China, TCM has never strongly rejected the theory of bacteria, but incorporated it into the new curriculum. The doctors of TCM mentioned in this book were good at explaining the physical changes caused by bacteria in the human body with various kinds of toxins. As for the biological role of bacteria, TCM emphasized that "bacteria are in the air". Bacteria can not grow without external factors such as air, seasons, temperature and moisture, and then put bacteriology into the category of Qi theory, which is the historical model of the convergence of Qi theory and bacteria theory in modern Chinese and Western medicine. In the history of TCM, the species of "bacteria" was not recognized, which makes it quite different from the physiological and anatomical debates between modern Chinese and Western medicine. The latter can be found in many examples in ancient Chinese medical history, and can even be explained by the view of "Western learning originates from China".[193]

During the Republic of China period, someone like Luo Xieyuan believed that bacteriology was a kind of "western knowledge learned from Asia", such as worm toxin, ghost abscess, worm-induced ulcer, roundworm and Yin-Yang toxins, which were all related to bacteria. However, the so-called "bacteria" were unheard of after all. Although there were doctors such as Zhang Taiyan or Luo who forced their interpretations, it was difficult to observe with the naked eyes after all. To TCM, it was a new species. Through the discussion, we can see that the vitality of modern Chinese medicine not only came from the absorption of western bacteriology, but also involved the dialogue of classical medical books of febrile diseases, including *Treatise on Typhoid Fever* and *Analysis on Febrile Diseases*. Except for some basic theories of Qi, in fact, modern Chinese medicine rarely uses *Internal Canon of Medicine* as the theoretical basis due to the fact that the effects in treatment are no less important than the theories when responding to bacteriology. It was the actual effect on infectious diseases that modern Chinese medicine relied on.

Through the discussion in this chapter, we can see that even though TCM had different views toward bacteria theory, its confidence in traditional medical treatment was as firm as a rock. Zhang Taiyan's "studying bacteria according to antiquity" is quite representative. He mixed the ancient knowledge of natural history, biology and medicine to respond to bacteriology. The discussion of Japanese Han medicine

---

193 Pi Kuoli, *Body View and Ideological Transformation of Modern TCM—Tang Zonghai and the Era of Convergence of TCM and Western Medicine*, Chapter 4, 5, 7.

provided strong supports to TCM to classify the classic therapies such as sweating, detoxification and purgation as "sterilization", which more or less strengthened the confidence of TCM in this discussion. In addition to absorbing the theory of Western medicine bacteriology, the other way to obtain "sterilization" knowledge was just to summarize the clinical experiences from the typhoid and warm disease systems of TCM and the mechanism of its drug application to find the possibility of "sterilization". Although the opinions of different doctors were cited, their theories of "discovery of sterilization" were all based on this.

However, the discussion of fever diseases in TCM during the Republic of China period was not limited to "sterilization", otherwise it can not explain why TCM did not develop bactericides, nor gave more thoughts on the treatment in this area. In addition to the fact that there were no laboratories and scientific methods discussed in this paper, what is more important is that even if there were bactericides, TCM would still abide by the "Qi theory", since TCM is based on the "Qi" of cold, heat and climate, rather than a kind of medicine for bacterial treatment. Obviously, based on the "Qi theory" and body view, modern Chinese medicine adopted an attitude of discussion, counter argumentation and highly selective acceptance of western bacteriology.

Lu Shige maintained: "If reforming Chinese medicine means translating a few western books of physiology, pathology, diagnostics, pharmacy or copying some Western medical terms, it would be too easy a job in improving TCM. It is the way to pack thousands of years of academic research of China in a different cover and claim it as one's own academic innovation. It is actually the narration of Western medicine in Chinese language, but not TCM."[194] Yun Tieqiao believed that once bacteria is studied, it is bound to learn serum injections. "If this is done, it is completely the Western medicine study which is irrelevant to Chinese medicine".[195] This embarrassing situation was reflected in Fu Sinian's criticism: TCM that accepted microbiology can not be called "TCM". Fu satirized that TCM "cannot be changed", unless the whole ideological system behind it is completely changed.[196] This highly one-sided and selective attitude of absorbing knowledge led to the situation that TCM during the Republic of China period could only choose some translated textbooks. Lu Yuanlei said: "There are so many translated Western medicine books (such as pathogenic bacteria) available that there is no need to compile them."[197] This selective acceptance, even for Lu who was at the forefront of the scientization of TCM, was the most "open" speech. It can be seen that the whole classical medical system represented by the "Qi theory" cannot be completely replaced by bacteriology.

---

[194] Lu Shige, Shige's Medical Talk My Views on the Improvement of Chinese Medicine, *General Views on Chinese Medicine in China*. p. 2068.

[195] Yun Tieqiao, *Collection on Medicine*, p. 35.

[196] Fu Sinian, On the So-called National Medicine, *Complete Works of Fu Sinian*, Vol. 6, pp. 316–317.

[197] Lu Yuanlei, Experience in the Academic Collation Meeting of the National Medical Museum,Lu's Collection of Medical Theories, *Two Kinds of Lu Yuanlei's Medical Books*, p. 166.

In retrospect, after the discussion of "scientization of TCM" in the 1930s, it is proved that the use of bacteriology was still less important than the use of western physiology. *The Lecture Notes on the Scientization of TCM*, written in 1955, advocates "explaining the theory of TCM according to modern scientific research". However, the pathological explanation was "based on the pathogen theory of TCM", rather than the bacterial theory of Western medicine.[198] Since modern times, TCM has not moved toward a path of pathological medicine based on bacteria. Exploring the positive and negative views of TCM during the Republic of China period makes up for the historical data of modern TCM, which may provide us with more understandings and reflections on the debate between TCM and Western medicine.

---

[198] Zhu Hegao & Lu Kuisheng (ed.), *Handouts on the Scientization of TCM*, Taipei: Xinwenfeng Publishing Company, 1987, Editor's Notes, p. 1.

Chapter 6
The Practice and Dilemma of New TCM: Yun Tieqiao's Talk on the *Treatise on Typhoid Fever* and Bacteriology

6.1 Quitting Literature and Becoming a Doctor

How did TCM doctors during the Republic of China period think about its own academic development and what did it think of bacteriology? Yun Tieqiao (1878–1935) is chosen here as the representative. It is undeniable that he could not represent the position of TCM for the Republic of China period, but his remarks can be just a microcosm of the previous chapters—the behavior of specific characters are the flesh and blood of "multi-dimensional medical history", and can also be used as a supplement to the extensive discussions in the previous chapters.

The protagonist of this chapter, Yun Shuyu, style named Tiejia, was born in Wujin, Jiangsu Province, into an average family. When he was young, he went to Fujian with his father who went there for his work. Being ill fated, he suffered from the grief of his parents' death before he was 15 years old. As Fujian was a sad place, he had to go back to his hometown Wujin and was raised by his relatives. Fortunately, life is always a story of sweet and sour. In the first spring right after he was 15 years old, he passed the county level imperial examination, but he didn't pursue his career by taking office. After all, in such an era, the imperial examination was not the only promising prospect for scholars. In the 22nd year of Guangxu (1896), Sheng Xuanhuai (1844–1916) raised funds to establish Nanyang Public College in Xujiahui, Shanghai, which was subordinate to both the China Merchants Steamship Company and Telegraph Bureau. Public schools were set up such as the Normal Department, Attached School, Secondary School and Upper School, which were the predecessors of Shanghai Jiaotong University today.[1] In 1899, more public schools were successively set up such as the Translation Academy and Eastern Literature

[1] For the content of classes at the beginning of Nanyang Public School and the curriculum arrangement of the coexistence of new, old, Chinese and Western schools, see Lu Fang, The Establishment of New Schools in the Late Qing Dynasty and the Connection Between Chinese and Western Academia—on the Case of Nanyang Public School (1896–1905), included in Lin Liyue (ed.), *The Strain and Innovation of Modern Countries*, Taipei: Tangshan Publishing House, 2006, pp. 103–126.

© Zhonghua Book Company 2026

K. Pi, *The Contest of Modern Chinese and Western Medicine*,
https://doi.org/10.1007/978-981-95-2832-5_6

School to cultivate translation talents. Later, the Translation Academy developed into the Commercial Press, a pioneer of China's modern publishing industry. Shanghai Nanyang Public School had a great reputation at that time. Sheng Xuanhuai himself was a rich businessman, so the school was well funded, with first-class teachers and equipment, as well as good job opportunities for the graduates. Having nobody's help, Yun Tieqiao had to plan for his future, thinking that as the imperial examination background was no longer glamorous, it would be better to pursue "practical learning", which could provide the potential in the new era, and a skill without depending on relatives. He entered Nanyang Public School in 1903 and graduated successfully in 1906. His skills in English reading and translation had greatly improved,[2] and later he turned to be versatile in editing, translating and writing.[3]

After graduation, he worked as a teacher in middle schools in Shanghai and Changsha, and had a fairly decent experience. In his spare time, he also tried to translate western novels. In the first half of his life, he was a writer. Due to his love of literature, he had a rigorous attitude toward writing, and his writing had also been polished more wonderfully and profoundly in the passage of years. It is hard to imagine that this doctor, who would occupy a place in the history of the integration of Chinese and Western medicine in the future, once had the experience of "doing nothing serious". In 1911, he entered the Commercial Press as a compiler. A year after, he was hired as the editor-in-chief of the *Monthly Novel* published by the Commercial Press, and took the lead in translating western novels. Although he did not lay a solid foundation for his medical attainments with several years of editing career, the translation of familiar Western knowledge prompted him to write books and establish his own theory in the future.

The origin of starting a career in TCM may have been Yun's greatest grief in his life. After 1916, his three sons were infected with typhoid fever (diphtheria). Yun Tieqiao had read medical books when he was young, but he was not proficient in medical skills due to the lack of clinical experiences, despite his profound learning and godly writings. At this time, he could only stand by and watch his three sons die one after another. Ordinary people, who were completely laymen in medical science, could do no more than lamenting on their own misery. However, a Chinese medicine learner as he was, his bewilderment probably hurt him more—his obsession in writing and his lack of expertise in medicine seemed to be a satire for him. Fortunately, it was not too late to mend. The successive pain of losing his sons didn't crush him. He began to pick up his medical books. On the basis of some of his previous work, he studied the *Treatise on Typhoid Fever* in depth, drew the energy and spirit of TCM from the classics, and consulted with the well-known typhoid expert Wang Lianshi (about 1848–1928) and the famous doctor Ding Ganren (1865–1926).

---

[2] Deng Tietao & Cheng Zhifan (ed.), *General History of Chinese Medicine Modern History*, Beijing: People's Health Publishing House, 1999, p. 285.

[3] Fan Boqun, From Lu Xun's Switching from Medicine to Literature to Yun Tieqiao's Switching from Literature to Medicine—the Theory of Yun Tieqiao, *Journal of Fudan University* (Social Science Edition), 2005 (01), p. 24.

The next year, his fourth son got typhoid fever, suffering from fever with chills, and dyspnea without sweat. The famous doctor they sent for, though having read the *Treatise on Typhoid Fever,* did not dare to use the prescription for typhoid fever, but only prescribed the drugs commonly used by the school of warm diseases, such as douchi, gardenia, soybean rolls, mulberry leaves, chrysanthemums, almonds, forsythia, which made it worse. Yun Tieqiao hesitated, and spent a sleepless night. As a last resort, he decisively prescribed a dose of ephedra soup, and said to his wife that as their three sons died of typhoid fever, and the doctors were helpless, he would rather this son take his medicine and die than let him sit and wait to die. As the result, the fourth son's skin turned moist after taking one dose, and his asthma was slightly lowered. After taking two doses, his sweating and fever subsided, and then he recovered. Since then, Yun was more convinced of the classical prescriptions for typhoid fever and studied the classics of TCM. It should be explained that Yun was by no means a partial doctor of TCM. He once said, "There was a special tradition in my hometown. All children who have completed their reading of Five Classics were often ordered to read medical books. Therefore, when I was young, I read the *Three Character Classic of Medicine*, *Basic Inquiries* and *Analysis on Febrile Diseases*".[4] He had long had some understandings of the basic theory of TCM, though lacking in clinical experience. Later, when relatives and friends got sick, they all came to ask him for a prescription, and most of them were effectively treated. So he decided to give up his editorial position and practice medicine. In 1920, he became a doctor in Shanghai, which was the beginning of Yun's leaving the Commercial Press and formally switching from literature to medical practice.[5] For him, TCM was the final choice of his life career and the beginning of his becoming an important figure in the medical history of the early Republic of China period.[6]

6.2 Yun Tieqiao's Historical Status and the Problematique of This Chapter

Yun Tieqiao once came into contact with western culture and learned Western medicine at the same time. He advocated that TCM should be taken as the main body and Western medicine should be properly introduced to improve TCM. He practiced medicine during the day and penned books at night. He was an author with many works and many of his medical works reveal the conflict and integration of Chinese

[4] Yun Tieqiao, *Research on Typhoid Fever*, Vol. 4, Taipei: Huading Publishing House, 1988, p. 77.

[5] The unhappiness and misunderstanding in editing work were also the inducement for him to quit literature and pursue medicine.See Fan Boqun, *From Lu Xun's Switching from Medicine to Literature to Yun Tieqiao's Switching from Literature to Medicine—the Theory of Yun Tieqiao*, pp. 24–25.

[6] For Yun Tieqiao's life and works, see Wu Yunbo, Yun Tieqiao's Life and Academic Thoughts, *Journal of Chinese Medical History*, Vol. 21, 1991 (02), pp. 88–93.

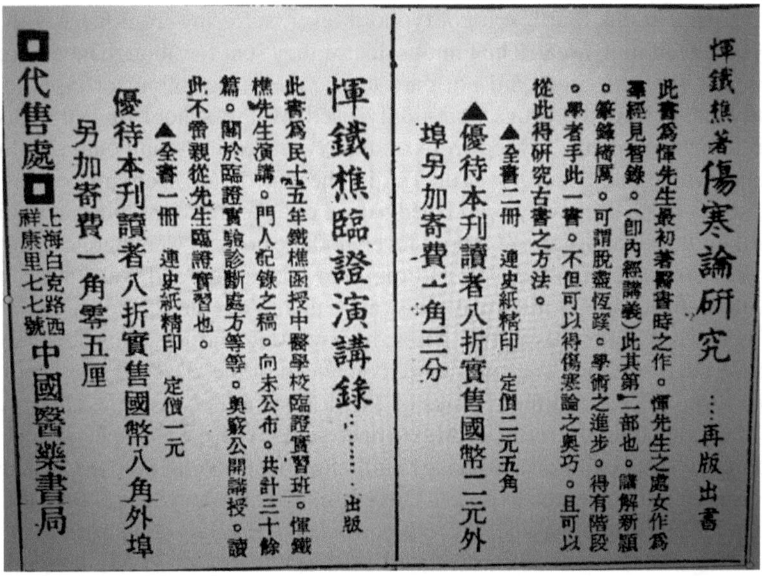

Fig. 6.1 Treatise on typhoid fever and clinical lectures by Yun Tieqiao

and Western medicine of the era,[7] which is an important reason why he occupies a place in the history of the integration of Chinese and Western medicine. His books are also mostly related to Zhongjing theory. He proposed to study ancient medical books and was one of the representatives of typhoid fever in the early Republic of China period (see Fig. 6.1).[8]

However, his preference of using the heavy dose of classic prescriptions was once attacked and questioned.[9] Fortunately, one thing that won him praise in the field of TCM was that he had written a book against Yu Yunxiu's theory. Yu also played a very important role in the medical history of the early Republic of China period, but it was just the opposite of Yun. Yu Yunxiu studied in Japan in his early years. Influenced by the abolition of Japanese Han during the Meiji Restoration, he published *A Frank Confession* in 1916, negating the TCM theory laid down in *Internal Canon of*

[7] All his works are mainly found in the Pharmaceutical Medical Series of (1928), including the 25 kinds of books such as *Collection of Medicine, The General Discussion of Medicine, The Wisdom of Experts, Research on the Treatise of Typhoid Fever, Understandings of Febrile Diseases, Febrile Diseases, Physiological Neologisms, The Development of Pulse, Introduction to Pathology, Theories of Pathology, Clinical Notes, Clinical Lectures, Selected Notes on the Supplemented Prescriptions of Golden Treatise, On Rheumatic Distention, Updated Pediatrics, A Survey of Gynaecology, On Medications, Summary of Symptoms of 12 Meridians, Pathological Treatment of Nervous System, Train of Thoughts, Notes on Febrile Diseases, Pharmaceutical Records.* He also had many translated novels, 20 issues of *Tieqiao Medical Monthly and a volume of Documents between the National Medical College and Yun Tieqiao.* See Zhen Zhiya (ed.), *A Brief History of Chinese Medicine*, Taipei: Zhiyin Press, 2003, p. 210.

[8] From the book advertisement of *Spring and Autumn of the Medical World*, 1936 (120), p. 2.

[9] This interesting and enlightening story comes from Chen Cunren: *My Medical Career*, pp. 13–14.

Medicine, which was hated by the Chinese medicine community. He was one of the anti-Chinese medicine leading figures in the early Republic of China period, and was also the general representative of the TCM abolition school at that time.[10] Yun, who wrote *The Wisdom of Experts* in 1922 and *Research on Typhoid Fever* the following year, proposed feasible reforms, explaining the misunderstandings of TCM and the aggressive words in *A Frank Confession*, which was one of the first challengers in the field of TCM to come forward and respond to Yu.[11]

If we think about Yun Tieqiao's remarks, we can see that Chinese and Western medicine were more than just being involved in controversies. He was not totally contemptuous of Yu Yunxiu's remarks as his profound criticism was exactly what made him believe that Yu Yunxiu had made great efforts in his study of *Internal Canon of Medicine*. He said, "Mr. Yu Junyun wrote *A Frank Confession* as a Western medicine doctor, and his knowledge of *Internal Canon of Medicine* is many times that of ordinary TCM doctors. An admirable scholar indeed!"[12] Researchers of medical history used to think from the perspective of "conflict between TCM and Western medicine". The conflict must have existed, but many attacks on Western medicine had not led to the reflection or reform of their own TCM academia. Moreover, just listing the theoretical views of each TCM doctors did not seem to highlight the close relationship between the real social life (such as the interaction between doctors and patients, the culture of daily medical life) and academic development at the time.

Yun Tieqiao believed that there was a "surging view" of Western medicine. However, those referring to Western medicine theories in the field of TCM were only "one branch, one leaf". A number of people under the banner of "preserving the quintessence of the nation" could not produce anything convincing.[13] According to his example, TCM should not just "fight back". Whether there could be more active reform and introspection was the key to the continued development of TCM. Moreover, the conservatism and retrogression in the field of TCM did not occur overnight, he said:

After the spread of Western learning to the East, Western medicine doctors made great strides forward, and TCM doctors stayed stagnant. Some people were eager to learn, but they didn't know where to start, so they either abandoned their medical career and went to school, or tried some sophistry... In short, since ancient times, no fundamental solution has been found in Chinese medicine works. In this case, Chinese people tend to resort to the ancients rather than go after innovation. A *Frank Confession* came into being in this context.[14]

---

[10] Zu Shuxian, *Research and Criticism of Yu Yunxiu's TCM*, Hefei: Anhui University, 2006.

[11] Jia Dedao, *Proceedings on TCM*, pp. 318–323. For this period of history, see Zhao Hongjun, *The History of Modern Debate between TCM and Western Medicine*, Shijiazhuang: Hebei Branch of Integrated TCM and Western Medicine Research Association, 1983, Deng Tietao & Cheng Zhifan (ed.), *General History of Chinese Medicine Modern History*, Op. cit; Deng Tietao (ed.), *Modern History of TCM*.

[12] Yun Tieqiao, *The Wisdom of Experts, Consultations to 'A Frank Confession'*, Taipei: Huading Publishing House, 1988, Vol. 3, p. 66.

[13] Yun Tieqiao, *Research on the Treatise of Typhoid Fever. General Introduction*, pp. 1–2.

[14] Yun Tieqiao, *The Wisdom of Experts, Consultations to 'A Frank Confession'*, pp. 66–67.

Yun believed that TCM had been questioned in the new era. If the only option for TCM to have was just "respecting the ancient" or "believing in the ancient", the TCM academic development was bound to be doomed. Sometimes the problem of TCM was not only the problem of its own academic development, but also the problem of the society, he added:

Recently, TCM witnessed its darkest era, and almost nine out ten people were totally unaware of what *Internal Canon of Medicine* was. One must have the common sense about different areas of science before being well versed in one particular area. It is true for westerner as well as for Chinese. Therefore, the "Golden Prescription" in *The Great Medical Practice* must be deeply rooted in the rules of heaven. *Five Classics,* intellect, history, astronomy, and Yi-ology are all what a doctor needs to pursue. It is particularly important for doctors to know *Tactful Strategies, Basic Inquiries, Sutra of Acupuncture, Typhoid Fever, Golden Treatise. Tactful Strategies* and *Basic Inquiries* have been taken as the unique learning all over the country during my whole life. No one can tell why. At the age of 20, one would be befuddled in the reading of *Internal Canon of Medicine, Classics on Medical Problems, Cavitation* and *On Qi Fu Acupoint,* not only being challenged by their complexity, but also wonder how all the different meridians can be so organized and unified. Inquiring to the old doctors, they often just shook their heads for not knowing. Some medical practitioners regarded *Ye Tianshi's Medical Cases* and *A Study on the Analysis on Febrile Diseases* as the secret sutra, read it, found it as incomprehensible as *Internal Canon of Medicine*, and then quit. After the reform movement of 1898, the Chinese classes at school occasionally involved five elements, which was scolded by teachers. From then on, TCM became a taboo, and it was a shame for ever having any TCM treatment. I know that thousands of Chinese people have shared this experience.[15]

The status of TCM had been deteriorating, and there were few successors. Many doctors were unable to tell the truth in the classics, and even senior doctors were not very clear about the theory of TCM. Impacted by the general social cognition, the theory of TCM had become a "relic" that does not conform to the trend of the times and was almost eliminated because no one was willing to discuss it. The situation of TCM can be imagined with these internal and external social pressures.[16]

In the new era, TCM must learn the strengths of Western medicine and face the west bravely. Yun said, "The assimilation of TCM and Western medicine should be improved by influence, not conquest".[17] Yun regarded the opposition of some Western medicine to TCM as the driving force for the improvement of TCM, which was the positive side of his remarks. He continued to appeal: "The opposition of Western medicine is not to be worried. All academic progress happens in adversity, not in prosperity. There should be many twists and turns. The opposition of Western

[15] Yun Tieqiao, *The Wisdom of Experts, Consultations to 'A Frank Confession'*, p. 66.

[16] The abolition of TCM, prostitution and opium were once regarded as the three major problems in modern Chinese society. See Deng Tietao (ed.), *Modern History of TCM*, Compiler's Introductions, p. 1.

[17] *Tieqiao Medical Monthly*, Vol. 2, 1935 (02), p. 1.; Fan Boqun, *From Lu Xun's Switching from Medicine to Literature to Yun Tieqiao's Switching from Literature to Medicine—the Theory of Yun Tieqiao*, p. 25.

medicine to TCM is due to its own corruption leading to its doom".[18] Yun believed that the value of Chinese medicine lies in its prescriptions, which can play a significant role in treatment, but it can only be called an effective "empirical prescription". It was criticized for not being clearly standardized by any academic theory, leading to the lamentation as "tens of millions of prescriptions turning out to be no prescription". It is truly an urgent task to study pathology and TCM theory.[19]

Yun Tieqiao did not think that Western medicine was completely undesirable, or that Western medicine viewed the encountering of Chinese and Western medicine from the perspective of colonial medicine as an "invader", just like those who believed in the departmentalism of TCM.[20] Same as Angela Ki Che Leung's view, modern TCM is actually the best example for us to be free of the colonial historical view and think about the impact of Western medical science and technology on China.[21] For example, Yun Tieqiao believed that Western medicine could play a role in interpreting, revising and correcting TCM ancient books, which is significant in the new era. He said, "Even Zhongjing should lend an ear to it if he were reborn".[22]

Furthermore, though the integration and conflict between TCM and Western medicine was an important topic in the medical community, the integration of TCM and Western medicine was not "a matter of using one or two kinds of Western medicine or a few Western medicine terms".[23] The views of a person should be understood in the great dynamic era. In discussing the history of the integration of TCM and Western medicine in the early Republic of China period, there were many views from different perspectives in the field of TCM besides the binary or opposing standpoints of "TCM verses Western medicine". The real focus should be on how Western medicine can promote the introspection and expression of TCM before checking what was left or changed in TCM.

Yun Tieqiao obviously felt that the TCM community was too concerned about the content of Western medicine knowledge, and was anxious to learn Western

[18] *Tieqiao Medical Monthly*, Vol. 2, 1935 (02), p. 1.

[19] *Tieqiao Medical Monthly*, Vol. 1, 1935 (01), p. 3.

[20] For the introduction to colonial medicine and postcolonial medicine, see David Arnold, translated by Jiang Zhushan, Medicine and Colonialism, Wu Jialing, Fu Dawei and Sean Hsiang-Lin Lei (eds.), *Science and Technology Yearns for Society—STS Reader I*, pp. 183–217; Li Shangren, Medicine, Imperialism and Modernity: Introduction to the Topic, *Taiwan Social Research Quarterly*, 2004 (54), pp. 1–16. For the research transference from colonial historical views to regional and alien cultural transmission, as well as the localization of (western) science and technology, see Warwick Anderson, Postcolonial Histories of Medicine, in Frank Huisman and John Harley Warner (eds.), *Locating Medical History: The Stories and Their Meanings,* Baltimore: Johns Hopkins University. Press, 2004, pp. 286–306. And Postcolonial Technoscience, *Social Studies of Science*, 2002 (32), pp. 643–658.

[21] Angela Ki Che Leung, Medical History and China's "Modernity", *China Social History Review,* 2007(08), p. 3.

[22] Yun Tieqiao, *Research on Typhoid Fever. The Difficulty of Mutual Proof between Chinese and Western Pathology*, Vol. 3, p. 51.

[23] Yun Tieqiao, *Research on Typhoid Fever. The Difficulty of Mutual Proof between Chinese and Western Pathology*, Vol. 3, p. 52.

medicine in terms of treatment methods. In response to Zhang Xichun's discussion[24] in the *Records of Western Medicine Reference*, he believed that: "Some TCM doctors claimed they can take advantage of Western medicine in TCM practices by using thermometers and enemas, referring to stroke as cerebral congestion, and convulsion as meningitis. It would be no more than a facade that has nothing to do with reform".[25] It can be seen that Yun had high requirements for the reference to the West by even pointing to the risk of changing and redefining the basic theory of TCM. Of course, he was quite different from Zhang. He held himself as not being well read in Western medicine and not daring enough to use Western medicine at will; his real strength was still in his constant writing and educating the new TCM doctors, just as what he used to be when being a writer of literature.

He tried twice to found the correspondence school of TCM. In 1925, he first founded "Tieqiao Correspondence School of TCM", with more than 600 graduates. It was closed in 1928 due to the opposition of some conservatives. At that time, the education of TCM doctors in the name of "school" must be approved by the government, otherwise it would be easily stopped. In 1933, he founded "Tieqiao Correspondence Medical Firm", and the number of employees increased from 364 in 1933 to 753 in 1936. In order to cooperate with correspondence teaching, he also set up *Tieqiao Medical Monthly* in 1934, which lasted till 1936. His school was quite successful. One of the students' father was an old TCM doctor. After reading his son's textbook *Yun's Correspondence Handouts* used in the school, he took the initiative to write to Yun, saying that he was "a man of great talent, a well learned doctor knowledgeable in both TCM and Western medicine". He said, "After reading medical books for 20 years, I am still perplexed with many problems that by no means could be solved. After reading the *Handouts*, I feel it was like finding a light in the dark, being guided in the right direction".[26] Many of Yun's works have become his textbooks, which shows that Yun was good at discussing difficult classical medical theories in understandable words in the new era.

Based on the above, this chapter has three problematique: the author once analyzed Tang Zonghai (1851–1897), the first TCM doctor who carried out the "integration of TCM and Western medicine".[27] As a representative of the integration of TCM and Western medicine in the early Republic of China period, Yun Tieqiao also deserves attention. This chapter attempts to trace Yun's theoretical core, as well as the differences and a new focus of the discussion between Chinese and Western medicine in the late Qing Dynasty. The history of modern Chinese and Western medicine is

---

[24] For the research of Zhang Xichun, see Wu Yunbo, A Review of Zhang Xichun's Thought of Connecting China and the West, *Journal of Chinese Medical History*, Vol. 14, 1984 (01), pp. 16–18; ZhaoHongjun, Annals of Zhang Xichun, *Journal of Chinese Medical History*, Vol. 21, 1991 (04), pp. 214–218.

[25] Yun Tieqiao, *Research on Typhoid Fever. The Difficulty of Mutual Proof between Chinese and Western Pathology*, Vol. 3, p. 52.

[26] Fan Boqun, *From Lu Xun's Switching from Medicine to Literature to Yun Tieqiao's Switching from Literature to Medicine—the Theory of Yun Tieqiao*, pp. 25–26.

[27] Pi Kuoli, *Body View and Ideological Transformation of Modern TCM—Tang Zonghai and the Era of Convergence of TCM and Western Medicine.*

mostly in the form of debate, and the integration of western theory has only been confirmed in a few knowledgeable views of TCM doctors. Can we sort out the development track that not only highlights the controversial issues, but also reflects the dialogue between China and the West? Finally, the difficulties faced by TCM at that time were discussed by Yun. Bacteriology was only one of them. From the historical perspective of febrile diseases, TCM faced a variety of academic problems, internal and external, and it had more interactive objects than just Western medicine. This chapter intends to explore the possibilities for TCM to reflect on the direction of academic development at that time.[28]

6.3 Seeking Inspiration from Ancient Medical Books—Reading and the Redefinition of Clinical Symptoms

The construction of medical theory and effective treatment methods are the problems of two different levels. The flaw of TCM development in the early Republic of China period obviously lied in the inability to convince those educated in science and Western medicine. When it comes to the academic debate between Chinese and Western medicine, Yun Tieqiao did think that Yu Yunxiu, who was anti-Chinese medicine, was picking on TCM on purpose. On the contrary, he believed that the theory of classical Chinese medicine was ambiguous, and it would be eventually criticized by Western medicine in the future even if no one doubted it. So, what tenable principles can TCM come up with in the communication with Western medicine? Yun made the comments based on the performance of most TCM doctors: "Few knew the truth of Chinese medicine, though many knew its efficacy. That is, even a quack would know a few effective prescriptions".[29] Those who were qualified to be called "doctors" did have some secret recipes that could heal. However, few people knew the real theory of TCM, nor the theory that can be put forward for discussion. He believed that "those who cannot read, or have no idea of theories except boasting of their 'experiences' can do nothing in curing diseases but to deceive themselves and

[28] Sean Hsiang-Lin Lei has a clear understanding of the debate and conflict between TCM and Western medicine, the interaction between the definition of disease and the "health concept" of the state and individuals in this period. For reference: Responsible Doctors and Patients with Faith—the Debate between Chinese and Western Medicine and the Transformation of the Relationship between Doctors and Patients during the Period of the Republic of China period, *New Historiography* 14.1 (2003), pp. 45–96; Why Hygiene Is Not Protecting Life—Alternative Hygiene, Self Being and Diseases in the Period of the Republic of China Period, *Taiwan Social Research Quarterly,* (2004.54), pp. 17–59;Sean Hsiang-lin Lei, *When Chinese Medicine Encountered the State:1910–1949*, PhD. University of Chicago.1999. For the transfer standard of the definition of diseases in TCM and Western medicine, see Bridie Andrews, Tuberculosis and the Assimilation of German Theory in China, 1895–1937, *Journal of the History of Medicine and Allied Sciences,* 1007(52), pp. 114–155.

[29] Yun Tieqiao, Ways to Improve TCM in the Future, *Physiological Neologisms*, Vol. 1, Taipei: Huading Press, 1988, p. 7.

others".[30] Reading is as important as clinical experiences. Clinical treatment would have no support without the book knowledge. At that time, the absolute standard of "experience" was prevalent in TCM practice. The TCM doctors, no matter those who became doctors through self-study or those who learned from their teachers, knew little about the principles of TCM.[31] The problem is just like what Yun said: there had been a lack of clarified explanations of TCM theory in physiology and pathology, including many terms. Taking TCM education as an example, teachers couldn't explain these difficult theories in the textbooks, and students were at a loss, and they could only muddle through this puzzle.[32] From the perspective of academic development, this rough inheritance will certainly have problems. So, how to improve it? Yun Tieqiao insisted that the development of TCM, in short, should be based on *Internal Canon of Medicine* and *Treatise on Typhoid Fever*, with reference to Western theories. He once purchased more than 20 works on typhoid fever from antique dealers, and believed that most of what Japanese medicine said was clear and better than what Chinese doctors said. However, he felt it was a pity that neither Chinese nor Japanese doctors who treated typhoid fever had ever discussed the inheritance relationship and knowledge system of *Internal Canon of Medicine* and *Treatise on Typhoid Fever*.[33]

Of course, the reason is that there are many difficulties in reading classical medical theories,[34] he said:

> There are some Western medical practitioners reading Chinese medical books, and many of them are my friends. However, Chinese medicine books are extremely difficult to understand and many of them were written after the Jin and Yuan Dynasties. My limited reading only covered dozens of this kind. However, it is enough for me to come to the generalization that they are full of nonsense with nothing worthwhile to use. The best books can be *Tactful Strategies* and *Basic Inquiries* from as early as the Song Dynasty, as well as *Internal Canon of Medicine* and *Typhoid Fever* after that. But *Internal Canon of Medicine* is all about Yin and Yang or five elements, while *Typhoid Fever* is of ancient style with a lot of erroneous words, plus it was confusing with different disorganized annotations. It's hard to believe that this incomplete old book can cope with ever-changing diseases. The six meridians in

---

[30] Yun Tieqiao, Neurolytic Relief Function, *Physiological Neologisms*, Vol. 3, p. 29.

[31] Sean Hsiang-Lin Lei had a good explanation for the problem of "experience". He commented that with all TCM's emphasis on "experience", when Western scientific medicine became an opponent that TCM had to face, the meaning of "experience" became a new term to be tested by Western science. It was no longer the so-called "practical" experience of ancient medicine. TCM must think about the problems and new challenges when its traditional "experiences" were being tested. See Sean Hsiang-lin Lei, *How did Chinese Medicine Become Experiential? The Political Epistemology of Jingyan, Positions: East Asian Culture Critique,*2002 (10:2), pp. 333–364.

[32] Yun Tieqiao, *Understandings of Febrile Diseases,* Taipei: Huading Publishing House, 1988, Vol. 2, p. 13.

[33] Yun Tieqiao, *Research on Typhoid Fever*, Preface, pp. 1–2.

[34] Pi Kuoli, The History of Exogenous Febrile Diseases in the Qing Dynasty—the Typhoid Fever Vs. Febrile Diseases and the Interpretation of the TCM History, included in the Office of Life and Medical History Research (ed.), *A New Theory of Chinese History. Medical History*, Taipei: Lianjing Publishing House, 2015, pp. 475–526. The content involves the differences between the reading of medical works and the actual operation technology of doctors in the Ming and Qing Dynasties.

> *Typhoid Fever* are particularly difficult to understand. It took a lot of time for readers to deal with its verbal complexities and they ended up in causing many misunderstandings, which is the case mentioned in the first volume of my book that famous doctors could not pass on their skills. Today, Western medical practitioners who volunteer to pursue Chinese ancient studies are mostly Europeanized, even though they are good at Chinese literature. Reading old Chinese books with a Europeanized brain is no other than to find order from the disorder. The five elements in *Internal Canon of Medicine* and the six meridians in the *Typhoid Fever* are incomprehensible for them, resulting in scandals and accusations from the arrogant medical practitioners When the five elements cannot be explained, the six meridians cannot be rationalized,[35] it is unlikely for the defense to be grounded.

From this earnest appeal, it can be seen that the texts of classical medical books is difficult, which put generations of TCM doctors at a loss. Among numerous medical books after the Jin and Yuan Dynasties, only a few of them were good. This view is quite consistent with Tang Zonghai's attitude of advocating antiquity.[36] Another significance is that the classics of TCM are full of puzzling theories of Yin-Yang and the five elements, which is the major reason for the incomprehension and attacks from the Western medicine. This shows that Yun no longer believed in TCM as the TCM doctors in the late Qing Dynasty, such as Tang Zonghai, who held that Yin-Yang and five elements contain all the truths.[37]

In this era of increasingly fierce debates between TCM and Western medicine, TCM must first be able to understand its own academic theory and express a set of principles that Western medicine and patients can "understand". Yun Tieqiao said: "The TCM practitioners, who don't know the value of *Tactful Strategies, Basic Inquiries, Typhoid Fever* and *Golden Treatise*, or never read the above four books, or feel at a loss after their reading, dared not use the prescriptions in them nor can use them flexibly according to circumstances."[38] Therefore, Yun stressed that the medical books that must be carefully read are not general prescriptions, but classics that lay out the foundation of TCM theory. This idea coincides with the views of many TCM doctors since the Qing Dynasty.[39] As for the development of the Republic of China period, as mentioned in the previous chapters, it was more or less going in the same direction. In the new era, TCM has to refer to and absorb the theories and

---

[35] Yun Tieqiao, *Research on Typhoid Fever. The Difficulty of Mutual Proof between Chinese and Western Pathology*, Vol. 3, pp. 53–54.

[36] Tang Zonghai once said: "*Internal Canon of Medicine, Classics on Medical Problems* and Zhong Jing's books handed down in the Qin and Han Dynasties are extremely accurate, they are far above Western medicine. "Tang Zonghai, *Five Kinds of Sino-Western Converged Medical Books. Essence of Medical Classics*, Taipei: Lixing Book Company, 1998, Preface, p. 1. For the rest, see Pi Kuoli, *Body View and Ideological Transformation of Modern TCM—Tang Zonghai and the Era of Convergence of TCM and Western Medicine*, Chapter 2.

[37] Tang Zonghai once said, "Although there is the Western medical book *Natural History* it didn't interpret the two words Yin and Yang separately and the governance of each is not defined". For Tang, "Yin-Yang" is not a misleading concept. It is the problem of Western medicine in not being able to understand its theory, rather than the crux caused by the theory of TCM itself. Tang Zonghai, *Five Kinds of Sino-Western Converged Medical Books. Essence of Medical Classics*, Vol. 1, p. 1.

[38] Yun Tieqiao, *The Wisdom of Experts*, Preface, p. 1.

[39] See the previous quoted article: *The Changing Jiangnan Medical Tradition—Modern Plague in Reading and Diagnosis*.

advantages of Western medicine instead of being conservative. He said: "Based on the understanding that the six meridians of *Typhoid Fever* are defined according to the symptoms of the human body, the meridians and acupoints of *Tactful Strategies* were inferred after the treatment of the diseases, it indicates that TCM was established upon the discovery of the origins and the development of diseases, which proves the research value of *Tactful Strategies*, *Basic Inquiries* and *Typhoid Fever. For* the erroneous words, there is a way to sort them out; for the distorted annotations, there is always a standard of correction. The attacks from Western medicine can serve for the improvement of TCM, which turned out to be what I call 'new TCM'."[40] In Yun's view, the basic skill of the practice of new TCM is to be familiar with the Chinese classics while taking references to Western medicine.

Yun Tieqiao's vigorous advocacy represented that TCM did not make enough efforts in reading and interpretation. From his translation and editing work, he was no stranger to Western medicine books. He once mentioned in his works that the Western medicine theory adopted by him comes from the Western medicine book translations published by the Commercial Press, such as the *Complete Book of Internal Medicine*, *Diagnostics*, as well as Professor Thomson's *Outline of Science.*[41] Many Chinese doctors couldn't read their own traditional medical books, let alone having the basic knowledge of Western medicine. They didn't even read any books. The fact that "those who are acquainted with both western books and TCM are down to zero" gave Chinese and Western medicine "no chance for the two theories to connect".[42] This is an interesting statement. In fact, it may highlight the fact that the "integration of TCM and Western medicine" reflects the thinking trend. It was not popular among most doctors, and there was no room for the development of medical knowledge. According to Yun Tieqiao's point of view, the two things that the new TCM should pay attention to were: reading both ancient classic medical books as well as Western medicine theories, and explaining the knowledge of TCM more explicitly so that it can be better understood.

6.4 To Fight Against the Outside, We Must First Settle Inside—The Pernicious Influence of "Ye School"[43] and Its Academic Reflection

From Yun Tieqiao's point of view, there was no academic development of TCM to be proud of at that time. Some of them were just modern doctors who made a living with a little knowledge of TCM. Yun once cited in his medical record that a woman

---

40 Yun Tieqiao, *Research on Typhoid Fever*, Preface, p. 2; Yun Tieqiao, *Research on Typhoid Fever. The Difficulty of Mutual Proof between Chinese and Western Pathology*, Vol. 3, p. 54.

41 Yun Tieqiao, On Glands, *Physiological Neologisms*, Vol. 4, p. 32.

42 Yun Tieqiao, Research on Typhoid Fever. The Difficulty of Mutual Proof between Chinese and Western Pathology, Vol. 3, p. 54.

43 A branch of TCM febrile disease studies founded by Ye Tianshi (1667–1746).

in her 30s, who had fever for more than 20 days with the symptoms of delirium, spasm and coma, sought medical advice from him. Yun found that the doctors she saw before were all famous doctors in Shanghai. One of them gave her more than 20 prescriptions, all of which were dendrobium, which simply robbed the patient who was from a family of no means. Yun Tieqiao thought that what she had was typhoid fever (of TCM). Dendrobium would only keep the fever in her body. It was totally ridiculous to use dendrobium only without a prescription. Later, a child suffering from rash with fever was treated with dendrobium by the same doctor, causing the unconsciousness of the child. Yun Tieqiao clenched his teeth and said, "I hate it so much that I'm ready to punch (him)".[44] The reason why Yun was so angry was related to the debate between typhoid and warm disease schools in the academic development of TCM, as well as their adherence to warm or cold drugs in clinical medication.[45] In other words, the interpretation of the disease caused by the six Qis in TCM did not necessarily involve only bacteriology. The views within the warm disease system was not unified and coordinated before the discussion.

Yun Tieqiao found a situation from his readings: the contents of the classics of TCM were difficult to understand and contradictory, but few doctors had discussed and questioned them. Accordingly, Shanghai, where he practiced, was located in the south of the Yangtze River. The medical market was a scene of "dealing with various warm diseases with fermented soya beans, bean roll and dendrobium",[46] which made Yun very sad. Most doctors followed the policy of using "chilly drugs" (dendrobium) advocated by the school of warm diseases to treat diseases, which caused the repeated mistreatment. What was the script on which these dramas were based? Actually, it was no other than the medical books written by the masters of the warm disease school. Yun said, "For the modern doctors, antelope and rhinoceros horn were used as daily necessities, and dendrobium was used as a safe drug. Regardless of typhoid or warm diseases, sweet and cool agents were mixed in one case. The most hateful thing is that dendrobium was used for the wind warm rash, which led to cough and fever, and eventually caused 90% of acute pneumonia". "The patient did not know the reason, nor did the doctors, and the mistreatment were repeated, all of which were caused by the sin committed by Wu Jutong and Wang Mengying".[47] Wu and Wang

---

[44] Yun Tieqiao, Ms. Jin's Typhoid Case, *Clinical Notes*, Taipei: Huading Publishing House, 1988, pp. 15–16.

[45] Warm disease is basically "heat pathogenic factor", which is treated with the herbs pungent in flavor and cool in property to clearing heat and detoxifying, but typhoid fever is "cold pathogenic factor", and the treatment is mainly pungent in flavor and warm in property, with cassia twigs and ephedra commonly used. For details, see Lu Mingjin, *Febrile Diseases*, Taipei: Zhengzhong Book Company, 1986, pp. 8–9.

[46] Yun Tieqiao, Understandings of Febrile Diseases, Vol. 1, p. 7.

[47] Yun Tieqiao, *Understandings of Febrile Diseases, Vol. 4,* p. 44. Yun Tieqiao may have made some mistakes in his observation. Febrile physicians such as Ye Tianshi did often use rhinoceros horn and antelope horn as important drugs for the treatment of febrile diseases (see (Qing) Ye Tianshi, *On Febrile Disease*, included in Li Shunbao (ed.), *Complete Book of Warm Diseases, Vol. I,* p. 3. However, neither Ye Tianshi nor Wu Tang advocated the use of dendrobium to treat warm diseases in their works, and even rarely added dendrobium to their prescriptions. So Yun Tieqiao's statement is very strange. Maybe doctors at that time really preferred using dendrobium in treating warm

were classified as among the four members of warm disease school, and another leader, Ye Tianshi, was also criticized.

Yun recalled his original intention and persistence when he first studied medicine, and lamented that over the past 15 years, many friends who studied the way of Qi and Huang with him had studied *Treatise on Typhoid Fever* before turning to be the followers of the "Ye Sect", so that "the modern doctors now are all Ye sect". Whenever there was a theory different from them, they attacked it all together.[48] Although Yun hated the "Ye Sect", he affirmed some effective prescriptions invented by Ye Tianshi in treating summer dampness. What he hated was that the Ye Sect had too much of sneaky characteristics. Yun himself did not deliberately want to distinguish between portal factions.[49] However, Yun's words revealed that typhoid and warm diseases did have the tendency of arguing and excluding others due to different academic views. Wasn't Yun involved in it? Doctors in south of the Yangtze River mostly believed in Ye's theory, so it was well known that "the shortcut to be a modern doctor is to be a follower of a book, that is, a disciple of the Ye Sect".[50]

It can be seen from the above discussion that Yun Tieqiao was definitely a physician of the typhoid school if there is a dichotomy between the theory and medication of the typhoid and warm disease school.[51] Basically, he believed that the debate on typhoid and warm diseases was confused by the nonsense of Wu Jutong, Wang Mengying and others. Medical study in the Ming and Qing Dynasties was locked in these two theoretical debates, without any conclusions and progress. "The more you talk about it, the more obscure it is". The more diligent one studied TCM, the less one would get. This situation needs the immediate change, because "as long as warm diseases and typhoid are not well defined, the so-called TCM scholars would eventually learn nothing".[52] Most importantly, the patients were at a loss. The doctors they inquired to could not give clear explanations about the names and prescriptions of the diseases. What they did was just to go through the motions and they obviously couldn't win the trust of their patients. Yun "deeply felt he is obligated to regulate

---

diseases, which could not be proved till after further historical research in the medication context. If the latter is true, it would be too arbitrary to blame Ye and Wang.

[48] Yun Tieqiao, Understandings of Febrile Diseases, Vol. 4, p. 35.

[49] Yun Tieqiao, Treatment of Fever, Febrile Diseases, p. 16, included in *The Wisdom of Experts*, op. cit.

[50] Yun Tieqiao, *Understandings of Febrile Diseases*, Vol. 3, p. 29. The debate about typhoid and warm diseases had been very heated since the Qing Dynasty. See my article: *The Changing Jiangnan Medical Tradition—Modern Epidemics as Reading and Diagnosis.*

[51] Yun Tieqiao followed most of the words of Lu Maoxiu (Jiuzhi, 1818–1886), who was the representative physician attacking the school of warm diseases in the late Qing Dynasty when it was prosperous. He believed that warm diseases were completely included in the typhoid system, and Yun Tieqiao's words were also similar. See Zheng Manqing and Lin Pinshi, *History of Chinese Medicine*, Taipei: Taiwan Commercial Press, 2000, p. 366. Lu Zhi's thoughts on typhoid and warm diseases are mostly included in his medical books. For details, see (Qing)Lu Jiuzhi, Fu Qingzhu &Dai Tianzhang, revised by Qin Bowei & Lin Zhiqing, *Complete Collection of Medical Books in Shibu Room*, Taipei: Wuzhou Publishing House, 1996, Anthology 2 and 6, pp. 36–46, 80–90.

[52] Yun Tieqiao, Understandings of Febrile Diseases, Preface, p. 1.

the names of the diseases". The first step of the plan is to distinguish typhoid and warm diseases.[53]

In South of the Yangtze River, doctors often use warm disease prescriptions, that is, to fight against "hot" diseases with "cool" drugs, which is an unbreakable rule. Yun talked about "the average doctors are afraid to read typhoid books, which is why prescriptions for typhoid were rarely used", and they even advocated the saying that 'there is no typhoid south of the Yangtze River". This was all due to the fact that after Ye Tianshi's medical books were published, "*Treatise on Typhoid* turned to be unheard of", which finally led to the situation that "typhoid was no longer known by the world".[54]

Yun said, "It's said that there is no true typhoid south of the Yangtze River. It's such a joke as they don't know that neither Nanyang nor Changsha belongs to the north".[55] Zhang Zhongjing cannot be regarded as a northern physician, so it is illogical to say that Zhongjing's prescriptions can only treat northern fevers.[56]Therefore, Wu Jutong's saying that "typhoid is the cold wind in the north, and warm disease is the warm wind in the South" is even more wrong.[57]

Yun also talked about his 30-year medical experience. Whenever he encountered the so-called warm diseases, he used typhoid prescriptions, which were "applicable for everyone, everywhere and all cases". All of the patients recovered in ten days.[58] There is no reason why the South should use the prescription for warm diseases.[59]

---

[53] Yun Tieqiao, Understandings of Febrile Diseases, Vol. 1, p. 1.

[54] Yun Tieqiao, *Understandings of Febrile Diseases*, Vol. 3, pp. 24–25.

[55] Yun Tieqiao, Understandings of Febrile Diseases, Vol. 4, p. 36.

[56] Lu Maoxiu also had the similar criticisms over regions, He criticized *Simplified Typhoid Fever* written by Qin Zhizhen (style name Huangshi), a doctor in the Qing Dynasty, and said: "It is said that the use of cinnamon and ephedra in Zhongjing was to cure the northern winter diseases in Hebei and Changsha. This disease was rare in the southeast of Jiangsu and Zhejiang. Therefore, it was divided into North and South and by the four seasons of spring, summer, autumn and winter, which was still the cliche in the Qing Dynasty. It teaches people to use cinnamon and ephedra, which can only be applied to the north in winter, not to the south in spring, summer and autumn. What is the so-called north? Changsha then was also today's Changsha, which is now the Changsha Government of Hunan Province, and is adjacent to Jiangsu and Zhejiang in terms of geography. There is no reason why Zhongjing prescriptions could be applied here rather than in the south of the Yangtze River. The place where Zhang Zhongjing lived was not far from Jiangsu and Zhejiang.So it is not feasible to use the North-South theory to distinguish the boundary between typhoid and warm diseases. This wonderful explanation is included in (Qing) Lu Jiuzhi, Fu Qingzhu, Dai Tianzhang, On Qin Huangshi's Simplified Typhoid Fever, included in *Complete Collection of Medical Books in Shibu Room*, p. 126.

[57] Yun Tieqiao, Understandings of Febrile Diseases, Vol. 2, p. 20.

[58] Yun Tieqiao, Understandings of Febrile Diseases, Vol. 3, p. 29.

[59] In fact, the boundary of south of Yangtze River (Jiangnan) had always been controversial, and is more difficult to define culturally. If we divide the North and the South with the warm or cool orientation in medication, it is only an overview, which is not accurate. To study the history of typhoid and warm disease prescriptions, we should focus on the effectiveness of local implementation and the cultural habits of medication. See Gao Yanyi, translated by Li Zhisheng, *Boudoir Teachers: the Culture of Talented Women in Jiangnan in the Late Ming and Early Qing Dynasties*, Nanjing: Jiangsu People's Publishing House, 2005, p. 24.

This is due to the fact that doctors didn't read *Treatise on Typhoid Fever.* However, *Analysis on Febrile Diseases* and *Ye's Medical Cases*, the books regarded as the standard by Southern doctors, are "evil books", which Yun honestly said that he did not have the patience to test their statements one by one.[60] When it comes to the theories of warm diseases, *Generalizations on Febrile Diseases* by Dai Beishan was the only book Yun Tieqiao praised, for its being simple and clear without many comments on pathology. The downside of it is: if this book is regarded as the only classic, it would have the disadvantage of over using the medication of cool property.[61] It can be seen that Yun didn't think much of the cooler medications of doctors south of the Yangtze River.

How to define "typhoid fever" properly? If the theory of warm diseases is groundless, how can it become a treasure book for doctors in the south of the Yangtze River? According to Yun Tieqiao, name matters. Name correction is needed if a disease is wrongly named. He said:

Warm disease means febrile disease; febrile disease means typhoid fever. When the cold hurts the outermost layer of the body, it causes taiyang disease, and the body temperature reacts by giving off heat, which is fever. There are fevers in spring, summer, autumn and winter. Winter fever is caused by the cold. Taiyang disease is presented with the body temperature gathering on the surface which turns into fever. It is thus said that the harm caused by cold is fever. The winter fever is typhoid, so is spring fever, summer fever and autumn fever. There is the saying: all fevers are typhoid.[62]

To sum up, Yun believed that warm disease is typhoid fever, and the fever in the four seasons basically belongs to "cold". Whether in academia or in the treatment criteria, it should be named "typhoid fever". However, from the perspective of TCM academic development, the warm disease system did exist. It still has a system of its own despite different arguments. After his comparative analysis, Yun said that in addition to the pulse, fever and sweating, the biggest difference between typhoid and warm diseases is:

> The same fever, if it happens in the middle of winter, or in unseasonal cold periods, it must be typhoid fever; if it happens in spring or unseasonal warm periods, it must be a warm disease. If it happens in the high mountains or deep water areas, all heat diseases are likely to be typhoid. In coastal areas, such as Jiangsu and Zhejiang, where the horizontal line in the water is not far from the land, all heat diseases are mostly warm diseases. When the time and place coincide where the disease occurred, the name of a disease can be confirmed and can be treated properly. All factors are related. When the disease varies in times and places, the efficacy is also different.[63]

Therefore, "warm diseases" do exist. If the weather conditions are "unseasonally warm", or in particular geographical locations, the occurrence laws of typhoid or

---

[60] Yun Tieqiao, *Research on Typhoid Fever. Typhoid Disease Types and Transmission of Classics*, Vol. 3, p. 60.

[61] For the above, see Yun Tieqiao, *Understandings of Febrile Diseases,* Vol. 1, pp. 2–3.

[62] Yun Tieqiao, *Understandings of Febrile Diseases*, Vol. 1, p. 8.

[63] Yun Tieqiao, Disease Names, *Febrile Diseases*, pp. 3–4.

warm disease can be seen. In particular, Yun classified diseases by its geographical environment, not for its being north or south, but for its being near mountain or sea, which is indeed different from previous doctors. As long as warm diseases are true, why should the medication of the warm disease system be attacked? Yun made it clear that typhoid, warm disease, damp and warm diseases, summer warmth (heatstroke) and spasm are the five most easily confused warm diseases.[64] Both typhoid and warm diseases are "caused by the cold" so that they still belong to one system. The so-called "warm diseases" in general should be renamed as "typhoid warm diseases" and treated within the typhoid system.[65] Yun concluded:"Typhoid should be subject to the *Treatise on Typhoid Fever*, and so should warm diseases. All ancient prescriptions in the *Treatise on Typhoid Fever*, which use cool property instead of warm property drugs, are prescriptions for treating warm diseases".[66] It can be seen that the southern doctors have doubts about the northern doctors' use of warm property drugs to treat fever. Instead of using warm drugs such as ephedra and cassia twigs, they only used cool herbal medicine to treat fever,[67] and all southern doctors abandoned *Treatise on Typhoid Fever*. Yun went the opposite way and said, "Doctors in Jiangsu and Zhejiang dared not use the typhoid prescription, which had been the way long before today. In fact, the typhoid prescription is extremely authoritative and it is the only therapy for a real typhoid case." "If you really identify a disease as typhoid fever, you can safely and boldly use the typhoid prescription. It lives up to the word of being 'steady'".[68] In Yun's view, typhoid prescription can also cure all the diseases cured by the warm disease prescription which is obviously redundant.

Yun Tieqiao was good at using drugs to treat throat diseases. You might as well see his experience in treating "scarlet fever", which was a newly emerging infectious disease in modern China.[69] John Dudgeon (1837–1901), a Western medicine doctor, once said: "Scarlet fever is a dangerous disease which should be treated quickly rather than taking slow pace. There is no surprise in this. An urgent case would close the throat and cause instant death".[70] It can be seen that the damage is severe. At that time, it was called "measles" in TCM. It mostly refers to strepped throat measles. Yun believed that doctors with the label of being a "throat expert" used "cold medicine", but they lost the skill of "using the pungent agent for activation" in *Treatise on Typhoid Fever* and caused many deaths.[71] Cold medicine can't be "activated". It needs the pungent and warm medicine in *Treatise on Typhoid Fever* to

[64] Yun Tieqiao, Disease Names, *Febrile Diseases*, p. 3.

[65] Yun Tieqiao, Disease Names, *Febrile Diseases*, p. 4.

[66] Yun Tieqiao, Treatment of Febrile Diseases, *Febrile Diseases*, p. 24.

[67] Yun Tieqiao, *Understandings of Febrile Diseases*, Vol. 4, p. 36.

[68] Yun Tieqiao, Treatment of Typhoid Fever, *Febrile Diseases*, p. 16.

[69] For modern laryngeal diseases, see Yu Xinzhong, A Preliminary Study on the Age of the Emergence of Strepped Throat Measles, *Journal of Chinese Medical History*, Vol. 31, 2001 (02), pp. 81–85; Yu Yongyan, A Brief History of Modern Chinese Medicine in the Prevention and Treatment of Diphtheria, *Journal of Chinese Medical History*, Vol. 34, 2004 (02), pp. 79–82.

[70] Dudge, *A Survey of Anatomy*, Guangxu 12th year, 1886, Preface, p. 2.

[71] Yun Tieqiao, Two Kinds of Physical Energy, *Physiological Neologisms*, Vol. 4, p. 36.

be "activated", which makes the sweat flow out of the body and forces the pathogens to withdraw from the body. When the symptoms of sore throat occur, the use of Yin nourishing drugs or cold herbal medicine will not "allow a way for the virus to be expelled", and the throat will become more infected.

He recalled that more than ten years ago, there was a popular medical book among doctors in Shanghai, taking the advice of avoiding "activation" in the treatment of laryngology as a treasure. As a result, it was "a deadly therapy", which was truly a disaster! Yun used such a harsh expression because his experience of using "maxing shigan decoction" in *Treatise on Typhoid Fever* to cure the epidemic told him that "sweating" (activation) of typhoid prescription could alleviate the symptoms of pain. Sweat left in the patient's body will lead to more serious symptoms.[72]

It was unknown as whether this means "sweating" can force germs out of the human body, but judging from Yun's inference, it is likely true. Sweating and bacteria, one is the TCM treatment of fever, and the other is the Western medicine theory introduced into China in modern times. The explanation of the connection between the two can give us a better understanding of Yun Tieqiao's theory, and the shift of the focus of the debate between Chinese and Western medicine in the early Republic of China period.

6.5 Yun Tieqiao's Understanding and Response to Bacteriology

The bacterial theory had been known in China by most doctors in the 1920s. Yu Yunxiu, who was regarded as a "leader of anti TCM", said: "Since the invention of bacteriology, all kinds of pathogens have been caused by bacteria, including tuberculosis, typhoid, larynx, dysentery, cholera, pestis, carbuncle and gangrene, inflammation of viscera and bones. It is the source of suppuration and fever. Most human diseases are caused by bacteria. With the development of bacteriology, fundamental changes have taken place in global health, medical treatment, as well as the theory of physiology and pathology."[73] No one can deny the existence of bacteria which is the foundation for the naming of diseases and the development of all medical and health work. Even Yun Tieqiao did not deny this. He said, "The spread of micro bacteria is everywhere, which is the origin of all kinds of infectious diseases".[74] Moreover, Yun Tieqiao stated openly, "Western medicine can test bacteria in treating diseases,

[72] Yun Tieqiao, Treatment of Febrile Diseases, *Febrile Diseases*, pp. 26–27.

[73] Yu Yunxiu, Chapter 9. Primary Disease-Diarrhea, A Frank Confession, included in *Selected Works on Medical Revolution*, Taipei: Yiwen Publishing House, 1976, p. 123;Yu Yunxiu: *Infectious Diseases*, Preface, p. 1.

[74] Yun Tieqiao, Overview of Western Medicine II, *New Physiological Discourse, Physiological Neologisms*, Vol. 2, p. 13.

but TCM can't, which is its weakness".[75] According to the situation at that time, the weakness of TCM was its lack of knowledge in bacteriology and the technology in testing bacteria. Yun also appealed: "Our medical community should associate the organizations, raise funds to buy instruments, western bacteriology books and anatomical models".[76] From this point of view, Yun was aware of current affairs and adaptable to changes. However, sometimes when the clinical syndrome encounters the problem of identifying diseases, the difference between TCM and Western medicine immediately showed up, which is not just a problem that can be solved by studying the bacteriology of Western medicine.

Yun Tieqiao treated several cases of acute miliary tuberculosis. He was asked to treat two children with Western medicine, which can be the example of integrating TCM and Western medicine in the early Republic of China period. However, as the disease was too advanced and the two children finally died. During such treatment, Yun believed that the disease did have similarities with the taiyang syndrome of typhoid at the beginning.[77] The ordinary "sweat method" could not relieve the symptoms, neither did the typhoid prescription. Yun had to rely on the spirit of "syndrome

---

[75] Yun Tieqiao, TCM and Western Medicine, *Clinical Lectures,* Taipei: Huading Publishing House, 1988, p. 35.

[76] Yun Tieqiao, *Research on Typhoid Fever.* Western Views on *Typhoid Fever*, Vol. 3, p. 56.

[77] Taiyang disease is the first disease in the syndrome differentiation and treatment of the "six meridians" in Zhang Zhongjing's *Treatise on Typhoid Fever*. It is due to the statements that "taiyang syndrome is featured with an irregular pulse, bad headache and sever cold", "taiyang disease with fever, sweating, pathogenic wind and slow pulse are called taiyang disease stroke" (Part I), "taiyang disease with fever or no fever, but definitely with bad cold, body pain, nausea and tight Yin-Yang pulses, is called typhoid" (Part 2) and other comprehensive symptoms. (see (Han) Zhang Zhongjing: Distinguishing the Pulse Syndrome of and Its Treatment, Part I, *Treatise on Typhoid Fever* (Gold Mirror of Medical Forbears Edition), Taipei: Lixing Publishing House, 1985, pp. 1–3, 51–52). The other five meridians are Yangming, Shaoyang, Taiyin, Shaoyin and Jueyin. Based on the syndrome differentiation and treatment of the six meridians, it is established in the book *Treatise on Typhoid Fever*, and its source can be traced back to the discussion in *Basic Inquiries. Febrile Diseases,* such as: "The first day of febrile disease is the day of major Yang when there is a bad headache and a stiff waist; the second day is the day of Yangming which dominates the body, of which the meridian stuffs the nose, extending to the eyes, leading to the increase of temperature in the body, painful eyes, dry nose, and difficulties in lying down. The third day is the day of Shaoyang which dominates the gallbladder, of which the meridian invades the ribs, further to the ears, causing the pain in chest and ribs, as well as deafness. The three Yang meridians are all affected except the viscera, so one can still sweat. The fourth day is a day of Taiyin which spread over the stomach, further reaching the throat, leading to a stuffed stomach and choking. The fifth day is a day of Shaoyin, of which the meridian passes through the kidney and reaches out to the lungs. Its origin is from the tongue, so the mouth is dry. The sixth day is a day of Jueyin, which passes through the Yin organ and was connected to the liver, leading to retracted scrotum when it is stressed. If three Yins and three Yangs, all viscera, Qi and blood are all blocked, it is time for death to occur." This represents the order of transmission and change of a disease in the human body, which is still the reference criterion of clinical syndrome differentiation of TCM until modern times. In short, "six meridians syndrome" is to summarize the various clinical manifestations and pathogenesis changes of exogenous febrile diseases into six categories, so as to facilitate the diagnosis of doctors. Ma Jianzhong, *Diagnostics of TCM,* p. 210;Guo Aichun (ed.), No. 31 of Heat Theory, included in *Interpretations to the Basic Inquiries of the Inner Canon of the Yellow Emperor,* p. 193.

differentiation and treatment" to relieve the discomfort of the patients. The deterioration of the disease was similar to the "Yin-Yang intersection" of death syndrome or the "spasm disease" in TCM.[78] The real spasm should be the "epidemic myelopathy" of Western medicine.[79] There are numerous different definitions. How to solve this problem? Yun couldn't give a definite answer. Many disease names "can't be found in old Chinese books", which may be the reason why Western medicine books should be studied.[80]

Such a dilemma shows that it is difficult for TCM and Western medicine to obtain consistency in the identification of disease names, and the judgment of disease names by TCM is not based on bacteria, which was caught on by those who wanted to abolish TCM. Yu Yunxiu believed that in the TCM classic *Basic Inquiries Counterpart Treatment*, the pathogenic factors invade the human body, reaching the viscera through the skin, sub pulse, collaterals and meridians. This kind of disease differentiation thought that starts from the outside to the inside, from the shallow to the deep, from minor to major, is the well cited classics in TCM disease discussion. However, he criticized that though some diseases began to invade from the skin, "diseases such as typhoid, tuberculosis, diseases of the digestive system, respiratory and urinary organs, as well as carbuncle and gangrene of muscles often enter from the mouth, nose and the lower private parts". The inference of diseases in TCM is full of "laymen's imagination".[81] Facing such criticism, it was very important for TCM to find ways to respond to the bacterial theory.

From Yun Tieqiao's point of view, internal causes (five emotions) and external causes (diet, sex) are often the pathogenic factors that TCM pays most attention to, while Western medicine focuses on external causes, that is, the influence of bacteria.[82] Each of these two ways of observation has their own merits. However, Yun started from "diseases enter through the mouth and nose" in the theory of warm diseases, and believed that "the pathogenic Qi of nature" would invade from people's skin, while "the cold and heat of water and grain" would invade the viscera from the mouth. What can really be introduced into the human body from the mouth and nose belongs to the more infectious cholera "filth" and the "micro bacteria" that infect various epidemics in the air.[83] However, Yun has always believed that "introducing pathogenic Qi from the mouth and nose" in the theory of warm diseases may not be flawless, because of the view that "typhoid enters from the skin is made clear in *Basic Inquiries*, and that it must be the weaknesses within the human body that external infection can take advantage, or there would be no harm done even there is cold".[84] TCM believes that a person with sufficient essence and Qi can resist the

---

[78] Yun Tieqiao, Research on Typhoid Fever, *Doubts on Syndromes*, Vol. 3, pp. 65–68.

[79] Yun Tieqiao, Research on Typhoid Fever, *Epidemic Myelitis and Spasm*, Vol. 3, p. 69.

[80] Yun Tieqiao, Research on Typhoid Fever, *Epidemic Myelitis and Spasm*, Vol. 3, p. 73.

[81] Yu Yunxiu, Progress of Disease No.8, A Frank Confession, included in *Selected Works on Medical Revolution*, p. 121.

[82] Yun Tieqiao, *The Wisdom of Experts Bian Que's Medical Case No. 11*, Vol. 2, p. 40.

[83] Yun Tieqiao, *Understandings of Febrile Diseases*, Vol. 2, p. 20.

[84] Yun Tieqiao, *Understandings of Febrile Diseases*, Vol. 3, p. 22.

invasion of foreign diseases, which is called "stored essence". Yun explained it with the "resistance" and "immunity" of Western medicine:

Upon further thinking, it can be realized that one won't get sick with only external causes without internal causes. During pandemic times when the dead lay all over, there were people free of infection, which is called immunity in Western medicine. For example, those who suffer from throat measles (scarlet fever) will no longer be infected if they recover from the disease. Nevertheless, if one's life style is irregular with no good appetite, one won't have enough vitality to resist external pathogens and would lose the immunity.[85]

In other words, bacteria are not absolutely equal to "disease". The physical condition is not the same for everyone. If the discussion is based on the disease itself, paying attention to the patient's own condition (internal causes) may be closer to the fact than analyzing bacteria or judging the disease by bacteria (external causes).

Western medicine judges diseases by bacteria. Yun Tieqiao believed that the name given by Western medicine were based on the classification of bacteria. "Rod shaped bacteria" was called typhoid; similar warm diseases with "similar bacteria, but a slightly curved shape" was called paratyphoid. What does this mean? Based on his own observation and experience, Yun believed that in terms of the ultimate goal of Western medicine in pursuing accurate disease names, it was impossible to judge what kind of disease it was clinically without blood and bacteria tests. The Japanese translated "typhoid" as the name of a disease, and mixed it up with Chinese "typhoid fever" for explanation soon after it was introduced into China, which was unaware of by neither Chinese doctors nor patients. It was difficult to tell if it was truly "typhoid fever" from the sick. When patients consulted Western medicine, they were often disappointed that Western medicine could not directly determine the name of a disease on the spot. When being questioned by the patients, the Western medicine doctors "were unwilling to resign by playing second fiddles", then turned to "despise the patients for their lack of common sense", and named it typhoid rashly. However, the story was still not over. The patient would choose to go to TCM doctors for diagnosis after seeing Western medicine doctors. However, TCM also had various problems as "echoing others", "lacking ideas" and "having no standard in their treatment or diagnosis". For a patient who had clearly got "wind warmth", they simply let go of the cassia twigs and ephedra prescriptions in *Typhoid Fever*, since it was defined by Western medicine as "typhoid", without knowing that this typhoid is different from the other typhoid fever, As a result, the patients died for this mistreatment.[86]

Another ridicularly situation occurred when Yun Tieqiao was treating a patient. Judging from the symptoms of "vomiting and diarrhea caused by drinking icy water in summer, feeling cold in autumn", it should be heatstroke. The patient complained to him, "The TCM doctor I saw said that I had cholera and it might turn into typhoid". This confused him, as cholera could never turn into typhoid at all, and there was no such strange theory in Chinese nor Western medicine. Thinking about it, Yun finally

[85] Yun Tieqiao, *The Wisdom of Experts Bian Que's Medical Case No. 11*, Vol. 2, p. 40.

[86] Yun Tieqiao, Conclusion, *Febrile Diseases*, p. 34.

realized that the doctor had been wrong in the first step of diagnosing the disease as cholera, and later said it would turn into typhoid, which was most likely due to his recognition that patients would seek the answers and definitions from Western medicine doctors. It was speculated that Western medicine would define it as typhoid, leading to his presumptuous statement that cholera will turn into typhoid, so he could never be wrong.[87] Finally, it was the patient himself, rather than TCM or Western medicine, that caused the death.

The above experience inspired Yun Tieqiao and conveyed him two important messages. First of all, the definition of disease is very important, and the correct judgment of a disease is the primary work of the treatment. The confusion and inconsistency between the names of Chinese and Western medicine caused trouble for doctors and patients in the early Republic of China period. Secondly, it was impossible for doctors to examine bacteria for each disease. He explained the comparison of infectious diseases between Chinese and Western medicine, and believed that: "Warm diseases and typhoid are collectively referred to as fever disease in the *Internal Canon of Medicine*, and acute infectious diseases in the Western medical books".[88] In Western medicine, they are classified as three kinds: typhoid, paratyphoid fever and influenza. Yun believed that the state of fever is most similar to the warm disease of TCM. However, there are more than ten kinds of infectious diseases that also have fever. The actual differences between these fever diseases should lie in the length of the incubation period and the type of fever, but Western medicine believes that the final judgment still depends on the type of bacteria after the test. Is it safe to determine the name of a disease by bacterial test? Yun believed that there are many diseases "are accompanied with fever". Even if the names are defined, such as influenza (severe cold), there are also different types of it such as bronchitis, gastrointestinal or neurological types. If doctors have to do "bacteria test" every time when diagnosing fever, the patients he can see each day would be no more than five. Important as bacteria testing is, it's not the only diagnostic method.[89]

In the treatment of warm diseases, Yun Tieqiao also raised his doubts about the bacterial theory: "It is questionable that the bacterial theory is regarded as an iron clad case by Westerners. I think the symptoms of a disease can also do well in making a diagnosis. The theory of bacteria might be totally out of date after 10 years".[90] Such an "elimination theory" of bacteriology seems too naive today. Why did he have this idea? It was due to his experiences of treating fever diphtheria. He cited the actual treatment as an example to illustrate that when a person suffered from diphtheria with the symptoms of taiyang disease as cited in *Treatise on Typhoid Fever*, he could have it cured by applying the typhoid prescription "Maxing Ganshi Decoction". He concluded: "No matter what kind of bacteria being the cause, taiyang

[87] Yun Tieqiao, Conclusion, *Febrile Diseases*, p. 35.

[88] Yun Tieqiao, *Understandings of Febrile Diseases*, Vol. 1, p. 4.

[89] Yun Tieqiao, *Understandings of Febrile Diseases*, Vol. 1, pp. 4–5.

[90] Yun Tieqiao, Comparison between Internal Canon of Medicine and the Evolution of Western Medicine in 2000 Years, *Physiological Neologisms*, Vol. 2, pp. 20–21.

disease will gradually disappear".[91] This conclusion is applicable to all kinds of warm diseases except tuberculosis. Of course, he maintained that this conclusion may also be overturned, but at least in terms of his clinical experiences, it is generally in line with the facts. If so, it is not the most important thing to judge the type of bacteria.[92]

Yun Tieqiao also believed that Maxing Ganshi Decoction can cure diphtheria within only one day. In terms of the bacteria theory, can this decoction really "sterilize"? Yun maintained that this is not entirely the case, because it can treat any fever with "fever, cold, no sweat" symptoms. As long as the symptoms are removed, no matter whether the fever is typhoid or laryngeal disease, it can be easily cured. However, once "the virus has established its base and made progress", there will be various other symptoms, such as five meridians symptoms in the typhoid fever system of TCM (except taiyang). Generally speaking, as the disease gets worse or the main symptoms change, it is called "transmission of menstruation"[93] in TCM. The classical theory of TCM is used to explain the pathogenic theory of bacteria, that is, "the virus takes the taiyang as the base, the starting point".[94] Most warm diseases can be cured as long as they can be treated with a typhoid formula when taiyang disease occurs. Yun came to this conclusion: "Germs can not survive unless in the conditions of fever, cold and no sweat, which are the main causes of the disease, rather than the presence of micro bacteria".[95]The conclusion of the whole discussion is that bacteria can not represent the characteristics of the disease, so that it should not be used as the standard for establishing the name of a disease.

After all, bacteria can be seen by the naked eye, or by using the instrument, which can not be truer. According to the theory of Western medicine, a fever disease must have a specific pathogen, but Yun Tieqiao thought that even though Western medicine says "different diseases have different bacteria", there are sometimes exceptions. Acute diseases often change, such as the symptoms of severe typhus, which further become typhoid, and finally turn into acute pneumonia or cerebrospinal inflammation. Yun's view that "after the change, this disease is no longer the same disease" is a logical reasoning. However, no matter how the disease changes, its bacteria should be the original cold bacteria. The essence of bacteria remains the same, but the symptoms may change rapidly, so the statement "the name of a disease is based on the type of bacteria" is not absolutely correct, and sometimes it will mislead the judgment of the patient's subsequent condition. It is not necessary for TCM to rush to learn the technology of "bacteria testing".[96] Sometimes bacteria can not reflect the dynamics of the disease, and the symptoms are ever-changing. Just identifying bacteria will not help the accuracy of TCM treatment. Hence comes Yun's saying: "A disease can't be named until after it is ascertained".[97]

---

[91] Yun Tieqiao, *Research on Typhoid Fever. Discussion on Medication*, Vol. 2, p. 39.

[92] Yun Tieqiao, *Research on Typhoid Fever. Discussion on Medication*, Vol. 2, p. 34.

[93] Yun Tieqiao, *General Introduction. Research on Typhoid Fever*, Vol. 1, pp. 28–29.

[94] Yun Tieqiao, *General Introduction. Research on Typhoid Fever*, Vol. 1, p. 30.

[95] Yun Tieqiao, Two Kinds of Physical Energy, *Physiological Neologisms*, Vol. 4, pp. 37–38.

[96] Yun Tieqiao, *Understandings of Febrile Diseases*, Vol. 1, p. 5.

[97] Yun Tieqiao, *Understandings of Febrile Diseases*, Vol. 1, pp. 10–11.

The symptoms of the disease are different in each person, the conditions that will change after treatment are also different, and the real name of the disease can only be judged according to the initial symptoms, which is the key to accurately identify the disease without testing bacteria. The only advantage of studying micro bacteria in TCM is that it can test whether the opinion "the understanding of taiyang disease is equal to the denial of bacteria being the key of a disease" is tenable.[98] For Yun, the technology of "bacteria testing" is another tool that can confirm the classical records of TCM.

Yun Tieqiao affirmed the achievements of Western examination of bacteria and the development of immunology.[99] But after observing the treatment of diphtheria by Western medicine, he said: "The Western treatment of this disease is to clean up the white rot of the throat with sterile cotton first, use serum to kill the throat bacteria in the blood, and then put ice at the back of the head to prevent fever and even the danger of spinal cord inflammation".[100] He also evaluated the cure ratio of serum as a specific drug for this disease: "According to Western medicine books, serum is a specific drug for this disease. The cure period is about six days, and the cure percentage is 75%. However, based on the field investigation I have conducted, it can't be so effective".[101] It can be seen from his report that the serum produced through bacterial testing may not be effective in treating this disease. Then what is the situation of TCM treatment? Yun stated: "Laryngology is a bacterial disease, and it is extremely effective to use apricot gypsum decoction. At the beginning of the dysentery, sweating can also reduce its potential. Most warm diseases have bacteria and can be decomposed in an appropriate period, because sweat is related to bacteria". He believed that the "sweating" of TCM can regulate metabolism and "glands", and the relationship between the physiological functions of various glands and diseases is a new medium for him to explain diseases with reference to Western medicine knowledge.[102] However, he did not explain the relationship between "sweat" and "bacteria" clearly except for taking it as a new discovery.[103] In short, his intention was to reconstruct the scientific and modern method of the classical medical theory on the basis of *Treatise on Typhoid Fever* by turning the Western theory of sterilization to sweating in the treatment of warm diseases. Unfortunately, no further research methods were proposed.

The theory of bacteria also enabled Yun Tieqiao to find a weapon to refute the theory of the warm disease school. Yun Tieqiao maintained that if it is certain that "typhoid" and "warm disease" are collectively referred to as acute infectious diseases,

---

98 Yun Tieqiao, Research on Typhoid Fever, *Epidemic Myelitis and Spasm*, Vol. 3, p. 73.

99 Yun Tieqiao, *Research on Typhoid Fever. Discussion on Medication*, Vol. 2, p. 39.

100 Yun Tieqiao Two Kinds of Physical Energy, *Physiological Neologisms*, Vol. 4, p. 36.

101 Yun Tieqiao, Two Kinds of Physical Energy, *Physiological Neologisms*, Vol. 4, p. 37.

102 Pi Kuoli, From "Tonifying the Kidney" to "Hormone" Therapy: Anti-disease Strategies and Daily Life History during the Republic of China Period, *International Symposium on "Diversity of Daily Life History in China"*, Tianjin: China Social History Research Center, Nankai University, September 26–29, 2011.

103 Yun Tieqiao, Treatment of Typhoid Fever, *Febrile Diseases*, pp. 18–21.

the so-called "incubation period" of acute infectious diseases in Western medicine is no more than 20 days, which just proves the ancient medical theory is wrong in stating "cold virus, hidden under the skin, does not come out in spring, and won't cause disease till after the summer solstice". Furthermore, the statement of Western medicine that all four seasonal infectious diseases will be prevalent can prove that the "hidden pathogens"[104] discussed in the theory of warm diseases is a wrong cognition.[105] The belief in *Treatise on Typhoid Feve*r made him use bacterial theory as a tool to defend his theory. However, it is a pity that he rejected the theory of warm diseases, which inevitably brought him some prejudices. For example, he believed that the "epidemic" mentioned by Wu Youke in the late Ming Dynasty came from the mouth and nose, which was different from the generally so-called warm diseases.[106] He did not go further to sort out the relationship between epidemics and typhoid fever in TCM classics, nor did he try to explain the various possibilities of bacteria and epidemics.

What sounds more fallacious is his thinking that health and epidemic prevention work is unnecessary. Yu Yunxiu once criticized the Chinese people's ignorance of epidemic prevention as follows: "There have been no epidemic prevention policies in this country. People have no knowledge, and doctors give no warnings, of epidemic prevention. When not being infected, people ignore it. They are close to the sick, with their food and clothes mixed up with those of the patients, spit all over the ground with messy feces and urine round, without even being unaware of it. When being infected, it is too late for a doctor to give treatment".[107] It can be seen from Yu's words that epidemic prevention itself is a policy to safeguard health with the idea of preventing "bacterial and viral infection". However, Yun countered this thinking and said, "According to the Western method, inflammation should be diminished,

[104] The theory of hidden pathogenic factor stemmed from the inference that "catching cold in winter will end up with warm disease in spring" stated in *Basis Inquiries. Qis of Nature.* That is, even if winter cold causes harm, one would not contract warm disease in spring if the body has sufficient vitality (also known as "hidden essence"). If not, the pathogenic factor of winter will be able to attack the human body in spring, which is called hidden pathogenic factor (warm disease). Relatively, "activation" and "hidden pathogenic factor" are the two most important and common types of warm disease. Being sick immediately after the invasion of pathogenic factor is "activation"; when the pathogenic Qi gets into the body without showing up for a while, it is called "hidden pathogenic factor". The former is also known as "new epidemic warm disease", or "exogenous warm disease";the latter is called "hidden Qi warm disease".So "hidden pathogenic factor" is also called "hidden Qi". For details, see *Research on Warm Diseases,* Taipei: Qiye Book Company, 1990, pp. 54–58.

[105] Yun Tieqiao, *Research on Typhoid Fever. The Incubation Period Proves the Fallacy of TCM's Not Being Ill*, Vol. 3, pp. 56–57.

[106] Yun Tieqiao, *Research on Typhoid Fever. The Incubation Period Proves the Fallacy of TCM's Not Being Ill* Vol. 3, p. 58.

[107] Yu Yunxiu, Admonition to Patients. Lack of Prevention, *Selected Works on Medical Revolution,* pp. 138–139.

bacteria be killed, infection be isolated and kept clean. It might be helpful in curing the disease, but its effect is very limited, and most of the results are not so desirable".[108]

From the perspective of antibacterial and epidemic prevention, it is simply unrealistic to view it from Yun's words. The overall health and epidemic prevention work may have achieved limited results in the early Republic of China period, but we can't measure the situation of the time with today's epidemic prevention work. The mentality of the people, the extent of cooperation and the implementation of the government may need to be studied and assessed.[109] As far as this is concerned, his view is:

> However, many Chinese can hardly follow suit, and it is particularly not easy for the poor to do so. For the most infectious diseases, the virus is spread in the air, which turns to be the vector of the disease, making it impossible to prevent. After all, there must be internal causes first, and then the bacteria can run rampant. Those who are immunized for life will not be infected even if they are by the sickbeds every day. Ordinary people who suffer from this disease (measles) once can be immunized for at least ten years. I think it is more feasible to study from the perspective of treatment. If the pathogens are clarified and the treatment is perfect, the infected are no more than being vaccinated. While in terms of prevention, it is definitely a work of more efforts with less effects, much ado about nothing.[110]

As for the methods of Western medicine to prevent infection, such as ward isolation or disinfection of patients' clothes, Yun held that it was unlikely for ordinary people to do a perfect job, and it was very complicated, especially for poor people. Some diseases have a long immune period after recovery. It is thus better to study the treatment methods rather than committing to prevention.[111] Moreover, strong immunity will prevent the infection of germs. Instead of constantly focusing on germs, it is better to take care of one's body first. Talking about the recuperation of diseases, Yun Tieqiao said that "food intake deserves the attention for all febrile disease prevention, which is the lesson of *Internal Canon of Medicine*". However, Westerners believe that as long as it is not a gastrointestinal disease, food is not the issue. In addition, Western medicine attaches importance to "sterilization", which does not have any rules for food, nor pays much attention to problems such as the conflict between the patients' constitution and food attributes. Therefore, the name of a disease determined by Western medicine is meaningless. Patients often have transferred symptoms and concurrent symptoms in its treatment because they do not control what they eat. Even if the name of a disease is determined, they still cannot

---

108 Yun Tieqiao, Influenza and Pertussis, *Theories of Pathology*, Taipei: Huading Publishing House, 1988, p. 24.

109 The epidemic prevention in some regions is different from the nationwide practice. It is too early to evaluate the epidemic prevention work in China at present. There have been some research results on local health work, such as Tianjin.Ruth Rogaski, *Hygienic Modernity: Meanings of Health and Disease in Treaty-port China,* Berkeley; London: University of California Press, c2004; Shanghai: Peng Shanmin, *Public Health and Shanghai Urban Civilization (1898–1949),* Shanghai: Shanghai People's Publishing House, 2007. There are also some fragmentary medical and health historical events found in series of local health chronicles, which will not be listed one by one.

110 Yun Tieqiao, Two Kinds of Physical Energy, *Physiological Neologisms*, Vol. 4, pp. 36–37.

111 About recuperation and prevention, in fact, TCM did not ignore it in the early Republic of China period. See the last two chapters for details.

be treated in the same way, which is the so-called "astray leads to astray".[112] From the perspective of TCM, this is one of the shortcomings of naming a disease based on bacteria.

6.6 Discussion on the Definition of Disease Names in TCM and Western Medicine

In the early Republic of China period, there had been a more thorough discussion on the significance of disease names to doctors and patients. By supplementing Yun's views, this chapter briefly discusses the controversy on Qi among the schools behind "diseases" during the Republic of China period. Yun Tieqiao said that when he was treating his daughter Huinan's illness, he went to a Western medicine doctor Lu Juxuan for treatment. Lu determined that his daughter had typhoid, but Yun diagnosed it as taiyang (disease), with the syndrome (severe fever, no sweat) consistent with those in the *Treatise on Typhoid Fever*. The Western medicine doctor wanted to use ice on her for three weeks to bring down the fever, but Yun's wife thought that she was too young of a child to stand it. Yun had to treat it himself. As he had never been involved in Western medicine, he was wondering if the typhoid in Western medicine was the same disease as the typhoid fever in TCM and if they could be treated in the same way? A treatment was needed immediately. Yun Tieqiao tried to use the prescription of "Gegen Qinlian Decoction plus 3.5g of ephedra" to treat his daughter. As a result, after taking two doses of it, which was "fever relieving and refreshing", his daughter clamored to drink milk, and her appetite also recovered. Later Doctor Lu was sent to see her again. He was surprised to find that the typhoid had been cured. Since then, Yun reflected on his contradictory and ridiculous thoughts of "feeling ashamed to say that he had read Chinese medical books" in the past, and believed that "Chinese medicine is not completely useless", which opened the door for his theory of comparing the names of Chinese and Western diseases.[113]

For some Western medicine doctors, TCM was incapable of discussing the names of the diseases in the context of "typhoid fever" in TCM. Yu Yunxiu once harshly criticized the theory that the early Republic of China period had entered the era of science. The theories of diseases by so-called old (Chinese) medicine "cannot be proved even if someone tries to, has nothing to prove even it can be proved. However, today's medicine has become a practical science and all statements need to be proved, otherwise it has no credibility".[114]

---

112 Yun Tieqiao, Influenza and Pertussis, *Theories of Pathology*, p. 23.

113 For the above examples, see Yun Tieqiao, *Research on Typhoid Fever—Proofs for the Non-passing Prescriptions of Taiyang Disease Therapy*, Vol. 4, pp. 76–77.

114 Yu Yunxiu, Chapter 9. Primary Disease-Diarrhea, A Frank Confession, included in *Selected Works on Medical Revolution*, p. 126.

He didn't think that TCM doctors could judge diseases, nor prove the theory they had learned. Tang Erhe (1878–1940),[115] a major anti TCM figure, said: "I venture to say that there are no grounds in TCM at all when it comes to medical theory. To put it in an easiest way, there is no possibility for TCM doctors to 'discuss diseases', let alone treat diseases'".[116] In this regard, the anti TCM school believed that TCM was totally incapable of explaining and defining diseases.

During early Republic of China period, patients took the initiative to "combine Chinese and Western medicine" when seeking treatment. In Yu Yunxiu's view, this is the patient's "intolerance" of the treatment process, and the delusion of "expecting a seven-year illness be cured by one treatment" is a sign of lacking confidence in doctors.[117] According to Yun Tieqiao, patients should not be blamed too much. He recalled that decades ago, he met an old TCM doctor who used a large number of aconite to cure stroke, as well as typhoid, febrile, spasmodic, summer heat and many other diseases. He felt puzzled and thought that the old TCM doctor must be a hidden expert. In addition to asking him for advice, he later recommended all patients who could not be cured to the old TCM doctor. As a result, the patients could "hardly survive" with his treatment. The son of Yun's colleague of the Commercial Press got the fever and went to the old TCM doctor for treatment. It was the same prescription of aconite. The patient took six or seven doses in a row, and his gums bled so much and even his quilt was soaked. Needless to say, the patient lost his life! The wife of Yun's other friend Shen, got "interstitial malaria". They went to the old TCM doctor more than 40 times in a row and took more than 200 prescriptions with aconite as the main ingredient. Just because Shen thought that average doctors did not dare to use aconite, he took it for granted that this old TCM doctor was a master of medicine. What was the result? His wife also died. Yun was in deep distress.[118]

This story reveals an interesting topic in the history of medicine. It shows us how doctors used special drugs to gain medical fame in the early Republic of China period, how to operate and sell their medical skills, and the doctor-patient relationship in the early Republic of China period, in which patients were greatly deceived. In addition, it can also be found that doctors were accustomed to using certain drugs to treat many tough diseases. Was it due to the doctor's not knowing the disease, or his using aconite on purpose just to win a good name? The author believed in

---

[115] Tang Erhe, formerly known as Nai, style named Tiaoding or Erhe, a native of Hangzhou, Zhejiang Province. He studied in Japan in 1907 and entered Kanazawa Medical School. After graduation, he went to Berlin University in Germany to study medicine. Returning to China in 1910, he served as a counsellor of the Advisory Board. He once served as the vice president and physician of Zhejiang Hospital, as well as the school doctor of Zhejiang University. In addition, he once served as the president of Beijing Medical College, director of the Academic Department of the Union Medical College, President of the Medical Association of the Republic of China Period, etc. His works include *Histology, Essence of Biology, Psychiatry, Parasitology*, etc. He had rich experiences in Western medicine. For details, see Xu Youchun (ed.), *A Dictionary of Figures of the Republic of China Period*, Shijiazhuang: Hebei People's Publishing House, 1991, p. 1188.

[116] Quoted from *The History of Modern Debate between TCM and Western Medicine*, pp. 118–120.

[117] Yu Yunxiu, Admonish the Patients. Being Unbearable, *Selected Works on Medical Revolution,* pp. 137–138.

[118] Yun Tieqiao, Disease Names, *Febrile Diseases*, pp. 6–7.

the former, because there was no medicine that can deal with all diseases, which TCM had never discussed. It can be seen that this quack just wanted to win a good name with aconite without being able to define diseases at all. Then, for patients who were at a loss, what if they tried another doctor? Yun said, "All crows under the sun are black. Particularly for doctors, this happened almost several times a month. As a result, it was a business to avoid the challenges by dealing with the cases with their verbal skills. No one has ever discussed it in detail about the twists and turns to inform the public".[119] Yun's experience really highlighted the patients' sufferings from the names of the diseases, by not being able to figure out what diseases they were suffering from.

Not only patients wanted to combine Chinese and Western medicine, the TCM doctors in the early republic China also wanted to have the "TCM with reference to Western medicine".[120] There were two difficulties in judging "disease names" and "pathological changes". For example, "typhoid" in the west was called typhus, but "typhoid fever" in China covers both the wide and narrow senses such as warm disease, wind warmth, dampness warmth, fever and so on. Western medicine distinguishes diseases based on the differences between disease types (nervous, digestive, glandular, etc.) and micro bacteria, which are not discussed in TCM. Yun had the view that only "Chinese taiyang disease" and "pre typhoid in western countries" could be defined "justifiably" as the same. Other changes such as "forward transmission, reverse transmission, combined disease, and concurrent disease" of typhoid fever in China and the similar syndrome of typhoid in western countries (paratyphoid) cannot be all together explained logically, which leads to more "confusion".[121] Even so, Yun still believed that the comparison of Chinese and Western medical names was still a work that can be further pursued. After combing the treatises of typhoid in western medicine and comparing them with TCM, he believed that some similarities between "prodrome syndrome" and "taiyang disease", "the rise of body temperature in the first week" and "warm disease", "thick tongue coating, constipation, high fever, pulse rate" and "Yangming meridians syndrome", "the third week heat is very relaxed, heart function is weak" and "Shaoyin syndrome", "intestinal hemorrhage and perforated peritonitis" and "peach blossom soup syndrome", can be used to make a preliminary comparison[122] and discuss the unification of disease names. To sum up, he came to the believe that the "syndrome" of typhoid fever in TCM could correspond to the "disease" of Western medicine.

From this comparison, we can see that the "typhoid" of Western medicine may include the definition of three syndrome types and warm disease in the *Treatise on Typhoid Fever* of TCM. In other words, the single disease name of Western medicine

[119] Yun Tieqiao, Disease Names, *Febrile Diseases*, pp. 2–3.

[120] Zheng Manqing & Lin Pinshi, *History of Chinese Medicine*, pp. 376–379. "TCM with reference to Western medicine" is further than "the convergence of TCM and Western medicine". For details, see Zhang Xichun, *Chinese Medicine with Reference to the West.*

[121] Yun Tieqiao, *Research on Typhoid Fever, The Difficulty of Mutual Proof between Chinese and Western Pathology*, Vol. 3, pp. 52–53.

[122] Yun Tieqiao, *Research on Typhoid Fever, Typhoid Disease Types and Transmission of Classics*, Vol. 3, pp. 59–60.

cannot be compared with that of TCM one-on-one. On the contrary, the disease names of TCM can sometimes be divided into many concepts to compare with the various symptoms of a single disease in Western medicine. Yun Tieqiao said, "The differences in the details are quite reasonable and can be deliberated".[123] Generally speaking, this theory is the "syndrome" of TCM and the "disease type" of Western medicine.[124] Yun deemed that the explanation of diseases can no longer rely solely on traditional terms such as Yin-Yang, five elements and six Qis. It is also necessary to examine and understand the "physical energy" of diseases. Only by combining the symptoms found in the syndrome differentiation of TCM and explaining them with the physiological terms of Western medicine can we truly reach the realm that "reading can bring you different understandings, and diagnosing diseases can give you the insight for the crux".[125]

If, according to Yun Tieqiao, Chinese and Western medicine were competing against each other in terms of disease, then why are we eager to integrate with Western medicine? The anti TCM response caused by bacteriology is reflected in the identification of diseases, as Yun said, "most people think that China's method of classifying diseases is not as good as foreign countries". It is manifested that TCM uses the viscera organs to determine the name of a disease, but it is criticized for not being knowledgeable about the viscera organs.[126] It is not as practical and accurate as Western medicine in terms of blood tests and bacteria testing.[127] These precise or rough classification methods of disease names had long been under control in Western medicine. Yu Yunxiu recognized that Western medicine doctors could also comment on the classification of internal and external causes of TCM in detail, such as protozoan parasites and bacterial parasites being "external causes", heredity and age being "internal factors".[128] The difference between China and the West is that Western medicine on diseases is all "down to earth, accurate, realistic, without any ambiguity. The diseases are classified by the hundreds, like a network headed by a key line, being totally under control and pointing to a direction like a path".[129] Yu ironically pointed out that the theory in the TCM classic *Basic Inquiries. Fundamental Truth* stated

---

[123] Yun Tieqiao, *Research on Typhoid Fever. Typhoid Disease Types and Transmission of Classics*, Vol. 3, p. 60.

[124] Yun Tieqiao, *Research on Typhoid Fever. Typhoid Disease Types and Transmission of Classics*, Vol. 3, p. 60.

[125] Yun Tieqiao, Changes in the Body after Blood Loss, *Physiological Neologisms*, Vol. 3, pp. 22–25.

[126] Yun Tieqiao criticized Tang Zonghai for mixing up the theory of triple energizers with the theory of peritoneum, which was totally confusing. Therefore, it is impossible for people to trust the names of diseases based on the viscera. See Yun Tieqiao, Influenza and Pertussis, *Theories of Pathology*, p. 19. For the discussion of Tang Zonghai's triple-energizer view, see Pi Kuoli, *Body View and Ideological Transformation of Modern TCM—Tang Zonghai and the Era of Convergence of TCM and Western Medicine*, Chapter 4.

[127] Yun Tieqiao, Influenza and Pertussis, *Theories of Pathology*, pp. 18–19.

[128] Yu Yunxiu, Chapter 9. Primary Disease-Diarrhea, A Frank Confession, *Selected Works on Medical Revolution,* pp. 121–125.

[129] Yu Yunxiu, Chapter 9. Primary Disease-Diarrhea, A Frank Confession, included in *Selected Works on Medical Revolution*, p. 124.

that "all diseases occur in the wind, cold, heat, humidity, dryness and fire", but they are not the real origin of diseases. For example, the "wind" will not bring diseases at all. The fundamental reason why real air can infect diseases is the bacteria in the wind, not the wind itself.[130] Bacteria can be "examined by using a microscope, tested with chemicals, and dissected by animals and humans, which is obvious. It is not as absurd as the theory of cold and heat, which cannot be tested".[131] Bacteria can be proved in many ways, but the pathogenic factors discussed in TCM can not, and its classification method is too rough and simple, which is the problem.

Although the existence of bacteria was not observed when discussing diseases, the classical syndrome differentiation and treatment that modern Chinese medicine had been proud of was still strongly advocated by Yun at that time. He said, "The effectiveness of the treatment is what really matters. If you want to treat a disease effectively, you must first know the disease". The "disease recognition" here is not to distinguish the name of a disease or define the name of a disease, but to "describe the symptoms in detail", that is, similar to the syndrome differentiation and "the study of pathology" in TCM.[132] This "pathology" is precisely the traditional way of looking, smelling, asking and feeling the pulse to explore the role of Yin and Yang, five elements and six Qis in the "syndrome" of the patients as the standard of treatment. In early Republic of China, though this theory was spurned by anti TCM school, people could still integrate it into the discourse when describing the diseases, using it as a bridge between patients and TCM. This made Yu Yunxiu quite angry. He said:

The patient seeing the doctor always started by saying: "I have internal heat, I have dampness." How can people know the theory of six Qis? Chinese people have been so much influenced that it's a household saying and everybody can talk with no grounds. Such strange phenomena are everywhere, alas! If the theory of six Qis is not clear, the society will never understand the concept of disease, the health and recuperation will go astray, leading to the likely accidents, which is a major problem for national health and an issue for discussion.[133]

Yu Yunxiu hated that patients still trusted the ridiculous statements of Chinese medicine, which led to many misunderstandings of disease interpretation or prevention. during the Republic of China period, where the pathogen of the disease was known, the "ancient theory" was still popular, which really made Yu Yunxiu lament on the "foolish loyalty" of people to the ancient Qi theory.[134] Although TCM had its own adherence on the interpretation of disease names, Western medicine was in the same medical market. Western medicine should learn to understand the terminology

[130] Yu Yunxiu, Chapter 9. Primary Disease-Diarrhea, A Frank Confession, included in *Selected Works on Medical Revolution*, pp. 124–125.

[131] Yu Yunxiu, Chapter 9. Primary Disease-Diarrhea. Ulcer, A Frank Confession, included in *Selected Works on Medical Revolution*, p. 126.

[132] Yun Tieqiao, Introduction, *Theories of Pathology*, p. 1.

[133] Yu Yunxiu, On Six Qis, *Selected Works on Medical Revolution*, p. 143.

[134] Yu Yunxiu, Chapter 9. Primary Disease-Diarrhea, A Frank Confession, included in *Selected Works on Medical Revolution*, p. 125.

of TCM. Similarly, TCM must also explain and respond to the disease differentiation of Western medicine. Yun Tieqiao examined the disease pedigree of TCM with the fine disease classifications of Western medicine, saying, "It is the habit of national medicine to put fever and typhoid as one category, summer heat and damp warmth in another. Other warm diseases and related diseases, such as measles, hemp, laryngosis, tianpox, convulsion, have their separate books, while malaria and dysentery are attached to warm diseases." It was quite chaotic, but the new disease classification method "cannot be used with the old books, nor to the Western medical books". The classification should be that "typhoid and warm diseases books should be separated as specialized books; convulsion (spasm) is listed as nervous system disease, and the word" pediatrics "be added to the book title to make a difference; measles, hemp, pox and rash are listed in pediatrics; malaria has the most variations; dysentery symptoms and concurrent diseases are the most complex, for which there should be discussions in special articles".[135] It can be seen that Yun had a preliminary idea of disease classification, after which he had to make the comparison with the disease names of Western medicine.

As mentioned earlier, Yun Tieqiao had some insights into *Treatise on Typhoid Fever*. Let's see how he compared Chinese and Western medicine with it. The naming of diseases in Western medicine gave Chinese medicine a lot of enlightenment. Yun Tieqiao said, "The treatment method of typhoid in Western countries can prove the truth of Zhongjing's theory on typhoid fever and the true features of typhoid disease".[136] Then, from the perspective of the general knowledge context of acute infectious warm diseases, starting from "all febrile diseases and the detailed classifications of Western medicine", he classified the disease names such as typhoid, paratyphoid, influenza, pneumonia, bronchitis, diaphragm, myelitis, pleurisy and so on. Yun used "precursor syndrome" to explain that nine out of ten of these diseases have symptoms of "headache, bone pain, limb fatigue, loss of appetite, or aversion to cold, followed by fever". The precursor of these diseases was the "taiyang disease" in *Treatise on Typhoid Fever*. It was concluded that: "The term typhoid fever in China has both broad and narrow meanings, and its range is extremely wide in the broad sense. The so-called 'all fever diseases, typhoid fever and the like' in the *Internal Canon of Medicine* are actually equivalent to the term of acute infectious diseases in western countries".[137] That is, the definition of typhoid fever in China can encompass many fever infectious diseases in Western medicine.

Then, all febrile diseases were defined as "typhoid fever". Why are there so many terms such as spring warmth, summer heat and autumn dampness? Yun believed that these are the characteristics of TCM when determining the name of diseases. The changes of Qi in the four seasons are different. People are affected by the changes of weather. Even if they are "harmed by cold", they also have different symptoms. Just like the four seasons, the name and symptoms of diseases are different, but they

[135] Yun Tieqiao, Malaria, *Theories of Pathology*, p. 55.

[136] Yun Tieqiao, Research on Typhoid Fever, *Discussion on Disease Types*, Vol. 3, p. 62.

[137] The above two paragraphs are quoted from Yun Tieqiao, *General Introduction. Research on Typhoid Fever*, Vol. 1, p. 28.

are always judged with references to nature. This is the essence of disease names in TCM.[138] To distinguish four seasons[139] and six Qis is to correctly judge the way of diagnosis and medication. Yun said: "For this purpose, we should distinguish wind, cold, heat, dampness, dryness and fire. The names of various febrile diseases vary with time, and we need to know the reasons. The *Internal Canon of Medicine* allocates four seasons to the five internal organs, and the six pathogenic factors (wind, cold, heat, dampness, dryness and fire-translator's note) are about the same".[140] Therefore, Yun believed that in comparing with Western medicine, we must still adhere to the six Qis and four seasons of TCM, and those terms are the framework of the classical Qi theory of TCM, which Yu Yunxiu severely attacked and tried his best to eliminate. In terms of the integration of TCM and Western medicine in terms of disease names, Yun thought that there was also a situation caused by the wrong understanding of doctors in the past when summarizing diseases in *Treatise on Typhoid Fever*, which can be reflected by the disease names of Western medicine. He said that "if scholars are obsessed with the belief that typhoid includes all diseases", it is also harmful.[141] The first thing is to separate the diseases that were mistakenly classified as febrile diseases in the past. As mentioned earlier, the so-called warm disease, "according to the Yangming treatment, the Gegen Qinlian can clear it up, which is the cure with no exception", that is, it can be cured with the "cooler" medicine in the typhoid prescription. However, Yun added, "this can be applied to typhoid warm diseases, but cannot be applied to typhoid with excessive dampness or heat stroke".[142] There are only three kinds of febrile diseases that can't be treated by the real typhoid prescription: spasm, dampness (dampness warmth) and heat stroke. Yun thought that spasms were actually epidemic cerebrospinal meningitis from Western medicine.[143] Heat stroke, namely heat warmth, is called "sunstroke" in Western medicine.[144] The damp warmth is due to "too few nutrients in the air and too much nitrogen, which makes the human body sick, all tissues lose their elasticity, and the lymphocytes cannot be fully absorbed, leading to excess water all over the body".[145] The above three kinds of disease names are all examples of Yun's analysis, reflections and clarifications on the names of TCM by invoking Western medicine.

In addition, there is another kind of fever that cannot be equated with typhoid, which is called influenza today. Yun Tieqiao held the view that the cold is similar

---

[138] Yun Tieqiao, *Understandings of Febrile Diseases*, Vol. 1, p. 9.

[139] Yun Tieqiao said, "The first step in the early stage of illness is really influenced by the time". "Therefore, *Internal Canon of Medicine* name diseases according to four seasons". See his book, New TCM, *Clinical Lectures*, p. 37.

[140] Yun Tieqiao, New TCM, *Clinical Lectures*, p. 36.

[141] Yun Tieqiao, Different Treatments of Typhoid Fever, Warm Diseases, Spasm, Dampness and Heat Stroke, *Febrile Diseases*, p. 15.

[142] The above two paragraphs are quoted from Yun Tieqiao, *Understandings of Febrile Diseases*, Vol. 4, p. 42.

[143] Yun Tieqiao, Disease Names, *Febrile Diseases*, p. 4.

[144] Yun Tieqiao, Disease Names, *Febrile Diseases*, p. 10.

[145] Yun Tieqiao, Different Treatments of Typhoid Fever, Warm Diseases, Spasm, Dampness and Heat Stroke, *Febrile Diseases*, p. 15.

to the spring wind warmth, but after all, the latter belongs to typhoid, which starts with "bone chilling" symptom at the beginning.[146] Yun defined the simple cold as Western influenza, of which "not much information was discovered in Chinese ancient books, probably for being too minor a disease to deserve any attention".[147] He believed that there are many kinds of influenza, which cannot be generalized by a single disease name. One of the most terrifying diseases is called "severe cold" in the definition of TCM. About 20 to 40 million people around the world have died of this disease, more than the death in the First World War during which 15 million people died.[148] Yun said sarcastically: "Westerners turn pale when talking about it, and there is no sound therapy till now".[149] He also held that few Chinese doctors knew the names of new Western medicine, such as the name of "severe cold", which Chinese doctors paid little attention to, and often mixed it up with influenza or whooping cough as cold or wind warmth.[150] It is not surprising that "TCM practioners ignored it".[151] This requires the TCM community to study and give it enough attention. Unfortunately, though many comparisons between Chinese and Western disease names were made, Yun did not actively discuss the epidemic of TCM. In fact, according to the development of the history of TCM, the epidemic did not seem to be within the typhoid system. Yun Tieqiao did not explain, nor compare the names of fever diseases in Western medicine with those of epidemics, but there was no doubt that TCM could treat infectious diseases.

6.7 Dilemma of TCM in the Early Republic of China Period

Cao Juren (1900–1972) said, "Probably in our father's generation, there were ideas of 'blending China and the West' and 'having a thorough knowledge of both western and TCM'. It was also common to make one son learn Western medicine and another learn TCM, so as to achieve the combination".[152] Chinese and Western medicine would think about each other's theories and naturally start learning from each other. However, the integration of TCM and Western medicine is by no means a matter of words. Finally, when we have to choose a correct theory, we found that the communication of medical theory was becoming more and more difficult, so many people had changed from the integration school to becoming debaters. This development

[146] Yun Tieqiao, Cold and Cough, *Theories of Pathology*, p. 8.

[147] Yun Tieqiao, Cold and Cough, *Theories of Pathology*, p. 2.

[148] Gina Kolata, translated by Huang John, *Influenza: Discovery of 1918 Influenza Pandemic and Fatal Virus*, Taipei: Shangzhou Press, 2002, pp. 15–40.

[149] Yun Tieqiao, Influenza and Pertussis, *Theories of Pathology*, p. 11.

[150] Yun Tieqiao, Medical Discussion, *Collection on Medicine*, Taipei: Huading Publishing House, 1988, pp. 33–34.

[151] Yun Tieqiao, Influenza and Pertussis, *Theories of Pathology*, p. 18.

[152] Cao Juren, *Ten Theories on New Things. II. Revealing the "Mystery"*, Hong Kong: Shengsheng Book Collection, Publication Year Unknown, p. 21.

had two sides, which were inseparable. Doctors who integrate TCM and Western medicine had different opinions. After the meeting between Chinese and Western medicine, when the debating situation became more and more clear, the so-called "focus of debate" was often the dilemma of the integration of Chinese and Western medicine.

In Yun Tieqiao's era, the debate between anatomic physiology and body Qi obviously turned to the theoretical confrontation between bacteriology and the Qis of natural environment (six Qis) for disease treatment. Moreover, the discussion of disease names in TCM and Western medicine had also surfaced, which was a new challenge that TCM in Tang Zonghai's era did not face,[153] and the change from the physical study of viscera to bacteria took place. It was more and more difficult to achieve an extensive medical intersection[154] of "being a family all over the world and five continents sharing the same path", as Tang said. On the other hand, Yun Tieqiao's problem was obviously more difficult, because the Qi of the viscera could be compared with and induced from Western medicine in terms of form and quality. However, bacteriology is in no way to be induced from six Qis. The number of human viscera can never be compared with the types of bacteria, and it was impossible to use TCM theory to discuss the integration of TCM and Western medicine one-on-one. The liver, heart, spleen, lung, kidney and other viscera could be at least developed from the context recorded in Chinese and Western medical books, while bacteriology had never been recorded in classical medicine at all.

Yun Tieqiao still insisted on the position of six Qis, four seasons or syndrome differentiation to respond to the fact that TCM was about to lose the right to define the name of a disease, but in fact he could not be free of the pressure of the time in "recognizing bacteria". In general, Yun's method was to ignore the noumenon of bacteria theory, take *Treatise on Typhoid Fever* as the keynote to find out any possibility of unifying and defining diseases, and oppose the proposal from the Central National Medical Institution to cancel the TCM disease names[155] and replace them with the disease names of Western medicine.

It has to be mentioned that Yun Tieqiao had some naive ideas and neglected areas. For example, he said, "The theory of bacteria will be forgotton one day, but the theory of six Qis won't".[156] His optimistic speculation is too ideal. However, it is not completely wrong, as the theory of "six Qis" still exists in the theory of modern Chinese medicine, but the bacteria theory is still booming, and there is no sign of being overthrown thus far. Another reason for Yun to be plausible and reasonable could be that TCM still had good curative effects in treating diseases, though Western

---

[153] Tang Zonghai encountered many convergent topics, such as "the Qi physiology and viscera of TCM" and how to face "the anatomic physiology and visible viscera of Western medicine". Pi Kuoli, *Body View and Ideological Transformation of Modern TCM—Tang Zonghai and the Era of Convergence of TCM and Western Medicine*, Conclusion.

[154] (Qing) Tang Zonghai, *Five Kinds of Sino-Western Converged Medical Books. Essence of Medical Classics*, Preface, p. 1.

[155] Yun Tieqiao, Discussion on the Proposal for Unified Disease Names, *Treatise on Medicine*, pp. 3–12.

[156] Yun Tieqiao, TCM and Western Medicine, *Clinical Lectures*, p. 35.

medicine is very precise in all aspects of pharmaceutical or pathological research. He said, "Those who can treat diseases can also possibly cure the diseases unless they are proved to be incurable". That is to say, it is more important to study treatment methods than to find bacteria.[157] In addition, according to Yu Yunxiu's words, TCM could still survive under the strong pressure of Western medicine, precisely because many patients still believed in TCM. Yu maintained that Western medicine had been introduced into China for some time, but Chinese people generally did not trust "new medicine" for many reasons. However, when discussing diseases, the new medicine "is not based on *Internal Canon of Medicine*, nor advocates *Treatise on Typhoid Fever*, Yin and Yang, five elements, nor distinguish wind, cold, dryness and dampness, but is based on science, which is difficult to understand. The names of the diseases are not related to Yin deficiency, Yang failure, liver fire nor stomach cold, which were novel, confusing and unheard of. It is very different from what the patient knows and expects".[158] Therefore, many patients still honored TCM theory without knowing much about Western medicine bacteria theory. In today's situation, if doctors do not pursue bacteriological research, I'm afraid they will only be a laughing stock. It is true that nowadays we are no longer as we used to be.

Yun Tieqiao saw that TCM was in a precarious situation after his medical practice began, and believed that the plight of TCM came from three aspects: the opposition of the government, the opposition of Western medicine and its own corruption.[159] The last two were what he attached importance to and called on the medical community for its attention to, while government intervention was not the urgent crisis of the time. It was precisely due to his scholarly character of seeking academic rather than political influence that he won the title of "founder of the Chinese medical revolution".[160] He also criticized his colleagues who launched the national salvation movement of TCM for their "bread crisis" to resort to resistance, fearing that TCM would be banned, by "gathering the mob to fight against the trends of time". He said that TCM was "the quintessence of the country" and could never be destroyed. These "rabble" were just having unnecessary worries.[161] These harsh words turned him into a "madman" and a "traitor" in the eyes of the TCM community.

In fact, the adherence and views of this respected and criticized medical celebrity on TCM academics may not be fully accepted by the TCM community. In particular, his theory that typhoid can cover all warm diseases is not a fact in academic development, because nowadays, the treatment of infectious diseases is still mainly based on warm diseases, rather than on typhoid.[162] He firmly believed in the medication and theory of the ancient prescription (typhoid fever prescription), which

[157] Yun Tieqiao, TCM and Western Medicine, *Clinical Lectures*, p. 36.

[158] Yu Yunxiu, Admonition to Patients. Fear and Doubts on New Medicine, *Selected Works on Medical Revolution*, pp. 141–142.

[159] Fan Boqun, *From Lu Xun's Switching from Medicine to Literature to Yun Tieqiao's Switching from Literature to Medicine—the Theory of Yun Tieqiao*, p. 26.

[160] Yun Tieqiao, *Understandings of Febrile Diseases*, Vol. 1, p. 4.

[161] Yun Tieqiao, *Understandings of Febrile Diseases*, Vol. 1, pp. 4–5.

[162] The study of both typhoid and warm diseases are effective guiding theories for the treatment of fever related diseases, but warm diseases are developed on the basis of typhoid. The theories

led to the death of some of his patients. For this medical dispute, he was almost sued.[163] Whether ancient prescriptions, modern prescriptions, typhoid prescriptions or epidemic febrile prescriptions, sticking to one standpoint will lead to criticism from the other side. Perhaps, the integration of typhology and warm diseases in the early Republic of China period and the switch to Western medicine should be reconsidered when studying the medical history of the Republic of China period in the future. Yun only pointed out the internal differences of TCM, but did not completely solve the disputes.

In the face of the declination and disturbance in traditional academia and the dual pressure of Western medicine, fighting back with the help of *Internal Canon of Medicine* would guarantee one's legitimate position, but blindly holding the *Treatise on Typhoid Fever* against all oppositions was not enough to convince the TCM doctors who held the theory of warm diseases in their discussion on the infectious diseases of Western medicine. If there was only a dispute between China and the West, the TCM world would easily have the consensus in opposing the outside world. But when it comes to bacteria and disease names, and the modern disputes involving typhoid and warm diseases, there might be a situation of "having different dreams in the same bed".[164] So Yun Tieqiao said, "The result of peer research is straying away from the ancient sayings. This is the so-called new TCM, which is neither Chinese nor Western."[165] Perhaps, the new development of TCM, which is "both Chinese and Western", had superficially taken shape, but the disputes between peers on academic development still needed to be resolved. After all, under the pressure of Western medicine taking the lead in the cause of unifying disease names, if the theory of TCM on warm diseases was just "between Chinese and Western" without first putting forward a set of standard and consistent theories of warm diseases, what could we do to regain the dominance of defining diseases? Yun Tieqiao's idea, which he himself might not feel so good, also highlights the TCM's awkward and tense relationship among bacteria, disease names and its own academic status.

---

may be different and need to be discussed in depth, but in terms of treatment methods, infectious diseases are still dominated by the theories of warm diseases. See Zhang Xiuhui (ed.), *Modern TCM Infectious Diseases*, pp. 2–5; Meng Shujiang (ed.), *Febrile Diseases*, pp. 1–3.

[163] Chen Cunren, *My Medical Career*, p. 14.

[164] In the exploration of modern academic transformation, the author found that any discipline, including medicine, actually faces a kind of "two-way reflections". That is, the response to new theories or Western learning, and the reflection on the positioning of traditional academia in the new era. The study of modern medical history should not only reflect on Western medicine and TCM with new and old ideas, but also reflect on the overall orientation of TCM "keeping up with the times" in its old ideology. About this idea, the author calls it "the reflection about two-way contemporary academic transition" (confronting West and traditional China).

[165] Yun Tieqiao, New TCM, *Clinical Lectures*, p. 37.

Chapter 7
Qi and the Individuals: The Discussion of Body, Disease and Living Space in the TCM Fever Diseases

7.1 Preface

This chapter will bring readers another perspective and ask a few questions: in the social background of TCM during the Republic of China period: what were the factors that retained their confidence in the traditional classics or treatment methods? In the view of Western medicine, what was the value of the traditional and conservative view of disease in daily life and how to put it into practice? Based on the concept of "multi-dimensional medical history", the next two chapters will examine the relationship between the knowledge of epidemic prevention in TCM and Western medical hygiene from the perspectives of social culture and daily life history, with literature and classics as a frame of reference, so as to explore the significance of Chinese medicine contexts (characteristics) of fever diseases. Although bacteriology has its "formidable" authenticity, it takes a long time for a theory to be put into practice from the laboratory. What's more, the introduction of Western medicine into China involves the entry of a different culture and science into a new society. In the process of adapting to the new society, it is bound to make some changes, which would inevitably lead to the convergence of science and culture between China and the West.

Viewing the antibacterial history of TCM from the perspective of the health history of TCM and Western medicine and the history of daily life, modern TCM, in addition to its own epidemic prevention strategies, may also include the health discourse of Western medicine and become a special integrated theory. Some traditions were taken as the practical daily health preservation and disease prevention. In fact, public health during the Republic of China period could not prevent the daily widespread exogenous fevers. It was mainly aimed at the epidemic situation of infectious diseases, the prevention and control of fevers that didn't belong to the legally acknowledged infectious diseases, which deprived them of the financial support at the national level, let alone the problems of regional differences. For most Chinese people, rather than worrying about invisible bacteria, they'd rather strengthen Qi replenishment and

© Zhonghua Book Company 2026

K. Pi, *The Contest of Modern Chinese and Western Medicine*,
https://doi.org/10.1007/978-981-95-2832-5_7

resistance in daily life, together with the fitness culture of modern China, which represents a modern Chinese medical health culture. Moreover, this chapter tries to discuss the view that the miasma theory of Western medicine formed a certain convergence in the Qi theory of modern Chinese medicine, presenting the "different theories with homogeneity" in public health. When the bacterial exposition became overwhelming, did the theory of TCM and the past epidemic prevention methods really disappear? How was it practiced repeatedly in daily life? What was the historical background that contributed to this phenomenon?

7.2 The Modernity of Microorganisms and the Social Background of the Birth of "Personal" Hygiene

Sean Hsiang-Lin of the Institute of Modern History of the "Academia Sinica" had noticed the dual interpretation of TCM and Western medicine of tuberculosis.[1] On the one hand, the diseases were based on the understanding of "bacteria" in Western medicine, which can derive various explanations. On the other hand, it was also affected by the concepts of "deficiency", "fatigue" and "loss" of TCM, and integrated into the disease narrative of daily life in Chinese society.[2] Sean Hsiang-Lin pointed out that even though bacteriology gained its status, or the concept of "one disease one cause" had been established, the traditional view of medicine and body was still present during the Republic of China period, leading to the coexistence of TCM and Western medicine. Such a context is also of great reference value in the TCM antibacterial history.

For Western medicine, the modernity represented by bacteriology as that China needed to use its power to promote public health to fight against infectious diseases.

---

[1] Sean Hsiang-Lin, Four Dimensions in Habit Formation: New Life Movement, Ethics, Family and Body in the Prevention and Treatment of Tuberculosis, *Collection of the Institute of Modern History, Academia Sinica,* No. 74, pp. 133–177. There are also many foreign studies, such as Davids.S.Barnes, *The Making of A Social Disease: Tuberculosis in Nineteenth Century France,* Berkeley: University of California Press, c1995. For the discussion on the relationship between bacteria and tuberculosis, see Bridie Andrews, Tuberculosis and the Assimilation of Germ Theory in China, 1895–1937, *Journal of the History of Medicine and Allied Sciences,*1997 (52), pp. 114–157. In terms of new public health, for the establishment and social impact of human behavior and infection theory, including the social and cultural history of tuberculosis, see Nancy Tomes, *The Gospel of Germs: Men, Women, and the Microbe in American Life,* Cambridge: Harvard University Press, 1988. Sean Hsiang-Lin also noted the relationship between tuberculosis and the unsanitary conditions of Chinese families and individuals, which is different from the view of foreign scholars that "tuberculosis is a social disease". See Sean Hsiang-lin Lei, Habituating Individuality: Framing Tuberculosis and Its Material Solutions in Republic of China Period, *Bulletin for the History of Medicine*, 2010 (84), pp. 248–279.

[2] Sean Hsiang-Lin, *Why Health Is Not Protecting Life—Alternative Health, Self and Disease During the Republic of China Period*, Taiwan Social Research Quarterly,2004 (54), p. 41.

In this regard, we take the extension of scientific knowledge established in the laboratory to daily life as an example.[3] Among them, the most important knowledge was to highlight the harm of microorganisms to people. The authenticity of bacterial science supports all the basic knowledge and prevention methods of infectious disease prevention measures, and it was also the starting point of public health. However, the Chinese people's knowledge of public health was limited Yu Yunxiu criticized, "Chinese people today are very naive when it comes to their health knowledge, and the most dangerous thing is that some never heard of pathogenic microorganisms".[4] The greatest influence of bacteriology in China in the early Republic of China period was probably not in therapeutics, but in preventive medicine. Yu said, "At present, the health administration pays much attention to the eradication of microorganisms. The sterilization methods and what is to be used in epidemic prevention, putrefaction, as well as disinfection, are of great significance".[5] He stated that all the methods killing microorganisms at that time were basically to kill those that can possibly cause the disease outside the human body before the disease occurred. Yu expressed in his *Microbiology*:

> (1) Body: one part of the body, such as the hands and feet, can be sterilized with disinfectants, but for the whole body, disinfectants can't be used, except for taking a bath with warm water and soap. The skin of children also absorbs drugs. When disinfecting the body, it is advisable to use disinfectants with caution. (2) Spit: use 5% salt water, with the same amount of spit and leave it for 24 h. It is also better to add a small amount of sodium carbonate to boil. (3) Defecation and diarrhea: add the same amount of lime milk and it should be left for 23 h, which is the most convenient and cheapest, or the same amount of carbolic acid and risol, etc. (4) WC: disinfecting walls, floors, portals with 5% carbolic acid water, and cleaning the toilet with lime milk. (5) Room ceilings: it is usually unnecessary to disinfect them, or at most wipe them with 2% carbolic acid water. The same applies to walls, doors and windows, cabinets, tables and chairs, etc. (6) Utensils: for those that can get wet, wipe them with 3% carbolic acid water. For food utensils, it's best to boil them with water. If disinfectant is used, it must still be washed with boiled water after disinfection. (7) Clothes and quilts: it is best to disinfect with steam. If the shirt is dirty, boil it in soap water. (8) Books: it is not easy to give them the perfect protection when cleaning the pages completely, but they can be exposed to sunlight. (9) Fur, leather and rubber: spray with 2% carbolic acid water. Disinfection by steaming is forbidden. (10) Dust and waste: it's best to disinfect by burning. (11) Bathing water: add 2% quicklime and discard it after several hours.[6]

What we have seen above is a positive way of disease prevention. I'm afraid we rarely "disinfect" like this nowadays. Carbolic acid, risol, lime, disinfectant, soap, etc., were commonly used in both cleaning and hygiene products at that time. They combined the modernity of commodity and consumption culture with the personal consumption behavior. For example, "Lihua Sanitary Soap" emphasized the use of soap to clean the body "with great bactericidal power", "remove dirt and sweat

---

[3] Cheng Hanzhang, *A Brief Introduction to Western Medicine,* Shanghai: The Commercial Press, 1933, p. 46.

[4] Yu Yunxiu, *Microbiology*, Preface, p. 1.

[5] Yu Yunxiu, *Microbiology,* p. 20.

[6] Yu Yunxiu, *Microbiology*, pp. 20–28.

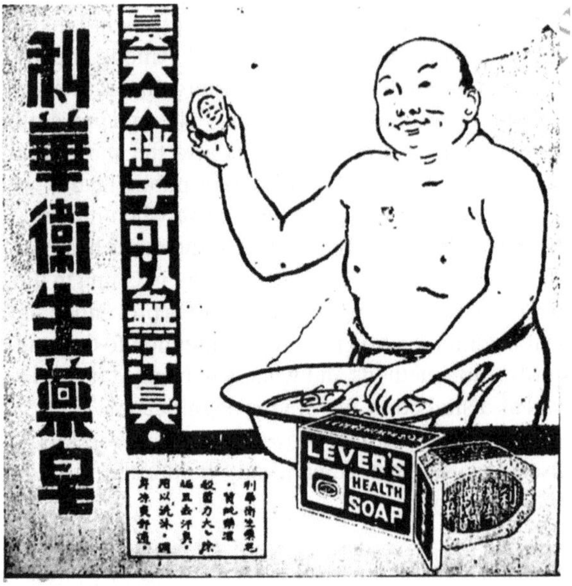

Fig. 7.1 Lihua sanitary soap

odor", "make germs inviolable" and so on (see Fig. 7.1).[7] The practical application of various disinfection methods in daily life focused on the idea of using external "substances" such as science and health "commodities" to eliminate bacteria (see Fig. 7.2).[8] This involves the prosperity of modern material culture, which is different from the thought of Qi in classical medicine.

Since the mid-nineteenth century, the occurrence of infectious diseases has been associated with social inequality, poor living conditions and poverty, even today. Moreover, the public trust in vaccinations had decreased, and the vaccination rate was extremely different among the areas.[9] We have legitimate reasons to suspect that in the early twentieth century, resource.

allocation and administrative effectiveness were poor and the living conditions in most regions still could not keep up with the pace of "modernization" in China, and the life protection line "armed" with bacteriological theory was extremely fragile. If we study the history of health without focusing on the "big cities" in modern China, we would see the big difference from past research. Even the health issue in rural areas of the Republic of China period has not been thoroughly studied.[10] Not being

[7] Shanghai Shen Bao Newspaper Office (ed.), *Shen Bao*, Shanghai: Shanghai Bookstore Press, 1982–1987. August 25, 1936, p. 3.

[8] Shanghai Shen Bao Newspaper Office (ed.), *Shen Bao*, September 30, 1936, 3rd picture of "Lysel Disinfecting Potions".

[9] Charlotte Roberts & Keith Manchester, et al., *Archaeology of Diseases,* pp. 182–183.

[10] The differences, mutual penetration and references between "state" and "locality" should be a topic that can be continuously explored, but the current research is still mostly from the perspective of "big cities" (Shanghai, Nanjing, Beijing, Guangzhou), e.g. Peng Shanmin, Public Health and Shanghai Urban Civilization (1898–1949), included in Yu Xinzhong (ed.), *Medical Treatment*

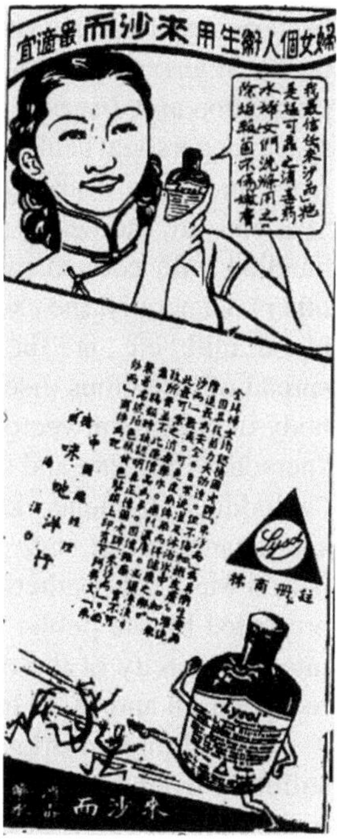

Fig. 7.2 Women's personal hygiene products Lysel

able to cover these relatively rural areas during the Republic of China period, this book is only revealing a few problems; the "public" health of the country has never been personal to the people, but emphasizes the use of group power to deal with these problems. Patients in the early Republic of China period often looked toward charities or local resources,[11] but rarely sought the help of the state. It must be noted that the

---

and Health since the Qing Dynasty, pp. 139–156, 357–370; Pan Shuhua, The Treatment of Fecal Pollution and Urban Life in Guangzhou during the Republic of China Period, *Proceedings of the Institute of Modern History, Academia Sinica*, 2008 (59), pp. 67–96. Only a few studies have started on the status of secondary regions or provinces, such as Wu Yuqin and Xu Maoming, A Review of Jiangxi Health and Epidemic Prevention System during the Nanjing National Government, *Journal of Jiangxi University of Finance and Economics*, 2010 (06), pp. 89–93.

[11] The relationship between medical treatment and charity actually involves the conditions of the government system of each dynasty and the local society. The works of Angela Ki Che Leung and Yu Xinzhong are very representative. Before the Republic of China period, especially in the Song, Yuan and Ming Dynasties, there had been remarkable research in the academic circles; Angela Ki Che Leung, A Preliminary Study of Local Medical Resources in the Song, Yuan and Ming Dynasties, included in *China Social History Review Vol. 3*, pp. 219–237; Yu Xinzhong, *Plague and Society in the South of the Yangtze River in the Qing Dynasty—A Study of Medical Social History*, pp. 249–288. As for the situation at the beginning of the Republic of China period, local society still relied on the strength of local gentry or fellow villagers' associations and merchants abroad to prepare for the annual epidemic prevention and the measures of the medical administration. See Feng Xiaocai, *Business is Business: Jiangsu and Zhejiang Businessmen in the Political Turbulence*, Shanghai: Shanghai Academy of Social Sciences Press, 2004, pp. 284–303. For charity, see Wang Chunxia, *Research on Modern Zhejiang Merchants, Charity and Public Welfare Undertakings* (1840–1938),

bacteriology of Western medicine has two different aspects. In addition to public health, it also emphasizes the relationship between "individual" and environmental interaction and disease. This dual nature sometimes finds a reasonable development space for personal health preservation. For example, Yu Yunxiu said, "Those suffering from infectious diseases must have the pathogenic microorganism in their body". "Patients are the headquarters of pathogenic microorganisms, and they need to be handled with care to prevent their microorganisms from spreading and harming others. Generally, the excreta of patients, such as stool, urination, sputum, spit, pus, blood, milk, etc., are the most dangerous".[12] Probably all the vectors that cause the spread of infectious diseases are created by dangerous "individuals", and the main body of parasitism vectors are also "individual", which highlight the importance of "personal" hygiene and self-management.[13] This might be indirectly give rise to the "individual" hygiene views in early Republic of China period, while the "public" significance of the state was ignored. To be a patient during the Republic of China period was truely pathetic. We are not here to explore the feasibility of the "morality presented by the public hygiene" during the Republic of China period by looking into the scarcity of the medical resource, which led to the reliance on the personal recuperation and TCM treatment.

In Xu Zhimo's works, there was a story about the protagonist Liu Shuhe who was suffering from "damp and warm diseases", which usually referred to typhoid fever in the early Republic of China period. At the beginning of his illness, Liu chose to go to a friend's home to recuperate. Later, his condition deteriorated to an irreparable situation, and he went to the hospital for treatment and finally died. Xu Zhimo said that "I knew the misery of not having a wife when I was in the hospital". In fact, it was an emotion that Liu couldn't have the care from his loved ones. Liu had to stay at a friend's home as a second choice, and then a hospital as the last choice.[14] During or after illness, many Chinese patients still chose to rest at home, or being taken care of by their closest family members. There seems to be little difference between ancient and modern times.

Self-caring at home is often the biggest challenge for patients and their families. Ancient medical and health care was underdeveloped, and many medical resources and medical information were not as accessible and popular as in modern times. Before the formation of medical knowledge, people relied on their common sense to seek ways to cure or recuperate from diseases, which was a very important phenomenon in Chinese medical culture. For example, Wang Ermin said, "When people are well fed and clothed, they would take better care of their health. However, they read the popular magazines which were handy, with references to various old

Beijing: China Social Sciences Press, 2009, pp. 229–238. For the legalization and institutionalization reform of philanthropy in the early Republic of China period, see Zhou Qiuguang & Zeng Guilin, *A Brief History of Philanthropy in China*, pp. 260–265.

[12] Yu Yunxiu, *Microbiology*, p. 37.

[13] Yu Yunxiu, *Infectious Diseases*, pp. 36–37.

[14] Xu Zhim, Condolence to Liu Shuhe, *Complete Works of Xu Zhimo*, Taichung: Baiqing Press, 1978, p. 88.

books about different symptoms, resulting in different preferences".[15] There have been a large number of books published on daily life after the Ming and Qing Dynasties involving disease and health preservation,[16] and the idea of treating diseases by oneself had long been rooted in people's life.

John Macgowan, a missionary of the London Missionary, who came to China in the late Qing Dynasty, lived and traveled around China for about 50 years. He said: "Almost every Chinese can become a doctor by virtue of having some medical knowledge. In fact, when you find someone who modestly claims to know little about medicine, that would turn out to be a big surprise to you. A Chinese man with a dirty face, in greasy, dirty clothes, so dirty that you don't want to touch him with a pair of pliers, would be someone you can not take your eyes away from. He is an ordinary worker, and doesn't have any superhuman intelligence, a man easily despised and ignored. At that time, someone will whisper in your ear that he is a very famous amateur doctor who has cured many diseases".[17] At the end of the Qing Dynasty, two foreign nuns in Xi'an complained: "Western medicine still can't beat TCM, and only a few people come to seek Western medicine treatment".[18]

In the early Republic of China period, more and more people went to see Western medicine doctors, but we must not overstate this change by taking the situations of several coastal commercial ports or large cities, such as Guangzhou, Shanghai, Beijing and Tianjin as those in other places of China. Although Western medicine became more popular during the Republic of China period, we should not forget that when Western medicine broke away from the service and charity nature of missionary medicine, the whole medical system had become the product of modern capitalism. In 1938, Chen Guofu said in his speech in Guiyang Medical College, "Foreign countries have more developed economy, so that ordinary people can enjoy modern medical treatment, while Chinese people are poor, and ordinary people can't enjoy these modern products. They are doomed in their poverty. Moreover, foreign drugs are not available in the mainland, and they must wait for Western medicine doctors to treat them. Isn't it like 'bringing the water of the Western river to rescue the fish in a dry pond of China'?"[19] It can be seen that the diagnosis and treatment costs of Western medicine were high at that time. In addition, the supply of Western medicine in modern times was still restricted by foreign countries, and there was a

---

[15] Wang Ermin, *Social and Cultural Ecology of the Ming and Qing Dynasties*, Taipei: Taiwan Commercial Press, 1997, p. 84.

[16] Zhang Zhejia, A Preliminary Study of Folk Popular Medicine in Traditional Society—A Discussion on Daily Books, included in Mei Jialing (ed.),*Enlightenment in the Changing World: Cultural Reconstruction and Educational Transformation (1895–1949)*, Taipei: Maitian Press, 2006, pp. 167–185.

[17] Macgowan, translated by Zhu Tao & Ni Jing, *The Brightness and Darkness of Chinese Life*, Beijing: Current Affairs Press, 1998, pp. 189–190.

[18] Alekseev Vasilii Mikhailovich (1881–1951), translated by Yan Guodong: *A Journey to China in 1907*, Kunming: Yunnan People's Publishing House, 2001, p. 213.

[19] Chen Guofu, Expectations for Medical Schools, included in Mr. Chen Guofu Scholarship Fund Management Committee(ed.), *Selected Works of Mr. Chen Guofu's Medical and Health Thoughts*, Taipei: Mr. Chen Guofu Scholarship Fund Management Committee, 1973, p. 285.

situation that "the price of Western medicine soared at the beginning of the European war, which frustrated many people".[20]In 1951, Chen Lifu recalled: "How many TCM doctors were there in the country? There are no accurate statistics, but it is estimated that there were about 100,000 people, who lived in different areas, going all over the countryside and serving the general public. As for Western medicine doctors, there was not even a single one available, except in metropolitan cities and Taiwan province. In many places of mainland China, Chinese farmers and ordinary poor people could hardly afford cheap Chinese medicine, let alone the expensive Western medicine".[21]

With the spread of modern Western medicine to the East, the founding of hospitals and the innovation of the medical system have made another choice available for treatment in people's daily life. Superficially, Chinese patients had more choices. After the Republic of China period, Western medicine and TCM competed and integrated with each other, and the medical resources that patients could have should have naturally increased, but this was only the wishful thinking. In 1936, Feng Yuxiang (1882–1948) said at a graduation ceremony for pharmaceutical students in a nursing school: "China is underdeveloped in all aspects. Science is underdeveloped, and education level is different in different regions. The medical care of the people is very poor in terms of 'quality' and 'quantity'. 89% of our compatriots are in the mainland and rural areas, and they are totally ignorant of scientific medicine, let alone the common sense of health. For example, according to the survey in Ding County, Hebei Province, 98% of the village doctors were TCM doctors. And what kind of TCM doctors were they? They were actually witches, amulet painters or ghost catchers, just ignorant swindlers. Moreover, in the villages of Ding County, almost one-third or even half of the villagers died of diseases without medical treatment. How pathetic! They could not even get the treatments of the swindlers! This was the situation in Ding County, and the situation of other rural areas that one can think of".[22] Under the condition that medicine was not popularized, Western medicine could not undertake the task of health care. The quality control of Western medicine was not as rigorous as it is today, resulting in many problems in Chinese medicine. Yang Xiling, a TCM doctor, criticized: "Since the reform, those who called themselves Western medicine doctors had abused the medical business even worse than the so-called TCM doctors. The orderlies in hospitals, the nurses in the army, the servants in pharmacies, who had never read the books of Western medicine nor attended any medical lectures and who were ignorant, regarded themselves as Western medicine doctors. If this continues, it would be unbearable to think about the future of Western medicine in China".[23] It can not be taken for granted that the western health system is in line with China's

[20] Chen Cunren, Popular Medical Discourse, included in Lu Zheng (ed.), *Collection of Rare Modern TCM. Medical Talk*, p. 993.

[21] Chen Guofu, Old Patients' Talk about TCM and Western Medicine, in *Selected Works of Mr. Chen Guofu's Medical and Health Thoughts*, p. 3.

[22] Feng Yuxiang, National Calamity and the Pharmaceutical Industry, *Selected Works of Feng Yuxiang*, Beijing: People's Publishing House, 1998, p. 359.

[23] Yang Xiling, Urgent Call to Ban Western Medicine, Medical Talk in Zhu Garden, included in Lu Zheng (ed.),*Collection of Rare Modern TCM. Medical Talks*, p. 590.

conditions. The regulations on infectious diseases in early Republic of China did not cover all infectious diseases in China. In addition to the incompleteness of the laws and regulations, there were many fever diseases, which could still be prevented by "personal" hygiene.[24]

In addition, there were vaccination activities organized by the government during the Republic of China period, but according to the research being done then, due to the high cost, the general public was simply unable to have injections. In addition, there was a lack of publicity and a lack of modern health knowledge for people who didn't think epidemic prevention to be important. Furthermore, people distrusted the vaccines. When the Sino Japanese War broke out, people were even afraid that the vaccine was part of Japan's bacterial war, which was their major concern.[25] Drug advertisements openly advocated buying drugs and taking them by oneself, which could prevent cholera, typhoid and other infectious diseases. The particular promotion of injections would cause sequelae. Those caring about hygiene could purchase drugs for treatment on their own (see Fig. 7.3).[26] Folk health commodities were also a way of strengthening personal health awareness.

What's more, due to the factors relevant to "people", even scientific Western medicine had become extremely unreliable in its quality, which turned out to be very stressful. In the early Republic of China period, it was much cheaper to find an acquaintance for a prescription than to go to the western hospital for diagnosis and treatment. One might also encounter a type of blackmail from western pharmacies. Lu Xun, a famous writer, once had a stomach disease. He asked a Western medicine doctor he knew for a prescription and asked his wife Xu Guangping to buy the medicine in a pharmacy far away from their home, but the medicine bought each time tasted different. How could it taste different if it was the same medicine? Later, Lu Xun sarcastically said that Chinese people were "penny wise, pound foolish". The truth is: "For the dose of only one day, two days of water was added, so the taste of the medicine was thinner than that of a proper dose".[27] It was not only the lack of accuracy, but could also be murderous. Moreover, Western medicine prescriptions were not understood by everyone. As Cheng Hanzhang said: the reason why there was no recognition of Western medicine was due to the fact that the treatment behavior of Western medicine was "too westernized". The prescriptions were all written in western language, which the patients could not understand. As Western medicine was not well explained to the patients, Chinese patients felt it to be very mysterious.[28]

---

[24] Huang Shengbai, *Commentaries on the Regulations on the Prevention of Infectious Diseases* (published in the official gazette on March 20, the Republic of China period), Tongji, 1918 (01,02), External, pp. 4–6, 169–170.

[25] Yu Deyuan, *History of Disasters in Beijing*, Vol. 1, Beijing: Tongxin Publishing House, 2008, p. 475.

[26] Shanghai Shen Bao Newspaper Office (ed.), *Shen Bao*, June 10, 1937, p. 3.

[27] Lu Xun, Instant Diary, Sequel to the Huagai Collection, included in the *Complete Works of Lu Xun*, Beijing: People's Literature Publishing House, 1996, Vol. 3, p. 312.

[28] Cheng Hanzhang, *A Brief Introduction to Western Medicine*, p. 36.

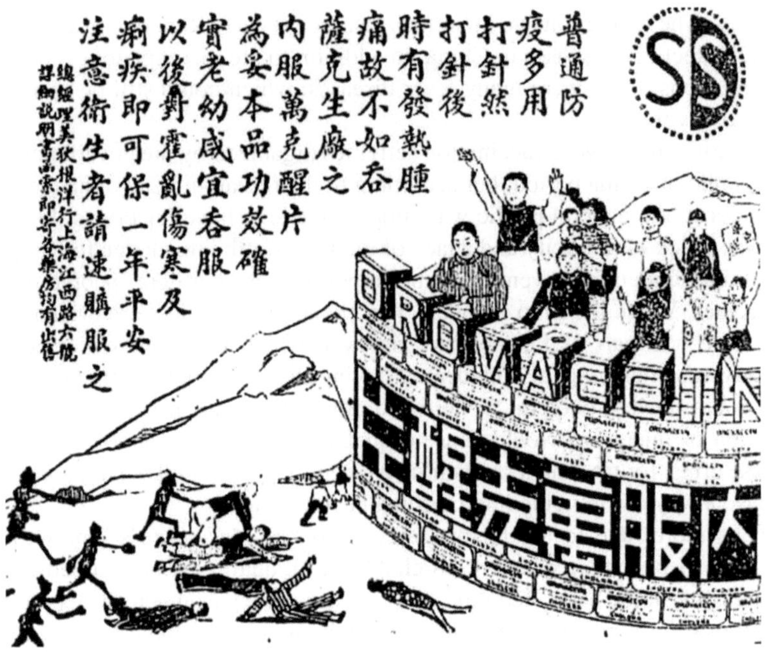

图 8 普通防疫药品——内服万克醒片

Fig. 7.3 Common epidemic prevention drug-Orovaccin

The shortage of Western medicine doctors was fatal to modern medicine in China at that time. A Western medicine doctor said, "There is one doctor for 800 people in Japan, one doctor for 1,700 people in the US, one doctor for more than 80,000 people in China, and they are all working in cities".[29] In 1929, Cheng Hanzhang, a Western medicine doctor, said that "there are very few qualified medical practitioners in China. Even the so-called Western medicine doctors, who graduated from medical schools at home and abroad, are far less than the doctors without a medical education, such as the self-taught, hospital interns, nurses, drugstore apprentices, and even nursing soldiers who served at their positions for several years claimed themselves to be Western medicine doctors so as to administer injections" At that time, the skills of Western medicine doctors were different, and the attitude toward patients gave people many negative impressions. Western medicine doctors also ignored diagnosis, presenting themselves as first-class sellers of drugs over time, so that the "whole society received no benefits of Western medicine which duly gained no credibility from the public". In addition, the promotion of Western medicine had led to the overflow of rights, leading to the opposition of Western medicine by many.[30]

---

[29] Feng Yuxiang, compiled by The 2nd Historical Archives of China, *Feng Yuxiang's Diary*, Nanjing: Jiangsu Ancient Books Publishing House, 1992, January 10, 1937, p. 10.

[30] Cheng Hanzhang, *A Brief Introduction to Western Medicine,* pp. 70–71.Therefore, patients during the Republic of China period had to seek their own blessings. Zhu Dongrun, a biographical writer, described the death of his child in his memoirs. This is what happened in 1930. Zhu was a professor at Wuhan University at that time.

Soon, Junda (Zhu's son) contracted meningitis, and the high fever did not subside for several days. He kept bending backwards, which shocked Lianfang (Zhu's wife). She held the baby in her arms all the time, but there was nothing she could do. Going to a Western medicine doctor, she was told that a spinal injection was needed but the doctor didn't have it. The doctor borrowed a rusty one, causing the child great pain but having no curative effect. Seeing it not working, they went to Sun Xiaxian, a TCM doctor who they used to visit often. As a responsible doctor, Xiaxian was anxious but helpless.

Meningitis was widespread, and Yun Tieqiao's medical prescription was posted in the *Shen Bao*. Tie Qiao was the senior employee of the Commercial Press. At this time, he was opening a correspondence school of TCM, which became quite famous. He believed that meningitis was a fever, and a large dose of cold medicine must be used to suppress the disease. Geng Naikuan copied the medical prescription and sent it to Lianfang. He said, "There is only one way, Sis. Do you want to try it?" Lianfang couldn't make up her mind and went to consult with Doctor Sun.

Holding this prescription, Mr. Sun's hand shivered. It was a disease of fever, as high as 40 degrees. The child's face was red and he kept on leaning backward. It was indeed very critical, but would the illness worsen and get out of control after taking cold medicine? Not being able to make up his mind, he said, "I'm afraid the cooling medicine won't work". He was extremely cautious and only prescribed some antipyretic Chinese medicine.

Doctor Ji, who was from Tangwan, Taizhou, was a famous pediatric TCM doctor. Lianfang hurriedly sent a car to pick him up, and said that he must be taken to them no matter what. Lianfang took out her 1,000 yuan savings and said, "Whoever cures the child's illness, this money is his". The situation was really critical. Mr. Sun dared not write a prescription and the medical prescription sent by Brother Naikuan was still on hold. The rusty needle of the Western medicine doctor didn't work. Dr. Ji could not be found after he left Tangwan. Lianfang and his mother-in-law were in a flood of tears. Finally, Doctor Zhang was introduced to them. As soon as Mr. Zhang took the pulse, he said calmly, "There is a way, don't worry". The child was very weak when Mr. Zhang's prescription was made. After taking this medicine, the child died.[31]

After all the twists and turns, Zhu's son died. Even though Zhu had a high social status and was financially well-off, there was no effective medical treatment. It is difficult to imagine how people of the lower class could deal with these daily diseases. Instead of "sending him to hospital", he treated his son at home in the traditional way of seeing TCM doctors. Western medicine was not helpful either. In fact, TCM was six of one and half a dozen of the other. "Meningitis" is basically the name of a disease defined by Western medicine. There was no such a name in ancient TCM. At most, it can only interpret the drug properties, and even find the appropriate prescriptions from the newspaper, and the patients could only resign themselves to their fate. We found that in the early Republic of China period, patients sometimes sought some

[31] Zhu Dongrun, Autobiography of Zhu Dongrun, *Complete Biographical Works of Zhu Dongrun*, Vol. 4, Shanghai: Oriental Publishing House, 1999, pp. 183–184.

feasible daily medical practice by themselves, rather than just enduring or waiting for a hard-to-find good doctor for treatment.

7.3 Beyond Bacteriology: The Relationship Between Exogenous Fever and "Qi" from the Perspective of TCM

Returning to the TCM context, the explanation of Qi took up the etiological discussion of TCM. Why is the position of "Qi" in modern medical history emphasized? In addition to the cultural and physical implications behind it, Qi is also highly related to "personal" health in modern times. Due to the fact that it does not need to be observed or defined by precise scientific instruments and national institutions, it is very easy to be integrated into daily language as a kind of body perception of life.[32] Whether typhoid or epidemic diseases, the names of the diseases were roughly determined by the corresponding relationship between the epidemic season and the current climate. Sometimes doctors may not reach a clinical consensus on the standard. After all, the climate cannot remain unchanged every year. It is certainly impossible to be precise to name them by seasons or calendar. The so-called doctors of the same school often differ in their interpretations of Qi and the mechanism of diseases. Chinese doctors generally believe that the severity of a person's fever can be determined by the nature of the Qi in him. Generally, seasonal diseases caused by seasonal Qis are the mildest. Any unpredictable miscellaneous Qi, severe cold and unseasonal Qis (that is, the Qi that does not follow the seasonal law and should not occur) are more severe after infection. During the Republic of China period, how did the understanding of seasonal Qi in TCM play the practical role in explaining diseases, treatment, prevention and recuperation when the actual epidemic broke out? Historical circles have done a lot of research on the pestis in 1910 and 1917[33] but little attention was paid to the

[32] Shigehisa Kuriyama, translated by Chen Xinhong, *The Language of the Body—the Mystery of the Body from the Perspective of Chinese and Western Culture*, Taipei: Jiujing Press, 2001, p. 7

[33] The classic monograph on the history of pestis in China is Carol Benedict, *Bubonic Plague in Nineteenth Century China,* Stanford:Stanford University Press, 1996. The earlier is Carlf Nathan. *Plague Prevention and Politics in Manchuria 1910–1931,* Cambridge:East Asian Research Center, Harvard University; distributed by Harvard University Press, 1967. A representative Japanese monograph is Inajima Wade, *Modern China—Health Institutionalization and Social Change*, Tokyo: Yanwen Press, 2000. More famous works with innovative perspectives includes such as by Hu Chengshan, who used the development of economy and transportation to observe the historical impact of the plague. See his publications: The Expansion of Modern Economy and the Cross Regional Epidemic of Severe Infectious Diseases—the Observation Centered on the Outbreak of Pestis and Cholera in Shanghai and Northeast China (1902–1932), *Collection of the Institute of Modern History, Academia Sinica,* No. 51 (2006.3), pp. 91–129, and Sino Japanese Confrontation and Competition for Leadership in Public Health—Observation of the Railway and Port Center City of 'Southern Manchuria' (1901–1911), *Modern History Research,* 2011 (01), pp. 31–46. Another school, the school of environmental disease history named by the author, takes Cao Shuji as its leader, and the publications are as follows: Cao Shuji & Li Yushang, *Pestis: War and Peace—China's Environment and Social*

situation of the world pandemic in 1918 in China. Let's take a look at it and see how much understanding we can get.[34]

Yu Yunxiu once recalled the pandemic: "Influenza is the most prevalent bad cold during the Republic of China period in July and August. Its cause is also a bacterium, discovered by Pfeiffer, which is called influenza. This bacterium is a short bacillus, which is the smallest among the bacteria. It is weak with a low resistance, easy to cause death when being dried up and can also be killed by 56 degrees of heat. This bacterium mostly exists in the mucous membrane and secretion of the respirator, propagates in the nasal cavity, trachea and other places, invades the lungs, and then produces purulent sputum".[35] Obviously, the cause of influenza is "Pheifferia", but it was proved that this bacterium was not the main cause of influenza at all after the invention of the electron microscope. At that time, it was considered to be the only cause of influenza. This may be related to the fact that bacterial exposition was very popular, and the observation instruments were not as advanced. As the disease was prevalent in all regions of China, it had attracted the attention of TCM circles. Cao Bingzhang, a TCM doctor, even wrote *Essentials of Autumn Epidemic Treatment*.

Cao's activities were mostly in his hometown of Shaoxing. He said that he learned about the epidemic situation in China from the newspapers published in Shanghai and Shaoxing at that time: "According to Chinese and Western medicine, it is called epidemic plague. It is said to be from the United States, and the epidemic was widespread, causing many deaths". "Why did Chinese and Western doctors name the influenza 'autumn epidemic'"? The reason is it is closely related to the seasons and climate, rather than on the focus of bacteria. Cao Bingzhang said, "In early autumn, there is intense drought and heat, and the heat is subdued inside; in late autumn, there is a sudden coolness, and dryness that effects the body. The disease caused by dryness starts after the Autumn Equinox and before Minor Snow".[36] Obviously, influenza is an epidemic that occurs in autumn. It is defined as "autumn epidemic" according to the characteristics of the season, and its Qi is characterized by "dry" Qi. Cao thought that to treat a certain epidemic correctly, we should read the books according to the characteristics of seasonal Qis.[37] The same is true even in the treatment that we must choose the appropriate drugs according to the characteristics of seasons, because the

Changes (1230–1960), Jinan: Shandong Pictorial Press, 2006. Cao Shuji, National and Local Public Health—on the Prevalence of Pestis in Shanxi Province in 1918, *Chinese Social Sciences*, Vol. 1, 2006, pp. 178–190.

[34] This book only discusses some prevention and treatment methods, as well as pathological explanations of Chinese and Western medicine at that time. For the outbreak of pandemic influenza, see Pi Kuoli, Epidemic and Social Response during the Republic of China period—A Comparative Study of the 1918 Pandemic in Beijing, Tianjin, Shanghai and Shaoxing, *New Historiography*, 27.4 (2016), pp. 57–107; Pi Kuoli, Pandemic Influenza in Modern China: A Study of the Epidemic Situation from 1919 to 1920, included in Liu Shiyong, *A New Vision of Health History: the Body, Disease and Historical Discourse of Chinese Society*, Taipei: Huayi Academic Press, 2016, pp. 117–142.

[35] Yu Yunxiu, *Infectious Diseases*, p. 35.

[36] Cao Bingzhang, Chapter 1 The Name of Autumn Epidemic, On the Essence of Typhoid and Miscellaneous Diseases, included in *Collection of Rare Modern TCM. Warm Disease*, pp. 749–750.

[37] Cao Bingzhang, Introduction, On the Essence of Typhoid and Miscellaneous Diseases, included in *Collection of Rare Modern TCM. Warm Disease*, pp. 749–750.

TCM therapeutic effect depends on its Qi and properties, rather than on its chemical components, which proves that the attributed knowledge of Qi is still practical.

In fact, similar examples are commonly seen in the works of warm diseases. It is expressed in *Treasure Raft of Epidemics* updated by He Lianchen: "The plagues can by caused by cold, dryness or dampness, depending on different seasons". "If the weather is dry for an extended time and the fever epidemic is prevalent, it is advisable to clear the fire, detoxify, and avoid using desiccant". On the contrary, "If it has been raining for a long time, and it is extremely damp, harm would be caused to the spleen, and many people would suffer from cold and epidemic diseases".[38] Climate change can affect the type of epidemic, so the treatment varies with the seasons. Cao also said, "Of all the harmful pathogenic factors, the wind is the leader, which can change with Qis. For example, when the weather is cold, the wind turns cold and causes typhoid; when it is warm, the wind causes heat; when it is cool and dry, the wind causes dryness".[39] Therefore, the "exogenous" Qi will affect the symptoms of the body, which is of clinical significance. Conforming to the changes of the four seasons is an important connotation of TCM health preservation, which makes its presence in the recuperation after the recovery from febrile diseases in modern times.[40]

The argument that "Qi" can lead to disease is not a nihilistic fact that cannot be speculated and observed, due to the fact that only when the external Qi has a causal relationship with the behavior of the patient (before the disease), that an epidemic will occur. In the Qing Dynasty, Cao Tingdong once said, "The body is exposed to the wind, cold and heat without knowing it. Before the occurrence of the disease, the pathogens can also be dispelled by sweat if one dresses warm and has hot drinks".[41] A patient can feel the invasion of external Qi and gets sick and his narration sometimes can serve as the reference for the doctor's diagnosis.[42] Even doctors can speculate

38 (Qing) Wu Zhen, updated by He Lianchen, *Treasure Raft of Epidemics,* p. 315.

39 Cao Bingzhang, Chapter 4: Diagnosis of Autumn Epidemic, On the Essence of Typhoid and Miscellaneous Diseases, included in *Collection of Rare Modern TCM. Warm Diseases*, pp. 755.

40 He Lianchen (ed.),revised by Wang Zhipu et al., *Updated Popular Treatise on Typhoid Fever*, Cao Bingzhang's preface, pp. 498–500.

41 (Qing) Cao Tingdong, et al., *Two Kinds of Traditional Chinese Health Preservation.Common Sayings of Lao Lao*, Beijing: Bibliography and Literature Press, 1993, p. 31.

42 For example, Wang Yanchang, a doctor in the late Qing Dynasty, who was from a doctors' family of seven generations, wrote a lot of medical books himself, but all of them were burned due to war. He once served as an aide to local officials in the Guangdong and Guangxi regions, and was sponsored to compile the medical books by his ancestors based on his memory, and his own writings were compiled into the book *Wang's Medical Records* (1871). In his book, he listed the possible classifications of "Qi" and daily materiality: "In the four seasons, cold air, cool nights, cold rooms, cold clothes, cold food, etc., are all chilliness; forest wind, mountain wind, alley wind, curtain wind, door wind, gap wind, fan wind, etc., are all winds; mud houses, damp lands, coated walls, water courts, sweat clothes, lacquer, sweat quilt, rain, etc., are all dampness; the lack of rain, a water shortage, smoking foreign cigarettes, tobacco, alcohol damage, or warm clothes, heat, scorching thirst, insufficient body fluid to moisten the mouth and intestines, etc., are all dryness; sunbathing and stove baking, hot pot, frying, stoves made of copper, iron, tin, silver, pans to cook oil, soup, vegetables, rice, etc., are all fire; lack of wind in midsummer, the abrupt entry into the cool room from the sunny and windy weather, the clothes newly dried, or hot water, etc., all belong to summer heat. Wearing the clothes dried in summer that are unpacked in autumn and winter, a person of deficiency

on the situation of the epidemic according to the climate at that time. For example, Cao Bingzhang said, "Most of the occurrences of autumn epidemic is due to the bad weather in summer and autumn, as well as a long drought. For example, right after the beginning of winter recently, it was extremely cold and rainy. For those who have the hidden warmth in the body, after going through cool and dry autumn before the severely cold winter, they would inevitably suffer from scarlet fever and winter febrile disease".[43] This shows that in many cases, the influence of weather, climate and temperature on the human body is more significant than that of microorganisms.[44]

Chen Guofu told a story: "In the 26th year (Republic of China period), Mr. Ge Hanlou, the chief engineer in charge of Channeling the Huaihe River into the Sea Project, suffered from typhus in Yangzhou". The weather was very cold at the beginning of his disease, and then it got hotter day by day. By the third week, when the typhus fever was at its peak, it was also the time when the weather was very hot. All the prescriptions made by the doctors failed, while his daily care was ignored. One morning, I realized it and said to Brother Jingtang, "It's very hot today. If Hanlou is still covered with a quilt and wears a sanitary coat, I'm afraid it's dangerous! "Saying so, he didn't ask to him to inform Mr. Ge's family. Even if he did so, I'm afraid it would be too late, because Mr. Ge died that afternoon. He used to be in good health and had never been ill, which is the reason for his lack of resistance. In addition, there was no way to recuperate. The doctor ignored the seasonal factor, and no one else reminded him. It occurred to me, but it was too late, and at the same time, I was not so sure. It's a pity that I can't finally save such a talent".[45] This indicates that the patient should take into account of the external factors like cold and heat, in order to find a proper way of recuperation, which is different from the theory of bacterial pathogenicity.

TCM probably uses "Qi" as a medium to "trigger" the occurrence of diseases. For example, Wu Youxing said, "There must be a cause of cold in typhoid fever, such as wind dew on one's clothes, the forced entry of water, undressing in windy air, or bathing on the eaves. The patient has trembling muscles, followed by tense limbs, suffering from bad wind and cold, with headache, body pain, fever and irregular pulse. The fast pulse with no sweat indicates typhoid fever, while the slow pulse

would suffer from heatstroke". It probably includes the relationship between the properties of many matters and Qi in daily life. Quoted from (Qin) Wang Yanchang, A Brief Introduction to the Six Immortals, *Wang's Medical Memos*, Jiangsu: Jiangsu Science and Technology Press, 1983, p. 68.

43 Cao Bingzhang, Chapter 7 Prevention of Autumn Epidemic, Essentials of Autumn Epidemic Treatment, included in Lu Zheng (ed.), *Collection of Rare Modern TCM. Medical Talk*, p. 771.

44 Ma Guangya, compiled by Liang Mingda, The Difficulties in Unifying the Names of Chinese and Western Diseases", *A Series of Chinese Medicine Clinicians for A Century.Ma Guangya*, Beijing: China TCM Press, 2001, pp. 10–11.

45 Chen Guofu, Abstracts on the Study of Illness, Choose the Proper Physician and Recuperation, included in Mr. Chen Guofu Scholarship Fund Management Committee: *Selected Works of Mr. Chen Guofu's Medical and Health Thoughts*, p. 234.

with no sweat indicates cold".[46] This theory of the disease being "triggered" by Qi is sometimes the most common expression and physical feeling in daily life. The famous writer Lao She (1899–1966) had such a description in his classic work *Camel Xiangzi*: "They (rickshaw pullers), children and adults, were looking for business on the street all day long, and the rainstorms in summer poured on their heads at any time. They all worked hard to earn money and are always sweating. The rainstorm in the north was violent and cold, sometimes with hail as big as walnuts. The cold rain, hitting their open sweaty pores, knocked them down into bed, with the fever lasting for a day or two. They had no money to buy medicine for their sick children. A rain brought up the corn and sorghum in the fields, but it could also drown many poor children in the city".[47] Generally, the lower class people suffering from these common fevers diseases during the Republic of China period never thought about bacteriology, laboratory analysis, scientific medicine and so on. For them, the most intuitive feeling may be that the body was invaded by external factors, including the "six Qis" that caused exogenous fever, and even all kinds of bad miscellaneous Qis, such as foul Qi, epidemic Qi.

Western medicine also pays attention to the individual symptoms presented by each patient. Just as influenza explained by Yu Yunxiu, it can also be divided into mucosal inflammation, gastroenteritis and nerves.[48] No matter how the symptoms change, the names of the disease will not change, because the "pathogen" causing the disease is very clear, which is a specific "bacteria" and the visible "organs" it invades. These classifications and definitions can not be defined only by the feelings of a doctor.

All the measures taken to prevent diseases were also to prevent the growth and spread of "pathogens"—the specific bacteria and viruses. This logic constitutes the whole Western medicine thinking on prevention and treatment. Therefore, in terms of Western medicine knowledge that Yu Yunxiu learned, influenza had nothing to do with autumn Qi. He said: "Patients with this disease should be isolated as soon as possible, and the expectoration should be disinfected". "When the disease is prevalent, keep yourself away from it. It's important to be cautious. In addition, if the disease is prevalent in schools, the schools should be suspended as soon as possible to avoid infection".[49] This is entirely based on preventing and blocking bacterial infection, and regulating the isolation methods among people. From the perspective of disease prevention or public health, the patients are the dangerous individuals, and their relationship with microorganisms is fundamentally different from the "Qi" in TCM or some theories of climate-induced diseases.

---

46 (Ming) Wu Youxing, supplemented by (Qing) Zheng Zhongguang, *Identifying Typhoid Epidemics, Supplementary Notes on Epidemics,* Vol. 1, Beijing: People's Health Publishing House, 1995, pp. 10–11.

47 Lao She, *Camel Xiangzi,* Beijing: People's Literature Publishing House, 2004, p. 267.

48 Yu Yunxiu, *Infectious Diseases*, p. 36.

49 Yu Yunxiu, *Infectious Diseases,* pp. 36–37.

7.4 A Profile from the Anti-Bacteria Perspective: Disease View Under the Integration of TCM and Western Medicine

Although the theory of bacteria has gradually established its status in the world of knowledge, TCM continues to challenge the theory of bacteria, believing that bacteria do not necessarily lead to the occurrence of fever. He Lianchen said, "If you catch a cold when being full, you will have cholera", which highlights a causal relationship of disease and an improper life style, rather than bacteria.[50] At the end of the Qing Dynasty, Chen Qiu discussed the "internal skill" of epidemic prevention. He said, "The most important thing is to raise one's spirit, but it is impossible to acquire it all of a sudden, and all that consumes one's spirit should be stopped. There are a few tips: no excessive alcohol, dry tobacco, and avoid hyperopia, long standing, long traveling, talking too much, overloading one's mind that may lead to insomnia. The most important tip is about sexual intercourse. If someone falls ill within seven days after excessive sex, the cure rate would hardly be one out ten."[51] Shi Yiren also had the similar statement, "Only the true Qi is kept inside, the flesh is closed and defensive. To use modern terms, it means there is sufficient antitoxin. Even though being confronted with bacteria, one cannot become sick". He also said: "This kind of antibiotic property must be based on spiritual tranquility". Emphasis of the spirit being strong enough to resist germs may be a very important aspect of TCM when discussing human immunization at that time.[52] Zhu Weiju questioned the most popular serum therapy in Western preventive medicine: "Western medicine not only takes bacteria as the pathogen, but also knows the location of the origin, so that its treatment method is no more than sterilization and excision. The latest and effective sterilization is serum". Zhu believed that the principle of serum therapy is to use the human body to produce an adaptability to the external environment, with a small amount of bacteria to nurture the adaptability of the human body to the environment (bacterial breeding), which is its strength.[53] However, during the incubation period of a general fever before the definite diagnose, the serum cannot be used. TCM decoction treatment can not only avoid this complexity, but also has a better curative effect. Zhu meant that when TCM treats patients with fever at the beginning, it was not needed to distinguish the types of bacteria, "Finding out that the inherent physiological function is hindered by the six pathogenic factors which

---

[50] He Lianchen (ed.), revised by Wang Zhipu et al., *Updated Popular Treatise on Typhoid Fever*, p. 499.

[51] Chen Qiu, et al.(eds), Collection of Liji Medicine Q & A to Epidemics and Cholera, included in Liu Shijue (ed.), *Wenzhou Literature Series Integration of Wenzhou Modern Medical Books*, p. 72.

[52] Shi Yiren, *Shi's Internal Canon of Medicine*, p. 30.

[53] Wang Shenxuan (ed.), Part VII Treatment, *Compilation of New Theories of TCM*,Shanghai: Shanghai Bookstore Press, pp. 3–4.

can be removed by decoction, and the natural immunization would duly be restored, how can the bacteria reproduce itself?".[54]

After the collision between TCM and Western medicine, the tradition had not remained static. As mentioned in the first chapter, at the beginning of modern times when bacteriology became dominant in the medical field, there was no great conflict of views between Chinese and Western Medicine on the etiology, and the discussion of fever in Western medicine was not as detailed as the classification of diseases after the emergence of bacteriology, the discussion of fever in Chinese and Western medicine even had some common ground to share. During this period, TCM, based on the combination of "exogenous" and "Qi theory" in the traditional treatise on febrile diseases, easily absorbed the miasma theory of Western medicine. Since modern times, the concepts of "air" and "nourishing Qi" in the chemical hygiene theory of Western medicine have affected the Qi theory of TCM. This sense of deja vu made TCM happy to accept it and carry a dialogue with the classical theory of Qi. For example, when Huang Zhuzhai wrote *Treatise on Typhoid and Miscellaneous Diseases* in 1948, similar to the theory in the era of Hobson, the relationship between "air" change and human muscle surface, as well as the comparison with the "exterior and interior" of the body in classical medicine, was still fundamentally influential.[55] Take cholera as another example. Zhang Guohua (1864–1933), one of the "three Zhangs in China" during the Republic of China period, adopted the names of Western medicine in his *Medical Changes.* Instead of giving attention to bacteria, he talked about the harm of the "carbon air" of Western medicine to the human body, and compared it to the "filthy Qi" of TCM. This is far from the thinking of Western medicine that bacteria determine the symptoms of the disease and health matters (see Fig. 7.4).[56] Westerners use the name of cholera, "nothing is more violent than cholera among the current epidemics", "In general, the most violent and abrupt diseases are no more than the two epidemics of typhoid and warm diseases"; the description of the two epidemics is just "absorbing carbon air and filthy Qi from the mouth and nose, mixing up with the body's nourishing Qi to turn into internal heat, instilling Qi into the blood, and upsetting the intestines and stomach".[57] Combining the various western scientific "Qi" research with the Qi theory of Chinese medicine had become a popular medical discourse in the early Republic of China period.

When the health care turned to hygiene during modern times, the discussion of focusing on "air" hygiene became prevalent in the health preservation fields of TCM. Wu Tingfang, a diplomat at the end of the Qing Dynasty and the beginning of the Republic of China period, said that human life depend entirely on air, so the air we

[54] Wang Shenxuan (ed.), Part VII Treatment, *Compilation of New Theories of TCM*, Shanghai: Shanghai Bookstore Press, p. 4.

[55] Huang Zhuzhai, *Treatise on Typhoid and Miscellaneous Diseases*, Xi'an: Shaanxi Academy of TCM, 1982, p. 161.

[56] Tianjin Special Municipal Health Bureau (ed.), *Epidemic Prevention Report of Tianjin Special Municipal Office in the Summer of the 27th Year of the Republic of China Period*, Vol. 18, Tianjin: Tianjin·Special Municipal Health Bureau, 1939, p. 124.

[57] Zhang Guohua, Epidemic Cholera, Medical Changes, included in Lu Zheng (ed.), *Collection of Rare Modern TCM. Medical Talk*, pp. 249–250.

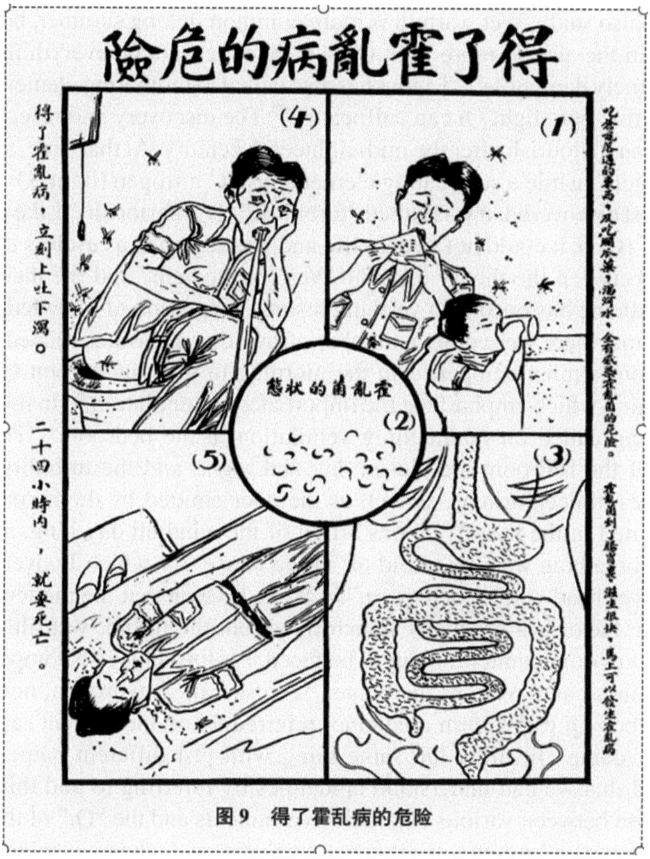

Fig. 7.4 Risk of Cholera

breathe must be clean. The study and bedroom where one lives should have windows for ventilation. For indoor crowds, the air is polluted and it is not safe to stay indoors for a long time.[58] Of course, some health experts believed that even though this saying is popular, Chinese people are used to closing the windows tightly while sleeping at night, resulting in tuberculosis from absorbing turbid air; but when you sleep with the windows open, you will only be attacked by the cold, which is more likely to cause tuberculosis. Thus you should not be confused by the saying of "air".[59] It can be seen that there were similarities and differences in the interpretation of Qi in Chinese and Western medicine at the beginning, which is thought-provoking. There are other Qis. For example, when discussing the "wet warmth" related to dampness,

[58] (Qing) Cao Tingdong, et al., *Two Kinds of Traditional Chinese Health Preservation. Common Sayings of Lao Lao*, p. 180.

[59] Jing Guansheng, Reference to "Zeng Wenzheng's Diary", included in Xiao Ping, Jing Guansheng (ed.), *Prevention of Diseases and Longevity. Health Preservation Series*, Shanghai: Shanghai Science and Technology Literature Press, 2013, p. 58.

Hu Anbang also said: "Wet warmth is more common in long summer, because there is less acid in the air and more light Qi, which can evaporate everything and cause mold rot, namely dampness". "Light Qi is also called a smothering element. If oxygen is removed, this pure light Qi can suffocate".[60] The discovery and research of these two airs began to flourish after the mid-eighteenth century. At that time, acid element meant "oxygen", while a suffocating element meant "nitrogen (light) Qi". When the latter was first discovered, it was called "turbid air" or "inferior air". Like the previous "carbon air" (CO), it could not sustain life and was regarded as useless to life.[61] The connection between the theory of air in Western medicine and the theory of Qi in Chinese medicine has become a very interesting integration of knowledge.

At that time, there were quite a number of hygienic measures related to Qi, such as "the windows must be opened in the morning to give out carbon Qi and let in nourishing air", which emphasized the importance of ventilation.[62] In modern times, Li Hongzhang called on maintaining ventilation in the bedroom: "The windows and doors of the bedroom are closed day and night, and the turbidity caused by lights, clothes, toilets, urinals, as well as the odor emitted by the human body, are all accumulated in the room". "I was afraid of the wind all day long, and the only thing I was breathing was the turbid air in the house, for which I covered with my comforter over head when I lied down".[63] It can be seen that the modern "wind" as a pathogenic factor has gradually transformed, but the turbid, wet filthy Qi in the house is the environmental problem to be faced. Lu Jinsheng also compared various "Qis" in Chinese and Western medicine: "The so-called hydrogen, nourishing Qi, light Qi, carbon Qi it (Western medicine) referred to are the ancient saying of cold Qi, heat Qi, damp Qi, filthy Qi, same thing with just different names".[64] Zhang Guohua said that we can understand epidemics by referring to and thinking about the interaction between various external environments and the "Qi" of the body. It is said: "In summer and autumn, there is more cholera, and when it is mixed with three Qis in summer and autumn, the carbon Qi is thin, with filthy fumigation, air soaring and breath blowing.... Scholars can integrate the weather, the Qis of the earth, time, season, body and diseases, to explain half of causes for the violent cholera of the epidemic". These discussions generally reflect the simplified interpretation method of this generalized TCM Qi theory.

When it comes to other knowledge about "infection", TCM mostly combines the ancient "unhealthy miscellaneous Qis" with the filth or odor produced by the

---

[60] Hu Anbang, *The Great Treatise on Damp Warm Diseases*, Shanghai: Chinese Medicine Guidance Society, 1935, pp. 6–7.

[61] Zhao Kuanghua, *General History of Chemistry, Vol. 1*, Hsinchu: Fanyi Publishing House, 1998, pp. 135–139.

[62] Shaoxing Medical Association, Treatment of Damp and Warm Epidemics, included in Li Shunbao (ed.), *Complete Book of Warm Diseases*, Vol. II, p. 2100.

[63] Jin Xiage (ed.), To the Fourth Younger Brother, Family Letters of Li Hongzhang, included in *Family Letters of Celebrities in the Qing Dynasty*, Vol. II, Yangzhou: Jiangsu Guangling Ancient Book Printing Society, 1997, p. 854.

[64] Qiu Qingyuan (ed.), Caution with Life, Collection of Medical Talks included in Lu Zheng (ed.), *Collection of Rare Modern Traditional Chinese.Medical Talks*, pp. 356–357.

spoiled material in Western medicine, which are quite consistent. However, though the external definition has changed, the interpretation method of TCM is still ancient in terms of the body view. For example, Zhang Guohua said, "The pathogens of epidemic diseases are inhaled by the mouth and nose, which is not only a membranous source, but can also spread all over the body. The *Classics on Medical Problems* says that it is spread out to the meridians, and the pulse is also unstable. The mouth connects the throat, the nose connects to the brain spine, the throat connects the heart, lungs, five internal organs, and the pharynx connects to the gastrointestinal and six viscera".[65] Zhang still uses the theory of membrane origin from the Qing Dynasty to explain the cause of disease.

How to understand the interaction between physical diseases and external "Qi" that people understand in their daily life? It is advisable to observe the five elements, the four seasons and the Qi in daily life. Hu Anbang, who wrote *The Great Treatise on Damp Warm Diseases* in the early Republic of China period, cited the medical case of Wu Jiaoshan, a physician in the Ming Dynasty, to illustrate the doctors' observation of "summer heat":

> Wu Jiaoshan treated a woman who was infected in winter. Wu felt her pulse, which was weak with the symptoms of heatstroke. Everybody was confused by it and asked her what happened. The woman said: because of the cold weather, I changed my cotton padded clothes, took a cotton padded comforter and covered herself. In a moment, I became thirsty, feverish and vomiting, till now. Wu said: it's true that she got heatstroke. Exposing the cotton padded comforter in the scorching summer sun and enclosing it in a container with the heat, there must be summer heat, which has not yet been released. Nowadays, people are deficient and easily invaded, so she is having the symptoms of heatstroke. The woman agreed.[66]

The "summer heat" infected to this woman came not from the season, but from the contact between people and objects in her daily life. The woman's affirmative answer represents that doctors and patients have a common discourse on the pathogenesis of summer heat. Then, Hu further explained that "heatstroke can also occur in winter", that is, there are summer diseases in winter. On the contrary, in summer, if you "spend the summer in a cold and dark big house, prefer drinking ice water, eating melons and fruits, you will have cold pathogens from the external, and you can be harmed by the internal cold. Summer time is limited, but the cold harm is done inside a person, hence comes typhoid in summer".[67] "Typhoid fever" can occur in summer, which interprets the occurrence of fever from the perspective of daily life. This set of cognition was still emphasized in the early Republic of China period. It was also said that heat toxin (Qi) from the outside world is harmful and there came a warning of keeping away from it: "When sweating, it is no good to wear clothes that were

---

[65] Zhang Guohua, Epidemic Cholera, Medical Changes, included in Lu Zheng (ed.), *Collection of Rare Modern TCM. Medical Talk*, pp. 249–250.

[66] Hu Anbang, 16. Medical Cases of Damp Warm Diseases,The Great Treatise on Damp Warm Diseases, included in Lu Zheng (ed.), *Collection of Rare Modern TCM. Warm Diseases*, p. 708.

[67] Hu Anbang, The Great Treatise on Damp Warm Diseases, included in Lu Zheng (ed.),*Collection of Rare Modern TCM. Warm Diseases*, pp. 708,743.

exposed to the scorching sun, or soaked in sweat".[68] All of them share the idea that the feeling of Qi (hot Qi) can be the cause of diseases, and "Qi" is accumulated from daily life objects, leading to human diseases. In addition, the previously mentioned theory of miasma in Western medicine has also affected the content of the traditional theory of Qi in TCM. For example, Cao Bingzhang said, "The pathogens of the epidemic is all from the wet soil, and the pathogenic factors of filth at ordinary times is transpiration with the air and sunlight, which is the mixture of miasma and fog. When it is touched, it is inhaled from the mouth and nose".[69] Although there have been many discussions on seasons and times of the "Autumn Epidemic" explained by Cao, its "transpiration with the air and sunlight is no different from the toxins of miasma and fog", which is obviously affected by the miasma theory. Entering from the "mouth and nose" is the view from the knowledge of Western epidemiology, and is more consistent with the plague discussion of TCM.

The concept that toxic air in the environment leads to diseases often appears in the theory of TCM. For example, Xu Runzhi (1855–1919), who was good at treating warm diseases, said that when compiling *Selected Sore Therapies of Hua Tuo*: "Houses and gardens have been closed for a long time, and toxic air was abundant. Caution should be taken before entering. When houses are closed for a long time, it is damp, the dampness is toxic and the air is stagnant. It may be haunted by pathogens".[70] He also said, "The burning coal is toxic, the earth pit stinks when it leaks fire, and people being fumigated by this will be dead without knowing... If you put a basin of water in the room and leave a window open, there will be no harm done even if the coal stinks".[71] Therefore, the toxins in TCM are actually related to the external environment or external factors. In a sensible way, it is logical that toxic air plays a role between disease and external environmental factors. Odor and fecal toxins are also related to the environment, as follows:

> Ze Country had five districts. It was mountainous and barren, and the farmers accumulated feces for fertilization. The family of Qi Shi, Gao Ping's student, had three people die in a row when they were emptying their manure pit. As fecal toxin was not contained in the *Record of Redressing Grievances,* Gao Ping had a lot of suspicions and eventually reported the case as the dead being beaten to death. Luo, the officer of Feng Tai, ordered the inspection of the three corpses, but only found that there were no scars, except the roots of their teeth were blue and black. The coroners discovered that the dung was accumulated in the pit from

---

[68] Or: "Fumigating the clothes in winter,drying them up to keep out the cold, the extra heat being accumulated, all of which would be released in spring, causing body heat, dizziness, cough, abdominal distress, and limb fatigue". It can be seen that Qi will accumulate on daily objects and make people sick. He Lianchen (ed.), revised by Wang Zhipu et al., *Updated Popular Treatise on Typhoid Fever*, pp. 498–499.

[69] Cao Bingzhang, Chapter 7: Pathology of Autumn Epidemic,On the Essence of Typhoid and Miscellaneous Diseases, included in *Collection of Rare Modern TCM. Warm Diseases*, p. 752.

[70] Xu Runzhi (ed.), Pathogenic Qi and Toxins in Empty Houses,Selected Sore Therapies of Hua Tuo, included in Liu Shijue (ed.), *Wenzhou Literature Series Collection of Wenzhou Modern Medical Books, Vol. II,* Shanghai: Shanghai Academy of Social Sciences Press, 2005, p. 995.

[71] Xu Runzhi (ed.), Coal Poisoning, Selected Sore Therapies of Hua Tuo, included in Liu Shijue, (ed.), *Wenzhou Literature Series Collection of Wenzhou Modern Medical Books, Vol. II,* Shanghai: Shanghai Academy of Social Sciences Press, 2005, p. 996.

> winter, till spring, summer and autumn, during which the toxic gas smothered. Once the pit was touched, it was most likely to cause death. The smell of covered dung water was so strong that the opening was fatal, no matter how deep the pit was. Those detoxified had black teeth and blue lips, which was as bad a death as if from other kinds of toxins. It was said that the detoxification method of the natives was to burn cypress incense, and throw cypress wood chips into the pit to dissolve the odor.[72]

In TCM, bad Qi is often called toxic air or filthy air. Whether in the field of internal medicine or surgery, "toxic air" is a common cause. "Summer sweat penetrates your clothes, and you must not bask in the hot sun. If the clothes are hastily put away at the time of drying up before a sudden rainstorm, the toxin of the hot sun will be confined inside. If it has the sweat in heat and is put on occasionally, the heat will be induced with the toxins directly in it. The symptoms are all typhoid fever, and if you mistakenly treat it with cold, it will cause madness and delirium".[73] "Toxin" sometimes refers to substances with form and quality, and sometimes refers to bad Qi in general. It is an important cause of exogenous fever. The "detoxification" mentioned in Chapter 4 is probably also a broad term as an extended interpretation in therapeutics.[74] As the "toxic" culture of TCM involves a wide range, it is only briefly introduced here. Next, we will focus on daily life to see how people's thoughts on fever changed during the Republic of China period.

---

[72] Another example: "In Wei Village of Gaoping, there was a pig dealer Zhang Min and others who were from Henan. When the piglets fell into a cesspit by mistake, the two sellers went down to the pit to rescue them, and died after being poisoned by feces. Their teeth were black, and their upper and lower lips were blue". All of them are from Xu Runzhi (ed.), Fecal Poison, included in Liu Shijue, (ed.), *Wenzhou Literature Series Collection of Wenzhou Modern Medical Books, Vol. II,* Shanghai: Shanghai Academy of Social Sciences Press, 2005, p. 996.

[73] Xu Runzhi (ed.),Selected Sore Therapies of Hua Tuo, included in Liu Shijue, (ed.),*Wenzhou Literature Series Collection of Wenzhou Modern Medical Books, Vol. II,* pp. 995–996.

[74] In addition, "toxin" may have the context of religious medicine and involve the problem of "insects". For example, *Authentic Surgery* contains: "In case of heavenly epidemic, numerous people were infected.Mahogany decoction can be used to rub into the nostrils, and taken a little at a time, so that one won't be infected when going into the patient's home". Mahogany had a restraining effect on pathogenic factors in ancient times. See Li Jianmin, *Therapic Craft.Medicine. History,* Taipei: Nantian Book Company, 2000, pp. 3–24. *Authentic Surgery* says that "Taiyi purple golden elixir" can treat plague, malaria, etc. As for the treatment of "tuberculosis, there was hardly any drugs. A necromancer said, grinding one tablet every morning, after three doses consecutively, the filth, bugs and monstrous pathogenic factors would be discharged. This therapy spread and saved the lives of countless people. A woman, who had been suffering from tuberculosis for a long time, took one dose and threw up more than ten small bugs right after. She then took Suhexiang pills, and the symptoms were gone. She was soon cured after recuperating for more than a month. It is really a treasure medicine for world health". It shows that the drug can also treat insects and "alien monsters". It can be seen that toxins, epidemics and insects can find highly related venation in the same drug. From (Ming) Chen Shigong, *Treatise on Acne No. 17, Authentic Surgery,* pp. 90, 92.

7.5 Discussions of Disease Prevention of TCM and Transformation of Daily Life

Even from the perspective of bacteriology, the concept of health during the Republic of China period just paid attention to the two aspects of "heterization" after bacteriology entered China: First, the importance of "personal" disease prevention and health was always placed in an important position, even outweighing the "public" perspective. Second, in the practice of disease resistance in general daily life, the knowledge of distinguishing bacterial species was not particularly important even though the authority of bacteriology had been established. Instead, it was emphasized that almost all warm diseases were covered by common disease prevention methods, such as disinfection, cleaning, isolation and other common knowledge. TCM was happy to integrate this "alienated" hygiene.[75] The combination of these two aspects of "heterization" also called the attention of TCM doctors during the Republic of China period to the corresponding relationship between "individuals" and "environment", and was inevitably mixed with a lot of Western medicine discourse. Lu Yuanlei, a TCM practitioner, said, "the Chinese medicine community should supplement scientific and health knowledge, such as implementing disinfection procedures, and abolishing all kinds of unhygienic habits".[76] It can be seen that in terms of health knowledge and measures, TCM was willing to learn. When setting up the course of TCM, Lu immediately thought about "stipulating the knowledge and skills necessary for all disciplines of national medicine. But no matter what discipline, it is necessary to provide the legal common knowledge of infectious diseases".[77] Subject to the state power, TCM did not actively participate in the administrative work of public health like Western medicine did. However, TCM was still undergoing changes.

Before modern times, "individuals" and "environment" did not completely intersect in medical knowledge. In the category of warm disease, it is a passive description. Under the cover of "Qi" between heaven and earth, individuals had no ability nor need to change the environment. They only needed to try to understand this set of disease theories and treatment methods[78]; in the classics of warm diseases, the discussion of "space" was relatively rare, and it began to increase gradually in modern times. For example, Wang Shixiong (style name Mengying) said, "Cholera and eruptive diseases became epidemics, which were caused by the brewing of heat and sick Qis. It should be known by everyone that there should never be too many people in the

[75] Jie Sheng, Prevention of Epidemic in the Future, *Weekly Supplement of Shaoxing Medical Journal,* 1920 (32), p. 3.

[76] Lu Yuanlei, Declaration upon Abolishing Classic Medicine in the Central Health Conference, Lu's Collection of Medical Theories, included in Zhang Yuping (ed.), *Two Kinds of Lu Yuanlei's Medical Books,* p. 90.

[77] Lu Yuanlei, Outline on Sorting Out the Academic Works of TCM, Lu's Collection of Medical Theories, included in Zhang Yuping (ed.), *Two Kinds of Lu Yuanlei's Medical Books,* p. 149.

[78] (Qing) Zhang Fengkui, additionally annotated by Ye Ziyu, Preface to the Engraved Version of Yu Jiayan's Theory of Epidemics, Supplement of Ye Ping's The Complete Book of Heatstroke, included in Cao Bingzhang (ed.), *Great Achievements in Chinese Medicine,* Vol. 16 (II), p. 39.

same room, never close the doors and windows tight so that the air can get through".[79] *Identification of Six Factors* explains the understanding of the influence of external "Qi" on fever:

"The summer disease caused by exogenous pathogenic factors is called malaria, and the disease caused by internal cold is called dysentery".[80] The Qi in the human body is closely related to the external factors that "trigger" diseases. They may vary from person to person and from one environment to another, and eventually lead to different warm diseases. Just like He Lianchen said, "Sleeping outside in summer to keep cool will cause malaria in autumn, if not cholera in summer".[81] It also shows the possibility of external Qi triggering physical diseases. In addition, Zheng Zhengguang said that the plague "could be from nature or from infection. In short, it starts from nature, becomes rampant by infection and declines at the transformation of Qi. This is generally the case with all epidemics".[82] The ancient theory of epidemics has its own set of rules and theories of its rise and falls. It can be predicted through a set of mathematical mechanisms. It is to be understood but not to be changed.

Since modern times, this knowledge has been transformed. Based on the foregoing, modern Chinese medicine combines the miasma theory of Western medicine with the traditional Qi theory, and the relationship between air, sunlight, water, soil and environment has become a major focus of the discussion of warm diseases in TCM. In his *Collection of Medical Talks,* Qiu Qingyuan combined the concept of "air" in Western medicine with the concept of "five Qis being the heavenly food for humans" in the *Internal Canon of Medicine* of TCM, which shows that these "Qis" are necessary for human survival: "The circulation of blood and the smoothness of meridians are all based on air". "Be with air means the air in the human body. If it

---

[79] For Wang Shixiong's life and new views on warm diseases, see Kim Taylor, Cholera and the Composition of the Wenre Jingwei (Complementing the Classics on Warmth and Heat, 1852) in East Asian History of Science, Technology and Medicine, included in Jiang Xiaoyuan (ed.), *History of Science in Multiculturalism: Proceedings of the 10th International Conference on the History of Science in East Asia,* Shanghai: Shanghai Jiaotong University Press, 2005, pp. 145–160. Kim Taylor didn't notice that Wang's contribution to the warm disease school and even the whole warm disease theory was to pay attention to the health of people, environment and space. Most of these observations were based on Wang's experience in observing cholera in the late Qing Dynasty. For citations, see (Qing) Wang Shixiong, Discipline, Updated Treatise on Cholera included in Sheng Zengxiu (ed.), *Wang Mengying's Complete Book of Medicine,* Beijing: China TCM Press, 1999, p. 156. For the study of cholera in the late Qing Dynasty, see Yu Xinzhong, The History of the Jiangnan Pandemic during Jiadao Period—An Investigation Based on the Changes of Modern Society, *Research on the History of the Qing Dynasty*, 2001(02), pp. 1–18; Li Yushang, Cholera Epidemic in China (1817–1821), *Historical Geography*, 2001 (17), pp. 316–336.

[80] (Qing) Lu Tingzhen, Identification of Summer Heat, Item 28 Identification of Summer Heat No.19, *Identification of Six Factors*, Li Shunbao (ed.), *Complete Book of Warm Diseases, Vol. I,* p. 2142.

[81] He Lianchen (ed.),revised by Wang Zhipu et al. *Updated Popular Treatise on Typhoid Fever*, Cao Bingzhang's preface, p. 499.

[82] (Ming) Wu Youxing supplemented by (Qing) Zheng Zhongguang, Supplementary Notes on the Names of Epidemic Diseases from the Paraphrase of Classics Part II, *Supplementary Notes on Epidemic Diseases,* p. 4.

is insufficient and cannot circulate, the essence won't spread and the six pathogenic factors will cause various diseases. I have seen some patients feeling happy to see the sun and trying to take advantage of the sun to carry forward Qi for the lack of it, that is, they didn't have enough nourishing Qi. In fact, it is due to the fact that the air is not circulating, wherever there is air, there is life, or vice versa. Air is the key for the human body".[83] This is just the beginning for the integration of theories.

In daily life, when discussing febrile diseases, TCM draws lessons from the thinking of changing the environment and pathogenic factors, that is, the concepts of "cleanliness" and "hygiene", and integrates into the theoretical framework of fighting against febrile diseases. For example, the typhoid fever prevention methods, discussed in the *Treatment of Damp and Warm Epidemics* which was compiled by Shaoxing Medical Association, are related to the chapter of "Health Preservation" in the *Internal Canon of Medicine.* But the ancient medical books have "all the words that are too profound to be put into practice". So the Association chose some rules that were easy to understand and implement for public reference. The new rules included the content of the Western miasma theory, as well as many cleaning measures: (1) Sweep the houses and make sure they are not polluted by dust. The four walls should be refreshed with lime, or sprinkled with decontamination liquid to prevent toxic dampness. (2) Garbage carries filthy air and it is not to be dumped freely. It should be dumped in a bucket, and held for the scavenger to pick up. Don't trample on it after it has been picked up. Keeping the streets and alleys clean would prevent all epidemics. (3) In the morning, the windows must be opened to let out carbon gas and let in the oxygen. Night time is different. Going to sleep without turning off the light or sleeping outside to stay cool should be forbidden. (4) All utensils like pots, jars, bottles and bowls are most likely to produce mosquitoes by being stored in overnight water. If tap water is available, it is advisable to quit using the above utensils. The gutter of the patio must be cleaned frequently and stay unblocked. It's better to pour burning kerosene into the gutter to get rid of filth and dampness. (5) Keeping a coffin at home is the easiest way to cause disease. Assuming that the deceased was suffering from an infectious disease, the consequence would be unimaginable, so the funeral home should bury the coffin as soon as possible. (6) Mosquitoes and flies can transmit diseases the most, so food must be covered to prevent mosquitoes and flies from spreading toxins. When using bowls and dishes, wash them first. When sleeping, one must hang the tent. Avoid mosquito bites as they can cause infectious diseases. (7) All kinds of raw and cold things contain microorganisms, so food must be thoroughly cooked. Don't eat overnight leftover food, and don't put them in the same room with the uncooked food, so that microorganisms won't invade. Drinking water must be boiled. Soda water and frozen water are harmful to people. Melons and fruits are also prone to disease, so it's better not to have much. (8) Spitting on the ground is the most immoral and an easy way to spread diseases. It is advisable to spit in a spittoon or a gutter in order to avoid the disease.

---

[83] Qiu Qingyuan(ed.), On Air, Medical Talks, included in Lu Zheng (ed.), *Collection of Rare Modern TCM,* p. 351.

Since 1909, non-governmental organizations such as the Shanghai Institute of Medicine and the China Health Association had health lectures to carry out initial education in public health, personal hygiene and disease prevention. Some concepts in these appeals were excerpted from the notice of Shanghai Medical Research Institute.[84] In fact, these concepts requiring cleanliness and hygiene were advocated as early as in the late Qing Dynasty.[85] Only in the discussion of fever in Chinese medicine is this appeal particularly notable, meanwhile it is quite different from classical medicine. These ideas of advocating hygiene and disease prevention are the new ideas that did not exist in the TCM treatment of "damp and warm diseases". Such health and disease prevention principles are often suitable for all febrile infectious diseases; Article (7) has noticed the position of microorganisms in the discussion of diseases, but as for the killing and preventative methods of specific bacteria, there had not been special classifications. As Cheng Hanzhang said, "Both the types of bacteria and the method of disinfection are based on the properties of the bacteria".[86] For public health experts who are proficient in bacteriology, the key is to prevent a certain fever and eliminate the properties and factors that are easy to breed specific pathogens.

During the early Republic of China period, people started to pay attention to disease prevention and sanitation measures with general significance, but bacteriology has no guiding significance for further practices in daily life. In the early Republic of China period, TCM took more of the practical operational knowledge according to the theory of malaria than the bacteriological theoretical framework behind them. In other words, even under the influence of bacteriology, it still focused on the theory of miasma. When the pandemic broke out in 1918, Cao Bingzhang said, "Some had it (Qi) deeply hidden and burst out abruptly, which was caused by the intake of dirty river water due to the dry weather, storing sewage in pools, or having unsanitory food. The epidemic duly occurred and lot of poor people died. There were also many people being infected because the clothes and feces of the infected patients were washed in the river water which was used by others to wash rice and vegetables".[87] Cao explained the change of Qi with the concept of incubation temperature in traditional febrile diseases, and believed that the outbreak of a serious influenza epidemic was related to dry weather, diet, water, cleaning, etc., but he did not emphasize the risk of "droplets" between people, which was the most important thing in the West to prevent influenza, and the related techniques of wearing masks and isolation. TCM advocated a wide range of environmental sanitation, which was based on the theory of miasma. In fact, the "miasma theory" is a broad expression.

[84] Shaoxing Medical Association (ed.), Treatment of Damp and Warm Epidemics, included in Li Shunbao (ed.),*Complete Book of Warm Diseases*, Vol. II, p. 2100.

[85] Yu Xinzhong,A Brief Exploration of the Evolution of the "Health" Concept in the Late Qing Dynasty, included in Research Center of Chinese Social History of Nankai University (ed.), *Collection of Social History of Nankai in the New Century*, Tianjin: China Social History Research Center, Nankai University, 2010. pp. 271–307.

[86] Cheng Hanzhang, *A Brief Introduction to Western Medicine*, p. 46.

[87] Cao Bingzhang, Chapter 2: Pathogeny of Autumn Epidemic, On the Essence of Typhoid and Miscellaneous Diseases, included in *Collection of Rare Modern TCM. Warm Diseases*, p. 751.

At the beginning, it attached importance to the clean environment, rather than bacterial characteristics and specific infectious routes. For example, Cao argued about "Autumn Epidemic":

> Since after the start of the epidemic, mosquitoes and flies are also the cause of much of the spread. This is due to abnormal weather conditions, the negligence of public health and people's uncontrolled health conditions, all of which attribute to the occurrence and spread of plagues. Now the weather is getting colder, the timely rain fell, the muddy water in the river will flow away, the septic tanks in the streets can relocate the filth to the hidden places, mosquitoes and flies are decreasing, the general vector of infection is gone, and the epidemic may decline.[88]

Abnormal seasonal weather is the pathogenic factor, but it should be noted here that if "Autumn Epidemic" is really the name of "flu" in TCM, as Cao said, then human droplets in contact with the air should be the most important way of transmission and prevention. In the period of pandemic influenza, foreign public health experts said repeatedly: put on a mask.[89] However, TCM held the view that mosquitoes, flies and dirty water are more related to environmental sanitation. This inconsistent confluence of the East and the West was a common discussion at that time. Only from the perspective of bacteria can the characteristics of "vector" infectious bacteria in the environment be meaningful.

Yu Yunxiu's example based on microbial cognition is very representative. He said, "Tetanus bacteria can live underground, soil is the source of infection. There are often typhoid, cholera and other bacteria in the water, so the cleanliness of the water is the most important thing in terms of sanitation". "Unclean tap water, river water and well water are often contaminated by patients' excrement and contain pathogenic microorganisms. This kind of water is the most dangerous, either as a drink or for washing cups and plates".[90] Western medicine tends to discuss the characteristics and types of "bacteria". During the Republic of China period, most TCM doctors did not have the technology to actually test bacteria even if they knew the classification of bacteria. TCM believed that almost all microorganisms were "foreign", and keeping clean would be enough. It's not so critical to test bacteria or understand the characteristics of bacteria. In other words, although it is a modern perspective to distinguish the types and characteristics of bacteria, TCM mostly discussed it in academic theories and books without putting it into practice.

As the most important of this miasma theory is the contact between humans and space, residence, material and body, it is still in line with bacteriology, though not focusing on the characteristics of bacteria. At the end of the Qing Dynasty and the beginning of the Republic of China period, the discussion of TCM mainly started with the hygiene and health of "individuals". "Clothes with sweat should be washed immediately. Make sure not to wear them after the sweat is dry, or it will lead

[88] Cao Bingzhang, Chapter 2: Pathogeny of Autumn Epidemic, On the Essence of Typhoid and Miscellaneous Diseases, included in *Collection of Rare Modern TCM. Warm Diseases*, p. 751.

[89] Howard Phillips & David Killingray (eds.), *The Spanish Influenza Pandemic of 1918–19*, London: Routledge, 2003.

[90] Yu Yunxiu, *Microbiology*, p. 38.

to disease". "Mountaineering, overlooking, wading in the wild, sightseeing, and breathing in the fresh air is the most important way to prevent epidemics".[91] These are the disease prevention rules of personal hygiene. Occasionally, there were also views extending to groups. For example, when it comes to epidemic diseases, it is recorded in *Compilation of Qing Dynasty Works:*

> Shanghai was densely populated and its residents did not pay attention to hygiene. The life in summer time can be divided into three periods a day. The sun was scorching outside the window by noon time. One can hardly breath when not having enough opium in the summer heat. In the afternoon, people gathered in taverns, tea houses, theaters and brothels. The room was stuffy, and dozens of people of indulgence gathered around as a flesh screen to eat rotten delicacies. At night, they drove to gardens in the open suburbs, going into reed sheds, mud fields, and straw pavilions, drenching with soda and ice cream, enjoying their revelries till the roosters started their morning crows. How could even an iron man keep up with this life style! Therefore, before the end of summer, dysentery prevailed, especially red dysentery, and nine out of ten died.[92]

Many scholars, such as Li Shangren, Yu Xinzhong and Hu Cheng, have gone through the discussion of this unhealthy life style and have a relatively clear understanding. In terms of Chinese people's disease discussions on living space, the prevention of "personal" diseases was often to hide at home to avoid the attack of bad "Qi" from the outside world. Before modern times, TCM had many disease prevention philosophies about the coexistence of people, space and residence. The following is the quote from *Common Sayings of Lao Lao* in explaining the daily practice of preventing exogenous fever.

> When the epidemic is prevalent, the unhealthy air of heaven and earth, which is infectious, mostly entered by mouth and nose. Like Wu says that "external pathogenic factors take advantage of breathing and enter the membrane". People infect each other through Qi which is carried by wind. It is the so-called "wind, the spirit of shifting and changing" in *Internal Canon of Medicine.* When going in and out, it is always advisable to cover one's mouth and nose with sleeves in order to avoid wind, which is a way to avoid the epidemic. There is gap wind between windows and doors. Tiny as it is, being forced out of the gap, it carries a special kind of cold air, which is particularly sharp, similar to a hidden arrow that is more hurtful in attacking the unprepared! Never lose caution to the concentrated wind!

For exogenous diseases, the wind was dangerous and terrifying, especially after Wu Youke's argument, the mouth and nose had become an important entry of external air to invade the human body. To avoid the blowing wind was an important task of health preservation. The best way to avoid all kinds of bad external Qi was to hide at home. "In a sudden heavy rain during the extremely hot weather, the heat in the yard is forced into the room. The fishy smell is the toxin from summer heat which is most harmful". It is said in *Internal Canon of Medicine*: 'Harm done in summer is followed by malaria in autumn.' The windows must be tightly closed to keep it

---

[91] Shaoxing Medical Association, Prevention of Diseases, Treatment of Damp and Warm Epidemics, included in Li Shunbao (ed.), *Complete Book of Warm Diseases*, Vol. II, pp. 2100.

[92] (Qing) Xu Ke, Fatal Diseases. Shanghai Summer, *Compilation of Qing Dynasty Works*, Beijing: Zhonghua Book Company, 1986, pp. 3524–3525.

away".[93] "Four situations of not going out: strong wind, heavy rain, severe cold, severe heat. No venturing outdoors unless it is totally necessary. That is, one should stay indoor quietly to cultivate heavenly peace; be silent and respectful particularly in big thunders and lightening to revere heavenly anger". In the living environment, the window had become an important barrier to isolate the external atmosphere or cold.

> The windows are to be tightly closed, but the needle gap leaks, and the breeze sneaks in. The Northerners keep out the cold by pasting paper all over the room in order to block wind and dust, which can also make the room clean and tidy. The bedrooms of the elderly are done in the same way. Papers must be re pasted in the early winter of each year.
>
> The sun is intense during a long summer, the heat lingers in the evening, and the wind brings heat. The bedroom window should only be opened in the morning to dispel the depression of the night. It must be closed after sunrise. The windows should be covered with heavy draperies, which are not light permeable, and the room should not be accessible all day. The air from the human body is also a source of heat, as all the heat is external, not internal. At bed time, the drapery can be rolled up and the windows should stay closed so that the pillow and mat can be as cool as they are in autumn.[94]

It can be seen that before the Republic of China period, the windows of many houses were closed. By the time of the Republic of China period, the focus of disease prevention measures called for attention by TCM had changed. Focusing on the perspective of individuals and residences, what we used to pay attention to was to turn the space into a secret room as much as possible to avoid the wind, cold and other external air attacking human bodies and causing diseases. Since the Republic of China period, people have gradually paid more attention to the circulation of air and emphasized the living conditions such as ventilation in spatial planning. It was stated by Shaoxing Medical Association: "According to the habits of sick families in Shaoxing, people were superstitious when they had typhoid diseases and other epidemics. Ghosts were such a terror that lights were put on not only at night but also during daytime. The room for the patient was full of people taking care of the sick, lying neck by neck, whispering, spitting and sweating. Nobody knew that the human body releases the most heat and that lights are the most toxic. There was more turbidity than clear air in this situation. Even if the non sick people staying in this room for long periods of time would feel dizzy, the chest and diaphragm stuffy, let alone the patient suffering from the epidemic! The inhaling from the mouth and nose, the immersion of the lungs and stomach, can turn a light case into a serious one, and a serious one into death, which is all due to these bad habits".[95] The problems of lights, turbid air, as well as the situation of indoor patients being poisoned by carbon air, sweat acid and filthy air, are all based on the Western miasma theory that the lack of ventilation and pollution will lead to disease; the inhaling from the mouth and nose causing epidemic disease is also bad Qis. Another tip is to call for the disbelieve

---

[93] (Qing) Cao Tingdong, *Common Sayings of Lao Lao*, pp. 42–43.

[94] (Qing) Cao Tingdong, *Common Sayings of Lao Lao*, pp. 33, 38, 78.

[95] Shaoxing Medical Association, Health and Prevention. Hygiene of the Sick, Treatment of Damp and Warm Epidemics, included in Li Shunbao (ed.), *Complete Book of Warm Diseases*, Vol. II, pp. 2099.

of disease being brought by ghosts, and that we should face up to the real problem of narrow space and poor air circulation in the house.

With the deepening influence of Western medicine, personal health preservation, which is more concerned in TCM, has gradually turned to the relationships among people. An individual is no longer just an individual, but a new "individual" who integrates into the environment, makes contact and has relationships with others. Ding Fubao said, "The transmission of infectious viruses is caused by the excreta of patients, feces, skin flakes, excreta secretion, expectoration, saliva, etc. or by the substances polluted by the above items, such as medicine, bedclothes, food, utensils, furniture, wards, air, water and soil, etc."[96] The focus has shifted from personal health preservation to the issue of symbiosis among people, materials and the environment.

7.6 The Space, Residence and Daily Care for Fever Diseases

In the early years of the Republic of China period, the debate between TCM and Western medicine was in the ascendant, and both sides were looking for ways to get more trust on their system from the public. TCM strove to be "scientific", while Western medicine was faced with merging the complex scientific theoretical concepts into "daily life", which can be understood by the general public and enhance the popularity of Western medicine. In *How Should Western Medicine Doctors Treat Patients*, Cheng Hanzhang called on Western medicine doctors not to be rigid toward patients, but to teach them "to correct their bad habits with hygienic methods". If the patient is a teenager, efforts need to be made for him to keep a pure mind and be free of desires, correct his outlook on life and fix the internal cause.[97] For the lack of medical resources, the patients often cherished all the knowledge that can help them recover. This unique demand was also noticed by Western medicine. In his *Elements and Virtues of Diagnosis*, Cheng Hanzhang said, "Treatment is served for the needs of the patients in getting more medical resources. The scope of treatment is very wide, like using equipment or drugs. The regulation of patients' diet, the guidance of sanitary conditions, and the correction of patients' temperament also have an impact on treatment. However, Western medicine must not play a high-profile role in all kinds of treatment, such as prescribing expensive drugs for the poor, which would only disappoint the patients."[98]

Care for the daily life of patients can not only meet the real needs of patients, but also reduce the negative impression of Western medicine as "a profit seeker". Chen Guofu said: "If the doctor and the patient have different views, the doctor had better honestly share his views with the patient, so as to make the patient feel at ease. If the patient who has been ill for a long time really has a deep understanding on his own disease, the doctor should accept them with an open mind, which will certainly help

[96] Ding Fubao, Chapter 9 Natural and Exposed Viruses, *New Internal Canon of Medicine*, p. 40.

[97] Cheng Hanzhang, *A Brief Introduction to Western Medicine*, p. 58.

[98] Cheng Hanzhang, *A Brief Introduction to Western Medicine*, p. 57.

him in his treatment, and may indirectly help develop his medical skills".[99] It would be best that doctors and patients can reach a consensus and learn more together. However, the appeal to Western medicine in the early Republic of China period was often full of contradictions and impeding doom. On the one hand, Western medicine should gain the recognition of patients, but on the other hand, it must still adhere to "science" with no compromising—it can never be wrong as long as the diagnosis and treatment are based on science, just like the saying of "science is never deceiving". Cheng Hanzhang believed that the reality is that doctors with formal qualifications left schools or hospitals to practice on their own, and gradually strayed away from the position of science. Although the medical technology was developed, the microscope was no longer used, and the treatment was also beginning to become perfunctory. Without scientific support, they eventually turned to be quacks.[100] Therefore, Western medicine should not be influenced by patients, nor should it make any "compromise" with patients' "wrong concepts" and their "reasoning without scientific basis". Cheng Hanzhang commented that Western medicine has a firm standpoint of "science": "The strength of Western medicine is completely derived from experimentation. Therefore, if we can follow scientific methods and conduct practical research, we will certainly be competitive by expounding on the details and the profound theories, and be more appealing. One needs to believe in one's own learning. Furthermore, a Western medicine doctor not only needs to believe in their expertise, but also need to be rational and be firmly against the irrational". If you have no faith in Western medicine or science, it's better to "stop practicing immediately, so as not to make mistakes for others and yourself".[101] He cited an example. If a patient wants a Western medicine doctor to just feel the pulse with TCM methods, the Western medicine doctor should teach the patient the correct concept and the reasons for having other examinations. If the patient does not listen to it, "it is better to call off the diagnosis and treatment", because without a complete examination, the effect of actual treatment cannot be achieved.[102] Generally speaking, it is better for a Western medicine doctor to persist in tedious diagnosis and scientific explanations than to ingratiate himself with patients. This highlights that a Western medicine doctor must put scientific norms in the first place, instead of fully conforming to the freedom of "individuals".

However, as a long-term patient, Chen Guofu spoke of the comfort that ordinary patients may need most: "Whenever I saw that my relatives and friends were sick and the doctors were helpless, I thought I could offer help. Although I didn't study medicine, I have my common knowledge, my ideals, my enthusiasm, and my

[99] Chen Guofu, Preface to 'Bitter Talk about Medicine', included in Mr. Chen Guofu Scholarship Fund Management Committee (ed.), *Selected Works of Mr. Chen Guofu's Medical and Health Thoughts*, Taipei: Mr. Chen Guofu Scholarship Fund Management Committee, 1973, p. 23.

[100] Cheng Hanzhang, *A Brief Introduction to Western Medicine*, pp. 72–73.

[101] Cheng Hanzhang, *A Brief Introduction to Western Medicine*, p. 58.

[102] Cheng Hanzhang, *A Brief Introduction to Western Medicine*, p. 57.

experience, which can make up for my shortcomings".[103] Common sense, ideals, enthusiasm and experience are all based on "personal" suggestions and views on medical treatment, which can not be proved by science. At the beginning of the Republic of China period, the patients' mind "converged with China and the West", and they might have learned a lot of new knowledge, but it is also possible that many traditional health care and medical concepts were deeply rooted in people's minds, which made it difficult for "Western medicine doctors with a scientific mind" to communicate with them. As a result, part of the fact is that it is the doctor's job to explain and diagnose diseases. In the end, it is the patient who still has to face the disease alone.

Even though there are so many gaps and contradictions between Chinese and Western medical concepts, as a patient, he may still cherish all the information that can be collected to fight against diseases, especially in such an era of insufficient and uneven medical resources. The patient's recuperation after the treatment is also a top priority, as it will be the main battlefield for the patient to fight against the disease. Chen Guofu wrote his thoughts in 1948: "There are few doctors in China, especially well trained doctors. When it is difficult for people like me to get proper treatment, one can imagine the situation of other people. Even if they are sick, it would be much better if they can treat themselves with their own medical knowledge without consulting a doctor, let alone using medicine. According to the current situation in China, everyone should have the common knowledge of medicine and health, so that the nation won't decline into poverty and illness".[104] According to this, the "personalization" of "medical knowledge" is the wish that patients can have the space to seek an explanation or treatment of diseases outside of formal medical care and

[103] Chen Guofu, Preface to 'Bitter Talk about Medicine',included in Mr. Chen Guofu Scholarship Fund Management Committee(ed.), *Selected Works of Mr. Chen Guofu's Medical and Health Thoughts*, Taipei: Mr. Chen Guofu Scholarship Fund Management Committee, 1973, p. 23.

[104] Article 10: Patients with acute infectious diseases shall not be accommodated in the same infectious disease room unless there is an isolated infectious disease room. Patients with different infectious diseases shall not be accommodated in the same room. Article 11:The infectious disease room shall be equipped with special utensils, bedding, toilet and medical instruments for infectious patients. Article 12: The utensils, bedding, excreta, residual food and drink, and other articles contaminated by viruses or suspected of contamination used by infectious patients shall be disinfected appropriately. Article 13: Items in infectious disease rooms shall not be moved to other places unless they are disinfected. Article 14: The sewage and excreta of the infectious disease room shall not be moved or discharged to other places without proper disinfection. Article 15: After an infectious patient withdraws from the ward, appropriate disinfection methods shall be applied in the room. Article 16: When a hospital accepts an infectious patient, it shall, within 48 h after the name of the patient is confirmed, submit the patient's name, age, residence, name of the disease, place and time of onset, the day, month, and year of the occurrence as well as the admission to the hospital to the administrative office and the Quarantine Committee in detail. However, pestis and cholera should also be reported even if they are suspected and the disease name has not been determined. When the patient referred to in the preceding paragraph dies or is cured, or is discharged from the hospital due to any other reasons, the name, cause, and time of the day, month, and year shall be promptly reported to the administrative office and the Quarantine Committee. From Cheng Hanzhang, *A Brief Introduction to Western Medicine*, pp. 100–101.

national health, rather than focusing on the level of "understanding modern medical care".

According to Sean Hsiang-Lin's research, one of the important transformations in the relationship between doctors and patients during the Republic of China period was to take hospitals as the main treatment places.[105] The ideal hospital in modern China is probably like this: "The ward is the place where the patients stay, which gives them the sense of comfort and pleasure, so that they can live happily and wait for an appropriate treatment. In addition, the medical equipment, the building and distribution of the whole hospital, the water closet, kitchen, bathroom, toilet, disinfection room, operating room, nursing room, repair workshop, sewing room and every other things needed can all be cleaned and disinfected according to the standard".[106] Most hospitals did not meet these requirements. Cheng Hanzhang couldn't help criticizing: "The establishment of the hospital is to accommodate the patients. However, the principle that patients need to stay in the hospital for recuperation after illness is that the hospital has sophisticated equipment, with nurses' care and doctors' inspection at any time. If the hospital equipment is not based on this principle, it is no different from the hostel; patients can recuperate in their own residence. Why bother staying in a hospital without equipment?"[107] At that time, the environment of most hospitals was not suitable for recuperation. As a result, Chinese patients were not willing to choose the western hospital as the first choice for recuperation. Even some counties and cities had to change the name of the "Western Medicine Clinic" to the "Chinese-Western Medicine Clinic" for the lack of business in "Western Medicine Clinics". However, this had aroused the opposition of the local Chinese medicine community, and the word "Chinese" had to be deleted. It can be seen that the signboard of "Western Medicine" at that time was not always popular.[108]

For infectious diseases such as pestis and cholera, the wards were divided into three types of living areas based on periods, i.e. observation period, diagnosing period and recovery period, which should not be mixed up. These requirements must be planned in advance and the hospital space must be divided, so as to achieve the goal of "isolation" as much as possible. However, even in Shanghai, the situation was not ideal: "The urban population is dense, the traffic is busy, and various infectious diseases are most likely to occur and spread. The health construction before the Marco Polo Bridge Incident had been destroyed. Therefore, there has been a bad shortage of the resources such as the Municipal Infectious Disease Hospital, the inspection and management of drinking water and food since the establishment of

---

[105] It is not easy for a province to have a large-scale infectious disease hospital. In addition, the funds are insufficient and the operation is hasty. It remains to be investigated how its functions can be brought into full play.

[106] Chen Wanli, The Process of the Establishment of Some Zhejiang Provincial Hospitals, *Zhejiang Provincial Hospital Quarterly,* Vol. 1, 1933 (01), pp. 1–2; Shangguan Wuchen, Report of the President, *Annual Report of Henan Provincial Hospital,* 1935 (01), photos at the beginning of the book and pp. 1–10.

[107] Cheng Hanzhang, *A Brief Introduction to Western Medicine*, p. 97.

[108] Cheng Hanzhang, *A Brief Introduction to Western Medicine*, p. 96.

this bureau".[109] In addition, since the war continued, there was no way to build. For average Chinese patients, it was really a dream impossible to enter an infectious disease hospital to recuperate from fever. Therefore, the western hospitals were not meant to be the main recuperation place for patients during the Republic of China period. For patients with fever, apart from seeing doctors and taking medicine, the most important recuperation place was still at home.

In the winter of 1936, Xia Ruitang, a doctor in the northeast, worked as a doctor in a Chinese pharmacy in Jinzhou. He was paid by the hour. This might mean that he was a junior or a newly placed doctor. However, because of his excellent medical skills, his name gradually spread. Soon after, he went out to patients' homes and was invited to treat the patients. A family member of a TCM doctor recalled: "It is very important for a doctor to be called by the patients, because the patients would pay the doctor directly. If the patient was satisfied and rich, the doctor would be paid very well. Some patients would buy generous gifts for the doctor during the new year's festival". As Xia visited more patients, he became rich. Once, the governor's wife suddenly went into a shock. Instead of sending her to the hospital immediately (regardless of traditional Chinese or Western Medicine), the governor's choice was to wait and invite a Chinese medicine practitioner to come to his home to treat the patient. Xia Ruitang cured his wife of her shock and skillfully solved the infertility problem of the governor himself. The governor later publicized his medical skills, and Xia became even more famous. The sick needed the superb skills of the doctors, but they hoped to implement them at home. Seeing a doctor at home often means that the sick can afford it—it was easier for the doctor to gain more fame and wealth if the family was rich or above average. If the rich chose this way, it is hard to believe that the poor would choose the more expensive western hospital for recuperation. Of course, charitable medical practice is not included.

If one relies on oneself instead of choosing a hospital for treatment, then the home care will become very important, and the caregivers around the patients also deserve the attention. The wet and warm epidemic treatment method collected by Shaoxing Medical Association explains the obligations of all people in the sick family: "The health care knowledge of the sick is not only needed for the patents' family, but is also the obligation of the patents' family. A good doctor who can cure the disease must first educate the family of the sick, so that all family members can take good care of the sick, help the doctors, instead of hindering the doctors, and blaming the doctors for their own mistakes".[110] Regarding this circumstance, there came the establishment of various nursing laws, which was not just to be learned by the nursing personnel. Ding Fubao, a translator of Japanese medical books, expressed that "In addition to medicine, it is particularly necessary for individuals to have health preservation".

---

[109] Shanghai Special Health Bureau, *Business Report of Shanghai Special Health Bureau,* Shanghai: Shanghai Special Health Bureau, 1941, p. 9.

[110] Shaoxing Medical Association, Health and Prevention. Hygiene of the Sick, Treatment of Damp and Warm Epidemics, included in Li Shunbao (ed.), *Complete Book of Warm Diseases*, Vol. II, pp. 2098–2099.

The care of patients with intestinal zhifus or tuberculosis is particularly important.[111] Yang Zemin further described:

> Nursing and treatment are closely related. Ideally, there should be special equipment, and there is no hospital for recuperation in China except Taoism or those in the big cities. When people got sick, they all depended on their families. It was the common knowledge of people to take care of the sick. Lu Xinwu of the Ming Dynasty discussed this in detail. He said that the way to treat diseases was to be careful in the room of the sick, no sneezing, coughing, walking, no noise made in dressing up, placing utensils, and breathing; properly adding or reducing the bedding without being felt by the sick. No inquiries about the severity of the disease, no request but just wait on the sick. It is not filial to keep on inquiring; no forcing food to the sick who has no appetite, no excessive food for the sick who wants food; eating while lying on bed is like swallowing a dagger, and the proper way is to eat with a spoon by lying on one side. Eating less is better than more as it is hard to swallow. No need to share timely with the sick of information that can cause sadness, anger, worry and detest. The sick are not to be woken up while sleeping, moved when they are in peace, corrected when they make mistakes, and stopped from fulfilling their wishes; greeting the doctors with courtesies, preparing the medicine according to the prescriptions. No frequent change of doctors nor prescriptions. Comforting the sick with the understatement of the situation when being asked.[112]

Compared with Western medicine after the nineteenth century, Chinese medicine in ancient times mainly focused on patients and the rehabilitation after illness. The same is true in modern times that the status of doctors themselves was not high and their focus was mostly on patients too. Newer Western medicine attaches great importance to the power of doctors. The (isolation) place and the responsibility of people also become important. For patients of infectious diseases, they need to be hospitalized, and even taken measures such as notification and isolation. The author has examined the course of Sun Yat Sen's treatment when he was ill. At that time, Western medicine believed that orthodox Western medicine treatment must be accepted in the hospital, while other treatments, including TCM, were not allowed. Therefore, Sun left the hospital and chose the Chinese traditional residential care, followed by massage, mental healing and TCM herbs.[113] To recuperate in a hospital, many TCM methods were not allowed. The latter is often the most important disease prevention strategy in the daily life of the general public.

In fact, recuperation is also to make up for the inadequacy of medical treatment. The father of Hu Linyi, a famous general in modern times, said: "How can today's doctors cure diseases? With the mistakes they made, it is better for them to do nothing. One would recover with some recuperation".[114] In the medical field at the beginning

---

[111] Miyamoto, translated by Ding Fubao, Chapter 1. Preliminary Typhoid Fever, *New Treatise on Typhoid Fever*, 1908, p. 2.

[112] Yang Zemin, 24. Nursing, *Medical Talk in Seclusion*: p. 166.

[113] Pi Kuoli, Medical Treatment, Doctors and Patients in the early Republic of China Period—the Death of Sun Yat-sen and the Controversy between Chinese and Western Medicine, included in Hu Chunhui & Tang Qihua (ed.), *Proceedings of the Postgraduate Seminar on History of Mainland, Taiwan and Hong Kong (2006)*, Hong Kong: Asian Research Center of Zhuhai Academy, Taipei: History Department of University of Politics, 2007, pp. 215–242.

[114] Jin Xiage (ed.), Hu Linyi's Home Letters, May 25, 21st Year of Daoguang Reign (to Mr. Moxi), *Home Letters of Celebrities in the Qing Dynasty*, Vol. I, p. 451.

of the Republic of China period, most Chinese patients still chose home as the place for recuperation. The connection between people and place started from the family. First, residential buildings have the function of security. Wang Ermin pointed out that in ancient times, the palace and the city, as Mencius and Xunzi clearly stated, could dispel dryness and dampness, avoid the harm of cunning insects, and prevent the city from being invaded. The construction of buildings and terraces has always been the focus of the government and the people since ancient times. However, in the private sectors, most of the simple and crude houses were built by themselves, by resorting to muddy work. Due to the above needs, folk magazines such as *Book of Treasure* and the *Complete Collection of Household Necessities* also had some writings on building houses, but they often fell into the theory of buildings rather than the construction methods, of which were repeatedly copied from one to another and of not much reference value.[115] It is worth mentioning that modern Chinese medicine also recorded some precautions to the healthcare in the residences in ancient times. He Lianchen said:

> It is said in the *Golden Prescriptions* that the residence should not be too fancy, which will make people greedy and detract from their ambitions. However, it is good to make it elegant, clean and that it can keep people from rain, heat and humidity. It is also said that in the room where ordinary people live, the sleeping area must be well insulated without any tiny gaps from which cold air can enter and cause a stroke without being felt. If there is a strong wind blowing in the rooms, try to avoid it rather than sitting against it for long. It is also said: do not set up a bed near the stove. Do not sit facing the stove. Something bad will happen after a long time of thinking. According to the *Book of Longevity Pills*, if the bed is two or three feet high, it is beyond the reach of the earth's Qi so that the pathogenic Qi can not invade. Don't stay in the room too long for the coolness, nor sit on the wet ground long so that the new pathogenic factor of cold and humidity can be avoided. The patient's bedroom should be spacious, the windows should be open, and the light should be plentiful. Pay attention to the indoor air, and make it fresh, which is the most important for health.[116]

This shows that although TCM has little connection with national public health, it has a long history of emphasizing family or personal care. In addition to some borrowed theories of Western medicine, it has some new features. As a contrast, when the state power intervened in the control of infectious diseases, the "isolation" of diseases was often not only out of biological factors, but also out of various complex social factors such as classes, gender and ethnic groups. For example, in the prevention and treatment of diseases in the early twentieth century, black people were often regarded as the headache as "refusing to mend their ways after being educated", and health institutions, mainly composed of white people, often formulated a discriminatory segregation policy to isolate black people.[117] This was not the case in the daily health of TCM, because the theory of TCM has been personal and of family related, which is less involved with national, ethnic and other factors.

---

[115] Wang Ermin, *Social and Cultural Ecology of the Ming and Qing Dynasties*, p. 85.

[116] He Lianchen (ed.), revised by Wang Zhipu et al., *Updated Popular Treatise on Typhoid Fever*, Cao Bingzhang's preface, p. 502. Samuel Kelton Roberts Jr., *Infectious Fear: Politics,Disease, and the Health Effects of Segregation*, Chapel Hill: University of Carolina, c2009, p. 148.

[117] Mai Huiting, *Problems of Family Transformation in China*, Shanghai: Shanghai Bookstore Press, 1990, pp. 119–121.

Problems of Family Transformation in China, published in 1935 recorded the unsanitary state of many Chinese families. For example, the food was rotten, the house was dark, humid and filled with foul air and odor. In addition, the author pointed out that "the relationship between family health and personal health is interrelated". "To improve family hygiene, we should start with personal hygiene".[118] This book still focuses on "personal" hygiene, including the air, food and other pathogenic factors. TCM practitioners of the Shaoxing Medical Association have explicated the problem of bacterial disease, but they have also emphasized the problems of space, air and sanitation in the family for the treatment of epidemic diseases. For example: "The bedrooms should be spacious and the windows should be open. Pay attention to the indoor air which is to be fresh. It is the most important for health. Mr. Wang Mengying said that in densely populated areas, when epidemic disease occurred, the air of the earth was hot and dirty. Regardless of the size of the house, it is necessary to let it open and get the clean air. When the wind blows, the epidemic Qi will naturally dissipate. On the contrary, the hot and turbid air will also be the signal flag of the epidemic Qi. This explains why those suffering from epidemic diseases were mostly the impoverished who didn't have decent food to eat nor a decent house to live.[119] Although the problems of "earth air" and "foul air" are mentioned here, the concept of "isolation" is not between people, but to isolate the bad air in the environment.

Some disease prevention thoughts of TCM miasma theory and the bacteria theory of Western medicine can be connected. Ding Fubao commented about isolating the pathogens of bacteria: "The sick room must have sufficient light and air circulation. This is not only for patients, but also for natural disinfection, which can kill the mold in the room". "There are infectious molds in the stool and urine. If you see a little stain on the white cloth, you can disinfect the spot, so that the surrounding areas won't be infected".[120] Although Ding's theory of focusing on sterilization and bacteria prevention is different from the above theory, the logic of isolating the pathogenic factor "air and bacteria" is very similar to the requirements and disinfection methods for keeping the air clean. Other general precautions in the home, such as "the room of the sick should be southward, quiet and clean, sunny, fresh and soothing, the room temperature should be moderate, and the layout should be tidy and comfortable"[121]; "if there are patients with epidemic diseases at home, how can the children be uncaring? They should wait on the patient for tea and medicine",

[118] Shaoxing Medical Association, Health and Prevention. Hygiene of the Sick, Treatment of Damp and Warm Epidemics, included in Li Shunbao (ed.), *Complete Book of Warm Diseases*, Vol. II, pp. 2099. In his comments, He Lianchen cited Wang Shixiong's view. Wang Shixiong's theory of earth air and foul air may have been influenced by the western theory of miasma, and it has been influencing the doctors of the Republic of China period.

[119] He Lianchen (ed.), revised by Wang Zhipu et al., *Updated Popular Treatise on Typhoid Fever*, p. 502.

[120] He Lianchen (ed.), revised by Wang Zhipu et al., *Updated Popular Treatise on Typhoid Fever*, Cao Bingzhang's preface, p. 502; Samuel Kelton Roberts Jr., *Infectious Fear: Politics,Disease, and the Health Effects of Segregation*, Chapel Hill: University of Carolina,c2009, p. 148.

[121] Mai Huiting, *Problems of Family Transformation in China,* Shanghai: Shanghai Bookstore Press, 1990, pp. 119–121.

"those who are sick should try to get treatment; those who are not sick should prevent themselves from being infected",[122] "it is advisable to change one's position in bed, so as to prevent local blood stasis and bedsores", etc.[123] He put forward suggestions on the planning of the room space and the care methods of the patients, generally in the category of taking care of each other between the patients and family members, which is also the theory of TCM.

Some disease prevention thoughts of TCM miasma theory and the bacteria theory of Western medicine can be connected. Ding Fubao commented about isolating the pathogens of bacteria: "The room of the sick must have sufficient light and air circulation. This is not only for patients, but also for natural disinfection, which can kill the mold in the room". "There are infectious molds in the stool and urine. If you see a little stain on the white cloth, you can disinfect the spot, so that the surrounding areas won't be infected".[124] Although Ding's theory of focusing on sterilization and bacteria prevention is different from the above theory, the logic of isolating the pathogenic factor "air and bacteria" is very similar to the requirements and disinfection methods for keeping the air clean. Other general precautions for home care are "the room of the sick should be southward, quiet and clean, sunny, fresh and soothing, the room temperature should be moderate, and the layout should be tidy and comfortable",[125] "if there are patients with epidemic diseases at home, how can the children be indifferent? They should wait on the patient for tea and medicine", "those who are sick should try to get treatment; those who are not sick should prevent themselves from being infected",[126] "it is advisable to change the position in bed, so as to prevent local blood stasis and bedsores", etc.[127] He put forward suggestions on the planning of the room space and the care methods of the patients, generally in the category of taking care of each other between the patients and family members, which is also the theory of TCM.

Although care among family members is important, once they have contracted infectious fever, the situation becomes more difficult. For Western medicine, "When visiting patients, they should first go to the dressing room to change clothes. Before leaving, they should be seriously disinfected and take off the clothes they put on during the visit. When returning to the room for rest, nurses can take off their clothes, take a bath and change their clothes. Meals are sent from the catering room to the ward.

---

122 Shaoxing Medical Association, Health and Prevention. Hygiene of the Sick, Treatment of Damp and Warm Epidemics, included in Li Shunbao (ed.),*Complete Book of Warm Diseases*, Vol. II, pp. 2099. In his comments, He Lianchen cited Wang Shixiong's view. Wang Shixiong's theory of earth air and foul air may have been influenced by the western theory of miasma, and it has been influencing the doctors of the Republic of China period.

123 He Lianchen (ed.), revised by Wang Zhipu et al., *Updated Popular Treatise on Typhoid Fever*, p. 502.

124 Miyamoto, translated by Ding Fubao, Chapter 1. Preliminary Typhoid Fever, *New Treatise on Typhoid Fever*, Shanghai: Medical Publishing House, 1908, pp. 13–14.

125 Mai Huiting, *Problems of Family Transformation in China*, p. 125.

126 Cao Bingzhang, Chapter 7 Prevention of Autumn Epidemic, Essentials of Autumn Epidemic Treatment, included in Lu Zheng (ed.), *Collection of Rare Modern TCM. Medical Talk*, p. 773.

127 Yang Zemin, 3. Discussion on Law (I) Governance, *Medical Talk in Seclusion*, p. 134.

When the ward returns the food utensils, they should first go through the food utensil disinfection station and then return them to the catering room. The operations done in the operating room are mainly for toxemia (diphtheria). It is particularly critical for the operation, along with the equipment, equipment room and preparation room".[128] With regard to visits to the sick of the infectious diseases, all technical operations to prevent infection must be completed in specialized hospitals, and family members were not allowed to take care of them at home. Hu Ding'an also pointed out that many Western medicine clinics are connected with families, which increases the risk of many infectious diseases. In addition to detailed inquiries during registration, disinfection procedures must also be carefully implemented.[129]

The ancient Chinese already knew about infection, but they didn't think it to be introduced by a virtuous gentleman though it was not wrong to take similar measures to avoid disease for the fear of infection. In the *Complete Works of Zhu Zi. A Rambling Record of Typhoid Fever,* there is an article entitled "On the Prevention of Epidemic Diseases", which expounds precisely this idea:

> The wise men's words should be passed in time to all people. It says: "It is said that epidemics are infectious. For the sick, their neighbors cut off their communications and even their family and close relatives left them. This is most hurtful and immoral. It was so hateful that someone wrote a book to inform people that the epidemic is not contagious and there is no need to avoid it. Well intended as it was, it is not true. It is not to be believed. Personally, I think it is better to tell them that it is out of kindness not to avoid it while knowing it is infectious, rather than telling people that it is not infectious and there is no need to avoid it. With the information of its danger, if one still has no intention of avoiding it, it means one believes in the luck of not being infected but not out of kindness. Once knowing the possible infection, one would run away as far as possible. It is out of kindness and righteousness to inform, but if one chooses not to avoid it, that means one is too kind too avoid it. Taking kindness and righteousness as priority and can not bear to avoid it, even if being infected, one learned the truth and knew it is the morality that one can not go against. There is no generalized rule as being infected or not, as it all depends on the pathogenic factors or righteous Qi, and asthenia or sthenia of one's body. When my grandfather Zhu was young, there was a family infected with epidemic disease in the neighborhood, and no one dared to be close to them. Grandfather went to cook medicine for them every day and didn't leave until everybody finished their doses. When Liu Bin was an official in Yongjia, there was a major epidemic in the county. He visited all places by feeling their pulses in person, inquiring about their symptoms and giving them the medications. He simply left without washing his hands after all was done. Scary as people would feel, he was safe and sound.[130]

It is a virtuous person who knows that the disease is contagious and "takes kindness as a priority rather than avoiding it". In the Song Dynasty, some people criticized the ruthlessness of "the family members isolating the infected in the south of the Yangtze River". They also cited the example of Wang Biao of the Jin Dynasty, criticizing the

---

[128] Cheng Hanzhang, *A Brief Introduction to Western Medicine*, pp. 96–97.

[129] Hu Ding'an, Concerns on the Risk of Infection Caused by the Contact between Family and Clinic, *Social Medical Journal,* Vol. 1, 1934 (08), pp. 1–3.

[130] Yang Zemin, (18) On Avoiding Epidemic Diseases of Zhu Hui'an, *Medical Talk in Seclusion*, pp. 261–262.

move of "avoiding the disease" as "inhumane".[131] The dominant power of one's own body in avoiding or not avoiding it may have changed under the control of "morality" since the Song Dynasty. Liang Zhangju (1775–1849) of the Qing Dynasty mentioned the custom that local families in Wenzhou had parents who died of epidemic diseases. After putting the corpse in the coffin, the whole family moved away. Liang criticized this kind of behavior of avoiding the epidemic as "being not kind nor filial. Such ignorant and reckless conduct in the poor countryside deserve the worst penalty. There were educated families who followed suit. It is really unbelievable. Clarion call is needed to awaken the public".[132] In modern times, the concern of the family for the sick "individuals" has replaced the fear of other healthy people caused by infectious diseases. There is also an interesting medical case recorded in *A Survey of Febrile Diseases*:

> The commander-in-chief was nearly 70 years old. He conquered Yangzhou in the south, captured more than 10,000 people, and selected beautiful maidens, with four of them placed on each of his sides. It is said: the newly captured people had their fear and worry kept inside plus disordered diet, which led to diseases. The pathogenic Qi was infectious to those who were close to them and it was the most risky. The elderly and the weak should take particular care. The commander-in-chief didn't listen. During the heavy snow in December, many new captivates caught cold, suffering from headaches, coughs, stomachaches, and many died. On the first month of the lunar calendar, the commander-in-chief went to a banquet and drank several rounds. He fell ill. His pulse was heavy and thin. It stopped after every three or four times of throbbing, with the same symptoms as the new captivates. He died on the third day. According to *Internal Canon of Medicine*, during the time of solar deficiency, lunar vacancy or unseasonal weather, the pathogens would permeate, reaching to the bones. Deadly indeed![133]

It can be seen that the infection of fever is the result of an irregular life style or the combination of various adverse factors (as climate and indulgence). Chen Guofu said: "It is not easy for a person with sound system and self-discipline to be infected by those diseases. On the contrary, a person who loses immunity and self-discipline can be attacked by germs easily, no matter where he tries to hide".[134] Therefore,

---

[131] According to the *Book of Jin Biography of Wang Biao*: "At the end of Yonghe reign, there were a lot of diseases. According to the old rules, the court officials, whose family members got sick with more than three infected, were not allowed to enter the palace for a hundred days even though they were not sick. For this, about a hundred officials were not allowed to enter the palace. Biao also said:" In the year of epidemics, all families were infected. If they were not allowed to enter the palace again, there would be a bad shortage of service, and the royal palace was almost empty. "The Emperor followed the advice". Quoted from Tao Yufeng (ed.), *Notes on Medical Affairs in Past Dynasties*, Beijing: People's Medical Publishing House, 2006, p. 749.

[132] (Qing) Liang Zhangju, *The Old Customs of Wenzhou, Casual Talk. Continuation.Third Talk,* Beijing: Zhonghua Book Company, 1997, pp. 284–285.

[133] Under the item of Luoqian Fuyun. From (Qing) Wang Shixiong (ed.), annotated by Chen Hui, Volume IV: Xue Shengbai's Damp Febrile Disease, *A Survey of Febrile Diseases*, p. 112.

[134] Chen Guofu, 90. The Cooperation of Good Friends and Good Medicine, 1st Edition of Medical Administration Ramble, included in Mr. Chen Guofu Scholarship Fund Management Committee(ed.) *Selected Works of Mr. Chen Guofu's Medical and Health Thoughts*, Taipei: Mr. Chen Guofu Scholarship Fund Management Committee, 1973, p. 249.

instead of just worrying about being infected, it is better to try to strengthen one's immunity or the discipline of one's life.

Since modern times, there has been no involvement of "morality" in the prevention of infection. In ancient times, the transmission of a parent's disease to their children was also known as "infection".[135] However, in modern times, "infection" mainly refers to infectious diseases, instead of prevention of infection. This represents the concept of Western medicine, and gradually influenced some Chinese medicine practitioners in accepting the concept of disinfection of Western medicine. For example, Cao Bingzhang said: "Whatever is used by infected patients, such as spittoons, urinals, towels, bowls and chopsticks, must be washed with carbolic acid water and lime water. The floors and windows of the houses where the infected live must be kept open at all times and cleaned. The vomit and excreted feces of the infected should be thrown with lime powder or charcoal acid water, poured into an open and sparsely populated place, and buried in the dirt. The toxins will be self absorbed by the earth to avoid infecting others. Before the patient dies of an epidemic, his mouth and nose should be covered with gauze so as not to infect others with immune bacteria".[136] Xu Renfu said: "No spitting on the ground. Disinfect spittoons. Keep good circulation of air in the room and make it clean".[137] These reminders laid particular emphasis on the disinfection, cleaning and bacteria prevention methods of Western medicine. Of course, the concept of toxin is very broad. In TCM technology, there are many detoxification methods. For example, "For the well water in summer, it is appropriate to put the whole piece of alum androgen into the water to detoxify the water and keep the snakes away. The water tank should be soaked with fresh acorus calamus root and dalbergia".[138] These measures penetrated into the daily life of the general public rather than being influence of Western medicine.

The author believes that such a theory is easy to resonate with the theory of miasma and even the disinfection method in the discussion of bacteria, which is probably the reason why these traditional concepts are often expressed in the modern medical books of febrile diseases. Cao Bingzhang once said: "For those who are already sick, it is urgent to seek proper treatment; for those who are not sick, they must be prepared for prevention".[139] But, what is the key to prevention? As far as Chinese medicine is concerned, there are many ways for individuals to avoid diseases when epidemics occur. Here we need to explain the "general theory" of disease prevention

---

[135] For example, it is said in *Authentic Surgery* that "The body Qi is also called fox Qi. It is due to the idea that the parents were infected and got the fox fetus, so its original temperament is kept". From (Ming) Chen Shigong, Body Qi No. 130, *Authentic Surgery*, p. 296. Chen Yinke once wrote an interesting essay on body odor. See his book *Fox Odor and Hu Odor, A Collection of the Cold Willow Hall*, Beijing: SDX Joint Publishing Company, 2001, pp. 157–160.

[136] Cao Bingzhang, Chapter 7 Prevention of Autumn Epidemic, Essentials of Autumn Epidemic Treatment, included in Lu Zheng (ed.), *Collection of Rare Modern TCM. Medical Talk*, p. 773.

[137] Xu Renfu, *Handouts on Practical Medicine*, p. 189.

[138] Shaoxing Medical Association, Treatment of Damp and Warm Epidemics, included in Li Shunbao (ed.), *Complete Book of Warm Diseases*, Vol. II, p. 2100.

[139] Cao Bingzhang, Chapter 7 Prevention of Autumn Epidemic, Essentials of Autumn Epidemic Treatment, included in Lu Zheng (ed.), *Collection of Rare Modern TCM. Medical Talk*, p. 771.

technology. For example, when the pandemic occurred, Cao said: "it is advisable to filter river water or well water and boil it. It is also necessary to use it for cooking porridge and rice. It is not allowed to drink the river water not in circulation, the water stored in the pool, the water being dirty and discolored, and the well water near the sewer toilet. Also, it is not allowed to drink tea that is not boiled, the tea that is left overnight, and the tea that is dirty and discolored".[140] He noticed the relationship between the environment and people, but the intermediary microorganisms had not been identified. The most important thing deserving attention was the health of the respiratory tract, such as droplet infection, isolated contact, sputum and other dangerous vectors. However, Cao listed the precautions for the prevention of gastrointestinal infectious diseases, such as typhoid fever and dysentery, which are mostly transmitted through drinking water. At that time, it was true that some people might suffer from gastrointestinal influenza, but the 1918 pandemic did cause more deadly pneumonia. This shows that the epidemic prevention theory discussed in TCM had actually absorbed the general miasma theory, rather than sticking to the pathological view that influenza bacteria would damage the lungs, which can be used as an observation of the difference between Chinese and Western medicine.

There are many "individual" epidemic prevention methods other than isolation in TCM procedures. At least from the Wei and Jin Dynasties, epidemic prevention methods[141] began to appear in typhoid studies and were used until the Republic of China period. For example: "when the epidemic is prevalent, it is advisable to burn incense in the room to dispel the pathogenic factors and unhealthy atmosphere. When entering the patient's room, it is advisable to eat a whole preserved egg. Those who can drink should drink a little sorghum wine. Men, women and children should wear a Taiyi pestilence pill, which should be wrapped in red silk. It's just to be hung on the neck without being touched".[142] These preventative drugs also appeared during several epidemics in the late Qing Dynasty.[143] By the time of the Republic of China period, there were even registered Chinese patent medicines being produced, such as "Anti Pestilence Super Powder". In fact, the main components of this medicine were menthol and borneol.[144] In addition, there was "Pure Yang Anti-plague Powder", with the main components as menthol, clove and Huoxiang. Its main function was "anti-plague".[145] Since the end of the Qing Dynasty, there have been various kinds

[140] Cao Bingzhang, Chapter 7 Prevention of Autumn Epidemic, Essentials of Autumn Epidemic Treatment, included in Lu Zheng (ed.), *Collection of Rare Modern TCM. Medical Talk*, p. 772.

[141] It is mainly published in "Prescriptions for Malaria, Pestilence and Febrile Toxin", with reference to (Jin) Ge Hong, supplemented by (Liang) Tao Hongjing,*Outstanding Prescriptions*, Vol. 2, Beijing: People's Health Publishing House, 2009, pp. 460–467.

[142] Shaoxing Medical Association, Treatment of Damp and Warm Epidemics, included in Li Shunbao (ed.), *Complete Book of Warm Diseases*, Vol. II, p. 2100.

[143] Lu Caixia, On the Evolution of Public Health Mechanism in Beijing and Tianjin in the Late Qing Dynasty (1900–1911), pp. 152–153.

[144] Department of Health of the Executive Yuan (ed.), *Monthly Bulletin of the Department of Health on Medical Licenses,* 1936 (02), p. 65.

[145] Department of Health of the Executive Yuan (ed.), *Monthly Bulletin of the Department of Health on Medical Licenses,* 1936 (08) p. 31.

of epidemic prevention pills, such as the Red Magic Pills and the Reviving White Pills in both the Chinese and French pharmacies, which claim to be "powerful tools for eliminating plagues" and could cure "epidemic diseases, cholera, heatstroke, enchantment and miasma".[146]

What's more, many perfume advertisements emphasized that it had the function of eliminating filth and preventing epidemic disease or waking up the brain. For example, Airo toilet water came into being at the end of the Qing Dynasty, which was "made of blossom concentrate". The advertisement declared that "A little added in rinsing water could prevent heat and damp, effective for healthcare. By sprinkling a few drops on bed, all foul smells will be vaporized".[147] It can be seen that the commodities at that time had a corresponding relationship between hygiene and fragrance. By the time of the Republic of China period, there were more such products, including the classic brand Twine Sis toilet water, Lin Wenyan perfume, which emphasized that they could "relieve heat and care for the skin, detoxify and deodorize".[148] "The sage fills the space with healthy Qi, so that the epidemic Qi is dissipated. This is the fundamental skill ! The ancients drank from a clear spring like fragrant medicine on New Year's day, and collected orchids and grasses to extract fragrant Qi to dispel the filth".[149] Even Twine Sis toilet water emphasized "sterilization and cleaning up filth", which was a "cosmetic and hygienic product".[150] "Fragrance" can dispel filth is an ancient argument. The relationship between "fragrance" and "sterilization" here is a grafting with Western medical theory. Of course, health consumption made the demand of such products possible, which was supported with cultural connotations. It is hard to believe that in addition to the "mask", the concept of TCM enabled perfume to play the role of disease prevention and epidemic prevention. For example, "in hot seasons, the epidemic air is all over, so is filth, which is very prone to transferring diseases. When you go out, you should sprinkle a few drops of 'epidemic prevention perfume' on a handkerchief to cover your mouth and nose to prevent diseases and filth. It is particularly needed when walking into a room of the sick and visiting patients" (see Fig. 7.5).[151]Perhaps this represents a kind of thinking different from "isolation". Perfume and the underlying disease resistance theory gave TCM epidemic prevention an alternative possibility.

There were more methods that were not focused on bacteriology and were "unscientific" in the eyes of Western medicine, which may still be adopted by the general public in modern times, showing a combined preventive culture of Chinese and

---

[146] Editorial Department of Globe News Agency (ed.), *Pictorial Daily,* Vol. 1, Shanghai: Shanghai Ancient Books Publishing House, 1999, p. 9.

[147] Editorial Department of Globe News Agency (ed.), *Pictorial Daily,* Vol. 2, p. 8.

[148] Shanghai Shen Bao Newspaper Office (ed.), *Shen Bao,* July 12, 1936, p. 4 and July 25, 1936, p. 4.

[149] (Qing) Zhang Fengkui, additionally annotated by Ye Ziyu, The Preface to Yu Jiayan's 'Theory of Epidemics', Supplement of Ye Ping's Complete Book of Heatstroke, included in Cao Bingzhang (ed.), *Great Achievements in Chinese Medicine*, Vol.16 (II), p. 39.

[150] Shanghai Shen Bao Newspaper Office (ed.), *Shen Bao,* August 6, 1936, p. 4.

[151] Shanghai Shen Bao Newspaper Office (ed.), *Shen Bao,* July 31, 1936, p. 3.

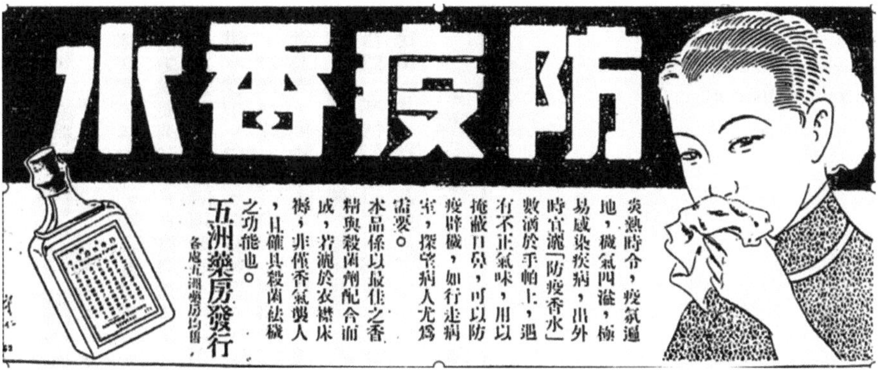

Fig. 7.5 Anti-plague Perfume

Western medicine (see Fig. 7.6).[152] For example, Yang Xiling recalled that once he was infected by an epidemic, and none of the family members, young and old, were spared. He remembered that the garlic spitting method in the *Outstanding Prescriptions* could prevent infection. When his wife first felt uncomfortable, she used the spitting method, and once she spit, she recovered and was prevented from infection.[153] Cao Bingzhang, on the other hand, said: "when the epidemic is prevalent, it is advisable to use a silk bag containing two liang (1 liang = 50g–translator's note) of alum, two liang of small black beans, and one or two androgens. It can be tied in a soaking tank to detoxify the water, and prevent the entry of snakes and cobras; incense can also be soaked to detoxify the water, or fern rhizome to absorb the micro organisms in the water. The same is true of putting the black beans into the well on the fifth watch (at dawn–translator's note)".[154] "Before going to bed on a spring night, you can soak your feet in the salty water up to the knees, which can dispel the wind".[155] Through external bathing, bad Qi can be washed away. These stories all point to thinking about disease prevention in addition to isolation and disinfection. Ordinary people still have many traditional methods to avoid contracting plague, and the old methods are still being used in the new era. There are more primitive methods, such as "in the remote places where no medication is available, one can drink cold water freely when the weather are extremely hot, and sickness would be gone with the sweat", and "it's particular effective to drink fresh plantain grass juice".[156] During early Republic of China period, TCM thought that these methods were still valuable, and they were

[152] *Spring and Autumn of the Medical World*, Book Advertisement.1936 (120), p. 53.

[153] Yang Xiling, Spitting As An Anti Plague Method, Medical Talk in Zhu Garden, included in Lu Zheng (ed.), *Collection of Rare Modern TCM. Medical Talk*, pp. 560–561.

[154] Cao Bingzhang, Chapter 7 Prevention of Autumn Epidemic, Essentials of Autumn Epidemic Treatment, included in Lu Zheng (ed.), *Collection of Rare Modern TCM. Medical Talk*, p. 772.

[155] He Lianchen (ed.), revised by Wang Zhipu et al., *Updated Popular Treatise on Typhoid Fever*, p. 499.

[156] This is quoted by Wu Xihuang from A Survey of Febrile Diseases. Wu Xihuang, *Interpretations of Chinese and Western Febrile Diseases*, p. 205.

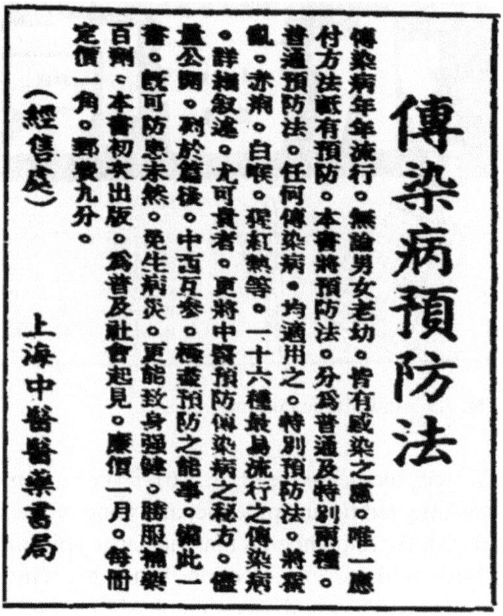

Fig. 7.6 Chinese and Western Converged Preventive Methods of Infectious Diseases

likely to be continuously used in rural areas lacking medicine. This is a part that can not be missed in the comprehensive review of modern medical history. There were also doctors advocating restoring or studying the "inherent epidemic prevention methods" and using science to explain the traditional Chinese epidemic prevention methods. For example, "burning incense and burning paper" means destroying the humid air where bacteria live to achieve the effect of epidemic prevention.[157] In the next chapter, the book will focus on the "epidemic prevention" of TCM to further the analysis of newspapers and periodicals in the early Republic of China period.

Modern doctors believe that the old idea that "a doctor takes the full responsibility for the treatment of a disease" should be corrected. As patients often fail to pay attention to self-care such as living in "improper places, inappropriate temperature and irregular diet with no idea of their own situations". It is said that "a doctor takes one, and a patient takes ten" of the responsibilities. Patients are more obligated in having self-care, let alone the variable febrile diseases of being "different from morning to the evening". Therefore, prevention and rehabilitation become very important, which is quite different from "public health".[158] In terms of health care, Western medicine tends to choose hospitals as the recuperation place. It is said in *Problems of Family Transformation in China*: "If the family's equipment for the

[157] Li Kehui, China's Inherent Epidemic Prevention Methods, *New Life of TCM*, 1936 (09), pp. 21–30.

[158] Shaoxing Medical Association, Health and Prevention. Hygiene of the Sick, Treatment of Damp and Warm Epidemics, included in Li Shunbao (ed.), *Complete Book of Warm Diseases*, Vol. II, pp. 2098–2099.

room of the sick is not perfect, or the patient is seriously ill, it is best to move to a hospital for medical treatment". Basically, the majority of fever patients were mainly recuperated at home, so "disinfection and isolation can be used for prevention".[159] Homes became the important place for practicing hygiene in the early Republic of China period. When explaining the method of epidemic prevention, Cao Bingzhang listed four key points—food, drink, clothing and domacile, which are all related to home care. He corresponded with the four characters "Yuan, Heng, Li and Zhen" in order. These four characters came from the first hexagram in the *Book of Changes*—"Qian". Why did he specify and make this correspondence? The biography of Zixia said: "Yuan is the beginning; Heng is the smoothness; Li is the harmony; and Zhen is the right. It is said that Qian is pure Yang, so it is extraordinary, logically followed by the beginning, smoothness, harmony, and righteousness. It is appropriate for a gentleman to follow the four virtues of Qian".[160] According to *Notes for the Book of Changes*: the beginning, smoothness, harmony and righteousness refer to spring, summer, autumn and winter, that is, the south, east, north and west, which also implies that the virtue of Qian is all inclusive. Therefore, it can also be interpreted as "Heavenly and human matters are all included".[161] In the practice of home, it reflects not a thinking of physical isolation between people, but the knowledge of nature and human beings, which is not under the planning of public health action.

Cao Bingzhang, a Chinese medicine practitioner, summed up his experience in the treatment of pandemic influenza and specifically mentioned the concept of isolation and epidemic prevention in Western medicine: "if someone in the family is infected with a disease, the children and women who share the same bed but are not sick must be in another bed in a separate room. They must not be allowed to get close to the sick person. No entry to the place with the epidemic Qi, nor letting in the people suffering from the epidemic elsewhere. Never eat the leftover food from the infected".[162] In addition to isolation, TCM has also learned the concept of "disinfection" of Western medicine and integrated into TCM disease prevention. This unique integration of Chinese and Western medicine was rarely noticed in the past. Cao Bingzhang once cited TCM methods of avoiding epidemic diseases to guide daily care.

> Visiting the infected or attending the funeral of the patient who died of an epidemic disease, one must keep tens of meters away. One should carry Sichuan pepper, camphor, realgar or rhubarb. If you are relatives and friends who must get close, you need to apply the powder of Sichuan peppers or realgar powder to your nostrils for prevention. Upon leaving, you can

[159] Mai Huiting, *Problems of Family Transformation in China*, p. 125.

[160] Li Dingzuo, *Interpretation of the Book of Changes*, Vol. 1. Cited from *Annotations and Corrections of the Book of Changes*, Taipei: World Book Company, 1987, p. 1.

[161] Yang Li, *The Book of Changes and TCM*, Beijing: Beijing Science and Technology Press, 1999, pp. 1096–1097.The relationship between Yi and medicine is quite close, and ancient physicians have continuously enriched the theory of TCM by explaining the relationship between *The Book of Changes*, medical principles, and body. Reference is made to He Shaochu (ed.), *Interpretations for the Book of Changes from Ancient Famous Doctors*, Beijing: China Medical Science and Technology Press, 1994.

[162] Cao Bingzhang, Chapter 7 Prevention of Autumn Epidemic, Essentials of Autumn Epidemic Treatment, included in Lu Zheng (ed.), *Collection of Rare Modern TCM. Medical Talk*, p. 773.

use paper to probe into your nose, which can make you sneeze better, so that the bacteria of filth will not be inhaled into your internal organs. If you accidentally inhale the stench of disease or the corpse, you can chew half of a purple gold tablet. After several hours of starvation, you can dissolve it. Do not eat quickly, particularly do not take supplements. If you smell the patient's sweat and odor, it will spread through your nose and brain, going all over the main and collateral channels. Once you feel the headache, you can grind the mustard powder with warm water and fill it in the umbilicus. Cover it with one or two layers of cloth, and put a kettle with hot water to iron it until you sweat.[163]

It is very interesting that the living can still offer condolences and make arrangements for the funeral of those who died of the disease. This is impossible in the "isolation" thinking of Western medicine. No matter whether these anti-epidemic laws of TCM are scientific or not, they provide a practical and feasible way, and humanly take into account the interpersonal culture of Chinese society. Cao's knowledge about the "isolation method" is not real "isolation". It is just to keep away from the patient's ill Qi and use some simple techniques and drugs to avoid being attacked by bad Qi. These are actually based on the traditional Qi theory, rather than the perspective of bacteriology.

As far as the environment is concerned, TCM attaches importance to the relationship between the weather, the Qi of the residence and the Qi of the human body, which are sufficient to affect the occurrence and treatment of fever. It is recorded in *Medical Talk in Zhu Garden* that in *Song Feng's Talk on Epidemics*, plague, pox, hair spots and fever toxin can be cured by lying in the shady wetland. " "Ge Qiansun, styled name Kejiu, was a Wu native in Pingjiang. He could not sweat when being under this treatment. He walked crazily along the river. The doctor kept him in the water and didn't let him out for quite a long time. Right after coming out and he was wrapped in a thick quilt, sweating and thus cured. Once upon a time, there was a felon who died of an epidemic in prison. The jailer reported his death. It was late in the evening, and his corpse was abandoned in the ravine. It was a cold day, he was naked and frozen overnight. He crawled to find a way to go back to the river, and as a result, he was exempt from punishment. Sun Fengting said: "The reason is similar to that of soaking in water and sweating." The plague is nothing more than a fever syndrome. The heat is confined in the body. When it meets cold, it will be resolved. This prisoner must have had some good deeds in his last life. "A man named Zhao Chao who suddenly died of fever on his way returning to land when there was a sea flood. His companions abandoned him on the coast and left. Zhao was blown by the sea breeze and recovered. Zang Anxi said that the chest and abdomen of a person suffering from fever were hot, which could be treated by painting mud from the bottom of the well on them. This is the case. Note: this is the principle of *Internal Canon of Medicine* in the statement of: "Keep on wearing light clothes, living in a cold place until you feel cold".[164] These traditional methods are indeed different from the disinfection and isolation knowledge of Western medicine. They emphasize

[163] Cao Bingzhang, Chapter 7 Prevention of Autumn Epidemic, Essentials of Autumn Epidemic Treatment, included in Lu Zheng (ed.), *Collection of Rare Modern TCM. Medical Talk*, p. 773.

[164] Yang Xiling, Fever Be Cured in Meeting Cold, Medical Talk in Zhu Garden, included in Lu Zheng (ed.) *Collection of Rare Modern TCM. Medical Talk*, pp. 553–554.

the possibility of conflict and reconciliation between the environment and sick Qi in the body and confirm that the Qi from the external environment has a good or bad effect on the recovery of fever. In addition, He Lianchen said: "In the pleasant spring time, it is good to walk in the spacious garden, with a mind open and free. It is no good sitting or lying for long that would prevent the depression from being relieved".[165] The moving, walking and the circulation of the body's Qi mechanism also involve the relationship between Qi and human health. It is important for daily recuperation.

An inappropriate living environment will aggravate a disease. Take Zheng Banqiao's family letter as an example: "On the 7th of May, I moved to the Deng's garden behind the office. The office was a building of the former dynasty. It was low and narrow. During the plum season, the humidity was severe, triggering my damp disease. The food was tasteless, and my feet were also ulcerated. I asked a doctor for treatment. I was advised to stay in a highrise".[166] "Wet" environment will lead to "damp disease", which points out the relationship between residence and disease. It is advised that in summer, "stay under the eaves, in a street shed, in the alley, or in a windowless house". Do not sleep in the open air for the coolness, nor sleep without a cover, sleep in the wind while sweating, nor fanning people to get cool. These are the secrets of disease prevention to avoid external bad Qi damage to the human body.[167] Chen Guofu said: "Throat diseases are mostly caused by heat. If we can properly regulate our body temperature and do not overheat it, it is easy to keep it from occurring".[168] What is "being caused by heat"? In daily life, excessive warm bedding, wrappings on the legs, spicy or hot food, sitting by the fire for too long are all that will lead to too much "heat". Even in the cold season, try not to make fire in a stove nor get too close to the stove unless it is necessary, or it will harm the throat. Chen said: "when treating a sore throat, doctors often tell patients not to approach the stove and sunlight. This is because this symptom is basically Yang, and it is not appropriate to use Yang to help Yang and aggravate the disease".[169] This appeal is not to kill microorganisms or prevent bacterial invasion, but to focus on the interaction between people and the environment, as well as physical fitness. Zhang Xichun said: "People affected by external factors always change with the constitution of a human body. For example, for the same epidemic infection, the patients in the same room or at the same time, may have different symptoms of cold or heat, or even be

---

165 He Lianchen (ed.), revised by Wang Zhipu et al., *Updated Popular Treatise on Typhoid Fever*, pp. 498–499.

166 Jin Xiage (ed.), Calligraphy to the Fourth Younger Brother from Fan County Office.Family Letters of Zheng Banqiao,included in *Family Letters of Celebrities in the Qing Dynasty*, Vol. p. 31.

167 He Lianchen (ed.),revised by Wang Zhipu et al., *Updated Popular Treatise on Typhoid Fever*, p. 499.

168 Chen Guofu, The Way Toward Health, included in Mr. Chen Guofu Scholarship Fund Management Committee(ed.), *Selected Works of Mr. Chen Guofu's Medical and Health Thoughts*, Taipei: Mr. Chen Guofu Scholarship Fund Management Committee, 1973, p. 154.

169 Chen Guofu,The Way Toward Health,included in Mr. Chen Guofu Scholarship Fund Management Committee (ed.), *Selected Works of Mr. Chen Guofu's Medical and Health Thoughts*, pp. 154–155.

completely different".[170] It can be seen that the transmission of sick Qi depends on the nature of Qi and the patient's constitution, not on the vector of bacteria.

During the Republic of China period, the Qi of the environment was no longer the most critical for the recuperation from diseases. Instead, the strength of individuals was emphasized. For example, Shaoxing Medical Association expounded:

> Hygiene is compulsory for the treatment of all diseases. If the disease is epidemic and unclean, it is dangerous and can harm the family and doctors of the patient. The sick must change their clothes and especially clean the bedding every day. All old clothes and quilts, all that can evaporate, must be placed in an empty room and locked in a box. If the coating is too warm, the disease can also aggravate. The death caused by a serious case is due to the heat being confined in the body and the Qi fails to be released. There were people who died of long term suffocation, but were mistaken as sleeping. They didn't answer the call and were found to be dead when the comforter was uncovered. It is said that they died of acute measles. It happened quite often in recent years.[171]

Also, Yang Zemin talked about the importance of bedroom space and air to recuperate from diseases: "Expand the bedroom: it is appropriate to expand the bedroom to make the air fresh for cases like scarlet fever and pox. For example, Wang Yipeng in the Ming Dynasty treated Yang's son, Fu Ji, for his continued cry for months. Wang set up his treatment in the hall by covering the floor with ashes in which the child was placed, and asked the nanny not to come close. The child went to sleep in a few minutes. He then asked the child to drink Elsholtzia, and the child recovered immediately. This is the same as the case of a certain child who was cured of pox. The child patient was placed in the sand to sleep. Shortly after that, the pox occurred. Those are all the cases for the reason of expanding the bedroom".[172]

Although Yang cited the examples of the ancients, his point was that the "fresh air" of the living place helped. This is to explain the behavior of the ancients with western scientific theories and rationalize it. It reflects that Chinese medicine during the Republic of China period used some ideas of Western medicine to construct and explain the theory of daily recuperation and disease prevention. In addition, in the discussion of TCM, "individuals" may reduce their own risk of illness by implementing some traditional medical techniques and rules. Cao Bingzhang said: "All the halls, bedrooms and kitchens should be cleaned, and no filth should be allowed. On a sunny day, the windows should be opened to let in fresh air and the sunlight to absorb dampness. For example, the stables of cattle, horses, pigs and sheep, and garbage should not be located near the houses and wells. It is also not allowed to wash meat, vegetables, and clothes beside the wells. In case of epidemic diseases and damp weather, it is advisable to burn incense, rhubarb, atractylodes, wormwood for

---

[170] Zhang Xichun, Sini Decoction of Yang Ming Disease, *Chinese Medicine with Reference to the West*, Vol. II, p. 733.

[171] Shaoxing Medical Association, Health and Prevention. Hygiene of the Sick, Treatment of Damp and Warm Epidemics, included in Li Shunbao (ed.), *Complete Book of Warm Diseases*, Vol. II, p. 2099.

[172] Shaoxing Medical Association, Health and Prevention. Hygiene of the Sick, Treatment of Damp and Warm Epidemics, included in Li Shunbao (ed.), *Complete Book of Warm Diseases*, Vol. II, p. 2099.

detoxification".[173] In addition to the traditional knowledge that "incense" can avoid diseases and the technology of burning incense to prevent diseases, the knowledge of Chinese and Western medicine in adjusting the room gave patients and non-patients an anti-disease "personal" technology for resistance. In these expositions, the significance of personal safeguarding life outweighs the significance of public health. For Western medicine, people who did not understand public health need to be re educated. Public health was more altruistic, but for TCM, the protection of life was implemented in the daily life of "individuals" in the private field. In fact, both of the two aspects were presented in the medical circles of the Republic of China period, but the latter was often ignored by critics.

In addition, Cao Bingzhang warned people in the epidemic "do not stay in bed near the patient, so as not to increase the patient's dryness-heat.Caution,caution!"[174] Cao's appeal was not directed at the fear of being infected by disease, but focuses on not aggravating the patient's condition. At that time, the different views and interpretations between Chinese and Western medicine for the course of infection can be seen. Shao Yingzhi once used malaria to illustrate the inadequacy of the bacterial theory.

> In the case of Shaoyang disease, it is aggravated by chest pain, which means that the chest tube and spleen are affected. It is also common for those with interior heat to have the dull pain on the left ribs. I also suspect that the spleen is affected by lymphatic suppression. Malaria is a disease which is caused by bacteria and protozoa in the West, and that it belongs to Shaoyang disease in TCM. The two are explained differently but I think they are the same. The left ribs of people is the blood manufacturing factory, which is also the base of detoxification. The pain naturally follows after bitter fighting. However, little bupleurum can not kill bacteria, but can cure the disease, just like apricot and calamine can not kill throat bacteria, but can cure throat syndrome. The same is true even for Zhongjing's thirteen prescriptions that can't kill typhoid bacilli, but can cure typhoid. Yu Fengbin cited the theory of "3-cause relationship" from a European physician, to explain the 3 causes leading to cholera. First, cholera bacteria sneaks into the intestines and stomach; Second, the climate is not suitable for human beings, but suitable for the survival of bacteria; Third, the weak immunity of individuals. Only when the above 3 factors get into a certain disposition can the disease be caused. One can not be sick by just having the first without the second. The same is true for having the second without the first. Therefore, Er Li, the teacher of Yu, once took cholera bacteria without getting sick. He was healthy and it happened in good weather. Yu also said that as we are exposed to germs in a bad environment every day, how do we know that cholera bacteria are not in our intestines and stomachs?We can be free of the diseases if our bodies are strong enough to resist them.[175]

Shao used the term "resist" to explain that Chinese medicine can enhance the disease resistance of the human body, which is quite similar to Yun Tieqiao's hypothesis that "Chinese medicine can treat the initial onset of all fever diseases". Shao quoted the theory cited by Yu Fengbin to reduce the key position of the bacteria

---

[173] Cao Bingzhang, Chapter 7 Prevention of Autumn Epidemic, Essentials of Autumn Epidemic Treatment, included in Lu Zheng (ed.), *Collection of Rare Modern TCM. Medical Talk*, p. 773.

[174] Cao Bingzhang, Chapter 7 Prevention of Autumn Epidemic, Essentials of Autumn Epidemic Treatment, included in Lu Zheng (ed.), *Collection of Rare Modern TCM. Medical Talk*, p. 773.

[175] Shao Canzhi, Impetus, *Suxuan Medical Talk*, included in Lu Zheng (ed.), *Collection of Rare Modern TCM. Medical Talk*, pp. 640–641.

in causing infectious diseases, avoid the confirmation of pathological anatomy that bacteria caused the damage of viscera and blood and explain infectious diseases by referring to the factor of "climate", which is often a concern in the discussion of heat diseases in TCM and traditional Qi theory. More importantly, the question of "personal resistance" raised by him inadvertently pointed out that the people at the time were concerned more about "personal" health than public health.

Attention to personal hygiene was actually an important feature of TCM during the Republic of China period. This was originally an area for health practitioners, and it was by no means the main content of the classics of febrile diseases in the Qing Dynasty and before. He Lianchen and Cao Bingzhang added a large number of factors about personal prevention of disease and health preservation in the medical book *Updated Popular Treatise on Typhoid Fever,* which was rare in the past. TCM during the Republic of China period added a lot of traditional health knowledge, as well as hygiene and disease prevention knowledge to the fever system. For example, it is stated in the article *Body Cleaning* which belongs to the ancient personal health knowledge:

> Patients after the discovery of a disease should clean up their face frequently to make the face shiny and promote blood circulation. The eyes should be wiped frequently, and kept closed at quiet times so as to have a peaceful mind, or rubbed with the backs of the two fingers to dispel the heat. The teeth should be washed and wiped frequently to remove the filth. The stomach should be rubbed often to digest food and dissolve the filth. The foot and the Yongquan point in the foot center should be rubbed frequently so as to remove rheumatism and walk well. Sleeping sideways with feet bent, so as not to lose one's essence and stagnate the Qi in the joints. Do not wash your face with cold water in summer, clean your body, and rub it frequently. These are the methods to harmonize blood and Qi after recovery.

These actions of cleaning the body not only focus on the narrow scope of "cleaning" in Western medicine, but also on cleaning the outside of the body, including cleaning the channels of Qi and blood to keep it flowing smoothly, focusing on Qi and blood. Other precautions, such as the protection of the body according to the changes of temperature, all emphasize on the prevention of bad air from the outside environment. Of course, the concept of pure cleanliness is also included. For example, "the clothes of patients must be changed every other day, and the bedding, in particular, must be clean".[176]

---

[176] For example: "The patient should not be overly covered. Being too warm can also cause disease. The seriously ill will die, due to the fact that the heat is confined in the internal Qi. The patient's back should be always warm, which will prevent the wind and cold from invasion; the chest should always be protected to keep away the cold. Never wear sweaty clothes when being cold, as it will hurt the back and the lungs; the clothes exposed to the sun for a long time will have heat toxicity. The clothes dried up by fire in winter may feel good but they will cause disease if they are put on for a long time. Before the ice melts in spring, the clothes should be light at the top and thick at the bottom, developing the Yin and curbing the Yang. Do not face the wind when taking off sweaty clothes in summer. Take it slow when adding clothes in winter; take them off temporarily if one feels a little warm. Observe the temperatures of the day, and keep the cotton padded clothes handy. Attention is needed for all individuals, for the healthy and the sick." He Lianchen (ed.), revised by Wang Zhipu et al. *Updated Popular Treatise Typhoid Fever*, pp. 502–503.

7.7 Reflection on "Personal Hygiene" in China

Since the nineteenth century, Western medicine has begun to transform. Li Shangren and Sean Hsiang-Lin maintained that the patients changed their roles but they were unable to change their own conditions. They could only wait passively.[177] This chapter and the next chapter involve the comparisons and supplements: after the introduction of new Western medicine into China, Chinese patients traditionally still had their independent interpretations and treatment of diseases. Although it is inconsistent with the purpose of modern medical care and health, for the exploration of the social and cultural history of Chinese grass-roots, we should look to the countryside instead of the big cities. This also shows the diversity of history and the possibility that the history of TCM itself brings various topics to global medical history. As a matter of fact, in modern times we are living, there is another utopia with all kinds of imaginations.

Is it better to talk about "individuals" or "public" in medical and health care? Lu Xun once sighed: "It is really difficult to preserve public properties in China. If the authorities are laymen, they will spoil them; if they are professionals, they will steal them".[178] The history of medical and health care is indeed a special case. Although most modern historians emphasized the birth of the modern health systems and institutions,[179] "health is important not because it is a personal matter, but because diseases can be transmitted from person to person, which will cause the public to suffer, 'individuals', 'groups' and 'nations' will be harmed and safety is lost".[180] The truth is the medical and health laws were a failure in modern China. The general public's mentality of seeking more for themselves has contributed to the spread of personal hygiene; the medical resources were far from enough to meet the needs of the patients. The quantity and quality were not up to standard. New medical care was more expensive and the medical process was complicated. If the patient felt something wrong, he would find another doctor. Even the books of Western medicine emphasize the "health preservation" (see Fig. 7.7)[181] of "individuals" for modern health, which is real life situation beyond public health.

The theory of Qi in TCM is a kind of philosophy. The argument that "Qi" causes disease is not groundless. "Exogenous Qi" can affect the symptoms of the body and has clinical significance. Qi plays a role of "triggering", and patients' feelings in

---

[177] Li Shangren, From Patients' Stories to Case Histories: the Transition of Western Medicine from the Mid-18th Century to the End of the 19th Century, *Discourse in Ancient and Modern Times* 2000 (05): 139–146; Sean Hsiang-Lin, *Responsible Doctors and Patients with Faith -- the Debate between Chinese and Western Medicine and the Transformation of the Relationship between Doctors and Patients during the Republic of China Period,* p. 76.

[178] Yue Nan, *Chen Yinke and Fu Sinian*, Xi'an: Shaanxi Normal University Press, 2008, p. 116.

[179] Perhaps since modern times, those who talk about health history have also pursued this progressive view of history. Jin Baoshan, "A Brief History of the Development of Health Care since the Republic of China Period", *Journal of Chinese Medical History* 2.1 (1948), pp. 18–25.

[180] Hu Songshan, *The Importance of Summer Hygiene Movement and Precautions for Summer Hygiene*, June 16, 1936, p. 4.

[181] *New Youth*, Volume 1,1915 (01), folder advertisement.

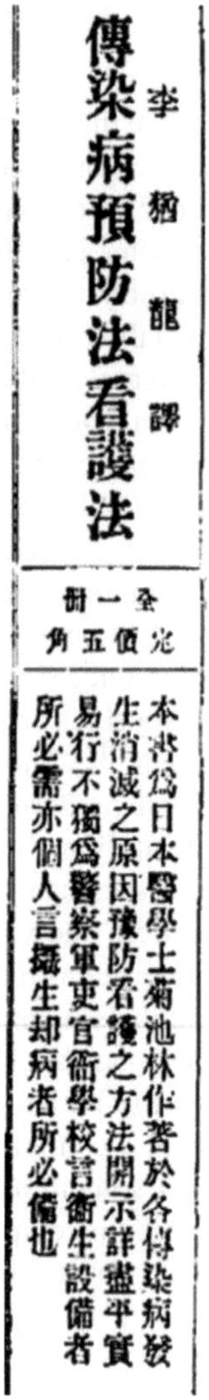

Fig. 7.7 The essential book of health preservation *Infectious Disease Prevention and Protection*

daily life often conform to the changes of Qi in the four seasons. The influence of weather, climate and temperature on the human body is more significant than that of microorganisms. When interpreting this underdeveloped science in modern China, Qian Mu said: "Abstract and logical ideas or theories were not very developed in China, and the Chinese people prefer understanding them through living and direct personal experience".[182] For ordinary people, bacteriology and laboratory analysis are not practical experiences of daily life. The most intuitive feeling may be that the

---

182 Qian Mu, Sino Western Contact and Cultural Renewal, *Introduction to Chinese Cultural History*, Taipei: Taiwan Commercial Press, 1994, pp. 214–215.

body is invaded by external factors, such as the "six Qis" that causes exogenous fever, and even various bad Qis, such as filth and epidemic Qi. The implementation of deep-seated science from the laboratory to society is indeed more difficult than traditional concepts. Of course, with the integration of Chinese and Western medicine, the essence of TCM's "Qi Theory" is also changed. The concepts of "air" and "nourishing Qi" in Western science have affected TCM's Qi theory. On the basis of the "miasma theory", TCM has absorbed Western medicine, which is prone to the knowledge of filth or stink in putrefaction. The rationale behind TCM's incorporation of modern health measures, such as cleaning and disinfection, into disease prevention measures is probably a mixture of miasma theory and traditional medical Qi theory, with less microbiology.

Influenced by Western medicine, TCM began to pay attention to the corresponding relationship between "individual" and "environment" in terms of disease prevention discourse and changes in daily life, and actively carried out clean and sanitary measures. This change involves the knowledge of space and air circulation. These discussions on the family recuperation space are different from those of Western medicine in the hospital. TCM has many methods to prevent infection in daily life. In addition to cleaning and hygiene, it also includes measures to regulate the "Qi" of poor living places, and even includes many ancient methods. For example, Fei Xiaotong said:

> The local society is a society of settlement. People were born, raised and died in the same area. Not only is population mobility very little, but also that the land people going for resources has rarely changed. In this stable environment, what individuals could trust was not only their own experience, but also the experience of their ancestors. An old farmer working in a rural society was only faced with the change of seasons, not the change of times. It recycles each year. The solutions used by predecessors to solve problems in life could be copied as a guide to their own lives. The more effective it had been proven in the lives of previous generations, the more it was worth preserving. Therefore, "The words of the saints Yao and Shun are the golden rules", and pursuing ancients was the guarantee of life.
>
> During the war of resistance against Japanese aggression, I was evacuated to the countryside of Kunming. My newly-born child cried all day and I could not find a doctor. I had to consult the landlady. As soon as she heard the cry, she knew that there were "false teeth" on the root of the baby's teeth, which were a kind of parasitic bacteria. It hurts during breast feeding, but the baby would be starved without being fed. She calmly asked us to wipe the baby's mouth with pickled vegetables and blue cloth. It stopped after a day or two. Every baby in this place had it, and every mother knew how to treat it. That's an effective therapy. As long as the environment remains unchanged and no new bacteria invades, this set of therapy without any theoretical support is always effective. As it is effective, there is no need to ask why.

For these kinds of traditions, the rule is to follow rather than to question, and life would be secure, naturally followed by a set of values. When we say "efficacious", we mean that there is an unknown magic behind it. If you follow the rules, you will be blessed. If you don't follow the rules, you will go wrong. Therefore, people gradually have a sense of awe for tradition.[183]

For ordinary patients, after all, bacteria were too ethereal, and the traditional Qi theory still prevailed. For example, avoiding infection with various external Qi was the center of TCM's disease prevention theory at that time. Chinese medicine did not deny that cleaning and hygiene was the "antibacterial" method, but its dialogue with Western medicine was on the basis of the original "miasma theory" of Western medicine. Later, though microorganisms were mentioned, TCM had not yet established a set of specific bacteria killing and prevention methods and classification system. After the prosperity of bacteriology, most TCM doctors showed a superficial agreement attitude but actually rejected it. In the next chapter, the infection of TCM will be discussed in depth. The disease prevention law overturns the previous view that TCM did not have the technology to prevent infectious diseases, and reviews the reasons why TCM could not establish a set of specific bacteria killing and prevention methods during the Republic of China period.

[183] Fei Xiaotong, *Local China and Local Reconstruction,* Taipei: Fengyun Times Press, 1993, pp. 52–53.

Chapter 8
Epidemic Prevention Technology and Antibacterial Thought of TCM During the Republic of China Period

8.1 Preface

If we lengthen the time span of modern Chinese medicine history and retrospectively look for ideas, we can find that China has emphasized the integration of TCM and Western medicine in the preventive treatment of infectious diseases since the 1950s, and has made certain achievements through the collection of unilateral and empirical prescriptions.[1] However, if we take a closer look at the achievements, we can find that the word "preventive treatment" should be taken apart. In fact, modern Chinese medicine has more "treatment" than "prevention", or more efforts were made to have breakthroughs in treatment, while leaving prevention to Western medicine.[2] In ancient times, there was no clear idea and method of epidemic prevention. In the Ming and Qing Dynasties, epidemic prevention mainly focused on treatment and medicine, without much "prevention", and most of them belonged to the category of "epidemic rescue".[3] In ancient times, the "preservation" of health care actually emphasized the prevention of disease in regard to eating and living styles, with little attention to the prevention of disease.[4] It is obvious that modern China witnesses the starting point for TCM to attach importance to epidemic prevention, the key point for TCM to be expelled from epidemic prevention work.

Regarding the public health history of modern Chinese and Western medicine, the pestis in the three northeastern provinces at the end of the Qing Dynasty and the beginning of the Republic of China period was a very obvious breaking point. After that, China completely adopted western public health and epidemic prevention laws. The discourse right from laws and regulations to daily measures was fully controlled

[1] Chen Bangxian, *History of Chinese Medicine*, Beijing: Commercial Press, 1957, pp. 376–379.

[2] Pi Kuoli, The Development of TCM in Shanghai (1950–1965)—An Investigation Centered on the People's Daily, *Sinology Research Newsletter*, Vol. 35, 2016 (04), pp. 1–12.

[3] Deng Tietao, *History of Epidemic Prevention in China*, pp. 140–150.

[4] Zhang Zanchen, *A Brief History of Chinese Medical History*, Shanghai: Shanghai: Qianqing Hall Publishing House, 1954, pp. 49–50.

© Zhonghua Book Company 2026

K. Pi, *The Contest of Modern Chinese and Western Medicine*,
https://doi.org/10.1007/978-981-95-2832-5_8

by Western medicine. TCM lost its status in public health, and faced the fate of being abandoned. It was too rough a time for it during the Republic of China period.[5] The above is a general understanding of Chinese medical history. What modern Chinese medicine did in preventing infectious diseases had been neglected by researchers or the Chinese medical community in the past.[6] The pestis in the three eastern provinces is an example. In fact, the epidemics had made the Chinese medicine community reflect on itself: "This disease is the most serious disaster, and priority should be given to prevention. In case of infection, it is better to treat it with Western medicine first. The prescription theory can be kept for reference." [7] As an important doctor in modern times, Zhang Zanchen had seen the importance of prevention in advance. However, he did not describe in detail how Chinese medicine prevented infectious diseases at that time. Many modern doctors and medical history scholars have ignored this issue, leading to the legacy of TCM in the prevention of infectious diseases being ignored in the discussion of the historical process of TCM.

This chapter focuses on the knowledge of TCM during the Republic of China period, mainly on the basis of newspapers and periodicals, supplemented by medical books, to explore the presentations, research and implementations of "TCM epidemic prevention" knowledge which was often ignored by researchers in the past, as well as a TCM style of daily sterilization, so as to make up for the missing part in the previous research in this area.[8] This chapter first discusses the awareness and importance of TCM on this issue, followed by the epidemic prevention knowledge inherited by TCM at that time. The discussion of medicine is the main topic. The daily preservation methods such as Qigong breathing, diet and mental health are too extensive to be discussed in detail here, so that the overall discussion can be more focused. Finally, it is my wish to put forward some historical studies based on the advantages and disadvantages of TCM in this respect.

---

[5] According to the author's research, TCM recognized it as the "quintessence of the country" and successfully shaped a force representing traditional culture. It presents a striking contrast with the imperialist and aggressive image represented by Western medicine. Pi Kuoli, The Connotation of "National Medicine"—on the Modern Transformation and Reconstruction of Chinese Medicine, *Journal of Zhongshan University* (Social Science Edition), 2009, Vol. 49 (1), pp. 64–77. For the transformation of TCM medicine during the Republic of China period, we can also see Sean Hsiang-Lin Lei, *Neither Donkey Nor Horse: Medicine in the Struggle over China's Modernity,* Chicago: University of Chicago Press,2014, and Bridie Andrews, *The Making of Modern Chinese Medicine, 1850–1960,*Vancouver: UBCP,2014.

[6] There were many measures for TCM epidemic prevention in the Qing Dynasty, and they continued to the Republic of China period. See Yu Xinzhong, *Health Epidemic Prevention Mechanism in the Qing Dynasty and Its Modern Evolution*, pp. 73–93.

[7] Zhang Zanchen, *A Brief History of Chinese Medical History*, p. 42.

[8] Some ideas can be found in the author's book: *Modern Chinese Medical History of "Qi" and "Bacteria"—Knowledge Transformation and Daily Life of Exogenous Fever*, Taipei: China Medical Research Institute, 2012, pp. 221–272. This chapter expands on the TCM epidemic prevention methods, and emphasizes the information found in the news media that is not contained in the books, so as to supplement the original ideas of TCM on "antibacterial".

8.2 Review of Epidemic Prevention by TCM During the Republic of China Period

In the late Qing Dynasty, officials and the public started to pay attention to the epidemic prevention system of Western medicine. In 1902, Chen Qiu (1851–1904), a TCM reformist intellectual, commented that the epidemic prevention laws of Western medicine was close to being perfect, and that western people "have a hygienic living style". However, China was not in any way on the track towards following modern medicine. If epidemic prevention was suddenly implemented, "it is not to serve towards a positive end, but would cause harm instead".[9] At that time, there were still opposing voices regarding the epidemic prevention laws as a nuisance and did not advocate its engagement in its research. After the founding of the Republic of China, in the social epidemic prevention affairs, TCM mostly participated in or organized "epidemic prevention meetings" and "clinics", but its business was still focused on "treatment" rather than "prevention". In terms of epidemic prevention in addition to absorbing the health knowledge of Western medicine, the Chinese medicine community mostly distributed "epidemic prevention drugs" or carried out treatment discussions, with less statements or developments in the area of prevention.[10]

When the northern pestis broke out in 1918, the government agreed to allow Chinese medicine to be applied at the scene of the outbreak for treatment. It was commented that this was a special "flexible method". It was officially declared that although people preferred TCM for epidemic prevention, the government must first explain to the Western medical quarantine officers that TCM would definitely abide by the relevant laws and regulations on infectious diseases and would not treat patients who had not been sent to the hospital or isolation centers at will. TCM could only treat them upon the confirmation and approval from the Western medical quarantine officers "to avoid disputes". It can be seen that at that time Chinese medicine could participate in its affairs, but the government did not trust Chinese medicine in its independent diagnosis and treatment.[11] Judging from the cholera epidemic at the turn of the summer and autumn in 1919, it was recorded that "the prevention of Western medicine was not as effective as the treatment of TCM", so the Beijing Police Department designated a group of TCM doctors including Yang Haoru, Chen Shizhen, Zhang Hanqing, to treat the disease in Langfang, and achieved good results.[12] Such achievements have actually shown that Chinese medicine was helpful in treating epidemic diseases, but not very particular about epidemic prevention.

---

[9] Chen Qiu, et al.(eds), Collection of Liji Medicine Q & A on Epidemics and Cholera, included in Liu Shijue (ed.), *Wenzhou Literature Series Integration of Wenzhou Modern Medical Books*, pp. 71–72.

[10] Unknown Author, Clinic of Epidemic Prevention Association (Anhui), *World of TCM*, Vol. 11, 1936 (01), p. 71.

[11] Unknown Author, President Jiang to Commander Zhang Datong, *Official Gazette*, Vol. 122, 1918, p. 143.

[12] Kong Bohua's Classic Study Office (ed.), *Answers to the Queries on the Treatment of Eight Infectious Diseases*, p. 106.

TCM's efforts in epidemic prevention can be seen in newspapers and leaflets. At that time, many newspapers and magazines set up notices or columns on "First Aid for the Current Disease" and published some prescriptions, so that people who had no time to see a doctor in case of an emergency could apply them according to the prescriptions. In 1934, Chen Zedong, a TCM doctor, said: "The weather in winter was very warm, the fog lasted for more than a month, and there was a bad smell. The climate was the source of most epidemics". The local Chinese Medicine Association specially published effective prescriptions in a magazine, so that those who had not been infected by the epidemic Qi could use them for prevention, and the infected could be improved. The published prescriptions were "black bean roll, Huoxiang leaf, perilla leaf and cyrtomium", which to be taken in the morning and evening every day to prevent and eliminate the epidemic.[13] *The Journal of Tianjin Chinese Medicine Association* had a special column on seasonal symptoms of spring, which mainly published prescriptions for diseases such as laryngeal disease and mumps.[14] TCM had been making efforts to publish prescriptions in this way, but the treatment was not satisfactory. According to the official magazine of the Ministry of health in 1930, someone from Changshu county reported that TCM had made money in the name of treating the epidemic.[15] This is actually a manifestation of the lack of public trust and authority in TCM epidemic prevention laws. Many TCM doctors were limited by schools of thought. They only treated epidemics according to or by adhering to the methods of a certain school of medicine. They were criticized as "a method of bluffing people to reap profits", which led to people's distrust of TCM in treating epidemics. Many of the treatments of ancient doctors might not be suitable for treating each specific epidemic, so the Tianjin Chinese Medicine Association called for collecting and sorting out ancient prescriptions.[16]

As early as the early 1930s, TCM doctors had realized that the treatment of infectious diseases by Chinese and Western medicine was not just a theoretical debate. The Ministry of health, led by Western medicine, had declared that it would not allow Chinese medicine to intervene in the prevention and treatment of infectious diseases[17] and criticized the TCM doctors for not knowing about infection and disinfection. They were simply called "the mother of infectious diseases". Patients who went to TCM doctors for infectious diseases were infected one after another, which was very dangerous, as the TCM doctors' rooms were full of germs. In other words,

---

[13] Chen Zedong, Column of First Aid for Current Diseases, *Authentic National Medicine*, 1934 (09), p. 18.

[14] Tianjin Institute of TCM (ed.), Column of First Aid for Current Diseases, *Authentic National Medicine*, 1934 (10), p. 34.

[15] Liu Ruiheng, Approval from Ministry of Health No. 71, *Health Bulletin*, Vol. 2, 1930 (04), p. 99.

[16] Tianjin Association of TCM, The Reply to Tianjin Association of TCM Submitted to the National Medical Center to Solicit TCM Health Facilities, *Authentic National Medicine*, 1936 (24), p. 5.

[17] Zhou Zhen, Soliciting Public Opinions on Implementing the Policy of Sharing Assignments Due to the Autocracy of Western Medicine Approved by the Ministry of Health, which Hinders the Development of TCM and Restricts the TCM from Treating Infectious Diseases, *Xinglin Medical Monthly*, 1930 (19), pp. 1–3.

traditional medicine could only be called the "special vector" of infectious diseases.[18] The Chinese medicine community had put forward a counterattack. Although the ancients did not see bacteria, they found that many ancient methods were effective from their research of ancient books and their own treatment process.[19]

Wang Hesan, a TCM doctor, said that if TCM could not cure infectious diseases, China would have become a "ghost country" for thousands of years. He believed that after Western medicine was introduced in China, the Western infectious diseases he was seeing were named in Chinese, but in fact, typhoid fever and cholera are the names of Chinese medicine diseases. There were many innovative treatments in history. How can we think that Chinese medicine has no medicine to cure infectious diseases?[20] Wang tried to highlight the effectiveness of TCM in the prevention and treatment of infectious diseases, but he did not further elaborate on how to proceed at the prevention level.

For example, Yang Zhiyi maintained that the interface of TCM should "give play to China's inherent academic knowledge of epidemic treatment and remedy the malpractice of Western medicine that emphasizes sterilization".[21] Does the inherent science of epidemic prevention include "prevention"? At that time, it was ignored by many people. Due to the fact that the focus of the debate between Chinese and Western medicine was still therapeutics, TCM acquired the knowledge of treating epidemics when reviewing the ancient academic, but it seemed to have forgotten the problem of epidemic prevention when sorting out the academic. The Chinese medicine community's indifference to epidemic prevention had its historical origins. Pestis, which affected the health process in modern China, is an example. Luo Xieyuan, a Chinese medicine practitioner in Sichuan Province, believed that Chinese medicine had therapies. From the beginning to its worst stage, there have been effective prescriptions for the treatment of pestis, "It is a futile effort for Western medicine to have the test and isolation, to have the items of the infected burned and traffic control. In the infected areas, a lot people died from being infected or not being infected, buried for being dead or not yet being dead! It was all due to the academic and political order of health. It had turned into a tool of slaughtering without living up to people's expectations. It was so inhuman that it is not to be blamed on the Westerners for their superstition about science!"[22] He criticized the fact that passive epidemic prevention methods such as rat catching, disinfection, and isolation were developed due to the incapability of Western medicine of curing it. It was a last resort. The highest level

---

18 Shou Bai, Attentions to the Special Vector of Infectious Diseases: Old Medicine, *Social Medical Journal*, 1933 (190), pp. 51–54.

19 Zhu Chenghan, Dysentery—An Introduction to Diseases, *Wuxing Medical Monthly*, 1947 (13), p. 16.

20 Wang Hesan, Can TCM Cure Infectious Diseases? *Modern Chinese Medicine*, Vol. 1, 1934 (03), p. 2.

21 Yang Zhiyi, My Views on "Epidemic Treatment" of TCM and Western Medicine, *Spring and Autumn of the Medical World*, 1930 (49), pp. 3–4.

22 Luo Xieyuan, On the Invention of Microbiology in Chinese Medicine, *Modern Chinese Medicine*, Vol. 2, 1941 (01), pp. 22, 24.

of real epidemic prevention is to cure the epidemics, rather than preventing it. In the same discussion, Lu Yuanlei said in 1928:

> Western medicine knows it (bacterial disease) but cannot treat it, which is no different from not knowing. They thus changed their tone, saying that when TCM treats diseases, they do not know the specific bacteria, and cannot determine what disease it is, so it cannot study the infectious diseases, and duly can not disinfect and prevent them. This means that if we want to study, disinfect and prevent diseases, we must use Western medicine… As for disinfection and prevention, it is particularly complicated. The Europeans and Americans have done their best in their disinfection and prevention, but infectious diseases are not gone. The disinfection and prevention of Chinese people had been neglected, but infectious diseases have not been widespread. According to the Europeans and Americans, Chinese people are highly resistant to toxins. The reason of this is that they have been often infected with germs without disinfection.[23]

Lu's remark that "infectious diseases have not been widespread in China" was by no means a fact. The key point is that most of the preventive injections of Western medicine are injections of bacterial liquid and bacteria, which are used to induce the human body's anti-virus ability. On the one hand, the disinfection of Western medicine is to stop natural infection, and on the other hand, it injects bacterial liquid and bacteria, which only makes bacteria more tenacious and diseases more difficult to be treated. It would be better not to disinfect or carry out preventive injections, but try to induce the body's resistance by natural infection. This idea is based on the fact that Chinese medicine can treat infectious diseases. In the following year, Lu stated: "The vigorous disinfection today can at best reduce the chances of infection of bacteria, but can never eliminate them. The anti-virus capacity of human body has been completely degraded due to the reduction of the chance of infection. Once the bacteria are infected, the disease is bound to get worse. The more emphasis the Westerners place on disinfection, the weaker their ability to resist infectious diseases, and the more difficult it is to prove the effectiveness of disinfection and prevention".[24] Lu's remarks were considered avant-garde in the Chinese medicine community, which indicates that the Chinese medicine community lacked the in-depth research on epidemic prevention compared with its study on therapeutics. In 1936, the Tianjin Association of TCM even criticized that "the preventive methods of Western medicine, such as cool air circulation and sprinkling medicine, are ineffective, and the treatment methods of isolation, freezing, injection and sterilization are harmful".[25] At the same time, Zhou Yuxi compiled the book about epidemics, which was written by Xiao Shangzhi. It clearly stated that the book had been approved by the National Medical Center. According to the author, in 1934, the book was revised and printed to prevent epidemics. It turned out to be a best seller, being reprinted repeatedly and even

---

[23] Lu Yuanlei, Answer to Zeng Yuying's Refutation, Lu's Collection on Medicine, Zhang Yuping (ed.), *Two Kinds of Lu Yuanlei's Medical Books,* pp. 72–73.

[24] Lu Yuanlei, Declaration upon Abolishing Classic Medicine in the Central Health Conference, Lu's Collection of Medical Theories, included in Zhang Yuping (ed.), *Two Kinds of Lu Yuanlei's Medical Books,* p. 87.

[25] Tianjin Association of TCM, The Reply to Tianjin Association of TCM Submitted to the National Medical Center to Solicit TCM Health Facilities, *Authentic National Medicine*, 1936 (24), p. 5.

being published in newspapers, with the total sales of more than 50,000 copies.[26] Zhou said: "Instead of discovering a therapy of the disease, their hygienists only use lime water to sterilize without speculating on its causes. In terms of prevention and detoxification, there is no good method, and the serum therapy is not reliable. The seemingly novel gains from Western medicine are no better than China's losses in disease treatment".[27] It is another criticism to the various unrealistic epidemic prevention measures of Western medicine.

Despite the above negations, it can not be said that the Chinese medicine community did not pay attention to the problems of epidemic prevention at that time. The remarks show that the Chinese medicine sector had fully understood the monumental weakness of Chinese medicine in epidemic prevention. In 1936, Huang Guocai, a Chinese medicine practitioner, maintained that the TCM knowledge of epidemic prevention was elementary. Even amid the prevailing trend, only about two tenths of the Chinese medicine community studied epidemic prevention, which was a very bad situation. He hoped that the National Medical Center would take up the responsibility of drafting regulations as soon as possible and issuing them to all localities for implementation. Huang proposed to establish a "TCM Epidemic Prevention School" as soon as possible by teaching the following: Firstly, to find out the transmission paths of various infectious diseases; secondly, understand the pathogen of the bacteria, learn to use the microscope to test the bacteria, make anti-epidemic slurry vaccines, and carry out vaccination. Finally, when an epidemic occurs, we should integrate the strengths of TCM and Western medicine, various health laws regarding bacteria, six Qis and seven emotions, and cultivate TCM epidemic prevention talents. Ten years later, the so-called "right to epidemic prevention" can be controlled by TCM doctors.[28] Li Xiaobi pointed out that Western medicine indeed had a better knowledge of sterilization than TCM. Although Chinese medicine was equipped with such medicines as aromatics with antiphlogistic agents, it still lagged behind Western medicine in terms of prevention technology. After all, there were only a few Chinese medicine practitioners who understood modern health and epidemic prevention laws. In particular, a large number of old Chinese medicine practitioners in the countryside shared the common weal and woe with the people. It is an important vision to concentrate on the training of old Chinese medicine practitioners as soon as possible, teaching scientific epidemic prevention measures and inventing epidemic prevention drugs.[29] Zhang Douyao commented that the Chinese medicine community should quickly set up an "Epidemic Prevention Committee" to impart epidemic prevention knowledge, and then set up epidemic prevention centers in all counties, so that the TCM doctors trained for epidemic prevention could take up this work. At times

[26] Zhou Yuxi (ed.), *Compilation of Epidemic Diseases*, Tianjin: Tianjin Chinese and Western Converged Medical Society, 1941, Casual Talk, pp. 1–2.

[27] Zhou Yuxi (ed.), *Compilation of Epidemic Diseases*, p. 12.

[28] Huang Guocai, The Methods Needed for TCM in the Training of Epidemic Prevention Knowledge, *Medical Journal*, 1936 (90), pp. 16–17.

[29] Li Xiaobi, The Methods Needed for TCM in the Training of Epidemic Prevention Knowledge, *Medical Journal*, 1936 (90), pp. 17–18.

of peace, they could learn epidemic prevention knowledge; when epidemics occur, they could assume the work of public health and give guidance to epidemic prevention. If a public hospital based on TCM could be established, it would not only treat epidemics, but also save the lives of the people of the lowest class. In addition, it was necessary to organize experts as soon as possible to study anti-epidemic drugs and distribute them to various places, or to "post the prescriptions" so that the public could use them whenever needed.[30] The above remarks show that the Chinese medicine community was still thinking about how to take back the power of "epidemic prevention" from the hands of Western doctors, mainly from the teaching of epidemic prevention knowledge.

From the perspective of historical documents, the TCM doctor Shang Fuhan went through the various ways of treating and curing epidemics in TCM, which also took exogenous febrile disease of TCM generally as a topic of discussion. He hoped that through this combing, we can verify the origin and development of TCM epidemic prevention. He said:

> At the beginning of an epidemic, it was quite similar to the current disease. It is difficult to determine from its diagnosis, so that it is difficult to begin the epidemic prevention work. Therefore, in case of a disease similar to the current disease, a bamboo stick was used to dip some dry tobacco oil on it and let the patient lick. If the patient could not tell its taste, it was an epidemic. Or raw soybeans could be used for the patient to chew. If it didn't taste fishy, it was also an epidemic disease. This method is the same as the method of testing furunculosis. For the test of epidemic diseases in Western medicine, all of the tests done with a microscope are more accurate than those in TCM, but the microscope was too expensive for rural doctors and the above methods seemed to be simpler.[31]

The epidemic testing technology described by Shang was completely TCM, which is different from Huang Guocai's discussion. The author believes that Huang wanted the Chinese medicine community to learn the epidemic prevention techniques of Western medicine as soon as possible, while Shang hoped to develop epidemic TCM prevention methods, each with its own emphasis. It can be said that this thinking is pluralistic, but it also reflects that there were more different opinions than the consensus from the Chinese medicine community, and the specific implementation and its methods were not analyzed in depth. If the Chinese medicine community were to come up with epidemic prevention measures, it must also face the problem of establishing the names of the diseases. Tian Erkang believed that TCM, based on the experience and rules of ancient medical books, had been quite effective in treating epidemics, but it had not been unified in diagnosing diseases. For one epidemic disease, the diagnosis of each doctor was often different, leaving patients at a loss.[32] He believed that special books on infectious diseases should be compiled as soon

---

[30] Zhang Douyao, Preface, *Medical Journal*, 1936 (90), pp. 18–19.

[31] Shang Fuhan, Research on Epidemic Prevention of Chinese Medicine, *Chinese Medicine Bulletin*, Vol. 4, 1936 (01), p. 31.

[32] Pi Kuoli, History of Exogenous Fevers in the Qing Dynasty—The History of Exogenous Febrile Diseases in the Qing Dynasty—the Typhoid Fever Vs. Warm Disease and the Interpretation of the TCM History, included in the Office of Life and Medical History Research (ed.), *A New Theory of Chinese History. Medical History*, Taipei: Lianjing Publishing House, 2015, pp. 475–526.

as possible, and the names of various infectious diseases in history should be sorted out so that doctors would know the names of the diseases as soon as they saw the symptoms.[33] In Western medicine, the name of a disease must be determined first, so that the specific pathogen could be prevented. As TCM had no testing technology, the discussion of disease names was inconsistent. Lu Yuanlei even thought that the disease names of Western medicine should be directly adopted, which triggered a debate in TCM circles. Hong Guanzhi pointed out that if the Chinese medicine community continued to adhere to the old disease names, "it would not be consistent with the original intention of the medical rule that the disease names should be recorded in the TCM diagnostic book, which is not helpful to the health administration and literature statistics. It is an indispensable part of the diagnose to determine a disease name, and there is no doubt it should adopt the modern disease names". He supported Lu's view, but it was no easy job to sort out the names of the diseases in the literature. Hong pointed out the dilemma by wondering "how many people can engage in literature research?"[34] Adopting western disease names may not be feasible, and it was more difficult to sort out the ancient disease names from the Chinese literature, which ended up in stagnation.[35] It can be seen that the "epidemic prevention" of TCM during the Republic of China period could only adopt the definition of diseases of Western medicine to carry out various health measures. This is an obvious disadvantage of TCM.

As early as 1934, the Medical Association of Peking collectively initiated the establishment of a National Infectious Disease Hospital. At that time, it was still in the planning stage, and the measures were first drawn up. It was initially planned to appoint Chinese medicine interns from the Peking National Medical College as service personnel, but the detailed organization had not yet taken shape.[36] Western medicine, on the other hand, had introduced epidemic prevention and health measures into the daily life of the general public through laws, regulations and school education. However, TCM measures were rarely introduced and studied. Of course, they were also excluded from the education system, and the overall development was slow. According to a method published in the municipal communique of Qingdao, Shandong Province in 1935, if TCM practitioners encountered infectious diseases, they must fill in weekly reports of infectious diseases. Although the specific implementation seems to have no assessment items, it can be seen that TCM had been

---

[33] Tian Erkang, TCM Enumerates Its Strengths and Corrects Its Weaknesses in the Diagnosis and Treatment of Acute Infectious Diseases, *Medical Journal,* 69 (1933), p. 5.

[34] Hong Guanzhi, Proposals to the Education Authorities and the TCM Education Enthusiasts for the Prerequisite of TCM Education, *New TCM,*1947, New Issue (1), p. 2.

[35] Yu Yunxiu, Preface to the "Interpretation to the Ancient Disease Names", *Interpretation to the Ancient Disease Names*, Beijing: People's Health Publishing House, 1953, pp. 1–6.

[36] Unknown Author, On the Founding of National Infectious Disease Hospital by Peking Medical Association, *Guanghua Medical Journal*, Vol. 2, 1934 (01), p. 93.

included in the prevention and treatment system of infectious diseases.[37] However, TCM did not have its own epidemic prevention laws.

As far back as 1932, Lu Yuanlei wrote *The Draft Outline of the Academic Standards for Chinese Medicine Organized by the National Medical Center*, and planned the basic discipline of "hygiene" in the outline of the subject division: "This discipline can give full play to the essence of China's inherent hygiene. The hygiene and epidemic prevention laws of modern times are also attached here".[38] It intends to sort out the existing hygiene and epidemic prevention technologies. Then, in 1936, the special health committee of the local autonomous planning committee under the Central Executive Committee of the Nationalist Party began to draw up a health facility plan, including public health, disease prevention management training and the publication of various special prescriptions, and urged the Chinese medicine community to offer ideas and suggestions, so that a plan could be made and circulated throughout the country. The National Medical Center also ordered the Chinese Medicine Associations in various provinces to "promptly collect plans on Chinese medicine health facilities" and send them to the TCM Centre for reorganization, before submitting them to the central government.[39] This was a good opportunity for TCM to collate the knowledge of epidemic prevention. Unfortunately, the Sino Japanese war broke out and the plan was stalled. In April of that year, Disease Prevention Laws in *TCM Hygien Implementation Draft* compiled by the Tianjin Chinese Medicine Association came out, in response to the solicitation of the National Medical Center. Rules are laid down as follows:

> The living room, courtyard, kitchen and toilet should be clean and dry. Dampness and filth bring about the pathogenic Qi that would lead to disease. Get up early in the morning, open the doors and windows of the house, clean up and release the turbid air accumulated at night, and then close the doors and windows tightly to prevent the invasion of pathogenic air such as miasma, fog and haze. Following the above advice, epidemic diseases can be avoided. When spring comes, it is advisable to burn anti epidemic herb in the house, put it close to the nose and do it daily to avoid epidemic disease. That is, when epidemic disease is prevalent, this method is used to avoid infection. Keep all rooms, as well as clothes, at the proper temperature in order to avoid typhoid and cold. Food should be simple and light with less fat, so as to avoid the toxin of sores. Take less tobacco and alcohol, so as to avoid blood consumption and lung damage. Opium and morphine should be particularly forbidden as they can damage the brain and absorb the marrow. Cultivating the spirit with less desire is the way to avoid tuberculosis, prostitution and sexual diseases.[40]

---

[37] Unknown Author, Guidance for Qingdao Hospital Practitioners and Chinese Medical Practitioners to Fill in the Weekly Report Form of Infectious Diseases, *Municipal Bulletin of Qingdao Municipal Government*, 1935 (68), pp. 11–12.

[38] Lu Yuanlei, Declaration upon Abolishing Classic Medicine in the Central Health Conference, Lu's Collection of Medical Theories, included in Zhang Yuping (ed.), *Two Kinds of Lu Yuanlei's Medical Books,* p. 156.

[39] Jiao Yitang, Instruction No. 3973 of National Medical Center, *Chinese Medical Literature*, Vol. 1, 1936 (02), p. 9.

[40] Tianjin Association of TCM, Health Facility Plan of TCM, *Authentic National Medicine*, 1936 (24), p. 38.

These TCM "health" methods were very extensive and not entirely aimed at infectious diseases. They should be regarded as a universal health and disease prevention method. The intention of the National Medical Center was to collect prescriptions, in addition to explain the popular disease prevention methods. Unfortunately, the time frame for the collection was limited and the results were not very effective.

By 1937, pestis was prevalent in Southern Fujian. Although the local government sent personnel to treat it, all the staff in the epidemic prevention center were Western medicine doctors, which was a shame toward Chinese medicine. Wu Quji said that TCM doctors should venture to go right into the epidemic area and face the lower class to carry out epidemic prevention work. However, TCM doctors were neither organized nor willing to enter the epidemic area.[41] In the summer and autumn of 1940, after the outbreak of the Sino Japanese War, enemy-occupied areas in all provinces reported cholera and typhoid epidemics. *New Voice of Chinese Medicine* published an article of introspection, elucidating that Western medicine had thoroughly studied the knowledge of epidemic prevention, but Chinese medicine had no special books on epidemic prevention and barely had any academic research. When the epidemic was prevalent, it was often helpless. The article clarifies that the knowledge of epidemic prevention is only a small part of bacteriology or hygiene, and it only needs two or three hours of training every day to deal with emergencies. He also criticized many Chinese medicine practitioners at that time for not even knowing the "disinfection method". If they really wanted to talk about preserving the quintessence of TCM, national medical education must keep up with times and abandon the conservative mentality of "using oil lamps or riding on unicycles".[42] After the outbreak of the Sino Japanese War, the Sichuan Branch of the National Medical Centre published the *Publicity Outline for the TCM Prevention and Treatment of Epidemic Diseases*, particularly publicizing the epidemic prevention methods with public credibility, and declaring that the treatment and experience of TCM have been handed down from generation to generation, "it is duty bound to guide the prevention and preparation of treatment", and calling on all medical branches and benevolent people to purchase and distribute the medicine.[43] Although it had successively posted the Publicity Outline for Prevention and Treatment of Epidemic Diseases, introducing many therapies, it is obvious that "treatment" was emphasized and "prevention" was neglected.[44] After the Sino Japanese war, TCM epidemic prevention was even worse. Most local health institutions were mainly based on Western medicine, and only when there was a shortage of manpower did they issue an announcement, calling for the joint efforts of the Chinese and Western doctors in organizing clinics, instead of taking Chinese

---

[41] Wu Quji, TCM and Epidemic Prevention, *Shenzhou National Medical Journal*, Vol. 5, 1937 (09), pp. 3–5.

[42] Zhuang Xuren, On the Necessity of Supplementing Epidemic Prevention Knowledge in TCM, *New Voice of Chinese Medicine*, 1940 (11), pp. 1–3.

[43] Cao Shushi, Liu Zishen & Kuang Hexiao, Instruction of Sichuan Branch of National Medical Center: Publicity Outline of TCM Prevention and Treatment of Epidemic Cholera, *Medical Improvement Monthly*, Vol. 1, 1941 (06), p. 16.

[44] Unknown Author, Publicity Outline of TCM Prevention and Treatment of Epidemic Cholera, Origin and Treatment of Dysentery, *Medical Improvement Monthly*, Vol. 1, 1941 (07), p. 18.

medicine into consideration in the initial stage when the local medical system was established. At that time, there was also a civil war between the Nationalist Party and the Communist Party, during which the Chinese medicine community had no specific vision in this regard.[45]

8.3 Cases in Taiyuan, Shanxi Province

After reviewing the reflection and dilemma of Chinese medicine during the Republic of China period on epidemic prevention, some examples were cited to illustrate the collective research on epidemic prevention in Chinese medical circle at that time. From August 1917 to the beginning of 1918, a serious pulmonary pestis broke out in Shanxi Province. From the spring of 1918 to 1919, an influenza[46] broke out. But the situation in Shanxi Province seemed to have been properly handled.[47] Although the government led by Yan Xishan then was successful in the prevention of infectious diseases, and its prevention methods undoubtedly focused on Western medicine. The official report even criticized the prescriptions of Chinese medicine as "useless".[48] However, when the pestis was in full swing in 1918, the official gazette recorded that some people in the Shanyin area recovered after taking the Chinese medicine prescribed and Lightning Powder was certified by the government. The report of the Wanguo Pestis Research Society of the three northeastern provinces indicated that there was no treatment for the disease, but this case makes people wonder what the role of TCM was? In fact, there was a so-called Committee of Chinese and Western Doctors in Shanxi, which provided effective prescriptions for Chinese and Western medicine that were the medicines provided just by Chinese medicine.[49]

Although the epidemic was put out by the cooperation of Chinese and Western doctors, it is obvious that Western medicine was still the main focus, and Chinese medicine was distributing Chinese drugs. There is no further evidence that Chinese and Western medicine had good communication or close cooperation.[50] Even without direct evidence, TCM did contribute to epidemic prevention. Yan Xishan was famous for supporting TCM development. In April 1919, when the well-known Chinese medicine group "Shanxi Chinese Medicine Improvement Research Association" was

---

[45] Unknown Author, No. 3 (3–1), *A Case of Improving Health Facilities and Strengthening Medical Efficiency--Requesting Health Center to Improve Their Institutions by Hiring More TCM Doctors to Assist in Diagnosis and Treatment*, Nanhui County Administration, Vol. 1, 1947 (01), p. 12.

[46] Pi Kuoli, Epidemic Diseases and Social Responses during the Republic of China Period—A Regional Comparative Study of the 1918 Pandemic in Beijing, Tianjin, Shanghai and Shaoxing, *New Historiography* 27.4 (2016), pp. 57–107.

[47] Cao Shuji, Public Health of the Nation and the Regions—A Case Study of 1918 Shanxi Epidemic, *Chinese Social Science,* 2006 (1), pp. 178–190.

[48] Wang Chengji (ed.), *Shanxi Epidemic Report*, Vol. 1, Taiyuan: Dalin Zhainan Paper Villiage, Shanghai: Zhonghua Book Company, 1919, pp. 145–156.

[49] Unknown Author, Telegragh of Yan Xishan from Taiyuan, *Official Gazette,* 1918 (726), p. 22.

[50] Wang Chengji (ed.), *Shanxi Epidemic Report*, Vol. 3, p. 13.

established in Taiyuan during the Republic of China period, Yan served as its president and led its fund-raising. Before the Sino Japanese War, the society was known as one of the best medical organizations in China, and the development fund could even support the textile industry and railway construction.[51] The research society even set up a medical training institute (a special school was established in 1921) and founded the *Medical Journal* in 1921, which played a pivotal role in the history of modern Chinese medicine. Unfortunately, it was suspended due to the outbreak of the Sino Japanese War in October 1937.[52]

During the Republic of China period, there were many epidemics in Shanxi Province. In 1922, the epidemic broke out again. The symptoms involved dizziness, abdominal pain, vomiting, swollen throat, sudden cold and sudden heat. Shanxi Chinese Medicine Improvement Research Association had to hold a meeting to work on the prevention and treatment methods to guide the public. When ancient Chinese medicine faced the epidemic, its interpretation would have been different according to different schools and regions. Since the early Republic of China period, the names of epidemics have been influenced by Western medicine, and there must be a definite and unified statement. It was not easy for Chinese medicine to propose unified prevention and treatment methods. It had to be discussed and decided at a meeting. This was also the dilemma of Chinese medicine in proposing the Epidemic Prevention Laws.[53] In 1924, pestis broke out in Linxian County. The *Medical Journal* published many treatment and prevention methods of Chinese and Western medicine. These preventive measures were jointly formulated by the association and Western medical practitioners. The actual outbreak of infectious diseases was also an opportunity for Chinese medicine to absorb Western medicine. It can be seen from the prevention methods published in the journal that Chinese and Western medicine were connected, and the isolation, burial, disinfection and other methods of Western medicine were widely known. In terms of the disinfection theory, TCM believed that fumigating and cleaning patients' houses with sulfur and atractylodes had the same effect as sprinkling lime water and lysol water to clean the ground as used by Western medicine. There are many kinds of epidemics, but for specific infectious diseases, Chinese medicine sometimes uses the preventive medicine "before their arrival". For example, for the pestis, someone who took "yellow earth epidemic dissolve decoction" for epidemic prevention said: "During the epidemic time, though not infected, I was feeling unwell, such as dizziness, fatigue, and lack of appetite, which was the omen of the onset of the disease. Taking one to three doses of the above medicine as soon as possible, and the various symptoms can be eliminated".[54] This is considered a preventive drug. TCM believes that the timing of taking medicine for prevention

[51] For details of the operation of the association, see Unknown Author, *The Contribution of Shanxi TCM Research Association, Chinese Medicine Bulletin*, Vol.2, 1935 (09), pp. 80–84.

[52] Deng Tietao, Cheng Zhifan (ed.), *General History of Chinese Medicine Modern History*, pp. 258–259.

[53] Unknown Author, A Study of Chinese Medicine Association on Epidemic Prevention Law, *Laifu*,1922 (228), p. 13.

[54] Unknown Author, Treatment: TCM Treatment, *Medical Journal*, 1924 (22), p. 76.

lies in the showing up of "slight symptoms", which can be regarded as preliminary "treatment". Its significance is different from that of Western medicine.

In the same year, epidemics were found in Xiejiagou village and other places in Shanxi Province. The Chinese Medicine Improvement Research Association in Taiyuan attributed it to the weather. "That summer, the hot and dry air was too intense". The patients all had the same symptoms, but it was impossible to determine what the disease was. TCM thought that it might be any one of meningitis, smallpox, pestis and cholera, and proposed the treatment methods of various diseases and some popular prevention methods. The general prevention methods of Western medicine were also elaborated during the improvement meeting; TCM suggested taking anti-epidemic pills and anti-epidemic balls in advance, and called for taking them as carry-ons, but the ingredients were not specified. "Purple Gold Tablet" was recommended whenever one felt discomfort. The report indicates that there were many preventive methods of Chinese medicine, and TCM doctors had also gone to various places to give their treatments.[55] This shows that TCM was still unable to establish the name of a disease at the outbreak of the epidemic. Most of the epidemic prevention methods they proposed were universal and popularized, rather than just targeting on one epidemic disease.

In 1928, another epidemic broke out in Shanxi Province. After investigating the epidemic situation, the local Chinese Medicine Improvement Research Association put forward the "Law on Preventing Epidemic Infectious Diseases" of Chinese medicine, which includes: cleaning streets and lanes, and instructing local police and street cleaners to carry out inspections. In terms of living, frequent cleaning of the environment was common, which indicates that western-style public health methods were accepted and western medical technology was adopted by TCM to prevent diseases. This was not the case in 1918, when TCM strove to promote TCM style techniques in treating epidemic diseases in organized groups. TCM style techniques include throwing into a water jar a piece of cyrtomium, a little raw alum and a handful of black beans, and changing them once every two or three days; rhubarb, realgar, atractylodes, mugwort leaves and other medicines should be burned indoors. They were to be burned slowly with smoke for disinfection and epidemic prevention. In terms of food and drink, people normally should "control all food and drink", "abstain from addictions" and "stay away from cold, heat and storms". In terms of medicine, it is advisable to grind "anti epidemic pills, red beans, euonymus, versipoellis, realgar and four compos" into powder and divide it into equal shares, making them into honey pills as big as small beans and stored them in porcelain bottles. Taking one per day would prevent the infection. There were other Chinese medicines such as Anti Epidemic Pill, Peace Powder, Miracle Cholera Medicine, Pass Powder and Wish Pill and Western medicines referred to as Anti Epidemic Balls and carbolic acid water.

[55] Unknown Author, Report Gate: Prevention and Treatment of Epidemic Diseases in Linxian County (letter): According to the Telegram of Linxian County, Epidemics Were Found in Xiejiagou and Other Villages in the County, *Medical Journal*, 1924 (22), pp. 68–69.

"There were many effective medicines that were distributed and made great contributions".[56] These medicines are mainly Chinese medicine, and most of them can be found in various prescriptions. Of course, there are also a few Western medicines, but it is not clear what the "Anti Epidemic Balls" were made of. In addition, the Chinese Medicine Research Association adopted Western medicine for the prevention and treatment of the disease, such as the use of odorant and lime for disinfection, the use of sulfur for fumigation of utensils, and some quarantine methods. There was no conflict between Chinese and Western medicine.[57]

Shanxi Chinese Medicine Improvement Research Association had made great contributions to the research and development in local TCM. Shi Yiren was the most meritorious. Shi was originally from Wuxi. In 1912, he studied medicine with Wang Yungong, a fellow townsman. In 1916, he officially started practicing medicine. He never stopped writing and studying medicine when he started his business. His articles were published in the *Journal of Shaoxing Medicine, Yuyao Health Bulletin, Hangzhou Sansan Medical Journal, Nanjing Medical and Health Journal* and other publications. As an author of a lot of technical papers and books, he was admired by the medical community for being "enthusiastic in medical research with persistence, and made amazing achievements". In 1928, he established the "Jiangzuo National Medical Institute" in Shanghai. In 1929, he published *The Problems of Chinese Medical Construction* and was employed as a teacher at the Shanghai Special School of TCM and China Medical College. In the same year, he went to Shanxi, where he served as the executive director and editorial director of Shanxi Chinese Medicine Improvement Research Association, and also the editor of *Medical Journal* for about 10 years. In addition, he was a professor at a medical school and a hospital doctor. He wrote books on seasonal diseases, infectious diseases, gynecology, pathology, prescriptions and examination of prescriptions. He also served as a member of the Shanxi Provincial Health Committee, the director of the Shanxi National Medical Branch, a member of the Taiyuan Medical Examination Committee, the chairman of the Taiyuan Chinese Medicine Association, and the director at the National Medical Center, director of the Implementation Department, full-time member and editorial member of the Chinese Medical Sorting Committee, member of the standing committee in the Chinese Medicine Committee of the Department of Health, and director of the Chinese Medical Education Society.[58] After the outbreak of the Sino Japanese War, Shi immediately left Shanxi to seek refuge in Hankou. After meeting with Jiao Yitang, he planned to put the School of TCM on file. In 1938, he moved to Wanxian county and lived in the residence of Li Chongren, a TCM doctor friend, for a short period. Later, he arrived in Chongqing and worked in the Chinese Medicine Committee of the Department of Health. He also joined the Chinese Medicine Relief

---

[56] Unknown Author, Shanxi Provincial Government's Express Mail Attachment: A Study of Shanxi Chinese Medicine Improvement Research Association on the Prevention Law for Epidemic Diseases, *Shanxi Provincial Political Bulletin*, 1928 (05), pp. 19–20.

[57] Unknown Author, Shanxi Provincial Government's Express Mail Attachment: A Study of Shanxi Chinese Medicine Improvement Research Association on the Prevention Law for Epidemic Diseases, *Medical Journal*, 1928 (45), pp. 85.

[58] Zhang Zanchen, A Brief Biography of President Shi, *Fuxing TCM*, Vol. 1, 1940 (01), p. 10.

Hospital attached to the Relief Committee and a member of the Medical Research Committee. Shi was the director of the China Medical Education Society. He was also a member of the Chinese Medical Textbook Compilation Committee attached to the Society, as well as a doctor of Chongqing National Hospital. Shi said that his career ambition was to "collate Chinese medicine and seek the independence of Chinese medicine". Shi was very knowledgeable about TCM reforms and believed that "sorting out theories and improving technology" was the most important goal of Chinese medicine then. If the Chinese medicine sector did not steady itself, the Western medicine would take over the responsibility of "reforming Chinese medicine". The time then was the most important transitional period of TCM. If they did not grasp it in a timely fashion, they would lose the opportunity of reform.[59]

The author believes that the development of medicine in various places has its own characteristics as China is a large country. Some local organizations need to come forward to sort out the academic work, but can not rely on the National Medical Center alone. There are numerous medical books from the past, and it is difficult to see the effect of academic collation only by relying on an immature organization that was still at its initial stage. Before the Sino Japanese War, the Shanxi Chinese Medicine Improvement Research Association had already collected medical books and prescriptions, sent members to various counties to pay on-the-spot visits, which were followed by the research and reviews. When infectious diseases were prevalent, it printed and distributed special publications to people from all walks of life for popularization.[60] However, Shi Yiren, who was idealistic, complained that there was nothing to do in Sichuan. In an exclusive interview, he criticized that TCM in Sichuan went up and down with the market. A lot of publicity was made for individual business, pursuing more profit than ideals. After Shi left Chongqing, the business of these people had a considerable increase. In other words, what they were following was nothing but the money. The "improvement of TCM" was just a cover signboard set up for business. Shi felt that this was shameful, and he did not want the nominal allowance provided without doing anything. It can be seen that those in charge of TCM in Sichuan did not seem to be serious in sorting out TCM.[61] In the autumn of 1939, Shi left Sichuan for Shanghai and founded the Fuxing TCM Magazine to carry out the idea of sorting out Chinese medicine. He founded Fuxing TCM College, and served as Provost (1940) and President (1941).[62] He was also a professor of Shanghai College of TCM, Chinese Medical College, New China Medical College and other schools.

In his early years, Shi had a lot of experiences in the treatment and prevention of infectious diseases.[63] In the process of editing the magazine, he also constantly paid

---

[59] Shi Yiren, A Few Words to the Graduates, *Fuxing TCM*. Vol. 1, 1940 (03), p. 1.

[60] Unknown Author, The Manuscript of Shanxi TCM Research Association, *Chinese Medicine Bulletin*,Vol.2, 1935 (09), p. 84.

[61] Yu Shenchu, Mr. Shi Yiren's Visit to Shanghai, *Fuxing TCM*. Vol. 2, 1940 (01), pp. 40–41.

[62] Unknown Author, Cover Photo, *Fuxing TCM*. Vol. 2, 1940 (06), p. 3.

[63] Shi Yiren, Advice for the Spread of Epidemic Diseases in Yizheng, *Shaoxing Medical Journal*, Vol. 9, 1919 (04), pp. 57–63.

attention to analyzing the outbreak of the epidemic, which helped him in his diagnosis and treatment of infectious diseases.[64] In 1933, he summarized his experience in the prevention and treatment of infectious diseases and wrote *Chinese Acute Infectious Diseases*, which was published and distributed by the Shanxi Chinese Medicine Improvement Research Association, with his careful revisions. Shi Yiren said that the book "can be used as a preparation for Chinese medicine to recover its sovereignty over the prevention and treatment of epidemic syndrome".[65] When discussing the prevention methods of pestis, he not only learned the experience of pestis prevention in modern times, but also learned the disinfection and isolation methods of Western medicine. The TCM prevention methods were mainly drug prevention. He listed dozens of prescriptions such as "eliminating filth and expelling drug addiction", "Fragrance Anti-epidemic Decoction" and "Antidote Panacea". Generally, the prescriptions in the medical books of the past were collected and the source was indicated, but they were still mainly based on treatment. Among them, the aromatic decontamination methods recorded in the "Mr. Xu Xiangren's medication of epidemic diseases" include "Zhuge Marching Powder" and "Eight-treasure Red Panacea", Shi added: "Although there are different views on the causes of the epidemic, it's mostly due to filth. In order to prevent epidemic disease, cleaning is more important, and the most appropriate medicine is fragrant agent. It is not difficult to eliminate filth immediately if it is implemented at the first place. So this prescription can be mainly used in the early stage of the disease, together with those such as clearing heat, promoting blood stasis, relieving constipation, and inducing resuscitation".[66]

The relationship between fragrance and cleanliness is an important thought of modern Chinese medicine epidemic prevention. As far as the daily prevention method is concerned, Shi Yiren did not talk about the content of epidemic prevention in TCM. Instead, they adopted the methods of Western medicine, including disinfection and isolation. TCM mainly focuses on the method of treatment, but many TCM practitioners, including Shi Yiren, misappropriated some concepts of treatment when discussing "prevention" to establish the TCM prevention discourse. For typhoid fever, Shi Yiren explained under the item "Antidote Magic Pill": "It is ranked at the top of the list of secret therapies, specially used to treat all kinds of toxins, deadly bacteria, toxins of cattle, horses, puffer fish, all kinds of epidemics diseases and mountain haze miasma". It is a "top medicine for sterilization" and was originally from Xu Huixi's prescription. The original annotation says that it can treat "deadly epidemic bacteria". Shi believed that the pathogenic bacteria refers to the toxic bacteria of Western medicine, and they are called bacteria because they are tiny. Therefore, Shi's inference is that as long as the disease is caused by bacteria, they should be treated in the

[64] Shi Yiren, Lun Shumen: The Course of Gengshen Epidemic, *Medical Journal*, 1922(08), pp. 20–21.

[65] Shi Yiren, *Chinese Acute Infectious Diseases*, Vol. 1, p. 18.

[66] Shi Yiren, *Chinese Acute Infectious Diseases*, Vol. 1, pp. 26–36. The medicine consists of realgar essence, mountain arrowhead mushroom, Sichuan meretrix, golden frost, red bud euphorbia, musk incense, and cinnabar.

same way.[67] Not only for treatment, the drugs transformed by Shi into "bactericidal" drugs became the basis for TCM to interpret "epidemic prevention" drugs. This is a remarkable example of the transformation of modern Chinese medicine into Western medicine terms.

8.4 Epidemic Prevention Drugs—Transformation of Disinfection and Sterilization Discourse

How should the Chinese medicine community respond to the sophisticated and progressive methods of Western medicine for epidemic prevention? In the late Qing Dynasty, Chen Qiu described the simple Chinese epidemic prevention methods: "The ditches and canals should be cleaned, the clothes should be starched, the springs should be drawn early and drained with sand, the fish and vegetables should not be kept for a long time, and better be kept in ice. The big houses should have more windows open, and the small ones should have a vent. The most important thing is to apply fine charcoal scraps to the dirty places in the toilets to keep away the filth". "A good meal should be followed by a cup of wine for preservation, which would enhance one's vitality, as if there is a general guarding the pass and all pathogenic spirits will retreat". On the whole, it includes several key points: cleaning, ventilation, fresh food, sufficient vitality and so on.[68] Although many Western-style epidemic prevention laws had been adopted, there were some differences in practice. In 1935, Huang Guocai, a Chinese medicine practitioner, reviewed the methods of TCM in preventing infectious diseases as follows:

(1) Maintain health: the most important thing is to preserve energy, control diet, and prevent colds, doing nothing against the nature of human body. Good immunity would protect the body from virus. (2) Strict cleaning: lime shall be sprinkled into all ditches and toilets to eliminate the source of mosquitoes and flies. Buy more pyrethrum to kill bedbugs, fleas, lice, mosquitoes, gnats, and rodents to eliminate the vectors of infection. The patient's bedroom should be fumigated with sulfur and closed for a long time. All the instruments and clothes used by the patients should be washed with boiling water to avoid infection. (3) The Infectious Disease Receptions and Treatment Centers shall be set up. Patients suspected of having infectious diseases shall be sent to the agencies for treatment to avoid infecting their family. Diseases such as measles, small pox, scarlet fever and diphtheria are all transmitted by air, which is introduced by breathing. If the patient is not strictly quarantined, infection is inevitable. This is the lesson learned from the past. Infections such as dysentery, cholera, intestinal zhifus are

[67] Shi Yiren, *Chinese Acute Infectious Diseases*, Vol. 1, pp. 123–124.

[68] Chen Qiu, et al.(eds.), Collection of Liji Medicine Questions and Answer about Epidemics and Cholera, included in Liu Shijue (ed.), *Wenzhou Literature Series Integration of Wenzhou Modern Medical Books*, p. 72.

mostly infected through the mouth. All food must be well cooked. The fruits on display in the market are not edible.[69]

On the whole, they have accepted the methods of Western medicine for epidemic prevention. Zhang Zhaolin, a TCM practitioner who published an article in the same journal, pointed out that "there are incurable diseases in the world, but there is no disease that is unpreventable. The ancients taught people to be prepared and to treat diseases before they got sick at work. This is not the way to enlighten people to prevent diseases". He believed that in the past, TCM lacked the research on disease prevention, and there were no special books. Most of them were oral legends or a few comments in the books. They were probably nothing more than "regulating living style, balancing work and rest, controlling diet, prohibiting alcohol and lust, adjusting temperature and taking tonic".[70] Although these appeals are necessary for health preservers, they are not the whole picture of modern hygiene after all. If doctors do not convey their knowledge, most of the patients would not know how to carry it out, and they would be nothing but empty talks. Tian Erkang, a TCM practitioner, believed that Chinese medicine does not lag behind Western medicine in the treatment of epidemic diseases, but Western medicine surpasses Chinese medicine in the prevention of epidemic diseases. "Aimless disinfection" and "unprepared prevention method" are the two major deficiencies of TCM, and even caused the infection and death of TCM doctors when treating infected patients.[71] At a critical juncture of competition between Chinese and Western medicine, Chinese medicine can no longer be as passive as it used to be. It is necessary to study ways to prevent infectious diseases. He said: "TCM has neither specialized knowledge nor knowledge about infection prevention. In clinical treatment, it is called cold, or catching cold. In addition to the prescription, there is the strict rule of shutting down the entry and exit, and the patient's natural recovery is completely cut off. The patient obeys the doctor's order, so the windows and room are closed, the air is blocked, the light is dim, the spitting is all over the floor, the feces and urine are messy, the humidity is steaming, and the filth is accumulated. The room is filled with the stimulation of amonia. The patient's fragile body is fumigated with the air of filth and toxins. Death might be a better choice." He criticized TCM for its disease resistance methods in the past, but the improvement strategies he proposed are basically the same as those by Huang Guocai. For example, keeping the environment and individuals clean, keeping the windows open for ventilation, keeping the food clean, do not eat together, and using lime to disinfect the unclean places and rooms. These measures were mostly from the knowledge of Western medicine.[72] It is said in *Compilation of Epidemic Diseases*: "With light diet, less desire, dredging the ditches, cleaning up the filth,

---

[69] Huang Guocai, Methods and Agents of TCM in Preventing Infectious Diseases, *Medical Journal*, 1935(86), p. 23.

[70] Methods and Agents of TCM in Preventing Infectious Diseases, *Medical Journal*, 1935(86), 23.

[71] Tian Erkang, TCM Enumerates Its Strengths and Corrects Its Weaknesses in the Diagnosis and Treatment of Acute Infectious Diseases, *Medical Journal*, 1935(86), pp. 4–5.

[72] Zhang Zhaolin, Methods and Agents of TCM in Preventing Infectious Diseases, *Medical Journal*, 1935(86), p. 24.

staying away from the hot spots, walking in the dense forests and bamboos, so as to prevent the epidemic before it happens. It is something everyone can do, and it is also an indispensable part of health".[73] To some extent, western knowledge of epidemic prevention have been learned. Other mental and psychological disease prevention methods are not to be elaborated here as it is focused on medicine prevention. From the general Chinese and Western medicine epidemic prevention publications, we can see the statements of similar knowledge such as cleaning, sanitation and isolation. However, in the newspapers and periodicals of Western medicine, it is very rare to introduce TCM methods. On the contrary, TCM has absorbed a lot of epidemic prevention knowledge of Western medicine. According to the *Medical Journal* of Shanxi Province, in addition to introducing the Western hygiene laws, it also introduced the knowledge of relevant vaccines.[74] During the time of the Republic of China period, the basic vaccinations of Western medicine had gradually gained the trust of the public. Take the summer typhoid vaccine injection in June 1936 as an example, about 7,786 people received the injection. It is reported that none of these people contracted typhoid fever. It can be seen that the vaccine injection for disease prevention was reliable.[75] Although Western medicine is not the core of this chapter, Western medicine did have internal epidemic medicine in the early Republic of China period. The "Edo Vaccins" published in the magazine in 1928 claimed that there were bacteria in the bottle, and there were four kinds of tablets to prevent cholera, typhoid, dysentery and pestis separately. They were taken before the occurrence of the epidemic, and the side effects were very small. They could be immunized for seven days.[76] Similar drugs were mainly antibacterial, such as "Panflavin" tablets, which was supposed to inhibit the growth of bacteria when being held in the mouth and throat, and could also prevent scarlet fever, bacilli infection, meningitis, erysipelas and pneumonia.[77] So, what was the preventive medicine of TCM?

As early as the late Qing Dynasty (1616–1911), *Questions and Answers about Epidemics and Cholera* compiled by Chen Qiu explained that peach leaves, pomegranate peel, purslane, Sichuan pepper, sophora flavescens, xiaolan, pangolin, otter meat, earthworm, mercury, realgar were all ancient insecticides, which could actually "sterilize bacteria" (they were called "micro insects" then), and there were also various similar drugs available in the past.[78] In February 1911, during the pestis in the three northeastern provinces, the official newspaper published the TCM prescriptions for public use and listed them in the column of the *Infectious Disease Prevention Law*. At that time, people in Dongguang County, Hebei Province presented an

---

[73] Zhou Yuxi (ed.), *Compilation of Epidemic Diseases*, p. 12.

[74] Unknown Author, Report Gate: Notice of the Central Epidemic Prevention Office on Prevention of Spring Epidemics, *Medical Journal*, 1924 (22), pp. 68–69.

[75] Shanghai Shen Bao Newspaper Office (ed.), *Shen Bao*, July 22, 1936, p. 4.

[76] Chen Peiji, Internal Medicine Vaccine for Epidemic Prevention, *Guangji Medical Journal*, Vol. 5, 1928 (07), pp. 11–12.

[77] Unknown Author, Prevention of Infection, *Family Annual Journal*, 1943 (01), pp. 221–223.

[78] Chen Qiu, et al.(eds.), Collection of Liji Medicine Q & A to Epidemics and Cholera, included in Liu Shijue (ed.), *Wenzhou Literature Series Integration of Wenzhou Modern Medical Books*, pp. 66–67.

prescription, saying that it was effective in their county, and *Beiyang Official Paper* had it published.

The original prescription Anti Epidemic Pill was tooth soap (10.85g), cinnabar (7.75g), realgar (7.75g), asarum (10.85g), costus root (6.3g), dried tangerine peel (6.3g), ageratum (3.1g), platycodon grandiflorum (6.3g), mint (6.3g), cyrtomium fortunei (6.3g), saposhnikovia divaricata (6.3g), pinellia ternata (6.3g), alum (7.85g), angelica dahurica (3.1g), and raw liquorice (6.3g). Grind them into fine powder and put into a bottle, which can be used to cure various acute diseases. The disease is presented with scattered pulse, clenched teeth, numb hands and feet, closed eyes, swollen throat and heartaches. Without knowing the causes, many doctors mistook it as laryngeal obstruction, which would definitely lead to the patients' death with their treatment. This syndrome is called cinnabar syndrome, also known as heart channel boil. Get 0.9g of the powder, blow it into the nose, and then take it with ginger soup. After that, use red paper to twist the front and rear heart pits. If you see red spots, you can puncture them with a needle and pick out the red tendons, which can ensure recovery.[79]

Upon the author's investigation, this prescription has a big problem. What broke out in that year was pestis, but this prescription was originally used to treat traditional "scarlet fever",[80] which does not share the symptoms of pestis at all. This kind of prescription for preventing and controlling epidemic diseases was not examined and approved by professionals before it was published, but it was quite popular in the early Republic of China period. It can at most treat cholera, acute gastroenteritis and heatstroke in the modern medical sense. However, people seemed to regard it as a panacea for epidemic prevention.[81] The government even offered it to the public as an epidemic prevention medicine.[82] In 1934, the Pinghan Railway Bureau issued "anti epidemic summer medicine" to its employees in summer. It is stated in the report that most of the drugs were ordered by the Drug Procurement Committee of the Bureau, apparently through legal and open channels. Each employee got a pack of "Rendan Pill" and two bottles of "Sha Medicine", which are traditional "Sha medicine" and often used as "anti epidemic medicine".[83] Some local agencies even asked people to take such drugs while getting vaccinated.[84]

Various TCM anti-epidemic prescriptions were spread through the mass media, such as newspapers and periodicals. For example, in 1924, *The Pursuit of Good Magazine* published the "Immortal Anti Epidemic Tea Prescription", which is

---

[79] Unknown Author, Governor Chen Zha's Issuing of Infectious Disease Prevention Methods and the Prescriptions, *Beiyang Official Journal*, 1911 (2692), pp. 6–7.

[80] Zhu Pingyi, Sha in the Qing Dynasty: the Birth of A Disease Category, *Sinological Research* 31.3 (2013), pp. 193–238.

[81] Pi Kuoli, Discourse of Chinese and Western Medicine and Modern Business Discussion: from the Example of "Sha Potion" in Shen Bao, *Shanghai Academic Monthly*, 2013 (1), pp. 149–164.

[82] Anonymous, Educational Affairs: Kuang Ji Report, *Xinghua*, 15, 1918 (21): 23.

[83] Unknown Author, Anti Epidemic Summer Medicine Purchased in Pinghan Road, *Railway Bulletin*, 1934 (906), p. 9.

[84] Shi Zhongyi, *The New Outlook of the Old Countryside*, Suzhou: Suzhou Chinese YMCA, 1933, p. 40.

composed of 34 drugs and it is said, "the immortal tea saves the world, taking instant effect", and it is "sent by good men with boundless virtue". This is by nature the same as the prescription from the folk donors. It can prevent epidemics, filth, cold or seasonal pathogenic factors, four unhealthy Qis, infection, fever, malaria, miasma, all kinds of dampness. It can be seen that most of those prescriptions have the effect of treating all kinds of common febrile infectious diseases.[85]The spread of these prescriptions also became a topic of discussion in TCM. For example, in 1920, the *Weekly Supplement of Shaoxing Medical Journal* published: "Acute diseases occur fast and are fatal. Any delay in going to the hospital or taking medicine would cause death... It is proposed that acute diseases be put into a special category in the future. Acute diseases can be marked on the prescriptions, with the word 'emergency' or a special stamp, in order to alert the pharmacies of the urgency and the priority of those prescriptions. For the scarce medicine, medical organizations should have it in storage when urgent needs arise. In this way, many lives can be saved if not all".[86]The drugstores should be knowledgeable of the emergency prescriptions so as to dispense the medicine quickly, which is to cope with the acute and fierce nature of infectious diseases. Some people also held that the prevention and treatment of epidemic diseases should be printed into leaflets or published in medical papers. This is the way "to prove that Chinese medicine in any era has the real value of being flexible and is able to meet the needs of the people".[87] In the past, most of the knowledge about epidemic prevention and control was scattered, so some TCM doctors proposed: "Special TCM books should be compiled and printed, so that all medical practitioners can have them as a guide".[88] It had become the consensus of some TCM doctors to compile their own special books on epidemic prevention and sort out the theories as the basis for the prevention and treatment of infectious diseases.

Shang Fuhan, a TCM doctor, believed that although there is no record of bacteria in Chinese medical books, most of the prescriptions for epidemic prevention and treatment have the functions of sterilization and detoxification. They should be gradually sorted out from the ancient books for further improvement and research, so that new drugs can be invented on the basis of tradition. In an article, he first took the "general epidemic prevention law" as an example, and compiled the Minor Golden Elixir prescription in *Basic Inquiries,* Tu Su Wine, Sui Dan Drink and Anti Febrile Disease in *Zhou Hou Prescriptions*, six prescriptions such as Epidemic Poltergeist Killing Pill, Ghost-evil-choking prescription and Realgar Pill in *Wings of the Thousand Gold Pieces Prescriptions*, Taiyi Holy Ice Pill and Taiyi Holy Pill in *Wings of the Thousand Gold Pieces Prescriptions*, Epidemic Cut-off Vermilion Pill in *The*

---

[85] Sun Weicai, Summary of Experiential Effective Prescriptions, *The Pursuit of Good Magazine*, 1924 (08), p. 42.

[86] Xiang Chen (Notice), Two Alerts to the National Medical Circles for Acute Epidemics, *Weekly Supplement of Shaoxing Medical Journal*, 1920 (22), p. 3.

[87] Zhou Yuxi (ed.), *Compilation of Epidemic Diseases*, p. 20.

[88] Huang Guocai, Methods and Agents of TCM in Preventing Infectious Diseases, *Medical Journal*, 1935(86), p. 25.

Secret Therapies of the Censors and Epidemic Prevention Therapy in the *Updated Compilation of Prescriptions*. He also said:

> All the above prescriptions are common anti epidemic agents for detoxification, sterilization and exorcism, and they are of great value. If there are different types of epidemic diseases, it is better to refer to the specific epidemic prevention prescriptions and drugs, and to select the simple and easy ones to use. With all the therapies treating epidemic diseases in the Jin, Yuan, Ming and Qing Dynasties, such as the Puji Disinfection Drink of Dongyuan, the Special Rhubarb of Yuan Boyan, the Original Drink of Ke Zhida, Ginseng Detoxification Powder of Yu Jiayan, my teacher used much gypsum, Pu Mingzi used much licorice, and Ye Tianshi tended to use a lot of Miraculous Bolus of Rhinoceros Horn Disinfection Drink, each having their own ways of treatment. Why should epidemic prevention be different? In addition, there are commonly used prescriptions from ancient to modern times, such as Marching Powder, Anti Epidemic Pill, Red Panacea, Wishful Pill, Peace Powder, Wolong Pill, Taiyi Yushu Pill and Taiyi Rescue Pill, Sha Panacea, Huoxiang Zhengqi Water, etc. Being the therapies for epidemics, they were also good for prevention.[89]

Shang Fuhan listed the prevention methods of various infectious diseases such as cold epidemic, natural pox, measles, diphtheria, scarlet fever, dysentery, pestis and Big Head Epidemics. It can be seen that TCM hoped to seek new prescriptions for epidemic prevention from ancient medical books. The prevention and treatment of epidemic diseases in TCM are often the same, but it is necessary to pay attention to the different types of epidemics and treat them according to each disease. The biggest difference between Chinese and Western medicine in epidemic prevention is that many Chinese medicines have the functions of prevention and treatment. They are "the heralds of an infected epidemic", that is, the symptoms before the epidemic, including cold back paralysis, dizziness, stuffiness, slight numbness of limbs, the irritation of five spots (heart, two arches and two palms–translator's note) and chest tightness, can be prevented with medicine. This is the idea of combining treatment and prevention.[90] Most of the anti-epidemic drugs mentioned by the Shang are generally for treatments, but regarding to all kinds of epidemics, can they really achieve the effect of prevention? This is the point many Chinese medicine practitioners questioned or examined. For example, Huang Guocai said:

> The ancient thin pox prescriptions and the anti-epidemic pills were all ineffective. The best medicine is no other than the imitation of cowpox, upon which the anti-epidemic serum was made and used as a vaccination, and it was effective.. The ancient anti epidemic methods, such as drinking Tusu wine and Jiaobai wine on New Year's day recorded in Chen Yanzhi's *Mini Prescriptions*, three or seven red beans and seven pockmarks hung in the well on New Year's day and the 15th of January recorded in *Five Elements,* taking black bean and white rice fluid, as well as purslane, abalone head ash, and cinnabar described in *Prescriptions of Master Mei*, etc.. The list of such ridiculous and useless methods is too long to be recorded in detail.[91]

Huang criticized that many methods of epidemic prevention in ancient times were ineffective. Zhang Zhaolin, a TCM practitioner, held the same position. He had the

---

[89] Shang Fuhan, Research on Epidemic Prevention of Chinese Medicine, *Chinese Medicine Bulletin*, Vol. 4, 1936 (01), pp. 31–35.

[90] Zhou Yuxi (ed.), *Compilation of Epidemic Diseases*, p. 32.

[91] Methods and Agents of TCM in Preventing Infectious Diseases, *Medical Journal*,1935(86), p. 23.

view that taking the elixir of epidemic prevention and carrying around the anti-epidemic powder were only temporary and backup measures, and they were mostly conservative.[92] Both of them openly expressed that the epidemic prevention methods which had not been tested and justified are doubtful. The author agrees on this point. How did people construct the "epidemic prevention" theory of these drugs at that time?

The theory of epidemic prevention in TCM was rooted in daily customs. Dong Lijuan pointed out in *The Mainstay of Chinese Medicine* that the earliest method of epidemic prevention in China was during the Dragon Boat Festival, "Mugwart is planted at every door. Men, women and children drink realgar wine during the Dragon Boat Festival. Realgar can kill bacteria and prevent summer diseases. Chemically, realgar is arsenic trioxide. Although arsenic trioxide is toxic, having a little of it can prevent diseases and can kill bacteria, which is significant to the human body. It is more meaningful than eating garlic. In addition, in climbing high on Double Nine Festival, there is a custom of having cornus wine, which is also a way to prevent disease. In this regard, the Chinese people have long had good methods in preventing epidemics, though they were not practical".[93] Dong believed that scientific research and popular traditional health customs should be taken into account, and only by combining science with tradition can we truly carry forward the quintessence of the nation. In terms of scientific interpretation, Dong has paid attention to the interpretation of chemistry and bacteriology, and the contemporaries have also played a role. When Zhou Yuxi introduced "cinnabar detoxification pill" in *Compilation of Epidemic Diseases*, he explained its prescription: "It (the pill) kills toxic bacteria and micro worms, preventing them from invading the mind and brain. Zhu Xiong is the special medicine for all emergency, just like Purple Gold Tablet, Marching Powder, Red Panacea, Treasure Panacea, which were repeatedly used. Allium macrostemon was the only therapy commended by Yuqian Hall, garlic is a common folk food, and peppermint can be extracted and frozen. It is a good medicine for modern health and daily use".[94] "Zhu Xiong" in the prescription refers to cinnabar and realgar, which are found in many modern epidemic prevention drugs. For example, *Three Chapters on the Integration of Chinese and Western Medicine in Infectious Diseases*, which advocates the integration of Chinese and Western medicine and uses science to verify the efficacy of TCM, quotes the *Zhou Hou Epidemic Prevention Prescriptions*: "Realgar is blown into the nostrils through water, or the red bean and sticky rice are soaked in a water tank, which are to be taken daily. Another drink is cyrtomium soaked in water. This is to prevent the disease from entering through the mouth and nose".[95] Most of the prevention methods adopted in this book are Western medicine

[92] Methods and Agents of TCM in Preventing Infectious Diseases, *Medical Journal*, 1935(86), p. 24.

[93] Dong Lijuan. Review of Epidemic Disease: (II) Prevention of Epidemic Disease, *Mainstay of Chinese Medicine*, Vol. 4, 1946 (10), p. 12.

[94] Zhou Yuxi (ed.), *Compilation of Epidemic Diseases*, pp. 17–18.

[95] Wang Zhizhou, *Three Chapters on the Integration of Chinese and Western Medicine in Infectious Diseases*, Tianjin: Institute of Chinese and Western Medicine, 1947, p. 18.

methods. TCM emphasizes more treatment than prevention. This is the only reference we can use, in addition to the data of realgar.

Shang Fuhan also mentioned the simple and convenient epidemic prevention method of Chinese medicine practitioners, for example, "when epidemics are prevalent, doctors must first eat a full meal, or drink a cup of realgar wine, or eat one or two cloves of garlic, or take a little Shaoxing liquor and preserved eggs before visiting a patient. No matter what kind of epidemic, they would not be infected. Author's note: satiety has the function of promoting metabolism, drinking has the function of stimulating nerves, realgar and garlic are also antibacterial products. It is a simple method of epidemic prevention. It would be perfect if the contact dis-infectious measures can be used at the same time". He also mentioned such details as the methods on guarding against epidemic diseases and preventing malaria in traveling.[96] Realgar, garlic, cinnabar and other drugs can also be found here. Shang believed that it can eliminate filth and bacteria, and also misappropriated the words of "sterilization". The introduction of other kinds of drugs is actually very similar. Zhou Yuxi pointed out in his *Compilation of Epidemic Diseases* that when the epidemic comes, it is urgent and severe. "It is appropriate to follow the maxim of the ancient sage not to cure the infected but to prevent people from being infected. The medicine of prevention can be of fresh and intense fragrant nature, to dispel the filth and detoxify". The author cited the "Fresh Fragrant Anti Epidemic Decoction" taken with Purple Gold Tablet. He explained: "When the epidemic is prevalent, the preventive treatment is to inhale the resuscitation and rescue pills to sneeze, swallow the epidemic prevention and rescue pills, check the pulse and scrape by oneself or prick the blood in serious cases. The worst thing is the pathogen of the epidemic is deeply hidden and can not be discovered". The pathogen of an epidemic is latent in the body, and it is kept internally. The decoction is boiled with water to clean the body. The medicine "swims in the meridians and enters the viscera, so that the visible and invisible epidemic virus can not be sheltered. Ordinary people can take several doses in advance to eliminate the unforeseen problems, and it is better if they can be spat out". In a remote area, it can be the mixed decoction of loquat leaves, acorus calamus, cyrtomium, loofah, which also has a preventive effect. The first three drugs mentioned above are similar to the epidemic prevention prescriptions described in the book, from which we can see the basic classification.[97]

The above drugs belong to a general treatment category. At the beginning of the Republic of China period, TCM prescriptions or drugs for the prevention and treatment of individual infectious diseases were also introduced. At present, according to the analysis of the journal data, besides pestis, cerebrospinal meningitis and cholera are the most introduced. For example, Liu Chongyin, a TCM doctor, said that there are a number of medicines that can prevent cerebrospinal meningitis, including schizonepeta spike (3.1g), soft saposhnikovia divaricata (3.1g), cicadas (3.1g), semen armeniacae amarae (6.3g), winter folium mori (6.3g), feverfew (6.3g),

[96] Shang Fuhan, Research on Epidemic Prevention of Chinese Medicine, *Chinese Medicine Bulletin*, Vol. 4, 1936 (01), p. 40.

[97] Zhou Yuxi (ed.), *Compilation of Epidemic Diseases*, pp. 31–32.

coptis chinensis (15.75g), gentian (25.2g) and raw licorice (3.1g). In case of epidemic cerebrospinal meningitis, each person should take two doses in advance to avoid infection. Liu explained that this can be added and subtracted on the basis of Zhongjing's prescription, and can be used for sweating, dispelling wind, killing worms, regulating Qi, detoxification and anti-inflammation. According to him, the epidemic broke out in the spring of 1943, and more than 300 patients died. After the treatment and prevention with the above prescription, the epidemic was controlled. This has been proved by repeated "clinical trials".[98] Another explanation is that the epidemic was caused by contact with miasma (Qi), and then bacteria and toxins were generated in the body, facilitating the formation of diplococcus or streptococcus, so that the bacteria and toxins are accumulated in the spinal cord and brain. The method to prevent cerebrospinal meningitis is: "Clean the room and drink enough fluid to adjust the body temperature, and use chamomile, mulberry leaves, honeysuckle, olive and rose as tea to clear away heat, detoxify, smoothen the intestines and disperse fire. Strong liquor, greasiness, sexual indulgence and hard work should be prohibited".[99] Generally speaking, it is also a combination of Western medical interpretation and thinking of sterilization and anti-inflammation. TCM has the concept of detoxification, dispersing heat, regulating Qi and so on. At that time, it had almost become an interpretation mode of integrating China and the West. As for cholera, Zhou Yuxi introduced the "epidemic prevention and emergency rescue pill" in his book *Compilation of Epidemic Diseases*, claiming that the prescription can cure all cholera. In fact, it generally refers to many gastrointestinal diseases. The medicine is "suitable for adjustment, without any hindrance, and can prevent epidemic and rescue emergencies". He said that this medicine is a variation of the "cinnabar detoxification pill", with two additional drugs of cyrtomium and artemisia annua leaves. Zhou said that he wasn't sure about the efficacy of the medicine until after it was made according to the prescription. He found that the main treatment was for "chest tightness and nausea, anxiety, excessive salivation, soft or slight numbness on limbs, which are the indications of being infected by a micro virus. This is particularly effective for prevention. After repeated trials and tests, he decided to publicize it to the society, and won charity from all walks of life. They eagerly made it and distributed it widely to the public, and popularized it for the treatment of summer and autumn diseases. The results were amazing. Mr.Xian thought that it was an unprecedented major new invention in the medical field in China. It has the functions of: activating Qi, detoxifying blood, clearing turbid water, detoxifying water, eliminating toxins, killing bacteria and micro worms and discharging them from the stool".[100] The terms of sterilization, detoxification and Qi activation combine the Chinese and Western explanations of pharmacology to achieve the preventive effect, just like the statements in the above-mentioned.

---

98 Liu Chongyin, TCM Treatment and Prevention of Cerebrospinal Meningitis, *Health Medical Journal*, 1947, March 17, 2nd Edition, p. 22.

99 Wang Lanyuan, Prevention and Treatment of Epidemic Diseases, *Weekly Supplement of Shaoxing Medical Journal*, 1920 (15), p. 4.

100 Zhou Yuxi (ed.), *Compilation of Epidemic Diseases*, pp. 18–19.

There are also some explanations of drug use for epidemic prevention, which do not use various TCM pathogenesis explanations instead of the term "sterilization", it is intended to eliminate the disease mechanism leading to the epidemic so as to achieve the effect of epidemic prevention. For example, Zhao Shuping, a TCM practitioner, explained in the column of "Q & A on TCM" in the newspaper, when answering the readers' questions on how to prevent children from being infected by epidemic diseases, that "meat should be moderated in diet", after dinner, "boil pear, lotus and green fruit for children to drink, which can not only clear away heat, but also increase immunity"; "If defecation is blocked, the cheeks are red or the palms feel the burning heat, some digestants can be taken with Jiaosanxian and rhubarb decoction". If the lips are slightly dry without other symptoms, use honeysuckle (6.3g) and chrysanthemum (6.3g) to clear away the heat before the treatment, which can be "a little remedy".[101] Most of the above-mentioned drugs are mainly for clearing away heat. In addition, diet control or the added digestant drugs are all related to the traditional Chinese medical concept of the body. Food accumulation in the stomach will lead to fever, resulting in a constitution prone to infection. The same thinking can be reflected from what Zhang Zhaolin said: "It is often said in my hometown that the person of deficiency do not suffer from epidemics, and the people of excess do not suffer from tuberculosis. It is based on the long time experiences and the effect is obvious. Pondering on it, it might imply that when one is full and filled with vitality, the smell must be turbid and unclear. The bacteria are prone to filth, making the infection more likely. Therefore, it is understood that the Westerners would have diarrhea once every ten days or half a month. It makes good sense. It is a particularly a good method for TCM to learn. Every half a month, you should take doctor Yan's tonic pills, to have slight diarrhea, which can not only prevent infectious diseases, but also promote the old to bring forth the new, which is important for health".[102] As "Bacteria" is prone to turbidity, TCM believed that satiety will lead to the increase of "turbid Qi" in the body. Therefore, drugs that have the effect of eliminating and purging the turbid Qi are used, so that the internal environment is not conducive to the growth of bacteria. Its focus is not just "sterilization".[103]

Other sporadic ideas that can be compared with the concept of sterilization also have their value. For example, in 1929, Xu Bingnan, a TCM doctor, found that a patient suffered from intestinal addiction (dysentery) and was not willing to accept serum therapy, so he chose angelica sinensis, codonopsis pilosula, white peony,

---

101 Zhao Shuping, Dr. Zhao Shuping's Answers to Mr. Liu Boyu's Question on the Prevention of Children's Diseases, *Liyan Pictorial*, 1939 (23), p. 31.

102 Zhang Zhaolin, Methods and Agents of TCM in Preventing Infectious Diseases, *Medical Journal*, 1935(86). pp. 24–25.

103 According to *Inner Canon of the Yellow Emperor. Acupuncture*: "The Yellow Emperor said: I would like to hear about the clarity and turbidity of human beings. Qi Bo said: grain produces turbidity, while air produces clarity. Clarity enhances Yin, and turbidity enhances Yang. Turbidity turns clarity by discharging it from pharynx, and clarity turns turbidity by discharging it from the lower part. When clarity and turbidity are intersected, it is called disordered Qi in human body". Quoted from Long Bojian's *The Collected Inner Canon of the Yellow Emperor*, Tianjin: Tianjin Science and Technology Press, 2004, p. 1761.

raw oyster, roasted turtle shell, roasted licorice, dashengdi, ophiopogon japonicus, dendrobium and other drugs for the treatment. He believed that the effect of these drugs was not "sterilization", but it was to fill the patient with vitality and "increase the antitoxins in the body". These traditional herbs could "have the same function as the serum" and can achieve the effect of epidemic prevention by strengthening vitality.[104] Another example is Zhang Ziying's affirmation that "the 113 prescriptions in Zhongjing's *Treatise on Typhoid Fever* were all made for killing bacteria". He explained that human diseases are nothing more than "stagnation of Qi and blood". Once stagnation of Qi and blood occurs, bacteria will multiply. "Zhongjing's prescriptions were made to remove stagnation, that is, to kill bacteria". He observed that when the farmers pile straw tents, the center would decay and produce micro bacteria over time. Farmers pull open the straw canopy, let the stagnant air out, or sunbath it, then the mold is killed, and the straw will not rot. He believed that this is the significance of TCM in treating bacteria by dispersing stasis. He also cited the causes of "stagnation of Qi and blood" such as drenching, cholera, diphtheria, and tuberculosis, which can be removed by TCM to prevent and treat bacteria.[105] All of these are to remove the pathogenesis of bacterial growth in the body, but not to sterilize. Of course, the core of their discussion is still inseparable from the influence of bacteria, only in different ways.

8.5 Incense: Air, Disinfection and Cleaning

Modern Chinese medicine has absorbed a lot of Western epidemic prevention knowledge. In previous epidemics, Chinese medicine has adopted this knowledge, as mentioned above. However, in the discussion of TCM, is there a hygienic law of TCM? In 1932, in response to the meningitis epidemic that spread from Macao to Guangzhou, Liu Qinxian held that both Chinese and Western medicine had good disinfection methods. Factors such as food, clothing, housing and air were most related to the prevention of infectious diseases. For example, clothes must be "disinfected" when they were clean. The simplest and the least costly way is to use "boiling water" to wash clothes; or the exposure to sunlight can also kill the toxic bacteria. In terms of food, Liu Ze held that it should be as light as possible since "disease comes from what enters the mouth". One should abstain from eating "stimulating" food such as barbecue and liquor. Water should be boiled before drinking, "making it impossible for toxic bacteria to grow".[106] From such appeals, it can be seen that TCM has been inspired by the modern health concept of Western medicine. The guiding ideology behind the hygiene concept of "cleaning" is actually the theory of

[104] Xu Bingnan,Efficacy of TCM in the Treatment of Bacteria, *Journal of Health*, Vol. 1, 1929 (04), pp. 4–5.

[105] Zhang Ziying, Bacterial Theory of Chinese Medicine, *Journal of Health*, 1932 (01), pp. 7–8.

[106] Liu Qinxian, On the Treatment and Prevention of Meningeal Inflammation in Chinese Medicine, *Xinglin Medical Monthly*, 1932 (41), pp. 14–15.

bacteria. The reason for "cleaning" is to eliminate the environment where bacteria breed and eventually eliminate bacteria.[107] The western-style cleaning products in the early Republic of China period were often connected with the Chinese term "disinfection".[108] In addition, as "healthy beauty" gradually became a fashionable term in the 1920s, the concept of clean and sanitary products often went with the image of "white" and "fragrant".[109] In old China, the sense of fragrant smell and aroma itself can be associated with cleaning and hygiene, and even with subsequent sterilization and disinfection.[110]

At that time, there was a saying that the "old-fashioned epidemic prevention" of the Dragon Boat Festival was generally "to make atractylodes, angelica root smoke to expel mosquito, and spray realgar. This practice is very interesting. As summer comes, the epidemic is prevalent, so it is necessary to have a thorough cleaning and use these drugs to disinfect; hanging the picture of the immortal 'Zhong Kui' also indicates the anti epidemic (ghost) action".[111] Although the latter involves superstition, the former is a TCM method to avoid disease by making Chinese medicine fragrant smoke. It was given a scientific explanation for the first time in modern times. In the Ming and Qing Dynasties, fragrance had proved its function of expelling filth and disinfection. For example, Yu Jiayan commented: "Before the treatment, drink fragrant and healthy medicine potion to the prevent the pathogen from entering. This is the best approach. Once the pathogen enters, it is urgent to expel the filth. The upper energizer is like fog, it rises and expels, so as to detoxify. The middle energizer is like retting, which is sparse and expelling, and it is also used to detoxify. The lower energizer is like blasphemy, which enhances the expelling, and it is also used to detoxify".[112] Aromatic drugs are followed by the antidote drugs to treat epidemics. This became the keynote of TCM in seeking traditional knowledge. After the early Republic of China period, Chinese medicine absorbed Western medicine. In the "Three Chapters on Chinese and Western Knowledge of Infectious Diseases", it is written that the ceiling and bed board can be disinfected with mercuric acid and carbolic acid, and the clothes can be disinfected with hot steam. Other appeals,

---

[107] Liu Shiyong, "Cleanliness", "Sanitation" and "Health Care"—the Change of Public Health Concepts in Taiwan during the Japanese Rule Period, *Research on Taiwan History*, 2001 (8.1), esp. pp. 66–67.

[108] See the cartoon of "Lysol" for external cleaning and disinfection, which is quoted from "*Shen Bao*" on June 27, 1936, p. 3.

[109] Peijun, Knowledge and Marketing: Cleaning and Hygiene Products in Advertisements during the Republic of China Period, *New Peking University History*, 2010 (08), pp. 61–76.

[110] Ruth Rogaski, translated by Xiang Lei, *The Modernity of Health: the Meaning of Health and Disease at China's Commercial Ports*, pp. 239–247.

[111] Zhong, The Old-fashioned Epidemic Prevention on the Dragon Boat Festival, *Life Knowledge*, 1946 (28), p. 16.

[112] (Qing) Zhang Fengkui, additionally annotated by Ye Ziyu, The Preface to Yu Jiayan's 'Theory of Epidemics', Supplement of Ye Ping's The Complete Book of Heatstroke, included in Cao Bingzhang (ed.), *Great Achievements in Chinese Medicine*, Vol.16 (II), pp. 43–44.

such as ventilation, mainly focus on Western-style health knowledge.[113] The knowledge of Western medicine about using boiling water, sulfur and other substances to kill bacteria was also learned by Chinese medicine very early.[114] Tian Erkang, a TCM doctor, recounted his experience: "In September of 1932, he undertook the mission of epidemic prevention in Wuzhai. Among the drugs in the epidemic prevention department, disinfection drugs were used the most. Later, he learned that this was the so-called epidemic prevention of Western medicine". He believed that we should be open-minded and thoroughly study the epidemic prevention methods of Western medicine. The study of disinfection drugs is another major subject. It can be seen that the awareness of "disinfection" is that Chinese medicine recognizes the greatest advantage of Western medicine, which urges some Chinese medicine to find traditional disinfection methods.[115]

Shang Fuhan maintained that TCM did not have the so-called "disinfection" as that of Western medicine, but there are some similarities in the use of certain drugs in the history of TCM. He cited the "six flavor lavender prescription" in *Zhou Hou Prescriptions* as the method of clothing disinfection. The drugs include aloe, musk, styrofoam, white gum, clove, Huoxiang, etc., by using the honey to glue them into incense to smoke the clothes. He also introduced the disinfection methods of the nasal cavity, skin and oral cavity. Among them, the disinfection of an oral cavity can be carried out by the "Fujian fragrant tea cake" in *The Complete Book of Jingyue,* which contains medicines such as aloe, white sandalwood, acacia catechu, licorice, musk and borneol. When these drugs are made into pills and put into the mouth, the pathogenic Qi can not invade. It is more convenient and practical than the mask of Western medicine.[116] It is also an external anti-epidemic medicine. Shanghai's *Herald Monthly* published the method of preventing throat disease by taking green olives (or salted olives) or eating raw radishes. There should be no hot nor spicy food. If there is redness, swelling, white spots or even faint pain in the throat, achyranthes bidentata juice with peppermint soup can be used to rinse the throat, or the dried rhizome of rehmannia and ophiopogon japonicus can be used to keep the throat clean and "make sure that the toxic bacteria can not stay".[117] Zhang Zhaolin, a TCM doctor, straightened out the strength of Chinese and Western medicine in disinfection: public health and the well-to-do families used medicine to prevent epidemics, such as cyrtomium and Xingfan (it should be alum-the author's note) in cleaning drinks, gas (which should refer to steam) to eliminate the toxins of clothes and quilts, atractylodes macrocephala and realgar mentioned repeatedly before are both famous cleaning and disinfection drugs in TCM. Atractylodes was used for fumigating rooms, carbolic

---

[113] Wang Zhizhou, Three Chapters on the Integration of Chinese and Western Medicine in Infectious Diseases, p. 40.

[114] Chen Shouzhen, The Power of Micro Bacteria, *Weekly Supplement of Shaoxing Medical Journal,* 1920 (22), p. 3.

[115] Tian Erkang, The Strengths and Weaknesses in the TCM Diagnosis and Treatment of Acute Infectious Diseases, *Medical Journal,* 69 (1933), p. 4 5.

[116] Shang Fuhan, Research on Epidemic Prevention of Chinese Medicine, *Chinese Medicine Bulletin,* Vol. 4, 1936 (01), p. 45.

[117] Xu Renfu, *Handouts on Practical Medicine,* 1997, p. 162.

acid for cleaning the floor and lime for eliminating the toxin of spitting and defecation.[118] Cyrtomium, Xingfan, atractylodes and realgar mentioned repeatedly before are all famous cleaning and disinfection drugs in TCM. In terms of drinking water disinfection, Shang Fuhan also mentioned cyrtomium, black beans, alum and took the TCM "eliminating filth and pathogenic factors" as the "disinfection and sterilization" in the Western medicine.[119] TCM has also opened a newspaper column to introduce the treatment and prevention of individual infectious diseases. In 1932, the National Medical and Epidemic Prevention Committee of Peking published the Law on the Prevention and Treatment of Cholera, with particular emphasis on the disinfection of drinking water. Liquorice, rhizoma coptidis from Sichuan, Shengqi granule, forsythia, Huoxiang, atractylod, mint and other drugs were used to make "public drinking drugs", or put cyrtomium, realgar, alum and other drugs into water tanks to dissolve the water toxin before supplying it to the public for drinking.[120]

In addition to the importance of clean drinking water, as many infectious diseases are transmitted through the air, air hygiene and epidemic prevention have also been highlighted, and ancient aromatic epidemic prevention methods have come into use. Shang Fuhan once proposed the "8 Prescriptions of Air Disinfection", which mostly used drugs to make powder sachets or burn herbal medicine in the air. He believed that:

> Bacterial life is generally good for dampness but bad for dryness. If the air is too dry, the water in the bacterial body evaporates without any residue. Being stopped from growing, it is prone to death. Among them, pathogenic bacteria are the most severe, such as tuberculosis and splenic gangrene spores, which can last for a long time. At the very least, it can prevent their development. The above methods have the function of decontamination, dehumidification, disinfection, sterilization, by means of fumigation or suspension in the dry air, much better than the simple dry disinfection method in Western medicine.[121]

Shang's integration of Chinese and Western medicine theories shows that burning Chinese medicine in the air may achieve epidemic prevention effects. There were many examples of this in the early Republic of China period, and the basic starting point was still the function of aromatic drugs in TCM. The word "epidemic" in the Anti Epidemic Pill often refers to infectious diseases in a broad sense. For example, Xu Renfu, a TCM doctor in Guangdong, explained under the item "Anti Epidemic Pill" that it is composed of several drugs and can be burned every morning, so that it can prevent infection.[122] The author found that during the whole period of the Republic of China, many daily necessities with fragrant smells were endowed with epidemic prevention functions, including perfume and cigarettes. For example, in 1926, the advertisement of "Giant White Dragon Cigarettes" published in *Shen Bao*

---

118 Shanghai Shen Bao Newspaper Office (ed.), *Shen Bao*, August 15, 1926, p. 19.

119 Ding Fubao, Notes on smoking, Collection of Medical Reviews, included in Shen Hongrui & Liang Xiuqing (eds.), *Medical Reviews in the Past Dynasties in China*, p. 1516.

120 Shanghai Shen Bao Newspaper Office (ed.), *Shen Bao*, August 15, 1936, p. 4.

121 Shang Fuhan, Research on Epidemic Prevention of Chinese Medicine, *Chinese Medicine Bulletin*, Vol. 4, 1936 (01), p. 45.

122 Xu Renfu, *Handouts on Practical Medicine*, 1997, p. 162.

indicated that smoking cigarettes can prevent infectious diseases and "kill worms and eliminate filth", which is based on the discussion of TCM.[123] Ding Fubao even believed that "tobacco contains a kind of disinfection substance, which can extinguish mold when it enters the mouth. Therefore, when infectious diseases are prevalent, smokers are immune from infection".[124] The anti-epidemic discourse of "fragrance" in TCM was compared with the disinfectant "smelly potion" in Western medicine, such as "Yalin Smelly potion" produced by Wuzhou Pharmacy, a disinfectant similar to bleach water. There was a sharp contrast between China and the West. The sense of smell indicates different anti-epidemic thinking.[125] The theory of ancient aromatic epidemic prevention was sorted out in *Compilation of Epidemic Diseases*:

> The Yellow Emperor asked: how can we stop the infection without having to resort to treatment? Qi Bo answered: for the uninfected, it owes to their positive Qi stored in the body, which keeps away the invasion of the pathogenic factors, so that the toxic Qi is avoided and prevented from the heavenly nose. Qi comes out of the brain, and it is not to be invaded by the pathogenic factors, that is, the mind is like the sun. It is said that epidemics are easy to infect. How to avoid it? There are four ways: First, it is appropriate to preserve the body by staying calm and free of lust, so that the healthy Qi can be consolidated inside, and the disease and pathogen can not overtake; second, to stay away from the infected so as to avoid the toxic Qi; third, it is good to use fragrant and appetizing agents to sneeze, so that the Qi comes out of the brain, and the heavenly nose. The heaven provides people with five Qis, which is what the nose receives and that's why it is called the heavenly nose. The pestilence Qi passes the brain through the nose. The brain is the pivot of the body, the gathering of the essence of the five viscera, and the headquarter of heavenly performance. The epidemic invades the brain, reaches the whole body quickly, goes in and out, rises and falls, stops and dies all of a sudden. Its death is the fastest. The use of fragrances for inducing sneezing is to let out the epidemic in the brain from the nose, the magic machine is activated so that the sick can recover in an instant. On one hand, when one sneezes with fragrance, the Qi comes out of the brain. Keeping in mind the sun to strengthen oneself, as the heart is the center of the holy power. Without the knowledge of this holy power, all the twelve organs would be in danger. Think of the heart as the sun, the holy power would come out of the Lord's brightness, like the sunshine in the beautiful sky, the haze is broken, the disease and pathogen have no place to hide. In this way, there goes the saying "the sage does not cure the disease, but prevents the disease from occurring".[126]

One of the most important concepts is that fragrant Qi can expel pathogenic and toxic Qi from the body through sneezing. It is a very special theory that pestilential Qi invades the brain, because most doctors use the concepts of air, breath and lungs to explain the path of pestilence. In addition to the concept of clean air, some TCM doctors also believed that aroma can excite nerves and enhance resistance. For example, Huang Guocai said, "When the epidemic is widespread, it can be used to touch the nose by reaching its nerves, maintaining its function and providing it with sufficient natural immunity, so that it can not be invaded by toxic germs. It

[123] Shanghai Shen Bao Newspaper Office (ed.), *Shen Bao*, August 15, 1926, p. 19.

[124] Ding Fubao, Notes on Smoking, Collection of Medical Reviews, included in Shen Hongrui & Liang Xiuqing (eds), *Medical Reviews in the Past Dynasties in China*, p. 1516.

[125] Shanghai Shen Bao Newspaper Office (ed.), *Shen Bao*, August 15, 1936, p. 4.

[126] Zhou Yuxi, *Compilation of Epidemic Diseases*, pp. 11–12.

is quite effective and can not be ignored".[127] Shang Fuhan also believed that using Marching Powder or Wolong Pill to twitch the nose was the so-called "nasal disinfection method", which could prevent epidemics.[128] For example, in 1941, the Sichuan Branch of the Central Chinese Medical College published the "Publicity Outline for Epidemic Prevention and Control of National Medical College", and the prevention methods include the restrictions of eating cold food, fruits and anything unsanitory. "Bitter Mustard" can be served at every meal to "increase the anti-virus function of the stomach"; "medicinal incense", such as ligusticum wallichii and atractylodes, can be carried around to "excite the nerves and relieve depression". In terms of air circulation, it was suggested to burn fragrant herbs, in addition to opening the window, so as to "circulate air and fumigate filth". In terms of "improving drinking water", cyrtomium, realgar, atractylodes rhizome and alum should be kept in storage to clear away water toxicity. It's obvious that keeping water clean is in line with the methods of TCM mentioned above, and the calls to avoid mosquitoes and flies are in line with Western medicine.[129]

Other calls for burning herbs to prevent epidemics were also recorded. For example, in response to the "meningitis" epidemic, Liu Qinxian believed that in terms of housing and air, in addition to paying attention to air circulation and exterminating mosquitoes and flies, the smoke of realgar or atractylodes would "produce indoor fragrance and eliminate toxin".[130] Many drugs are recurrent, such as realgar. Shanxi Chinese Medicine Improvement Research Association also expressed that applying realgar to the nostrils can disinfect and prevent epidemics. If there are wounds on hands and feet, the wiping of realgar can disinfect and prevent the invasion of epidemic virus from the wounds.[131] The Central Epidemic Prevention Office had also introduced the use of stemona soaked in liquor to wipe wounds, which can also kill lice and prevent typhus. This can be regarded as an example of a few Western medicine methods that led to health agencies using Chinese medicine for epidemic prevention.[132] Shang Fuhan listed "methods of eliminating vermin", including exterminating snakes, scorpions, rats, mosquitoes, flies and bedbugs. Most of them used incense. He believed that apart from paying attention to the tidiness and cleanliness of the environment, TCM was not very clear about worm-led infectious diseases. At that time, Western medicine also lacked good extermination methods. This was a

---

[127] Huang Guocai, Methods and Agents of TCM in Preventing Infectious Diseases, *Medical Journal*, 1935(86), p. 23.

[128] Shang Fuhan, Research on Epidemic Prevention of Chinese Medicine, *Chinese Medicine Bulletin*, Vol. 4, 1936 (01), p. 42.

[129] Cao Shushi, Liu Zishen & Kuang Hexiao, Instruction of Sichuan Branch of National Medical Center: Publicity Outline of TCM Prevention and Treatment of Epidemic Cholera, *Medical Improvement Monthly*, Vol. 1, 1941 (06), p. 17.

[130] Liu Qinxian, On the Treatment and Prevention of Meningeal Inflammation in Chinese Medicine, *Xinglin Medical Monthly*, 1932 (41), p. 15.

[131] Xu Renfu, *Handouts on Practical Medicine*, 1997, p. 162.

[132] Unknown Author, Report Gate: Notice of Spring Epidemic Prevention Issued by the Central Epidemic Prevention Office, *Medical Journal*, 1924 (22), pp. 85–87.

part in need of further development. Such a discussion was not given much attention by the Chinese Medicine community.[133]

8.6 Exploration on the Lost TCM Epidemic Prevention Technology

The modern health system is a kind of public affair based on state power and institutional setup, with a brand-new vision.[134] However, if we analyze the concepts of "epidemic prevention", "cleaning" and "disinfection", we will find that Chinese medical history has equally given us a brand-new vision: that is, TCM had those knowledge connotations in ancient times, but with different expressions. Ever since modern times, it needs to be sorted out, innovated and reproduced in a different way. TCM summarized many epidemic prevention drugs, prescriptions and methods, which is practically very significant. Many drugs appeared repeatedly, such as realgar, atractylodes rhizome, cyrtomium, Huoxiang, garlic and cinnabar. Only by sorting out the accumulated experience of the ancients on drugs can it be served as the foundation for creating new drugs.

Doctors had compiled a number of prescriptions, and if these drugs could be tested, there might be surprising discoveries. From the "523 Mission" in the late 1960s to Tu Youyou's experience in winning the Nobel Prize, we can explore an effective path from sorting out drugs from ancient books to scientific experiments.[135] Unfortunately, the so-called sorting out work during the Republic of China period was not a success. The foregoing depends on the historians' hindsight and the collection of numerous materials. However, the collection and discussion of such epidemic prevention prescriptions by the Chinese medicine community were in fact quite scattered. And compared with the discussions on typhoid and warm diseases, it seemed that "epidemic treatment", rather than "epidemic prevention", was the mainstream of discussion in the Chinese medicine community. In addition, TCM during the Republic of China period had lost its leading power of epidemic prevention, and many epidemic prevention prescriptions could not be "experimented" (or "tested"—to be more accurate) by TCM in a planned way during the pandemic.

The concept of epidemic prevention in modern Chinese medicine is a general rule. Although there are differences in the use of drugs for individual diseases, it is highly related to the prevention of infectious diseases and epidemics in a broad sense. Of

133 Shang Fuhan, Research on Epidemic Prevention of Chinese Medicine, *Chinese Medicine Bulletin*, Vol. 4, 1936 (01), pp. 47–48. Yu Xinzhong commented: "What disappoints me is that it lacks a sense of history. It often uses historical materials from the perspective of modern health and concepts, with little investigation and understanding of different health concepts and behaviors in the specific historical contexts in different times and spaces".

134 Yu Xinzhong, Historical Contexts and the Concern of Reality—Research on the History of Modern Health in China and Myself, *Anhui History*, 2011 (04), p. 10.

135 Rao Yi, Zhang Daqing & Li Runhong, *Artemisia of Youyou: Tu Youyou and Artemisinin*, Beijing: China Science and Technology Press, 2015, pp. 31–38, 108–110.

course, it can not be denied that this is a rough general rule developed by the inability to determine the precise name of a disease. New infectious diseases are constantly emerging and knowledge is constantly subdivided. Many diseases may not be found in ancient books, or the names of diseases can not be matched. How to deal with this situation of "new diseases emerging beyond the old frame"?[136] Are those general preventive drugs really effective for every infectious disease? This is rather doubtful. TCM was still in the process of discussion and development in epidemic prevention methods. It seemed that there were a lot of voices, and many drugs and methods for epidemic prevention were proposed. There was no unified epidemic treatment administration nor regular patterns in using drugs, and most of them were obtained from the personal opinions of the doctors or from medical books. With the overall discussion, the TCM community has not developed its own methods in the actual epidemic prevention work, nor conducted corresponding experiments. Most of the drugs discussed and published in this paper are of unknown origin and have not been differentiated. Compared with the traditional theory of exogenous febrile diseases, TCM also demonstrates less epidemic prevention theories, and even has no statistics on epidemic prevention efficacy. The credibility of prescriptions is questionable. At least, it is a fact that not enough attention was given to epidemic prevention, no matter what effect it had. Yang Zhiyi, a Chinese medicine practitioner, once commented: "In the past, TCM focused on preserving healthy Qi. When special drugs were invented, experiments were not widely carried out and the results were not publicized. Given more study and implementations, they would be recognized by the world".[137] He revealed the problems at that time and the direction of future development. TCM has discussed the methods and prescriptions for epidemic prevention more systematically, but it had not yet become a national consensus, and there was no desire of reaching a consensus. As Shang Fuhan urged: most of the anti-epidemic and anti-epidemic prescriptions in Chinese medical books contain bactericidal effects, and the detoxification and anti filth functions of various medicines are more unique than those of Western medicine which specializes in sterilization. If we studied hard and tried to improve on them, the TCM style of hygiene and epidemic prevention would certainly be a unique school.[138] At present, it is still an unaccomplished ideal and cause. The direction of the reform of modern Chinese medicine is a myriad, and we can't criticize it for its performance during certain periods. In the history of TCM, there are still many "lost" technologies worthy of exploration. It depends on whether TCM realizes this historical enlightenment in the future.

---

[136] Fan Xingzhun, *A Brief History of Chinese Medicine*, Beijing: Ancient Books of TCM Press, 1986. p. 221.

[137] Yang Zhiyi, My Views on "Epidemic Treatment" of TCM and Western Medicine, *Spring and Autumn of the Medical World,* 1930 (49), p. 4.

[138] Shang Fuhan, Research on Epidemic Prevention of Chinese Medicine, *Chinese Medicine Bulletin*, Vol. 4, 1936 (01), p. 31.

Chapter 9
Recuperation, Diet and Taboo: The Transformation of Classical Theory in the World of the Sick

9.1 Introduction

Modern Chinese and Western medicine have very different views on the treatment of fever caused by bacteria. For today's people, headache, cough, fever and other minor illnesses do not last for long. In order to cope with a heavy work load and busy life, the course of an illness lasting two or three days is probably acceptable. Even if one does not recover quickly, most of the patients work during their illness, change doctors frequently or even blame it on the poor effects of the drugs they take. However, little attention is paid to "recuperation" after illness. It is a fact that the ancients took care of themselves after the febrile disease. Jiang Hanhuang in the Qing Dynasty said, "Those who suffer from typhoid fever related diseases all have the symptoms of typhoid fever. Some were delayed in getting treatment, some were not recuperated properly, some got complications after being infected, all of which were treated with different therapies."[1] That is to say, there are many concurrent diseases of febrile disease. Among them, improper recuperation is one of the important reasons for their deterioration. *Analysis on Febrile Diseases* in the Qing Dynasty quotes Wu Youke:

> Recuperation after the initial recovery is easier than treating a disease. How can it be possible that one can treat a disease without being able to recuperate! However, recuperation after illness is not less important than the treatment. At the beginning of the disease, if it is properly treated without violating the rules, one will recover in three to five days for a light case, seven or eight days for a sever case. No residual pathogens would be left. If the patient is not seriously ill, it may not be necessary to be treated with medicine, and the proper diet would be good enough to help. This is the "all food and nourishment therapy" in the *Canon*.[2]

[1] (Qing) Jiang Hanhuang, Typhoid Fever and Its Complications, Principles for the Compliance with Times, Beijing: China TCM Press, 1993 (02), p. 28.

[2] (Qing) Wu Tang, Systematic Differentiation of Warm Diseases, Li Liukun (ed.), Complete Medical Works of Wu Jutong, Beijing: China TCM Press, 1999, p. 85.

© Zhonghua Book Company 2026

K. Pi, *The Contest of Modern Chinese and Western Medicine*,
https://doi.org/10.1007/978-981-95-2832-5_9

This shows the importance of dietary conditioning, which is also one of the focuses of this chapter. Food has the Qi and flavor of matter. The nature of Qi is changeable and varies according to people, seasons and regions. The ancient sages said that "food itself can connect Qi, just like clothing can cover the body". "Food" and "Qi" have a strong internal connection to the body. Food can be transformed into Qi of the human body, and this process is very important. On the other hand, the knowledge involved in bacteriology supported by science is unified and regular. It standardizes people's behavior, unifies the details of daily life and takes combating the infection of bacteria as the highest guiding principle. In this knowledge context, food also has specific references, as what Yu Yunxiu said: "Vegetables, milk or fish polluted by the patient's excrement but are not well cooked would be invaded by the microorganisms and will enter the abdomen."[3] It can be seen that uncooked food is unsanitary and may carry germs. Chinese and Western medicine also have different views on food pathogenicity. When talking about the relationship between diet and microorganisms, Lu Jinsheng, a TCM doctor, said that there are many explanations for people's diarrhea, "some are due to cold and some are due to heat". However, Western medicine retorted: "The cause of diarrhea is that microorganisms are brought into people's stomach and intestines due to an unclean diet. When microorganisms spread in the stomach and intestines, the pathogenic factors grow prevalent and then there comes disease. What matters with cold and heat? It's totally unscientific!" In this regard, Lu responded that the term TCM originally used had been "spleen and stomach" rather than "stomach and intestines". This is the difference in the interpretation of anatomical shapes and qualities. Although microorganisms are related to diseases, it can not be said that every disease is caused by "germs". He cited a vivid story: a relative of his raised monkeys who got diarrhea. It was confirmed that it ate cooked food that was sterilized during cooking instead of raw food that was likely to contain microorganisms. Monkeys used to eat raw fruit, but they were given the "cooked food" which was thought to have less microorganisms when being raised by humans. The monkeys were not "acclimatized". The relative followed the advice by feeding the monkeys raw food again. Within three days, the monkeys recovered.[4]

---

[3] Yu Yunxiu, *Microorganisms*, p. 39.

[4] Lu Jinsheng said: "… monkeys are accustomed to eating fruit, and raw food that is not cooked. Of course, there are many microorganisms in uncooked fruit. It is reasonable that monkeys should have diarrhea at ordinary times. Why has this never happened? If the physiology of monkeys is different from that of humans. A human's resistance is weak,while a monkeys' resistance is strong.So general microorganisms will cause diarrhea when they reach the human intestines and stomachs, but will not cause diarrhea when reaching the monkey's intestines and stomachs. Fruit with microorganisms will not cause diarrhea because of the strong resistance. Once food is cooked, microorganisms will be killed. Nothing can be safer then. Even people with weak resistance will not have diarrhea if they eat it. Of course, the intestines and stomachs like those of monkeys will not have diarrhea. As a matter of fact, it is proved that monkeys will have diarrhea immediately after eating cooked food. Does it mean that microorganisms are attached to raw food for humans and cooked food for monkeys? According to our TCM, different reactions would occur from different habituation when food enters the intestine and stomach. People are used to cooked food, monkeys are used to raw food, and if they eat what they are not used to, they will have diarrhea. So I advised the relative that he should only give raw food to monkeys and prohibit them from eating cooked food. My relative followed

Compared with TCM cold and heat, diarrhea caused by "irregular diets" is called "food damage". Therefore, the relationship between diet and disease in TCM is still mainly based on the relationship between the attributes of food and the human body,[5] which is different from the relationship between human beings and microorganisms in Western medicine. When talking about modern medical and health history, historians often pay attention to the disease itself and the measures of the health system, but neglect the post illness rehabilitation, which is extremely relevant and important to the history of daily life. The integration and conflict of concepts between Chinese and Western medicine involved is also significant. With the focus on "recuperation" of febrile diseases, this chapter combs some expositions involving Qi and bacteria in modern febrile diseases in view of diet, drugs, taboos, with the wish to draw a clearer outline for the daily life subdivision of "multi-dimensional medical history".

9.2 Relationship Between Classical Food Taboo Theory and Ferile Diseases

In ancient China, there was a wealth of knowledge about the recuperation of patients. The method of health preservation and longevity is purely a reference for daily life. It is pursued by people both rich and poor.[6] However, there is little discussion about the connotation of classical health preservation during modern transformation, or the combination of disease history and patients' daily life. The previous chapter has discussed residence and space, and this chapter will discuss the relationship between febrile disease recuperation and diet, and even the introduction of new drugs during the Republic of China period.

The food diets of modern hospitals are mostly controlled according to the patient's physique, but for the majority of people in the early Republic of China period who were unable to recuperate in the hospital due to insufficient medical resources, they must take their home as the main venue for recuperation. In most cases, the cultivation of modern Western medicine was on the right track of school education, but in addition to school education, the propagation of medical knowledge in TCM was originally carried out in daily life, and continued through oral transmission and textual experience. The daily diet precautions of patients during illness occupied an important part of medical knowledge. This idea of "diet as medicine" is difficult for westerners to understand. A missionary in the late Qing Dynasty said, "Raw pears are a commonly used antipyretic. Even though sharing the same appearance, these

---

my advice, and in less than three days, both monkeys recovered.My humble questions is: what on earth is the relationship between diarrhea and microorganisms? " Quoted from Lu Jinsheng's On Diarrhea, Collection of Medical Manuscripts in Jingjing, included in Shen Hongrui & Liang Xiuqing (eds.), *General Medical Views on Chinese Medicine in China,* pp. 2066–2067.

[5] Lu Jinsheng's On Diarrhea, Collection of Medical Manuscripts in Jingjing, included in Shen Hongrui & Liang Xiuqing (eds.), General Medical Views *on Chinese Medicine in China,* p. 2066.

[6] Wang Ermin, *The Cultural Life of the Common People in the Ming and Qing Dynasties,* Taipei: Institute of Modern History, Academia Sinica, 1996, pp. 54–62.

pears are very different from those in our hometown. They are almost tasteless and hard enough to be chopped with an axe. It is really pitiful to see a patient with a red face and bloodshot eyes, powerlessly trying to bite this rock hard pear to quench their thirst and reduce fever".[7] In fact, the "pear syrup" and the "five-gravies" in the *Analysis on Febrile Diseases* all take water pears as an important prescription,[8] which is puzzling to Westerners. Perhaps western people are more familiar with their popular orange juice or mandarin oranges when they are hot and thirsty.[9] In addition, it is explained in *Analysis on Febrile Diseases*: "In reference to diet, no prescription was given (by Zhongjing). It said that if you are seriously ill and don't take medicine, 'diet' is the key term, from which one can see that the stomach Qi is critical".[10] It can be seen that there is an important set of cultural and empirical knowledge behind eating pears to treat fever (such as storing body fluid and taking care of stomach Qi). Ancient doctors also attached importance to the role of diet in treating diseases, without taking medicine as the only treatment.

As for food and disease, Yu Xinzhong elucidated in his research: since traditional medicine has not explained the role of food in the spread of epidemic diseases in theory, the understanding of this aspect also stays at the level of experience and intuition, and not enough attention was paid from the society to the close relationship between food and epidemic diseases. Yu examined ancient medicine from the perspective of food hygiene control and management. He believed that even though food hygiene inspections were gradually done by the police at the end of the Qing Dynasty, their practical role was still questionable: "Although the system was of great significance for a long time, its initial practical effects can hardly be complimented".[11] Classical medicine did not attach importance to the relationship between food hygiene and epidemics, but for many epidemics or exogenous fevers, there have been a set of dietary norms and taboos, especially the recuperation period after recovery. Chen Guofu once called: "It is no good to eat cold, salty or sour food right after recovery. Sometimes it may bring out the disease. More attention is particularly needed to the weak periods of one's body. In the past, children didn't read, and they had the opportunity to practice nursing at home. Now children read books, but there is no such truth available in the books to inform them, so they turned out having neither knowledge nor experience. This is a great regret for the health of our nation".[12] Attaching importance to the content of food and "personal" care belongs to "self-care methods" and is a precious asset. However, this knowledge seems to

---

[7] Macgowan, translated by Zhu Tao and Ni Jing, *Men and Manners of Modern China*, p. 197.

[8] (Qing) Wu Tang, Systematic Differentiation of Warm Diseases, Li Liukun (ed.), Complete Medical Works of Wu Jutong, Beijing: China TCM Press, 1999, p. 24.

[9] Ding Fubao, *Communication between Chinese and Western Prescriptions*, Beijing: Commercial Press, 1929, p. 100.

[10] (Qing) Wu Tang, Systematic Differentiation of Warm Diseases, Li Liukun (ed.),Complete Medical Works of Wu Jutong, Beijing: China TCM Press, 1999, p. 36.

[11] Yu Xinzhong, Epidemics and Society in the South of the Yangtze River in the Qing Dynasty—A Study of Medical Social History, p. 214.

[12] Chen Guofu, The Way of Health, included in Selected Works of Mr. Chen Guofu's Medical and Health Thoughts, p. 144.

have gone from the textbooks of the Republic of China period under the influence of the West.[13] These traditions have some influence in daily life. In contrast, the new knowledge technically lacks corresponding supporting measures in society at the level of daily practice. These traditions are deeply rooted historical concepts, which are not regulated by external forces, such as the regulations of medical institutions. It is the knowledge that people practiced in their life. This is an area that has been neglected in past medical history research.

Food taboo traditions of exogenous fever can be traced back to the period from the *Internal Canon of Medicine* to the completion of the *Treatise on Typhoid Fever. "Basis Inquiries · A Chronicle of Six Elements*" states that "eating the seasonal grain to get its true essence", that is, choosing food according to the season of the year can avoid specific diseases caused by the Qi of special seasons.[14] The formation of the theory of food taboos for febrile diseases was initially reflected in the discussion of the criteria for treating diseases. It is necessary to abide by the norms of "treating heat with cold, starting with warmth; treating cold with heat, starting with coolness; treating warmth with clearness, starting with cold; treating clearness with warmth, starting with heat". From this, we can see the law of using cold medicine to treat fever diseases. Another example is: "In the treatment of febrile diseases, cold water is used to stimulate. Putting on less clothes and staying in a cold place, the disease will be gone when the body is cold".[15] That is, it is necessary to treat them with "cold" as it is the opposite nature. Similarly, it is no good to have hot food.[16] In addition, *Basis Inquiries* records that "the feeling of the pathogenic Qi from heaven is harmful to people's five internal organs; the feeling of cold and heat from water and grain is harmful to the six viscera".[17] The theory of disease is closely related to the Qi of the viscera and the body. The theoretical basis of the discussion on food taboos are: "Heaven provides people with five Qis, and earth provides people with five tastes... The five tastes are imported, hidden in the stomach, and the tastes are hidden, so as to nourish the five Qis. The Qis are born in harmony, the body fluid is produced, and the spirit comes into being".[18] It explains the process of food being internalized into essence and Qis in the human body through the correspondence with the Yin and Yang and the five elements, as well as the coordination between the viscera and the

[13] Scholars such as Li Zhende of the Institute of History and Philology of the Academia Sinica and Zhang Zhongmin of Fudan University have both studied the physiology textbooks of the Republic of China period. See Wang Youpeng (ed.), *General Contents of Textbooks for Primary and Secondary Schools in Modern China*, Shanghai: Shanghai Dictionary Publishing House, 2010.

[14] Guo Aichun(ed.), No. 71 of A Chronicle of Six Elements, *Interpretations to the Inner Canon of the Yellow Emperor*, pp. 461–484.

[15] Guo Aichun(ed.),No. 32 of Heat Syndrome, Interpretations to the Inner Canon of the Yellow Emperor, p. 199.

[16] Guo Aichun(ed.), No. 70 of A Chronicle of Five Elements, *Interpretations to the Inner Canon of the Yellow Emperor*, p. 458.

[17] Guo Aichun(ed.), No. 70 of A Chronicle of Images Corresponding to Yin and Yang, *Interpretations to the Inner Canon of the Yellow Emperor*, p. 32.

[18] Guo Aichun (ed.), No. 31 of Viscera in Six Periods, included in Interpretations to the Basic Inquiries of the Inner Canon of the Yellow Emperor, pp. 64–65.

nature or tastes of food. The "taste" of food itself contains the meaning of Qis. The sayings "taste is from shape, shape from Qi, and Qi from essence" and "essence is due to Qi, shape to taste" indicate that the taste of food is related to the body, Qis and essence.[19] When food is taken, it is called "Qi enters the stomach". Its essence will undergo a set of established procedures to nourish the meridians and viscera, which is the basis of establishing a classical body view of diet for its importance to the body.[20]

The *Internal Canon* has only completed a rough guiding principle, and food taboos for individual diseases have not yet been fully formed. However, at least, for a major disease in the ancient history of diseases, there are many food taboo clues to follow in the *Heat Theory. Basic Inquiries.* For example:

> The Emperor asked, 'Why is there still fever remaining after the recovery of febrile diseases?' Qi Bo said, 'Those who have remaining fever is due to their overindulgence in food before the recovery period, which turns into a remaining fever.' This is the case that the heat pathogen is stored even when the disease weakens. When grain meets fever, the pathogen is retained. The Emperor said: 'I can understand. How to cure the remaining fever?' Qi Bo replied: 'Depending on the level of deficiency. Some adjustments can be made by adding nutrition or releasing the intake, which can be the cure. The Emperor asked, 'Are there any taboos in taking care of the sick?' Qi Bo said, "Eating meat right after the recovery will bring the disease back. This is the taboo".[21]

Febrile disease is one of the few diseases that ancient medicine had developed therapeutic criteria and established relatively complete dietary taboos. Overeating will produce heat similar to the heat in the body. If the body heats up, it will be difficult to cure the disease; meat in a broad sense is not conducive to fever, which is another major taboo. Li Jianmin believed that even eating meat was gradually common in the Han Dynasty, the daily diet of ordinary people in the Qin and Han Dynasties was still dominated by vegetables, water and drink,[22] especially to the general public, who could not afford meat.[23] So "eating meat, bringing back the disease" may not be a common situation, and most of this belongs to the upper class. This kind of knowledge accumulated through some micro experience can only be a rough and simple understanding. What kind of meat can or can not be eaten is not explained in detail in the classics. T*reatise on Typhoid Fever* by Zhang Zhongjing is even more important, because the principle of food taboos put forward by him for exogenous febrile diseases was still restated in medical books until the Republic of

---

[19] Guo Aichun (ed.), No. 5 of On Yin and Yang, included in Interpretations to the Basic Inquiries of the Inner Canon of the Yellow Emperor, p. 31.

[20] Guo Aichun (ed.), No. 21 of On Meridians, included in Interpretations to the Basic Inquiries of the Inner Canon of the Yellow Emperor, p. 142. Another reference can be made to my book: Medical Communication between China and the West: Tang Zonghai and the Crisis of Modern Chinese Medicine, Taipei: Dongda Book Company, 2006, Chapter 5.

[21] Guo Aichun (ed.), No. 31 of Heat Theory, included in Interpretations to the Basic Inquiries of the Inner Canon of the Yellow Emperor, pp. 194–195.

[22] Li Jianmin,The Diet of the Ancients from the Perspective of "70-year-olds Can Eat Meat", *Recipes · Medicine · History*, Taipei: Nantian Book Company, 2000, pp. 323–324.

[23] Lin Naishen,*Chinese Food Culture,* Taipei: Nantian Book Company, 1992, pp. 76–77.

China period. For example: the amount of food and drink can reflect the severity of febrile disease in most cases. Generally speaking, eating means that the body has "heat", and "Yang (heat) pathogenic factor" itself will "offset the grain",[24] so it is said that "heat will consume the grain and cause hunger".[25] In addition, "having heat" is not a good thing for "heat diseases" of the same nature: "Typhoid fever starts with fever for the first six days, which won't get better until after the ninth day. Appetite is not supposed to be back along during the recovery, otherwise it is a sign of disease residue. If food like bread doesn't bring the fever back, it is an indication of stomach Qi being retained, which ensures recovery".[26] According to the interpretation of Cheng Wuji (about 1066–1156), "disease residue" means stomach Qi that is not totally exhausted by the disease. It is normally understood that "the sick can hardly eat, but if they eat a lot, fever will definitely follow".[27] During the time of fever, sudden appetite or overeating are both signs of deterioration of the disease, which is also consistent with the statement of "excessive food brings the disease back" in the *Internal Canon.* On the contrary, if the heat in the body can be removed, the appetite will come back, which is a good condition. It is said, "appetite comes with the removal of heat is a sign of recovery".[28]

In general, eating is not recommended before the recovery of febrile disease. It is recorded in *Treatise on Typhoid Fever*: "The symptom of typhoid fever is relieved, but the patient is still not feeling well at the beginning of recovery. It is hard to digest food with the weak stomach Qi. With less food, the sick would feel better and recover sooner... This is why the newly recovered can not digest food".[29] Due to the fact that the stomach Qi has not been completely recovered, eating too much food is not conducive to the recuperation after the fever, which is the most important fever food taboo since the Qin and Han Dynasties. It is also called "food damage" in medical books, and it is quite clearly explained:

---

[24] (Han) Zhang Zhongjing, annotated by (Song) Cheng Wuji, collated by Wang Yong, Differentiating Pulse and Syndrome of Yang Ming Disease and Therapy VIII, *Annotations of Treatise on Typhoid Fever*, Beijing: People's Health Publishing House, 2005, p. 198.

[25] (Han) Zhang Zhongjing, annotated by (Song) Cheng Wuji, collated by Wang Yong, Differentiating Pulse and Syndrome of Yang Ming Disease and Therapy VIII, *Annotations of Treatise on Typhoid Fever*, p. 226.

[26] (Han) Zhang Zhongjing,compiled by (Jin) Wang Shuhe, annotated by Li Shunbao, Differentiation of Vomit and Therapy X, *Golden Treatise Pulse Canon*, Beijing: Xueyuan Publishing House, 2006, p. 58.

[27] (Han) Zhang Zhongjing, annotated by (Song) Cheng Wuji, collated by Wang Yong, Differentiating Pulse and Syndrome of Yang Ming Disease and Therapy XII, *Annotations of Treatise on Typhoid Fever*, pp. 256–257.

[28] The foundation of "essence" in the body comes from the grain Qi. "Those who can't eat have no essence". Food is not prohibited, but it is only good to have a restored appetite after the fever is removed. Quoted from (Han) Zhang Zhongjing,compiled by (Jin) Wang Shuhe, annotated by Li Shunbao, Differentiation of Febrile Disease with Yin Plus Yang and Therapy XXIX, *Golden Treatise Pulse Canon*, pp. 59, 108.

[29] (Han) Zhang Zhongjing, compiled by (Jin) Wang Shuhe, annotated by Li Shunbao, Differentiation on the Fatigue Syndrome Due to Yin-Yang Disorder and Therapy XII, *Golden Treatise Pulse Canon*, p. 65.

> "If the newly recovered patient forces down food, heat will be stored, resulting in the double Yangs of grain Qi and heat, the so called "food damage".[30] Before the heat pathogen is expelled from the body, the grain Qi will fight against it, causing the old disease to recur. This is a generalized dietary taboo after illness. Although we can't eat too much at a time, it's not an absolute "fast". As the saying goes, "fasting kills many ". Instead of indulging in food, patients should control their intake.[31] If the taboo is accidentally violated, there is also a solution: "Overeating would cause the accumulation of food in the stomach, which can be released by Chinese rhubarb".[32] In this case, the best way to recuperate is to "damage the grain", and the most appropriate drug is rhubarb that can purge the grain Qi.[33]

There are many related taboos that can not be listed in detail here.[34] The relatively complete taboos on recuperation after a fever first appeared in the *Treatise on the Origin of Various Diseases*. Similar books are commonly seen in TCM publications, such as the *Medical Notes in the Awakening Room*, which recorded: "After typhoid fever, meat and sex are forbidden. Those who go against it will not be cured".[35] In modern times, He Lianchen concentrated on the taboos in ancient books, and extracted them as follows: (1) Fatigue symptoms: at the beginning of the recovery from febrile disease, the body fluid has not recovered, the blood and Qi are still weak. Early labor would generate internal heat, which would get into the main and collateral channels, leading to disease. So all kinds of work, from combing hair to bathing, should be carefully handled. (2) Food damage: a person with a new fever has a weak spleen and stomach, and has not recovered the grain Qi. Any red meat, intestinal blood, or greasy fish would result in sever dysentery, which is incurable. Baked bread, fried meat, chestnuts and dates are all hard to digest, which would bring about stuffing into the stomach and cause constipation, eventually causing fever and leading to disease.[36] These expositions are an important knowledge in Chinese febrile

---

[30] This is a note by Cheng Wuji. (Han) Zhang Zhongjing, compiled by (Jin) Wang Shuhe, annotated by Li Shunbao, Differentiation on the Fatigue Syndrome Due to Yin-Yang Disorder and Therapy XIV, *Annotations of Treatise on Typhoid Fever*, p. 280.

[31] (Qing) Chen Menglei (ed.), compiled by Yang Jialuo, *Food Taboos, Ancient and Modern Book Collection. Art Dictionary.Epidemic Gate, Vol. 45,* Taipei: Dingwen Book Company, 1985, p. 3317.

[32] "Overnight food accumulation" is called "overnight food" by Zhongjing, and "overnight grain " by Cheng Wuji, all of which share the same meanings. (Han) Zhang Zhongjing, compiled by (Jin) Wang Shuhe, annotated by Li Shunbao, Differentiation on the Fatigue Syndrome Due to Yin-Yang Disorder and Therapy XIV, *Annotations of Treatise on Typhoid Fever*, p. 280.

[33] However, rhubarb is too strong a laxative, which is also bad for recuperation after illness. For example, "If you consume rice porridge for a few days and are still constipated, add angelica, aster and ophiopogon japonicus into the prescription. If you have enough stool fluid, dry feces will get through. If rhubarb is misused, the blood and Yin fluid will be damaged.It is to be watched closely." Quoted from He Lianchen (ed.), revised by Wang Zhipu et al., *Updated Popular Treatise on Typhoid Fever,* p. 495.

[34] For the study of early taboos, see Pi Kuoli, *Pedigree of "Food Taboos"—on Fever in the Qin and Han Dynasties,* 2008 (4.1), pp. 81–114.

[35] (Ming) Miao Xiyong, Doomed to Death upon Breaking the Taboos, *Medical Notes in the Awakening Room.* Beijing: Ancient Chinese Medicine Publishing House, 2000, p. 163.

[36] (Qing) Dai Tianzhang,revised by He Lianchen, Vol. 1. General Theory of Febrile Diseases.Therapies of Febrile Diseases Syndrome, included in *Revised Generalizations on Febrile Diseases*, p. 33.

disease studies. The point is that patients suffering from febrile diseases must have the control of meat intake and have sufficient rest. As for sexual behavior, we will discuss it at the end of this chapter. The focus here is just the problem of diet. The details of the knowledge that has been constantly supplemented and derived since after the writing of *Internal Canon* are different, but the content is consistent with those taboos. Until the Qing Dynasty, this knowledge was still very important for patients suffering from fever. A story in *A Dream of Red Mansions* shows that "fasting" is helpful for fever recuperation.

... Doctor Wang came and felt his pulse. He was puzzled and asked: "Yesterday was better. How can it get weaker today? Is it from overeating, or anxiety? The external symptoms have cleared up. The lack of recuperation after sweating is no good". Saying so, he went out and wrote a prescription. When Baoyu looked at it, he found exorcising medicines being removed and poria cocos, rehmannia, angelica and other mental and blood nourishing medicines being added... Later that day, he came back with the excuse of not feeling well. Although Qingwen suffers from severe disease, it is fortunate that she has always been a hard worker without much stress on her mind. Moreover, she has always been a light eater, and no damage was done from food. The custom and secret therapy of Jia's Mansion is fasting first, followed by some medicine, whenever a cold or cough occurred. So when falling ill the day before, she starved for two or three days, and then picked some medicine to take. Now by doing some work and with a few days of recuperation, she is getting better.[37]

The woman in the story suffered from a fever, which had already improved a lot, but her illness came back, and the doctor suspected that she was "overeating". The so-called Jia's secret recipe, "fasting", was also a way to control diet. This is the knowledge derived from the taboo of the knowledge of febrile diseases, which originates from the ever lasting TCM classics. Perhaps the febrile diseases in the Ming and Qing Dynasties mostly revolved around the debate between typhoid and warm disease, but the food taboo theory of the warm disease school still largely inherited the connotation of the typhoid fever school. After the Republic of China period, the theory of dietary taboos were still in medical books. He Lianchen said, "In either typhoid fever or febrile disease, even the major pathogen has to be retreated, the heat still remains and the vitality has been weakened. The stomach is deficient and the spleen is stagnant. The disease would come back anytime when the recuperation is improper, and the taboos are ignored."[38]

---

[37] (Qin) Cao Xueqin, annotated by Gao Er, *A Dream of Red Mansions, Vol, 2, Episode 53,* Taipei: Li Ren Bookstore, 1984, p. 819. From the narrative of the text, Qingwen felt feverish with a headache and stuffy nose due to frequent access to cold and warm environments (see Chapter 51, pp. 791–792, and Chapter 52, p. 805). Qingwen finally died of "girl phthisis".But Chen Cunren speculated that what she got was called "lung phlegm and asthma", which is "lobar pneumonia" in Western medicine. See Chen Cunren & Song Qi, *Medical Examination of the Dream of Red Mansions*, Guilin: Guangxi Normal University Press, 2006, p. 111.

[38] He Lianchen (ed.), revised by Wang Zhipu et al.,*Updated Popular Treatise on Typhoid Fever,* p. 487.

The contents of these taboos are mostly copied from medical books of the past.[39] Drinks, fat delicacies, raw and cold food should be eliminated, otherwise it will lead to "blocked meridians by greasiness and pathogenic heat being kept inside". Although the spirit is vigorous for a while, it is still far from a full recovery. However, grains and some dishes can be ingested in a measured way. "How happy it is to gradually transport the pathogenic heat stored in the body out of the pores!".[40]

During the Republic of China period, Western medicine became more influential. Although medical institutions were still not popularized throughout the country, the medical knowledge of Western medicine had played an important role in home diet. In his book *On Infectious Diseases*, Yu Yunxiu introduced many famous infectious diseases. Besides the diagnosis and treatment methods, the most noteworthy part is that there is the unique knowledge area such as "tips for rest in peace", "tips during recovery" and "tips for the caring of the sick", which covers most of the precautions for recuperation after illness.[41] This detailed classification is likely to prompt TCM to attach importance to the knowledge of recuperation in classical theories, reinterpret and elaborate it and start a dialogue with Western medicine. Some TCM followers began to believe that medical theory must be put into daily practice. If patients could not understand it, it would lose the significance of medicine as a practical science. Jiang Wenfang said, "Medical knowledge is purely a practical knowledge. It is a review of Chinese medicine. With thousands of years of experience, it is far more magical in curing diseases than mechanical Western medicine. The mystery of this theory is really difficult for the public to understand. The beginners feel that they are at a loss as how to get the essence. This is a key part that is being attacked by the Western medicine, and is also one of the major reasons why TCM study stagnated".[42] So the integration of classical theory into daily practice is one of the efforts made by TCM during the Republic of China period. Yang Zemin also pointed out that the new Chinese medicine should develop all the methods needed when serving the treatment of diseases. There is an old saying: "In today's Chinese medicine, taking the medicine orally is the only way we know. What we don't know is that decoction is only one of the therapeutic methods, rather than the only method. Xu Lingtai held that "decoction itself is not enough to cure all the diseases". Bianque had a theory that "ordinary people worry about all kinds of diseases, while doctors worry about not having enough therapies". As the result of scientific prosperity, modern

[39] For example, "Pang An often said:After the recovery from a disease, people should first eat clear porridge soup, followed by thicker porridge soup, and eventually thick porridge. They should also eat less, and never overeat. Alcohol and meat should particularly be forbidden.The fever would come back if there is a lack of care.This is called 'food damage'. Wang Shixiong said that the recovered was not supposed to eat porridge, crucian carp, puffer fish and the like unless the urine was clear and the tongue coating was clean. Alcohol,greasy, sweet, fresh or nutritious food are to be gradually taken after the first solid defecation. Hasty eating would bring the disease back. "He Lianchen (ed.),revised by Wang Zhipu et al., *Updated Treatise on Typhoid Fever,* p. 495.

[40] He Lianchen (ed.),revised by Wang Zhipu et al., *Updated Treatise on Typhoid Fever,* pp. 495–496.

[41] Yu Yunxiu, *On Infectious Diseases*, pp. 14–15.

[42] Qin Bowei, *Practical Chinese Medicine,* Taipei: New Wenfeng Publishing Company, 1987, Jiang Wenfang's preface, p. 3.

medicine has more therapies, but Chinese medicine not only stopped evolving, even the old therapeutic methods invented by predecessors have no longer been in use. In today's world, when transportation is convenient and the competition for survival is fierce, the diseases of humans are increasing, while the TCM therapies tend to be decreasing."[43] This means that in the past, there were many effective ways to treat diseases in addition to oral decoction, which should be actively elaborated and developed. Western medicine has gradually been accepted in Chinese society, which also has a positive stimulus for Chinese medicine. In terms of knowledge of recuperating febrile diseases, Chinese medicine has begun to pay attention to practical theories and techniques in the daily recuperation of patients. Among them, the core knowledge related to disease and diet belongs to the category of nutrition in Western medicine, which has attracted the attention of TCM. Yang Zemin said:

> The continuity of life depends on the intake of nutrients, and the intake of nutrients depends entirely on the supply of dietary materials. Therefore, the amount and the appropriateness of food taken have a profound impact on individual health. Those who study diet to keep healthy are called food doctors in ancient times and dietetics in modern times. The study of the food taboos for diseases is called food therapy in ancient times and dietotherapy in modern times...Diet and disease are as inseparable as a figure and its shadow. Water can carry a boat, and it can also capsize a boat. Diet can be beneficial, and it can also be harmful. Only those who are knowledgeable about medicine are good enough to discuss diagnosis and treatment. Only those who are knowledgeable about the function of food are qualified enough to discuss medicine.[44]

The importance of diet in medical treatment, after the popularization of western nutrition related knowledge, has partly affected the thinking of the development of traditional medicine. Chinese medicine also recalled the ancient "food medicine", to find the support from classical knowledge in the dialogue with the nutrition of modern science.

9.3 An Example of the Transformation of Modern Body View—Qi and Resistance

The previous chapter discusses the personal hygiene aspect of TCM. Although personal health is the basis of public health, overemphasizing "individuals" is not the modern goal that public health experts would like to see.[45] It was a fact that the public power of national health was not in play during the Republic of China period. What's more, the New Life Movement, a large-scale health movement known as the Golden Decade, actually focused on individuals. Many research achievements were also made. Instead of emphasizing how good personal hygiene is, the author tries to explain that the background and atmosphere of this era might have helped to the

[43] Yang Zemin, III.Therapies (3) On External Treatment, *Medical Talk in Seclusion*, pp. 140–141.

[44] Yang Zemin, (18) Diet Therapy,*Medical Talk in Seclusion*, pp. 158–159.

[45] Bi Rugang, *Public Health*, p. 1.

improvement of TCM hygiene. In addition, in the process of development, TCM has been influenced by many western medical concepts, more or less bringing many traditional concepts, such as blood Qi and essence Qi, into the modern scope.

TCM attached great importance to the theory of personal hygiene and disease resistance. In addition to some connections between residence and space in the theory of miasma, the most important one is the "healthy Qi" in the traditional body view. Before modern times, there had been plenty of discussions on preserving vital energy to resist diseases in the TCM theory of febrile diseases. Wu Youxing said:

> The pathogenic factors can be from nature or infection. The same disease might have different symptoms. The breath of ordinary people is connected with nature. When the Qi is full, it is not easy for the pathogenic factors to enter. If the Qi happens to be deficient, external pathogenic factors may take advantage when breathing. Once upon a time, there were three people who walked early in the fog, the one with an empty stomach died, the one who drank fell ill, and the one who was well-fed was fine. What difference does it make for the epidemic pathogenic factors? For people of prime age with vitality, no matter strong or weak, the disease would be triggered if his healthy Qi is not sufficient, but this is not exclusive. Those extensively exposed to pathogenic factors would definitely contract the disease, the less exposed might contract it later when the pathogenic factors overcome the health Qi. It also depends on if people are hungry or full, worried and angry. When the healthy Qi is harmed, the pathogenic factors will spread out and the blood circulation is blocked. The Yang Qi of the body is restrained by pathogenic factors, resulting in fever diseases.[46]

Epidemics can be infectious, but their "transmission" is closely related to individuals. If one is full of "healthy Qi", it is not easy for the pathogenic factors to invade. On the contrary, when the "healthy Qi" declines, the pathogenic factors can take advantage. After the pathogenic factors invade the human body, it may also "defeat the healthy" and temporarily hide in the human body. The pathogenic factors will reappear only when people do not pay attention to it or violate the taboos in their daily life, which eventually leads to fever. The epidemic knowledge of TCM does not pay special attention to the problem of "groups", considering the individual healthy Qi as the premise to avoid infection. Another example is Jiang Hantun's saying: "When the five epidemics come, it is easy for them to infect each other. The healthy Qi stored in the body can prevent the pathogenic factors from its toxicity".[47] It shows that enough healthy Qi can keep one from being infected. In addition, it is said in *A Study on Epidemic Rash*: "In ancient times, there was no epidemic rash or chicken pox until the beginning of the Han Dynasty. Why? This was because the world was opened up in Zichou and humans were born at dawn. People at that time were simple, with a primitive life style of eating raw meat, with less harm from emotions and desires, and there was no extravagant greasy food. It was a small world, so there was no epidemic nor rash. All happened during the Han Dynasty, which was planned by Heaven".[48]

---

46 (Ming) Wu Youxing,annotated by (Qing) Zheng Zhongguang, *The Origins of Diseases, Additional Annotations On Warm Epidemics*, Vol.I. p. 9.

47 (Qing) Jiang Hantun, Epidemic Diseases, *Principles for the Compliance with Times*, Beijing: China TCM Press, 1993 (04), p. 58.

48 (Qing) Yu Shiyu, The Origin of Epidemic Eruption, An Experience of Epidemic Eruption, included in Li Shunbao (ed.), *Complete Book of Warm Diseases, Vol. III*, p. 118.

This shows that people in ancient times paid attention to diet, life, emotional and other aspects of recuperation, so as not to be infected with epidemic rash, pox and other diseases.

In addition to emphasizing healthy Qi, these discourses also emphasize the "personal" hygiene methods and precautions of daily life. Personal negligence in daily life is often worse than epidemic infections. "Even those who get the worst (of the epidemic) will not die with proper treatment. If one is seriously sick, exhausted, old, it is hopeless. Plus when its an epidemic, it is particularly incurable".[49] This shows the importance of self health management and (classical) hygiene when epidemics occurs. Chen Guofu said, "It is said that in treating this disease (infectious disease), TCM pays more attention to prevention than killing worms. For example, when there are no theft, either in the city or countryside, it shows that the police are doing a good job, not that there are physically no thieves. There are still thieves hiding, but they have no chance to take action when there is a good police department around. It makes sense. There are all kinds of microorganisms in the air. Why do some people get sick and others don't ? Of course, it is not all due to the number of micro worms, but the health condition of one's own body."[50] This kind of body view not only has the thought of isolation and disinfection, but also inclines to the thinking of self-reliance. This "personal" hygiene is the management of a person's individual daily life that insulates itself from the group and the public. For example, Cao Bingzhang pointed out the importance of preventing autumn epidemic:

> It is advisable to abstain from drinking, because alcohol can damage the blood. If one is feeling dry, coughing and choking before being ill, it is recommended to have half a cup of pear juice and radish juice together, having them mixed up evenly, and stewed. If one's nose is hot and the stool is dry, it is recommended to have the decoction of 3.5 oz of jellyfish and five waternuts. For a slight sore throat, it is to have the decoction of 1.8 oz of black ginseng and 0.26 oz of mint leaves. If the syndrome is too severe, it is advised to refer to the previous treatment and ask a doctor for a diagnosis and treatment. Not all the diseases can be cured with a few herbs.[51]

Before the disease occurred, Cao had provided effective and feasible simple treatment. This kind of technology, which is between treatment and diet, was the asset of TCM epidemic resistance at that time. In addition, Cao talked about the way of dressing: "When the epidemic is prevalent, clothes and bed quilts should be washed and changed frequently and be kept clean. Clothes should be loose, as tight clothes will affect blood circulation and it is easy to cause the body to sweat, so it must be appropriate. Clothes should not be too warm, or it would cause sweat, and one's pores

---

[49] (Ming) Wu Youxing, supplemented by (Qing) Zheng Zhongguang, The Difference between the Hidden Pathogenic Factor and the Active Pathogenic Factor, *Supplementary Notes on Epidemics*, Vol. I, p. 46.

[50] Chen Guofu, The Way of Health, included in Mr. Chen Guofu Scholarship Fund Management Committee (ed.), *Selected Works of Mr. Chen Guofu's Medical and Health Thoughts*, p. 180.

[51] Cao Bingzhang,Chapter VII: Prevention of Autumn Epidemic, On the Essence of Typhoid and Miscellaneous Diseases,included in *Collection of Rare Modern TCM. Warm Diseases*, pp. 772.

would be open, which would contract external pathogenic factors".[52] The external pathogenic factors emphasized here are diseases and pathogens caused by external climate, not bacteria. This is very important, due to the fact that when the theory of bacteria gradually became popular, TCM attached more importance to recuperation than preventing the harm of bacteria. Chen Cunren also took the prevention of tuberculosis as an example, illustrating the individual effort of disease prevention: "The way to prevent tuberculosis is to be sanitary and clean, which is still a passive way to prevent tuberculosis. To nourish Yin is the only positive way to prevent tuberculosis. If we want to prevent the disease from the environment in which we live, it is impossible, and there is no way to prevent it. The only option is to nourish one's Yin and cultivate the essence to fundamentally increase the body's resistance against germs. That is, it can be infected by tuberculosis and also be eliminated naturally. Therefore, if there is enough Yin, even if the husband suffers from tuberculosis, the wife will not be infected for several years. From this point of view, blind fear and crazy cleaning is a ridiculous and passive way."[53] Interestingly, strengthening the physical qualities according to the characteristics of the disease (the concept of "nourishing Yin and cultivating the essence") is a shortcut to disease resistance, which may be enlightening to modern Chinese medicine and is worth further study. In addition, Chen Guofu took diphtheria as an example and said: "Diphtheria is an infectious disease, which is caused by the invasion of diphtheria bacteria. Laryngeal pain is an inevitable symptom of this disease. When talking and swallowing, the pain often worsens, even with head swimming, which is very sad. Those with a poor physique, maladjustment of cold and heat, inflammation of tonsils, and weak resistance are most likely to be infected. Without these causes of infection, they will never be infected."[54] He emphasized that the "cause" of being infected was not bacteria, but the weakness of resistance caused by the superposition of various adverse factors, which were highly related to the so-called body view of Qi in TCM, the feeling and imbalance of a person's constitution and external Qi. There was also an advertisement in the early Republic of China period that added vitality to the body, which could resist germs and prevent infectious diseases. When it is unnecessary to explain the pharmacology, "invigorating Qi" is often a very useful term, including for treating exogenous fever (see Fig. 9.1).[55]

---

[52] Cao Bingzhang, Chapter VII: Prevention of Autumn Epidemic, On the Essence of Typhoid and Miscellaneous Diseases, included in *Collection of Rare Modern TCM. Warm Diseases*, pp. 772.

[53] Although tuberculosis is not strictly an exogenous disease, it involves bacteria and body constitution, and it is a major disease during the Republic of China period, which is why this is cited as an example. Quoted from Chen Cunren, Popular Medical Discourse, included in Lu Zheng(ed.), *Collection of Rare Modern TCM.Medical Talk*, p. 1000. In addition, during the Republic of China period, pulmonary tuberculosis was considered to be caused by prolonged exogenous cold, which is also noteworthy. Chen Guofu said: "Most lung diseases are mostly caused by colds, without which it is hard for lung disease to develop".

[54] Chen Guofu, The Way of Health, included in Mr. Chen Guofu Scholarship Fund Management Committee (ed.), *Selected Works of Mr. Chen Guofu's Medical and Health Thoughts*, p. 155.

[55] Shanghai Shen Bao Newspaper Office (ed.), *Shen Bao*,(Shanghai: Shanghai Bookstore Publishing House, 1982–1987), May 31, 1918, p. 4.

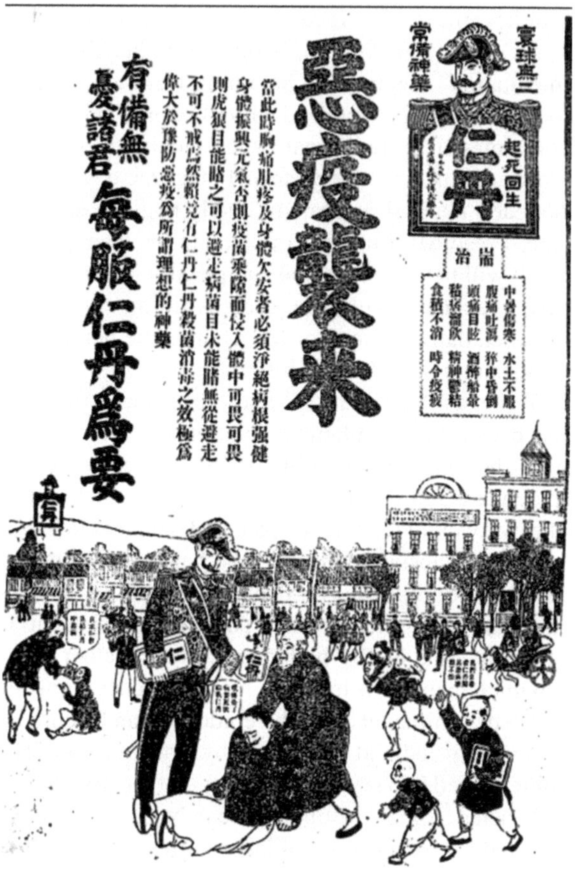

Fig. 9.1 Benevolent pill against the epidemic

There are many ways to strengthen the physique, and a large number of examples can be found in traditional medical records. *The Collection of Chinese Health Preservation Theories* (1930) expounds: "The main points of health preservation are spirit, material and daily life. In terms of the spirit, we should be super happy; in terms of material, we should be comfortable with clothing, food and living; in terms of daily life, we should be quiet and dynamic with moderation, understand truth, find fun, so that we can be wise and maintain our health, eventually achieving the goal of longevity".[56] This kind of health concept during the Republic of China period is usually related to Chinese traditional health science, and the knowledge involved is the recuperation technology that individuals can pursue in their daily life. Most people also use "health preservation" to correspond to the popular "health" discourse at that time, and explain the traditional content from the perspective of modernity, but still on the basis of tradition. Moreover: "Nowadays, people who are concerned

[56] Shen Zongyuan, et al.(eds.), Two Kinds of Chinese Traditional Health Preservation. The Collection of Chinese Health Preservation Theories, p. 79.

with hygiene mostly focus on sitting in silence. The skill of sitting in silence, that is, the skill of meditation, is the key to health".[57] It probably reflects the idea that "meditation" is related to breathing fresh air, which can help prevent lung disease, cough, etc. Ding Fubao had a lot of related publications.[58] Another example is Qian Mu, a master of traditional Chinese culture, who said, "I was weak. I became sick every autumn since the year of 1911. One day, I read a little Japanese book, saying that early death is a great sin. Daily hygiene deserves much attention. In my spare time, I read Mr. Lu Fang's poems in his later years, which were quite inspiring to me. It will be a great shame and penalty if I don't have a long life, but it is a pain to have a regulated daily life, such as sitting still, walking in the countryside."[59] The so-called daily hygiene of Mr. Qian is the pursuit of a healthy lifestyle, rather than the meaning of public health.

Terms as "constitution" and "resistance" that are not mentioned in TCM have also been used to explain the relationship between body state and disease prevention since the Republic of China period. For example, Cao Bingzhang believed that an epidemic is relevant to people's physique, such as being fat or thin, strong or weak. The overweight tend to be "pale and deficient in Yang", with phlegm and dampness, and easy to absorb dampness and heat, leading to "persistent stickiness". Physique can only be improved by enhancing Yang Qi and resolve dampness. On the other hand, the skinny tend to be "pale and deficient in Yin". Yin deficiency is easy to cause "internal fire", which plays a role together with dampness. So body fluid must be supplemented to improve Yin deficiency constitution.[60] One's physique is the key to determine whether the epidemic can be cured, and physique, like healthy Qi, can be adjusted and controlled by drugs or diet. This is a technology that can be implemented in daily life space beyond the use of hospitals, the public health system and bacteriological testing, and can be easily mastered by ordinary people, without the need for bacteriological laboratories or professional testing techniques. As early as the Qing Dynasty, Cao Tingdong said, "Every disease must be first examined from its symptoms, to find the original causes. From the top to the heel, what causes the cold, heat, and itching? From morning to evening, what are the living and eating habits? As long as the data of the disease is collected, it is easy to have it cured".[61] He emphasized that the patient's self diagnosis, diet, living condition, sense of body were easily perceived by oneself. Another example is what Qin Bo said in modern times:

---

[57] Qiu Qingyuan (ed.), On Meditation Heal Preservation, Medical Talks, included in Lu Zheng (ed.),*Collection of Rare Modern Traditional Chinese*, p. 366.

[58] Ding Fubao, *Essence of Meditation*, Shanghai: Shanghai Medical Book Company, 1920, pp. 57–58.

[59] Qian Mu, IV. Private Model School and the Fourth Higher Primary School in Wuxi County, *Memoirs of Parents and Teachers in My 80s*, Beijing: SDX Joint Publishing Company, 2006, p. 91.

[60] Cao Bingzhang, Chapter IV: Diagnosis of Autumn Epidemic, On the Essence of Typhoid and Miscellaneous Diseases, included in *Collection of Rare Modern TCM. Warm Diseases*, p. 752.

[61] (Qing) Cao Tingdong, et al., Two Kinds of Traditional Chinese Health Preservation. Common Sayings of Lao Lao, p. 30.

> The resistance to pathogens varies with the development of the body. In judging diseases, we should pay more attention to the constitution. Those with a strong physique are less likely to fall ill, and are easy to recover even if they do. Those who are physically weak have weak resistance to the inducements, and are easy to suffer from diseases which eventually become chronic. There are also people whose physique are changeable. Some are strong when they are young, but become weak without recuperation in their lives. Others can be weak when young, but would become strong with recuperation later in life. Once the body is fully developed, the physique is not easy to change.[62]

We can see that, though there were still some statements about supplementing "Healthy Qi" during the Republic of China period, the words and statements with the same meaning were actually partially replaced by terms like "resisting pathogens", "physique" or "supplementing nutrients". For example, it was contained in the research that the functions of various "vitamins" and clarified that the lack of certain nutrients would lead to the weakness of organs, especially digestive organs, thus reducing "the vitality of the body", and germs and microorganisms would invade easily.[63] Another example is the advertisement of "cod-liver oil", which also shows that it can resist germs and prevent exogenous diseases (see Fig. 9.2).[64] At that time, such information was quite diverse, and might also contain a lot of exaggerations and lies. For example, *Vitamins and Life* criticized many people for claiming that vitamin A was a "vitamin against infectious diseases". Taking more of this component can prevent cold, cough and other common infectious diseases. Even for fever, "take a dose of vitamin A, and you can recover immediately".[65] This kind of book was introduced to China, where personal health preservation is emphasized. Its title directly uses the word "health", and puts forward a body of knowledge that deserves the attention of individuals, without referring to the responsibility of the state and policy planning at all.

In addition, the so-called "constitution" discussion, in the knowledge of Chinese medicine during the Republic of China period, was exclusively related to the discussion of individual body Qi. Cao Bingzhang explained the relationship between human body strength and epidemic disease. He said: "Between the strong and the weak, the strong can not easy to be attacked by the pathogenic factors, while the weak are. It is easy for those having strong Qi to recover as they are less likely to be attacked by the pathogenic factors; while for those who are weak in their Qi, it is hard to recover and they are more likely to be attacked by the pathogenic factors". Wu Jutong said: "In the summer heat, those strong in spirit will not be affected by the pathogenic factors; the less strong would have temporary dizziness, which might last half a day and the

---

62 Qin Bowei, Practical Chinese Medicine, p. 60.

63 There are also quite a few studies on the influence of organs or glands on the interpretation of diseases related to the Chinese and Western body views. What is presented here is only part of it due to the limited space. Regarding the relationship between food and health preservation, see Du Yaquan et al.'s translation, compiled by Oriental Magazine (ed.), *Food and Health*, Shanghai: Commercial Press, 1924, pp. 95–96.

64 Shanghai Shen Bao Newspaper Office (ed.), *Shen Bao,* January. 10, 1937, p. 3.

65 L.J. Harris, Translated by Huang Feng & Lin Jieniang, *Vitamins and Life*, Changsha: Commercial Press, 1938, pp. 165–166.

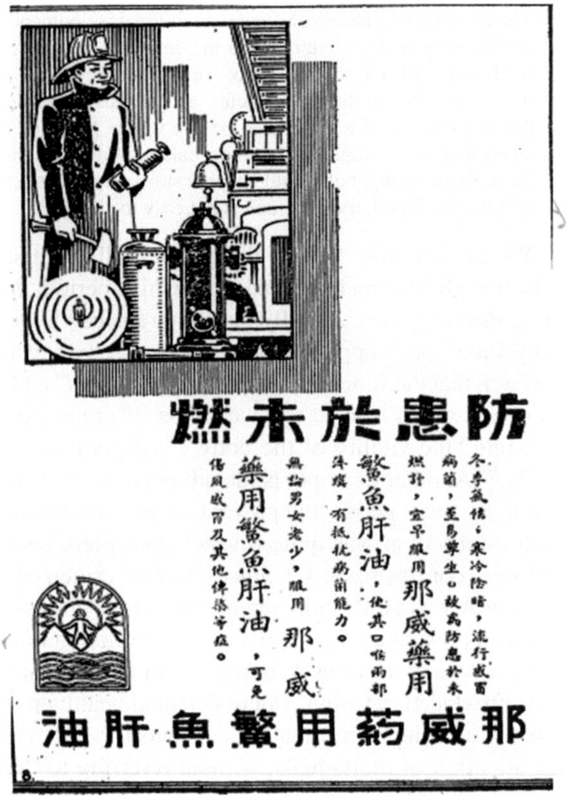

Fig. 9.2 Nawei medicinal cod liver oil

weak would be sick. Some may not instantly fall ill, but the sickness is contained in the bones and flesh, which is a sign of Qi deficiency. The heat pathogen cannot be transmitted until the cooling down of the golden autumn, which is also the time for the occurrence of summer diseases. This process would be postponed till late autumn or early winter for those who are deficient in Qi and the symptoms would be more severe".[66] The more deficient in Qi, the later the disease occurs, and the deeper it lies in the body. When the external seasons change, the combination of the Qi of the body and the external Qi will induce it, followed by an epidemic after. These arguments point out that if a person is strong and healthy enough, it is less likely for epidemic to invade. Furthermore, TCM also discusses the Qi of the body and the resistance together, as Shao Yanzhi explained:

> From Zhongjing's prescriptions, it can be seen that soaking in hot water is to sweat, warming up the meridians is to regain Yang, and vomiting is to dispel toxins. These are all the ways to keep the human body away from germs to enable the body's resistance. Germs are villains, and the resistance is a gentleman. When the gentleman is prevailing, the villains are retreating. This is the way it should be. In biological terms, the body is a field that germs try to live in.

---

[66] Cao Bingzhang, Chapter 4: Diagnosis of Autumn Plague, On the Essence of Typhoid and Miscellaneous Diseases, included in *Collection of Rare Modern TCM. Warm Diseases*, pp. 752–753.

If the environment is more suitable for human than for germs, the germs will decline, which is called natural selection.[67]

"Resistance" is often discussed together with "healthy Qi". At that time, China's statement about being strong and able to produce resistance means a lot. In modern Chinese politics, how to rid China of the image of "a sick man" who is physically weak has always been a popular and important research topic.[68] In the scope of discussion on the history of febrile diseases in TCM, having a strong body also means having a good spirit and resistance at the same time, which can resist exogenous febrile diseases and even beat germs. For example, Yang Xiling said:

The Japanese Gensai Fujita shared the secret of physical and mental health on the relationship between mental function and infectious diseases. It is said that infectious diseases are caused by micro bacteria, which seems to have nothing to do with one's mental state, but this is not true. The relevance between them is extremely high. If one is mentally strong with good blood circulation, there is no room for micro bacteria to reproduce. The cells in the body are active and strong in resistance and one's lungs, stomach, and intestine have the ability to kill bacteria. However, if one is mentally weak, the fear of micro bacteria would slow down blood circulation and cell activity is reduced. Although there are few micro bacterias invading, all parts of the body tend to collapse and withdraw without fighting. So the white flag is raised and micro bacteria takes control. It definitely makes sense to look into the physical-mental- relationship of the body, and the prevention of strong mentality from the invasion of bacteria.[69]

In fact, Yang also focuses on the resistance of "individuals", including mental and physical strength, smooth blood circulation and regards it as an element of resisting germs. Even western science can be used to affirm the traditional health preservation of Chinese medicine, such as: "Meditation can regulate blood and spirit scientifically". This regulation can "strengthen the resistance" and eliminate the disease.[70] When it comes to diet, supplementary nutrition is the basis for developing resistance, which means both modern Chinese and Western medicine attach great importance to the knowledge of diet. Generally speaking, there are some different interpretations of the relationship between the nature of food and the body between China and the West, so there comes the different preferences of food. Yang Zemin said:

Chinese and Western people hold the opposite view of health preservation, that is, the dispute over vegetable and meat. Chinese sages believed in the nourishment of vegetables and the meaty delicacies were the toxins leading to rottenness. The key to health preservation lies in a sound spirit, unlike westerners who often hunt for bloody food to get fatty protein. The immortals take longevity as their goal of life and their food list is all of plants. In

---

[67] Shao Canzhi, The Impetus, Suxuan Medical Talk, included in Lu Zheng (ed.),*Collection of Rare Modern TCM.Medical Talk*, p. 641.

[68] Karl Gerth is a representative. He believed that modern Chinese consumer culture is closely linked with nationalism. See Karl Gerth, *China Made: Consumer Culture and the Creation of the Nation.*(Cambridge: Harvard University Asia Center, Harvard University Press, 2003).

[69] Yang Xiling, The Power of Mental Strength against Infectious Diseases, Medical Talk in the Garden. TCM Is Not Useless, *Collection of Rare Modern TCM.Medical Talk*, pp. 568–569.

[70] Yang Zemin, 3. Discussion on Law (I) Governance, *Medical Talk in Seclusion*, p. 133.

> the Song Dynasty, the Confucianists, in addition to their theoretical achievements, had also some sayings on health preservation, which were all about vegetables, let alone Buddhism that abstains from killing animals. Since Metchnikoff of Russia advocated the theory of self toxification in the intestines, Europeans have also gradually become vegetarians, particularly Germans nowadays. The maniacal Hitler was a lifelong vegetarian.[71]

Yang believed that the western diet culture emphasizes meat, while the Chinese diet is dominated by light vegetables as is commonly understood. In the early Taoist health literature, it was also advocated to take herbal medicine, rather than meat, for immortality.[72] In modern times, it has absorbed the knowledge of Western medicine, that is, chlorophyll in vegetables can "increase the resistance of cells and prohibit bacteria from growing".[73] Yang finally mentioned that Westerners have turned to vegetarianism in recent years, which in fact highlights his own recognition of the benefits of vegetarianism as is a Chinese staple class of food. Yang expressed in his article on diet therapy: "In modern times, nutritionists focus on the rich taste of flesh and blood, while our ancestors focus on the thin taste of self nourishment, which seems to be conflicting. However, flesh and blood can increase weight and bone can refresh the spirit. Therefore, the fat tend to be turbid, the skinny tend to be lucid, and those who prefer delicate food to coarse grain often have the stuffed stomachs, while those who prefer vegetables normally have healthy stomachs."[74] However, some Chinese doctors believe that the Chinese and Western diets are different, and the resulting physique, diseases and therapies should be different too. Shen Lin, a healer of epidemic febrile diseases, wrote in the book *On the Differences between Chinese and Western Pathogenesis:* "Westerners establish their countries by nomadism, who feed on mostly meat. The meat is warm by nature and tastes thick. Its temperature reaches to the skin, so Westerners often bathe in cold water. The cold can't harm the outside skin, but the disease comes from the inside. The Chinese diet is based on agriculture and grains are their major food. The grain is clear and tastes thin. Its temperature is lower than the skin, so that the cold invades. When the westerners bath in cold water, the cold gets into the meridian and causes pain. Western medicine smears it with iodine and takes aspirin, and the pain is gone. When the Chinese feel the wind pathogen outside, the wind heat hurts the muscles and causes pain. If they smear it with iodine, it will be treating heat with heat."[75] These are some

---

[71] Yang Zemin, 15.Vegetarianism,*Medical Talk in Seclusion*, p. 258.

[72] As stated by Peng Zu in the *Stories of Immortals,* "Immortals either enter the clouds with their bodies, fly without wings, ride dragons and clouds to soar; or transform into birds and beasts, floating in the green clouds; or sneak through the rivers and oceans, soaring in famous mountains; or intake vitality and Zhicao". Zhicao is also known as Lingzhi, which ancient people believed to be the drugs only second to the treasures like gold, silver, and cinnabar. Taking multiple doses can make one immortal. There are a large number of records about Zhicao in the *Baopu Zi Inner Chapter—Immortal Medicine.* (Jin) Ge Hong, annotated by Zhou Qicheng, *Updated Translated Biography of Immortals*, Taipei: Sanmin Book Company, 2009, pp. 18–19.

[73] Yang Zemin, 15.Vegetarianism,*Medical Talk in Seclusion,* p. 259.

[74] Yang Zemin,18. Diet Therapy,*Medical Talk in Seclusion*, p. 161.

[75] Shen Lin, Interpretations of Febrile Diseases, included in Cao Bingzhang(ed.), *Great Achievements in Chinese Medicine*, Vol. 18, p. 81.

interesting differences between Chinese and Western views on disease, diet and body constitution.

Fever is the beginning of a series of complications. In the treatment process of these diseases, even though there are different priorities or conditions, we can always see some related terms frequently reoccurring for their diagnosis and treatment, typically "nourishing Yin and clearing away heat", "light taste" or "promoting fluid and nourishing Qi".[76] The Chinese medicine treatment and recuperation system represented by these words is quite different from the recuperation methods commonly used by Western medicine to treat various febrile diseases, like taking supplements such as beef broth and iron liquor. Wu Xihuang once said:

> The Western medicine therapy for this disease (typhoid fever) is to use milk, beef, mutton, chicken, duck, white pigeon porridge and the like, which would only add heat to aggravate the disease. For a severe febrile disease, it is applicable at the beginning, which is hardly what I am knowledgeable about. To summarize it accurately, for this disease, fluid food is the only option. The rough hard food, or whatever food that is difficult to digest, is prohibited.[77]

Wu Xihuang also compared the severe febrile disease in western medicine (referring to the febrile disease with rapid fever) with typhoid fever. The western medicine also used more tonic foods, such as chicken, duck, cattle, sheep, pigeons and other supplements, which were different from the TCM treatment. Generally speaking, TCM advocates fasting and eating less when suffering from fever. Many foods have been clearly and specifically stipulated in the medical books of the past to prevent various new complications, such as "the newly recovered should steam the food if they were to eat dogs and mutton" or "raw dates", and "those who drink alcohol and eat leeks will have the disease reoccur".[78] In contrast, Western medicine advocates nourishing the body with "nutritious" food, which is in great conflict with TCM. Chen Guofu brought up the academic theory of TCM and western medicine by suggesting that people must eat less when suffering from exogenous cold, because rich and fat food would "increase the fecundity of bacteria", and also "make it difficult to drive out the invading cold".[79] Yang Zemin cited the theory of nutrition to explain the reason that nutrition and food intake must be reduced for the sick. He said:

---

[76] As for the key in recuperating febrile disease, Wu Tang once said, "Recovering from warm diseases, Yin is the most important thing to nourish Yin. It is not to have hard rich food too soon. For the constitution of Yang deficiency, it will be revealed right after the recovery from warm disease. In this case, the nourishment of Yin is not applicable, or the Yang fire would be extinguished". (Qing) Wu Tang, *Systematic Differentiation of Warm Diseases*, included in Li Liukun (ed.), *Complete Medical Works of Wu Jutong*, p. 85. Probably, the residual heat after the disease is not cleared out yet, and many taboos should be observed. The body can't be nourished until after the heat subsides. However, as the time division of the course for the disease is very unclear, rules are supposed to be observed generally.

[77] Wu Xihuang, On Febrile Diseases, Plague and Warm Toxin– the Light and Severe Syndromes of Febrile Diseases in Western Medicine, Interpretations of Chinese and Western Febrile Diseases, p. 24.

[78] (Ming) Miao Xiyong, Doomed to Death upon Breaking the Taboos, *Medical Notes in the Awakening Room*. Beijing: Ancient Chinese Medicine Publishing House, 2000, p. 163.

[79] Chen Guofu said, "Diet matters if we want to avoid cold. If we eat too much, the blood will go into the stomach to help digestion and concentrate inside. The defensive power against the external

The human body needs a certain amount of nutrients, which is the case for each average person in terms of the amount of food. When one is sick, the amount of nutrition required will change, and thus the appetite will also change, by increasing or decreasing or having no appetite at all. If one still keeps the diet as before, due to carelessness, the digestive organs as the stomach and intestines would be swollen and painful, and even vomiting would occur. If the food is stagnated in the intestines too long, it would rot and ferment, and become toxic, which would stimulate the stomach and intestines, causing not only pain and vomiting, but also toxic fever, delirium, and even convulsions (common in children). These are all the consequences of overeating, which is commonly seen.[80]

Probably, the TCM doctors who absorbed western medical theories would also agree that diet and nutrition intake or the prevention of excessive intake deserve attention. Western medicine may share the understanding, but the taboos of eating after a fever are still a part of the concern for TCM. The following is a further review of this aspect.

9.4 The Immortality of Typhoid in Hunger

Even in the new era, the connotation of "typhoid fever", a classical disease name, also integrates the traditional food taboo and preservation theory into a new concept of disease recuperation. However, as Yu Xinzhong said, TCM did not pay attention to the so-called food hygiene concept in modern times. In particular, typhoid fever is a kind of fever disease originally transmitted from the digestive tract, which has a lot to do with drinking water. It was an important project of Western medicine at that time to regulate the hygiene of food and the identification of the pathogenic factors. For example, the statement "typhoid bacillus, which has flagella, is active and invades the human body by using food and drink as its media",[81] is based on the understanding of microorganisms and disease vectors. However, TCM pays more attention to the body's adjustment when suffering from typhoid fever. During the Republic of China period, it was first proposed to treat typhoid fever in the *Treatment of Damp and Warm Epidemics*, which is similar to the convergence of TCM and Western medicine.

The damp febrile epidemic disease is caused by the hidden pathogenic factors in the stomach and intestines, which disables the digestive function. It is best to bear hunger and lie down quietly. It is easily hurt by not only greasy and fishy food, but also the food that burns and broils the viscera, which should be forbidden. The same is true for cold fruits and melons which chill the spleen and stomach. It's best to have radish soup and dried vegetable soup to dredge the stomach and intestines. It

is weakened. So we should temporarily reduce our appetite if we have a cold. Less food is helpful for recovery. It is well known that we should not eat fishy food, but we should also stay away from greasy food because it can increase the fecundity of bacteria and make it difficult to drive out the invading cold. That's why Chinese people always clean up first before taking supplements. " Chen Guofu, The Way of Health, included in Mr. Chen Guofu Scholarship Fund Management Committee (ed.), *Selected Works of Mr. Chen Guofu's Medical and Health Thoughts*, p. 156.

[80] Yang Zemin, 18. Diet Therapy, *Medical Talk in Seclusion*, pp. 159–160.

[81] Xu Renfu, Handouts on Practical Medicine, pp. 188–189.

would be helpful to have some Clearing Dew with some boiled water, or some fine bud tea to transport their body fluid. When it gets better, one can take some liquid nourishment, such as thin porridge, thin lotus root starch, and boiled beaten eggs. It's preferred to eat more often a day and less each time, only to appease hunger. It's not proper to have any kind of unripe fruit, oil or solid food until after the recovery. The sage Mr. Pang Anchang, said that the newly recovered should only have thin rice porridge, followed by thicker porridge, with less amount. It is not advised to have meat, liquor or any cold and greasy food too early. Mr. Wang Mengying said, "The newly recovered are not to have porridge nor fish until they have clear urine and a clean tongue coating; neither should they have greasy, sweet, highly nutritious food or liquor until they have a solid stool. It should only move forward slowly. Haste is likely to bring the disease back".[82]

He Lianchen, the editor in chief of this book, cited the theories of scholars of febrile diseases such as Pang Anchang in the Song Dynasty and Wang Mengying in the Qing Dynasty to strengthen his theory that illness must be controlled by diet. Greasiness, meat, wine, melons and fruits, raw and cold food, etc., are all taboos, while some liquid foods can be taken in moderation. When suffering from diseases, all "spleen nourishing drugs such as ginseng, astragalus, poria cocos and white atractylodes rhizome" can only promote the pathogenic heat in the body, and should be prohibited. If you eat the food with "greasy and sweet taste", it will only lead to "meridians being blocked by greasiness and pathogenic heat being kept inside". The best recuperation food in the early stages of the disease is "thin white porridge". Cautions should also be taken to the amount and meat is absolutely prohibited, which is completely consistent with the classical theory.[83]

Another important book on humidity and temperature is Hu Anbang's *The Great Treatise on Damp Warm Diseases*, which uses the food taboo theory of classical medicine to explain:

> Those with damp and warm diseases should be particularly cautious. Light food is good. When the fever is severe, there is no problem of having no food that might enhance the fever. When the fever abates and the patient has the appetite, it is proper to have fried rice soup, rice coke, porridge soup, lotus root flour served with boiled water, Bergamot Dew or malt tea. It is strictly forbidden to eat raw and cold meat, eggs, milk, spice or stinky food. It is not only applicable to damp warm diseases, but also to all fever related diseases. This is what is stated in the *Inner Canon*", overeating will retain the disease, while meat will bring back the disease".[84]

Hu pointed out that most of the edible things were light or liquid food. Foods like fish, eggs, milk, five spices, meat are prohibited. These food taboos are not

---

[82] Shaoxing Medical Association, Health and Prevention.Hygiene of the Sick, Treatment of Damp and Warm Epidemics, included in Li Shunbao (ed.), *Complete Book of Warm Diseases*, Vol. II, pp. 2099.

[83] (Qing) Dai Tianzhang,revised by He Lianchen, Vol. 1. General Theory of Febrile Diseases. Therapies of Febrile Diseases Syndrome, included in *Revised Generalizations on Febrile Diseases*, p. 77.

[84] Hu Anbang, 15. Mdcical Cases of Damp Warm Diseases, The Great Treatise on Damp Warm Diseases, included in Lu Zheng (ed.), *Collection of Rare Modern TCM. Warm Diseasess*, p. 672.

only applicable to damp febrile disease, but also to the recuperation of all febrile diseases. He explained in another medical case that this knowledge is important not only for patients, but also for family members in charge of care at home. An 18-year-old patient surnamed Zhou suffered from an external infection. After treatment, he gradually recovered, and his appetite also increased. One day, his mother went out and his brother and sister were entrusted to take care of him. "Out of his own wish, the patient had ten bowls of porridge and fifteen pieces of peach cake a day, still feeling it was not enough". As a result, the so-called food damage in classical medicine occurred, and his stomach was distended and his chest was stuffy, so he hurried to see the doctor again. Hu prescribed some medicine for him again, but the patient didn't come back any more. I'm afraid it was more ominous than propitious.[85] The morality of this instructive case is, in addition to warning patients of the importance of diet, to emphasize that since TCM recuperation is home based, the caregivers must also be well acquainted with the practical operation of this knowledge in daily life, so as not to worsen the patient's situation.

Another Chinese doctor noted for his emphasis on the knowledge of daily diet for typhoid fever should be Chen Cunren. He had done a thorough research on typhoid fever. He believed that typhoid fever was not difficult to treat, and it is all about the recuperation. He said: "Recently, typhoid fever is more prevalent than ever in spreading all over. The fever period of this disease is extremely long, which truly frustrated the patients. However, it is not a ferocious disease. Those not being cured were due to the three reasons: 1. Being physically weak and having too many variables. 2. overworking and refusing to rest. 3. lacking regulation in diet during and after the disease. Of the above three, the last one leads to the worst deterioration of the disease.[86] Physical weakness and unwillingness to rest and recuperate can cause the symptoms to reoccur, with the most cases caused by 'food deprivation'. He also pointed out that factors such as "catching cold" or "liver fire and anger" can also lead to the recurrence of typhoid fever, but none of it is as harmful as "food damage", which shows the importance of diet taboos".[87]

On the guiding ideology on dietary taboos of typhoid fever, Chen Cunren said: "The dietary procedure of typhoid fever can be summarized into four standards. When there is a fever, one must strictly observe the word 'hunger', when the fever subsides, one must observe the word 'cautiousness'; when appetite grows upon recovery, one must observe the word 'moderation'; when still being weak right after the recovery, one must observe the word 'recuperation'. Make sure to starve during the time of a fever. Whether typhoid fever can be cured depends partly on the treatment of the doctor, and partly depending on whether the patient can observe the word 'hunger'. As the saying goes, typhoid fever can never get worse with starvation, which is to

---

[85] Hu Anbang, 16. Medical Cases of Damp Warm Diseases, The Great Treatise on Damp Warm Diseases, included in Lu Zheng (ed.), *Collection of Rare Modern TCM. Warm Diseases*, pp. 674–675.

[86] Chen Cunren, Popular Medical Discourse, included in Lu Zheng(ed.), *Collection of Rare Modern TCM. Medical Talk*, p. 1012.

[87] Chen Cunren, Popular Medical Discourse, included in Lu Zheng(ed.), *Collection of Rare Modern TCM. Medical Talk*, p. 1021.

advise the family of the sick with typhoid fever that long periods of starvation is less likely to cause death than no starvation. There should be no worry about the lack of nutrition."[88] In short, typhoid fever can only be cured without the fear of hunger. The more the hunger can last, the better. No need to worry about starving to death. The reason is: "In typhoid fever, the digestive function has been completely stopped due to intestinal obstruction, and there is no need to have food for its consumption. Therefore, the patient doesn't feel hungry for a very long time. The duration of the time depends on the disease. It is very common not to eat for a month".[89] Chen Geng further stated that countless patients died every year due to the ignorance of the importance of "starvation".[90] There is a saying: "The most hateful thing for the treatment of typhoid fever is careless eating".[91]

So why do we need food taboos? Although the interpretation of TCM during the Republic of China period was based on the spirit of the "fasting" theory of classical medicine, it was still influenced by a number of western medical theories with many new elements added. First of all, the new pathogenic theory focuses on human organs, that is, the organs in the body attacked by diseased bacteria. As far as typhoid fever is concerned, it refers to the large intestine and small intestine. Chen Cunren said: "It is known that typhoid fever is caused by the cold pathogenic factor, but it is also due to a careless diet. The disease enters from the mouth, turning the large intestine into the source of the disease, so there should be the taboo of eating."[92] The theory of fasting in the classical *Treatise on Typhoid Fever* does not involve the intestines, but typhoid germs can obviously cause intestinal inflammation, which serves as the theoretical basis for the fasting theory beyond classical medicine. Chen also said, "The heat of typhoid fever is caused by intestinal congestion. The intestine in the abdomen is stagnant and inflamed, and the stuffiness is like a sausage. The pathogenic factors in the intestine won't be cleared unless the heat caused by cold recedes. One must take medicine to clear it up, and stay hungry to eliminate retention, which would greatly reduced typhoid fever and help in recovery".[93] Chen added that food taken during the fever period would rub the intestinal surface, causing diarrhea, which is commonly known as "leaking typhoid". Therefore, there is no joking when discussing the appeal

[88] Chen Cunren, Popular Medical Discourse, included in Lu Zheng(ed.), *Collection of Rare Modern TCM.Medical Talk*, p. 1015.

[89] Chen Cunren, Popular Medical Discourse, included in Lu Zheng(ed.), *Collection of Rare Modern TCM.Medical Talk*, p. 1016.

[90] Chen Cunren, Popular Medical Discourse, included in Lu Zheng(ed.), *Collection of Rare Modern TCM.Medical Talk*, p. 1012.

[91] Chen Cunren, Popular Medical Discourse, included in Lu Zheng(ed.), *Collection of Rare Modern TCM.Medical Talk*, p. 1017.

[92] Chen Cunren, Popular Medical Discourse, included in Lu Zheng(ed.), *Collection of Rare Modern TCM.Medical Talk*, p. 1012.

[93] Chen Cunren, Popular Medical Discourse, included in Lu Zheng (ed.), *Collection of Rare Modern TCM.Medical Talk*, p. 1016.

for fasting. "No doctor, even if he is hard working, ranked on top, can cure a typhoid patient who keeps on eating. Death would eventually be caused by diarrhea".[94]

Yang Zemin called this "starving" way of curing diseases "hunger method", by saying: "There should be one or two days of fasting, because food may stimulate gastroenteritis or increase the toxins that make it worse due to food fermentation".[95] The theories of inflammation and toxin fermentation caused by stimulating the intestines and stomach are originated from TCM, but they are also obviously the examples of absorbing the theories of Western medicine. In addition, Chen Guofu believed that eating less can avoid the risk of infection. He said: "For some febrile infectious diseases, if you want to avoid infection or reduce the risk of infection, you'd better clear your intestines first, and then eat less or something easy to digest. If you have smooth blood flow and sound health, you can reduce many unnecessary risks".[96] This explanation of the TCM fasting theory is obviously influenced by Western medicine theories.

With regard to typhoid fever, Western medicine focuses on the theory that diet is the cause of the disease. The point of its discussion is that it is caused by unclean food or water, and the origin of the disease is in the intestine. On the basis of this theory, TCM discussed the inflammation of intestines, using "digestion" to explain the condition of the affected part (intestine).[97] As for the unhygienic experience of typhoid fever, TCM focuses more on overeating or a disordered life, but less on the factors caused by germs. Chen Cunren said: "The majority of patients with this disease are men in their twenties and thirties. They are extraordinary healthy, used to resisting cold better and eating freely. For years they don't contract an immediate fever, and it is only to be accumulated gradually. Once it occurs, it is bound to be very serious, bringing them to the juncture of life and death in one or two months".[98] The problem of bacteria is not mentioned here, but it is indicated that the free eating by the patients can cause disease. The control of the disease depends not on cleaning the environment, but on personal awareness and the support of others (caregivers). Chen believed that when typhoid fever is about to go to the recovery stage, the patient would feel the extreme hunger. Chen reminded: "At this time, the patient is not in a normal state and must be restricted".[99] In the process of nursing and

[94] Chen Cunren, Popular Medical Discourse, included in Lu Zheng (ed.), *Collection of Rare Modern TCM.Medical Talk*, p. 1017.

[95] Yang Zemin, 3. Discussion on Law (I) Governance, *Medical Talk in Seclusion*, p. 134.

[96] Chen Guofu,The Way of Health, included in Mr. Chen Guofu Scholarship Fund Management Committee (ed.),*Selected Works of Mr. Chen Guofu's Medical and Health Thoughts*, p. 181.

[97] For example: "Typhoid fever and warm diseases are mostly caused by stomach and intestines, which have long lost their digestive power. It is best to bear hunger, lie down and be quiet. When the tongue is clean without coating, it is the time to have soup, from thin to thick, and the disease won't come back." He Lianchen and Wang Zhipu (ed.), *Updated Treatise on Popular Typhoid Fever*, p. 494.

[98] Chen Cunren, Popular Medical Discourse, included in Lu Zheng (ed.), *Collection of Rare Modern TCM.Medical Talk*, p. 1012.

[99] Chen Cunren, Popular Medical Discourse, included in Lu Zheng (ed.), *Collection of Rare Modern TCM.Medical Talk*, p. 1017.

recuperation, patients do not need to have many doctors involved. It mostly relies on the patient's consciousness, confidence and the assistance of others (mostly family members). Chen also said, "One should be free of worries about one's physical condition or frustrations. It is said confidence helps survival. Doctors give the regular treatment, patients accordingly build up their resistance continuously, the febrile disease would subside and the sick would surely be the winner of the game. Even if the sick become bony, they would still gain weight and become stronger than ever with proper recuperation".[100] Patients should have confidence in themselves and the fasting theory in classical medicine, be responsible for themselves, and eventually they will recover.

Chen Cunren listed the number of medical cases in his book, mostly to illustrate the importance of fasting for typhoid patients. Let's read this profound medical case first:

> Shen Shanqian, an employee of Yuanfengrun Candle Store in New East Bridge, had been suffering from typhoid fever for 50 days, sleepless at night with extreme fever for about a month. He also had dizziness and different variables, being on the verge of death. The disease went through a few changes with a number of compound medicines. It was difficult to handle and would take a long time. By observing the fasting rule, he stopped eating for about 40 days during the fever and eventually recovered. Many patients of sick children with the same disease came to see the doctor.

In addition, Chen cited the article *One Cake, One Life* published in the newspaper:

> There was a child in the neighborhood who suffered from typhoid fever. The fever was gone and there should have been no problem if he was taken good care of. Unexpectedly, his relatives had a wedding and sent over some cakes, and the child would like to eat. Being the only child, he was spoiled by his parents and was allowed to have one piece. Surprisingly, the cake caused trouble right after getting into his stomach. The disease came back repeatedly and became very dangerous. Many famous Chinese and Western doctors have been invited to consult with each other. With the cost of four or five hundred gold coins for the treatment from all possible therapies, the sick boy ended his life in bed. A life was lost by a piece of cake. It was obviously a wrongful death.[101]

Compared with the concerns of Western medicine for food hygiene, the tidiness and cleanliness of patients' rooms and the disinfection of water, TCM plays a key role here. Other medical records also show stories of the same nature: even patients with severe typhoid fever can often recover unexpectedly if they strictly observe the rule of fasting. If not, there will be no way for a cure, resulting in the recurrences of the disease or death.[102] This medical case is intended to highlight that "the child's parents were too ignorant" and "it is a pity that the child's parents, out of love for their child, had caused such a terrible disaster". It is also quite different from the ancient regimen that the harmony between human body and nature, which is more

---

[100] Chen Cunren: Popular Medical Discourse, included in Lu Zheng (ed.), *Collection of Rare Modern TCM. Medical Talk*, p. 1015.

[101] Chen Cunren, Popular Medical Discourse, included in Lu Zheng (ed.), *Collection of Rare Modern TCM.Medical Talk*, pp. 1017–1018.

[102] Chen Cunren, Popular Medical Discourse, included in Lu Zheng (ed.), *Collection of Rare Modern TCM.Medical Talk*, pp. 1023–1027.

emphasized, is less related to the people and the surrounding environment. Being influenced by the western medical care thought, it is also slowly moving toward the responsibility of the people around the patient in their care work. The responsibility of relatives at home is just like that of the nurses in the hospital.[103]

Chen Cunren made great efforts in the operation of specific diet. In his book, he divided the typhoid fever periods into several stages, from the "fever period" to the days of illness, and even the recuperation period after illness, listing beneficial diet and taboos one by one, and explaining the reasons. The old saying goes: "Those who have a light fever and a flat appetite for food can have thick soup, which is commonly known as crusted rice soup, burnt rice soup, rice crust porridge. They are supposed to be the only food for the sick with fever. Scorched black crusted rice soup is the best. It is intended to help the stomach and is easy to digest. The thick soups are nutritious. They can be made of carrot, tomato or taro, of which the fluid can nourish the body without stagnating the stomach as it is mobile. It is also a treasure for typhoid fever".[104] He also suggested that patients should have more liquid food or drink, which is consistent with the concept that fever consumes human body fluid, which should be made up in recuperation. For example, "plain boiled water is the best drink for typhoid fever". In addition, thin lotus root powder soup, cereal soup, watermelon dew are also recommended. He also reminded that the most important thing is to "follow the principle of hunger and never eat till feeling full". As the course of disease changes and the fever resides, more food and drink can follow, but caution is still important.[105]

Careful readers can find that most of the foods listed by Chen Cunren are liquid or beverage, and there is no meat, which is completely in accordance with the ideas of classical medicine. However, with the absorption of the recuperation theory of Western medicine, the boundaries of some taboos have also been loosened. Interestingly, the reason for loosening is to return to the creed established by classical medicine, as Yang Zemin said:

---

[103] Another example is in the *Updated Popular Treatise on Typhoid Fever:* "At the beginning of typhoid fever, eating is most difficult. If the remaining heat in the stomach is not clear and eating is too early, then the pathogenic heat will recur. When the stomach heat is clear and the tongue coating is also clean, yet no food is taken, the remaining vitality would be gone. How can one survive?At this time, it is mainly to test the tongue coating. If there is heat in the stomach, the tongue must have the coating, which could be dry, scorched and even prickly. During this period, it is to be only adjusted with plain boiled soup. It is necessary to eliminate the grain Qi, so that the stomach is empty, which makes it easy for the pathogenic heat to retreat. Today's parents have no idea of typhoid food damage, but they do addict to the rules from the past that typhoid patients do not eat porridge and rice, while keeping sour and sweet fruits at the bedside with no rules. What they do not know is that once they get into the stomach and intestines, they will become sticky, which will promote pathogenic fire in the stomach and which is more harmful than the grain Qi. " He Lianchen (ed.),revised by Wang Zhipu et al.,*Updated Popular Treatise on Typhoid Fever,* p. 495.

[104] Chen Cunren, Popular Medical Discourse, included in Lu Zheng(ed.), *Collection of Rare Modern TCM.Medical Talk*, p. 1018.

[105] Chen Cunren, Popular Medical Discourse, included in Lu Zheng(ed.), *Collection of Rare Modern TCM.Medical Talk*, p. 1019.

> The principle that both Chinese and Western medicine believe in and abide by is that people suffering from typhoid fever should not take pastry. According to Western medicine, typhoid fever is a kind of intestinal fever. Food fed into the intestines will increase the peristalsis of the intestines, and make it severe. In addition, the digestive and absorption functions of patients with intestinal fever will decline. The food will become abnormal due to indigestion. The stimulation of the intestinal lining would cause even more intestinal fever. According to the TCM, typhoid fever is featured with warm and heat. Adding food into the intestine would increase the stagnation of warm and heat, from which it is referred to as food damage. Both statements are valid and reasonable. There was a saying that a typhoid patient never dies of hunger. Therefore, for patients of this disease, all food is on the list of prohibition, a rule I don't think much of. When typhoid fever occurs, the patient does not want to eat, even when food is offered. When the heat gradually fades, the tongue coating is thin, the stomach and intestines are clear, the dampness toxin is transformed, the intestinal heat is reduced, and the physiology becomes hyperactive, it is the time to feed on flowing nourishment, which can not only supplement nutrition, stimulate vitality, but also improve the healing, unless it is overdone. In my clinical experience, I'd rather 'honoring the wish of the patients' than sticking to the fasting principle. Food can be offered to those who can eat but not to those who can not, regardless of stages of the disease.[106]

Yang's words not only highlight that food taboos can not just follow a certain golden rule, but also prove that some food taboo theories are quite influential. They often come from the repeated narration and education of TCM classics and medical cases. The flexibility Yang emphasized still follows the classic guiding principle of "honoring the wishes of the patients". As long as the classics are followed, the bottom line of taboos can be loosened in different situations.

One can't help feeling curious and make an inquiry: since the Republic of China period, there have been quite a number of supplements, not traditional Chinese, but imported from the West, such as milk, beef broth and even medicine. How can this be explained by the theory of classical medicine, or is there any possibility of integration?

---

[106] Yang Zemin quoted: "Jiang Yingsu's medical case is consistent with my opinion, which is recorded as follows: In the 16th year of Wanli, there was a very severe epidemic in the south. There were a lot of deaths when I was living in Jiming Temple. The chief monk had been suffering from the epidemic for more than ten days. A number of doctors said that food should be forbidden. Being not allowed to eat,the sick were hungry and begged for food. I said that it would be presumptuous to deprive the sick of food. Being grounded as it is, the fasting is applicable for those hurt by food. The saying 'a typhoid patient never dies of hunger' means the good prevails over heat pathogenic factor.Starvation won't lead to death. It is said in the classics that 'good diet keeps good health'. As the internal deficiency is caused by the disease, and fasting is only to deteriorate it. How can the patient survive then? If soup is taken in a proper amount, it can be a supplementing decoction to help recovery. In many cases, quite a lot of patients survived without fasting. It was recalled that 15 years ago, cholera was prevalent in Xuzhou. A local hospital gathered cholera patients for treatment, and they were not allowed to drink according to the rules. At that time, all patients were thirsty and asked for water. Even with lot of normal saline injected, they were thirsty as usual. At night, patients were so thirsty that they drank cold water from the tap and all recovered. Those who followed the doctors' advice by not drinking water died. This is the case of cholera,how can you imagine the situation of other epidemics? It is the classic theory of "going with the feeling of the patients", which remains true for thousands of years. " Quoted from Yang Zemin, 25. Problems of Typhoid Fever Fasting, *Medical Talk in Seclusion*, pp. 166–167.

9.5 Western Nutrition and Chinese Taboos

In terms of specific foods, milk can be a key role in the recuperation of westerners for fever, even for most diseases. Ding Fubao, when introducing the recuperation knowledge about typhoid fever in the Japanese medical community, also emphasized "food hygiene", including milk, porridge, juice and other liquid foods.[107] Although milk is on the list, it is a problem food. Missionaries in the late Qing Dynasty recorded: "If you suggest that patients have more delicious and nutritious milk, someone will remind you that milk is hot in its property, and it will promote heat in the patient's body. As Chinese people often believed that nutritious food will cause fatal consequences, many people thus slowly starved to death."[108] In the eyes of foreign missionaries, the Chinese people recuperate with "fasting" and even refuse to drink milk, which is a strange act of self destruction. On the other hand, Western medicine believes that "typhoid bacteria can reproduce most in cow's milk, which contains pathogenic microorganisms when it is not clean. At the turn of summer and autumn, there are many kinds of microorganisms in other foods, which can be harmful to people who are not careful".[109] If germs can be removed, there should be no doubt about the cold or hot properties of food. For another example, in the United States at the beginning of the twentieth century, some people even worried that tuberculosis would pollute milk and beef. How to eliminate bacteria from food was a great concern in Western society at that time.[110]

In fact, milk may not be feared by Chinese patients, because milk is a good food and a helpful medicine during the recuperation period of epidemic febrile diseases. For example, *Analysis on Febrile Diseases* records that "after the recovery of epidemic febrile diseases, it would take a month or a year for one to have a pink face, fast pulse, feeling hot in the evening, thirsty but no appetite for food. The five juices are to be the main drink, including cow milk".[111] There is also a saying that "human milk is the divine product for nourishing blood",[112] confirming the value of dairy drinks, which can be found in both rehabilitation and sex culture.[113] But Chen Cunren didn't think much of the idea of "milk" being used for the recuperation of febrile

---

[107] Miyamoto, translated by Ding Fubao, Chapter 1. Preliminary Typhoid Fever, *New Treatise on Typhoid Fever*, Shanghai: Medical Publishing House, 1908, p. 11.

[108] Macgowan, translated by Zhu Tao & Ni Jing, *The Brightness and Darkness of Chinese Life*, Beijing: Current Affairs Press, 1998, p. 197.

[109] Yu Yunxiu, *Microbiology*, p. 38.

[110] Bayne Joness, translated by Chen Zhaoxi, *Microorganisms and Human Life* (1931 original), pp. 92–93.

[111] (Qing) Wu Tang, Systematic Differentiation of Warm Diseases, Li Liukun (ed.), Complete Medical Works of Wu Jutong, Beijing: China TCM Press, 1999, p. 84.

[112] He Lianchen (ed.),revised by Wang Zhipu et al.:*Updated Popular Treatise on Typhoid Fever*, p. 496.

[113] Zheng Jinsheng, *A History of the Medicinal Forest,* Taipei: Dongda Book Company, 2005, pp. 157–158.

diseases. Although upon the absorption of western nutrition knowledge, he added[114] "no food is forbidden if it is of proper nutrition" under the premise of "food is forbidden even in hunger", and pointed out that liquid nutrients can be used to recuperate febrile diseases. However, he still had doubts about milk. He said: "During the typhoid fever period, those who are not used to milk should not drink milk. This is a critical point I seriously put forward. This view of milk fasting, which truly makes sense, would certainly be opposed by the whole western medical community." Chen cited the famous Western medicine doctor Zhou Zongyi's paper on typhoid fever, which disapproves of milk (Minsheng Medicine, Issue.31), to support his opinion. Interestingly, the focus of this article is not to say that the sick can not drink milk for typhoid recuperation. Zhou maintained that "recently, western scholars have divided patients with fever into two groups, one group has rich nourishment supplies, and the other group has only light supplies. As a result, there is no significant difference between the two groups in the course of recovery",[115] which confirmed that the essence of diet does not have any difference in the recuperation of fever, and milk is certainly proper. Although Chen still suspected that milk might be the culprit of intestinal bleeding during the convalescence of typhoid fever, he finally concluded that the real reason why milk was "not suitable for patients with fever" was that the Chinese patients' dietary habits were incompatible with Western milk, not the food (milk) itself. He said:

> When I was a medical student at university, foreign teachers often said that when I was feverish, my body's consumption would increase, and I would be unable to support it without extra nutrients. This sounds reasonable and pleasant. So I told the patients with fever to sleep well and have milk. What was the result? Of the ten patients, nine were worried and kindly declined my advice. I could not help feeling that they really didn't know how to appreciate this favor. When I was giving myself the favor (that is, when I was ill), I knew that this favor was really like kidnapping. No wonder they didn't appreciate it. Me either. As a result, I could no longer follow the teacher's instructions and had to replace milk with home-made porridge soup and tea.[116]

The doctor not only thought that fasting should be strictly observed, but also suggested that the food the patient ate should fit the Chinese diet. Milk was not really bad for the recuperation after typhoid fever, but many people were not used to drinking milk, which was not conducive to the disease. Another example was "sugar". Sugar had been widely used in soups of classical medicine, so when Western medicine says that glucose has a nourishing effect on fever, Chinese medicine can easily accept it. For example, Yang Zemin said: "Some TCMs are used for dietotherapy, and the most popular food is sugar. In the past, Western medicine regarded sugar as a taste correcting agent rather than a therapeutic agent. Since the invention of glucose therapy, it has been ignored. Sugar is often added to ordinary antipyretics, oral

[114] Chen Cunren, Popular Medical Discourse, included in Lu Zheng(ed.), *Collection of Rare Modern TCM.Medical Talk*, p. 1012.

[115] Chen Cunren, Popular Medical Discourse, included in Lu Zheng(ed.), *Collection of Rare Modern TCM.Medical Talk*, p. 1020.

[116] Chen Cunren, Popular Medical Discourse, included in Lu Zheng (ed.), *Collection of Rare Modern TCM.Medical Talk*, pp. 1019–1020.

administration and injection, which is also a TCM treatment. Sugar can replenish the body without complex digestion, which has been known by today's nutritionists".[117] In the sense of treatment, both Zhang Zhongjing and Ye Tianshi noticed the role of sweeteners, which are the same as glucose therapy in Western medicine. Sugar is rich in lubrication, and it can relieve irritation and inflammation pain. Finally, it has the "stomach strengthening" function of recuperation after illness, which is particularly valued by epidemic febrile disease experts. Yang also gave a scientific explanation: "After a fever or after a long period of stomach disease, the appetite fails to perk up, and the ancients called it "high liver fire" instead of "stomach Yin deficiency", which is hard to interpret. In today's understanding, it is actually due to the lack of stomach power and stomach acid. Stimulating drugs should not be used for the lack of stomach power. Ye Tianshi founded a theory of "nourishing the stomach with sweetness and blandness", which mainly uses radix adenophorae, ophiopogon japonicus, pollen, rice kernels, yams, and licorice. Such drugs contain sugar and starch, which can be taken orally after long simmering without digestion. It is a good way to strengthen the body and recover stomach strength gradually after resting. "Medicines with sugar such as starch, or Ye Tianshi's "sweet and sour Yin medicine", such as black plum, white peony, and shengdi, can improve weak digestion caused by the lack of stomach acid after a fever, which is to seek scientific evidence for the nature and taste of food.[118] Since the late Qing Dynasty, various "fruit sugar juices" have emerged, for the functions of taking sugar juice to replenish blood, invigorate the spleen or as an appetizer, and to moisten the intestines.[119] After the Republic of China period, there were more advertisements for hygienic fruit juices. Of such drinks, there was more communication than conflict with Chinese medical theories.[120]

One side of the conflict is the prohibition of "meat" in the classical food taboo theory, which was discussed earlier, has triggered many discussions in modern times. Qiu Qingyuan once pointed out the harm of meat to the recuperation of fever. It was recorded in a medical case: "The nephew of He Mei, after the fever, became weak with less appetite, which was called stomach asthenia. The same can be said in Western medicine. After being hospitalized for recuperation, he recovered in a month. He drank chicken broth and beef broth every day. Upon hearing about it, I said it was dangerous. The deficiency was in the stomach Yin, not in the stomach Yang. It was better to use pork broth and duck broth. After a month, he died of the fever".[121] The patients in this medical case were obviously "replenished" by Western medicine.

---

[117] The original text: "Zhongjing was the first person to use sugar therapy in TCM, such as Ganmai Jujube, Xiaojianzhong decoction, and Zhilicorice decoction, all of which used sugar as the main agent. In recent times, Ye Tianshi was the best user of sugar therapy, such as sweet acidification for Yin, sweet to regulate Yang, and sweet to moisten dryness, all of which used sugar as the main therapy". Quoted from Yang Zemin. X. On Saccharide, *Medical Talk in Seclusion*, pp. 185–186.

[118] Yang Zemin, 10. On Saccharide, *Medical Talk in Seclusion*, pp. 186–187.

[119] Editorial Department of Globe News Agency(ed.), *Pictorial Daily*, Vol. 7, pp. 12.

[120] Shanghai Shen Bao Newspaper Office (ed.), *Shen Bao*, August 7, 1936, p. 3.

[121] Qiu Qingyuan(ed.), Caution for Life, included in Lu Zheng (ed.),*Collection of Rare Modern Traditional Chinese*, p. 359.

The cold and hot nature of food was not emphasized by Western medicine. Cao Bingzhang, a TCM doctor, proposed to eat more cold food and less meat. However, it can be replaced by seafood, and smoking is not allowed, because "Tobacco contains toxic substances, which can promote the flame of toxic fire, and can damage the blood and brain nerves".[122] This is greatly influenced by the physical outlook of Western medicine, but the standard of food taboos are basically still the TCM theory, especially eating more cold food, which seems to be an important principle of food therapy for heat diseases.[123] Li Hongzhang said that meat is toxic: "By having meat all year round, the blood and flesh would be toxified. Once being attacked by an external disease or an infectious disease, the mild disease will become severe and cause death."[124] It can be seen that there is a close relationship between meat intake and serious exogenous diseases. Yang Zemin explicated the effect of "watermelon", and compared it with the TCM "gypsum", as both of them have antipyretic effect.[125] He explained that the medical herbs that are sweet, cold and nourish Yin, including

---

[122] Cao Bingzhang said: "When the autumn epidemic occurs, it is better to eat, not too much, raw radish, pear and other cool things, even when nobody is sick yet. It is better to eat more plant foods, such as water chestnuts, sugar cane, mung beans, whip bamboo shoots, spinach, artemisia, woad (cabbage);eat less animal meat, such as pork, lamb, beef, chickens, geese, ducks, fish, shrimps, crabs, and all greasy foods; there are also edible food from animals, such as salted eggs, jellyfish, kelp, sea crucian carp, local fish, etc. It is advisable to give up smoking paper cigarettes and dry tobacco, because both contains toxic substances. " Caobing Zhang, Chapter 7 Prevention of Autumn Epidemic, Essentials of Autumn Epidemic Treatment, included in Lu Zheng (ed.), *Collection of Rare Modern TCM.Medical Talk*, p. 772.

[123] Chen Guofu also said: "If the sore throat (diphtheria) is not very severe, as long as the stool is smooth, have more salty soup, eat more vegetables, carrots, pears and other cool things, it can be alleviated or even healed". Chen Guofu, The Way of Health, included in Mr. Chen Guofu Scholarship Fund Management Committee (ed.), *Selected Works of Mr. Chen Guofu's Medical and Health Thoughts*, p. 155.

[124] Jin Xiage (ed.), To the Fourth Younger Brother, Family Letters of Li Hongzhang, included in *Family Letters of Celebrities in the Qing Dynasty*, Vol.II, p. 854.

[125] For example, Yang Zemin said: "When body temperature continues to increase, those with persistent fever are often thirsty, sweaty, and in a state of coma,which is the so-called yangming stomach heat in *Treatise of Typhoid Fever*. Gypsum or watermelon would have a wonderful effect. This disease is common during the summer. Yuan Zhicai recorded a medical case to prove it: In September, when I was ill with summer malaria, I drank Doctor Lv's medicine in the morning, and when I got out of bed, I suddenly vomited and felt dizzy. My mother held me up and I felt my blood was rising from my chest and my life was hanging in the air. Suddenly, Zhao Chencun, a friend of mine, came to visit, and my family tried to turn him away by telling him I was ill. He said: 'I know some medicine.' He felt my pulse, smiled and said, 'It's an easy case.' He had gypsum and other drugs ordered immediately. With a spoonful of it, I felt like a stone of great weight was pressing down on my stomach and intestines, and all the blood and Qi were gone. At the end of the day, I fell asleep, sweating slightly on the forehead, hearing in my half sleep that my mother was sighing: 'Isn't it an elixir?' After another moment's sleep, he was still sitting around and asked if I wanted some watermelon? I said, 'I think so.' Then he had melons bought and said, 'Eat as much as you can and I am leaving.' After having a few slices of melon, I felt my head was enlightened. I ate porridge at night. The next day, he came and said: 'You got yangming malaria. Doctor Lv mistook it as the taiyang meridian by using cohosh and Qiang Huo to pushed your blood upstream. Only white tiger soup could cure it, but it is also dangerous!'" Yang Zemin, 34. The Great Effect of Gypsum Watermelon on Reducing Fever, *Medical Talk in Seclusion*, p. 234.

habitat, ophiopogon japonicus, reed root, dendrobium, watermelon pollen, all have the effect of cooling and antipyretic, which is why they have been favored by scholars of febrile diseases.[126]

Chen Cunren, who raised doubts about milk with another example, said: "Upon the recovery (of typhoid fever), one should not avoid meat and veggies. Those who have good digestion for supplements should not avoid meat, while those who don't can not even have veggies. One should not take tonics immediately after recovery because of the weak appetite, as tonic stagnates the stomach. Taking too much of it would harm the body instead of benefiting it. Chicken broth and beef broth are not greasy, and the taste is extremely delicious. They are not only popular with patients, but also free from the negatives of tonic".[127] Chen held that broth is better than some tonics. It is more suitable for recuperation after having a fever. His theory highlights a question: Is it feasible to have broth for recuperation from fever while there is a prohibition of meat?

Since the late Qing Dynasty, there have been quite a lot of meat nutrition preparations on the market. For example, the advertisement of "Sanxing chick broth" highlights the contribution of Western medicine in toxifying patients' weak bodies with chicken broth, and says that "it is nonsense that chickens can cause deficiency",[128] and also responds to the doubts of TCM about hot tonics. Another brand "earth beef broth" from the China France Pharmacy stated that human beings are originally composed of flesh and blood, so it must be more effective to nourish the body with nutriments made of flesh and blood than TCM, which uses grass roots and bark to nourish the body. The pharmacy also sold several kinds of beef broth, even a beef and chicken mixture, all of which were quiet about the food prohibition knowledge of TCM.[129] "Sanxing nourishing venison broth" was said to have the effect of "greatly replenishing blood and flesh", but the pharmacy also knew what the Chinese were afraid of. In this case, it used the method of emphasizing that Western medicine had used scientific refining methods to make broth, so that it was no longer in the taboo list of TCM herbal literature, such as "too hot in overdose" or "limited dose for the young" of deer meat. In other words, venison broth is a new and scientific product, which is different from traditional venison.[130]

During the Republic of China period, more and more delicate "beef essence", "chicken essence" and other nourishing drinks were made from meat. For example, "Lion Power" beef broth and chicken broth (see Fig. 9.3),[131] manufactured by the German Maher Pharmaceutical Factory, emphasized that protein was a nutrient element of the human body, and of course, it was also integrated with the Chinese

---

[126] Yang Zemin, X. On Saccharide, *Medical Talk in Seclusion*, p. 186.

[127] Chen Cunren, Popular Medical Discourse, included in Lu Zheng(ed.), *Collection ofRare Modern TCM.Medical Talk*, p. 1022.

[128] Editorial Department of Globe News Agency (ed.), *Pictorial Daily,* Vol. 3, p. 71.

[129] Editorial Department of Globe News Agency(ed.), *Pictorial Daily,* Vol. 6, p. 36.

[130] Editorial Department of Globe News Agency(ed.), *Pictorial Daily,* Vol. 5, p. 6.

[131] Shanghai Shen Bao Newspaper Office (ed.), *Shen Bao*, September 30, 1936, front page advertisement. August 15.

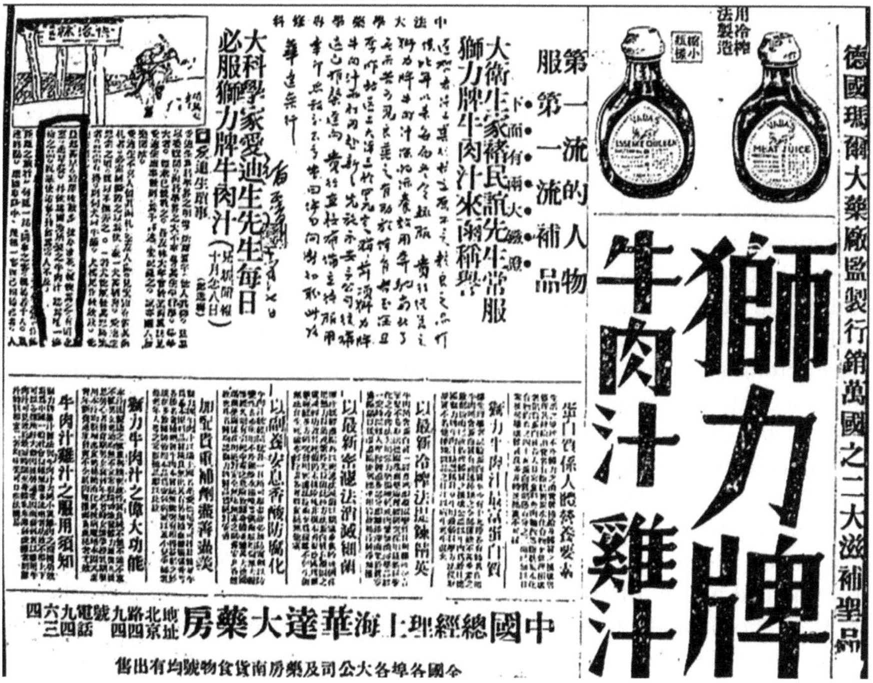

Fig. 9.3 Lion power beef broth and chicken broth

"tonic" element, indicating that the drug could "help digestion, resist diseases, and promote vitality".

The advertisement also made use of the experience of celebrities to show that the broth had outstanding effects. First, Chu Minyi and Edison were chosen. No need to introduce the former. As an important member of the Nationalist Party, he went to Germany to study medicine at an early age and obtained a doctor's degree specializing in rabbit mating. He was branded a traitor and was shot.[132] As for the latter, he was a famous inventor. The advertisement quoted reports that Edison drank the broth every morning. No wonder he had clear thoughts and infinite creativity. In fact, the medicine is at most similar to today's chicken essence. These drugs actually highlight the Chinese people's idea of pursuing "body tonic" to cure all diseases, which has been repeatedly copied in the context of health culture.

Since there was no such tonic in ancient times, the discussion of TCM often presented different polarization reactions. Wu Xihuang said, "Western people also use chicken soup, beef and mutton broth to cure toxic heat, nourish the viscera, and wait for the antipyretic, which is the same as the Chinese method of nourishing the positive by subduing the negative".[133] This is one aspect of western tonics, but he

[132] Chen Cunren, *Life During the Anti Japanese War*, Shanghai: Shanghai People's Publishing House, 2001, pp. 56–76.

[133] Wu Xihuang, *Introduction, Interpretations of Chinese and Western Febrile Diseases*, p. 6.

also gave an example: "In the autumn of 1917, a woman in Gulangyu Islet was sick and had a fever. She was diagnosed by a Western medicine doctor who could speak Chinese. She had been ill for more than ten days. The doctor recommended iron liquor, Quinine and beef broth to her, saying that she could recover after four weeks of recuperation. I said, This can be cured in a few days by using Chinese medicine. By taking the taste-reducing and pulse restoring soup with Zhimu as I prescribed, she recovered in three days".[134] He believed that the TCM treatment still had its advantages, and it was not necessary to use the western method of tonics. Another example is Xu Renfu's saying: "The sick having typhoid fever should not eat anything solid, which would stagnant in the intestines and stomach. The typhoid fever patients would never die of hunger, and the hunger can be eased with liquid substances, such as beef broth, lotus root starch, potato and taro, leaf mustard, and rice noodles".[135] This is a confirmation for the use of nourishing fluid food, seemingly conflicting with the classical medical theory, but it is a complement. There is also a condition for free meat broth intake: "If the patient has been eating for many days and moves freely, he can also eat freely".[136]

Opponents believed that meat is not conducive to the recuperation of fever, even if it is boiled into soup or broth. Chen Guofu said that a friend suffered from typhoid fever and had a fever of 102 degrees (Fahrenheit-the author's note). After he was sent to the hospital, the fever rose to 105 degrees. The doctor was puzzled. It took him a while to find out that the hospital had given the patient chicken soup. When the chicken soup was stopped, the fever dropped. Chen said, "It is said in China that chickens are a stimulating food, which is probably true". The implied meaning is: "Many doctors only know that the medicine is effective. What they do not know is that certain foods conflict with certain medicines. If they do not have enough common sense, how can they avoid the mistreatment?"[137] This can also be used to compare the differences between TCM and Western medicine in terms of diet and recuperation of a fever. Western medicine believes that what we need is to supplement the nutrition of food when suffering from fever, so it is said: "If we are malnourished, our resistance is weakened, the bactericide in the blood is thin, and virus infection is easy. Therefore, when infectious diseases are prevalent, we should pay more attention to nutrition,

---

134 Wu Xihuang, Introduction, Interpretations of Chinese and Western Febrile Diseases, p. 5.

135 Xu Renfu,Handouts on Practical Medicine, pp. 188–189.

136 For example, "Huso or sturgeon swim bladder and fish glue (the same as pig hooves, bird's nest, sea cucumber, or chicken and duck, which are to be boiled and the gravies are better) can enrich the marrow; chicken headed white duck and black-bone white chicken are used to replenish Yin and remove heat; pig lungs dipped in bletilla powder can protect the lungs and stop bleeding. If patients have eaten for many days and can move freely, they can also eat freely. This is an important method of dietary tonic". He Lianchen (ed.),revised by Wang Zhipu et al., *Updated Popular Treatise Typhoid Fever*, p. 496.

137 Chen Guofu, "61.Don't Believe It Or Not Believe It At All", 1st Edition of Medical Administration Ramble, included in Mr. Chen Guofu Scholarship Fund Management Committee(ed.), *Selected Works of Mr. Chen Guofu's Medical and Health Thoughts*, pp. 241–242.

which can enhance the sterilization of the blood to prevent virus infections."[138] However, TCM believes that people who suffer from fever should stand "hunger", eat light food or even fast. In fact, during the recuperation period of febrile diseases, meat is not clearly defined in TCM. Although it was widely accepted not to eat meat, Dai Tianzhang said: "At the beginning of a febrile disease, the sick can have porridge, but it is better to eat less and stay hungry, and make sure not to become full. They should not be offered food even if they want it. After a while, they can gradually eat mutton, rice porridge, but not pheasant, rabbit, deer meat nor pork and dog meat".[139] Most meats were not recommended, it was not to the extent of taking "meat" as a taboo, and some tonics similar to shredded meat soup was fine. Some Chinese doctors were in favor of these body building new tonics. When talking about the "post disease convalescence period" of typhoid fever, Chen Cunren said:

> During the disease, the best food should be the nutritious and digestible fluids. Upon recovering from typhoid fever, chicken broth and beef broth are indispensable for a patients health care, even if meat is included. Some patients think that it is not appropriate to eat meat right after recovery. Chicken broth and beef broth are mistaken as stimulating, which they dare not eat at the early stage of recovery. In fact, it is totally wrong. As typhoid fever is a non surgical disease, there should be no prohibition of consuming meat or chicken upon recovery. At this time, broth supplement is needed. Beef broth and chicken broth are the only proper foods. Nothing is better or more effective. Those who have been ill for one month need to have beef broth and chicken broth for two months. It is obvious that those who have been ill for one and a half months need to have broth for three months to recover their vitality, to enrich their physical strength and enhance their Qi and blood.[140]

Chen Cunren's opinion is obviously different from Chen Guofu's experiences of disease. The former advocates that broth be a supplement. Instead of focusing on the taboo of "meat", the focus should be on the easy digestion and non greasiness of broth that caters to a patient's taste, which is similar to the notion of "honoring the wishes of a patient". The pluralistic development of the "tonic" culture since the Republic of China period has actually loosened some "taboos" in classical medicine, and the aforementioned rules of meat are an example. Many TCM doctors have put forward the concept opposite to classical medicine, which guides us to think about the possible perspective of connecting the two knowledge systems.

[138] Qiu Jun, Introduction to Infectious Disease Prevention, *Social Medical Journal*, 1933 (190), p. 51.

[139] (Qing) Dai Tianzhang,revised by He Lianchen, Vol. 1. General Theory of Febrile Diseases.Therapies of Febrile Diseases Syndrome, included in *Revised Generalizations on Febrile Diseases*, p. 37.

[140] Chen Cunren, Popular Medical Discourse, included in Lu Zheng(ed.), *Collection of Rare Modern TCM.Medical Talk*, p. 1022.

9.6 "Deficiency" and "Recovery" After Fever

TCM includes the concept of "tonic", especially for post disease care. Although there are many taboos and rules, there are also many "tonic" methods, of various kinds. Generally, "food tonic" is better than "medicine tonic",[141] because it is convenient and suitable for daily recuperation.[142] What is the relationship between tonic and fever? Probably "deficiency" is a very important factor, especially the recuperation of the deficiency syndrome after a fever, as deficiency can easily cause exogenous diseases. *A Dream of Red Mansions* records such a story:

> Baoyu said, "You may not know that Sister Lin (Daiyu) has an internal disease. She was born weak, and easily catches cold, but it's better to take pills after taking two doses of decoction to relieve the cold". Mrs Wang said, "The doctor mentioned the name of the pill a while ago, and I forgot it". Baoyu said, "I know those pills, nothing but some ginseng nourishing pills." Mrs Wang said, "No". Baoyu then said, "The eight-treasure motherwort pill? Left or right?(different ingredients-translator's note) Or is it wheat flavored rehmannia glutinosa pill?" Mrs Wang said: "Neither. I only remember the word 'Vajra'". Baoyu smiled and said, "I've never heard of a 'Vajra pill'. If there is a 'Vajra pill', there should be 'Bodhisattva powder'!" Everyone in the room laughed. Baochai smiled and said, "I think it's the heavenly king's heart pill". Mrs. Wang smiled and said, "That's the name. Now I'm confused". Baoyu said, "Not really. Just being confused by 'Vajra' and 'Bodhisattva'.[143]

Lin Daiyu was obviously suffering from exogenous cold, but the main cause was "internal disease", that is, she was born weak and was prone to diseases such as catching a cold. Therefore, the "deficiency" of the patient's body was also one of the reasons why she was prone to exogenous diseases. There are more daily tonics, basically all of which are listed. It can be seen that Cao Xueqin was knowledgeable about the culture of nourishing when it came to diseases. This is not surprising. It seems that all Chinese at that time knew a little about this kind of nourishing culture and often gave foreigners a feeling that Chinese people were taking tonic medicine all the time. Missionaries in the late Qing Dynasty commented that:

> On one hand, it seems that the Chinese are extremely in short of medical resources, but on the other hand, everyone is a doctor who can diagnose and prescribe for others' diseases at any time. The medical society has evolved for hundreds or thousands of years. Maybe everyone can say something about medical theory, which is also due to the lack of medical resources. The Chinese people trust doctors very much and have the ability to absorb large doses of drugs, as if they are enjoying themselves away from illness and taking a lot of TCM

[141] According to the *Updated Popular Treatise on Typhoid Fever*, Cheng Zhongling said:" The medical remedy is not as good as the food remedy. If the disease and pathogenic factors are not exhausted, and the vitality is weak, the strong remedy is not as good as the light and mild remedies. Depending on the situation, they should be taken gradually. As the pulse settles, the medicine should be reduced, and the food, meat, fruits and vegetables should be fully served. " He Lianchen (ed.),revised by Wang Zhipu et al.,*Updated Popular Treatise on Typhoid Fever,* Cao Bingzhang's preface, p. 496.

[142] For example, Yang Zemin said, "Food therapy is easy for digestion and rich in nutrients. If the taste is catered and time is adjusted, the disease will be easily cured". Quoted from Yang Zemin, 3. Discussion on Law (I) Governance, *Medical Talk in Seclusion*, p. 133.

[143] Cao Xueqin & Gao E, *Annotations of A Dream of Red Mansions*, Vol.I, Chapter 28, pp. 435–436.

> herbs. As we all know, the physique of the Chinese is weak, making the business of amateur doctors possible. A sick Chinese is always ready to take any medicine and listen to anyone's advice. Despite untrained doctors, quacks, amateur doctors and some deceptive means, the people of this empire are as healthy and as strong as people of today, which undoubtedly proves that Chinese people are in good health. China is a typical example that people rely on the overwhelming power of nature to maintain their health, rather than those untrained doctors and those stupid and rude treatment methods that take people's lives prematurely.[144]

Everyone knows a little about medical knowledge. In fact, from another angle, isn't it the best footnote that this knowledge of drug recuperation is deeply rooted in every patient's daily life?[145] The Chinese people are very worried about various complications after a fever. These complications are not necessarily caused by the disease itself, but by the irregular performances in recuperation by violating taboos, leading to the recurrences of the disease, and even contracting new diseases. He Lianchen said:

> After a severe febrile disease, one should be careful in drinking, eating, and other daily life activities before regaining one's vitality. Moreover, one's Qi and blood inevitably become weak and any excessive joy, anger, talks or movements would bring back the disease due to fatigue damage. The fatigue activate the blood Qi that is already deficient and the remaining heat is generated. The disease is cured when heat pathogen subsides, and the disease comes back when the heat pathogenic factor returns. This is true for all diseases, particularly febrile diseases.[146]

Generally speaking, it is just about food and living styles. In addition to food prohibition, there are many appeals that must be observed, such as resting or avoiding moodiness. If you do not pay attention to "hygiene", you will induce "recurrence" of various fever diseases. Like He Lianchen said: "The four recurrences, namely, the recurrences of fatigue, food, disease itself and anger, are easy to cure for the sthenia, but not for the asthenia. They can be cured for the first recurrence, not for the second. According to my experience, it is mostly caused by the fatigue and also sex which leads to death. Over eating is likely to cause recurrence and drinking is the worst; anger is likely to cause recurrence and outrage is the worst. These repeated recurrences would result in overall damages. For asthenia, the time for the severe cases to stay alive would be only 10 to 15 days, and prolonged for the less severe. Even for those who luckily recovered with proper medical treatment and recuperation, they are still fragile, and can easily have a severe cold. It is the most critical for the doctors

---

[144] Macgowan, translated by Zhu Tao and Ni Jing, *Men and Manners of Modern China*, pp. 197, 200.

[145] However, everyone can express a set of TCM theories. I'm afraid it's not just for TCM doctors, but also Western medicine doctors. For example, Liang Shiqiu said, "I know some tactful doctors. Before the treatment, they would first practice a set of physiognomy by identifying the patients, and try to please the patients. By being a Western medicine doctor, he can still quote a set of *Treatise on Typhoid Fever* with Yin, Yang and five elements to an old woman". Liang Shiqiu, Doctors, included in *Essays of Yashe*, Taipei: Zhengzhong Book Company, 1981, p. 134.

[146] (Qing) Dai Tianzhang,revised by He Lianchen, Vol. 1. General Theory of Febrile Diseases. Therapies of Febrile Diseases Sequela, included in *Revised Generalizations on Febrile Diseases*, p. 77.

to give advice, and the sick to be aware of the rules of recuperation!"[147] We can see that, besides participating in the treatment process, doctors must also be serious in facing the problems of recuperation, and remind patients of their cooperation so as not to violate these daily care taboos. Dai Tianzhang also said:

> The recurrence of febrile disease, if it's repeated several times, is normally due to the lack of hygiene and the negligence of care for the patients. After repeated recoveries, there are often four damages and four deficiencies. There are four possible causes for the recurrence. One is overwork when the vitality has not been restored and the remaining pathogenic factors have not been cleared right after the recovery. A little bit of labor would cause the recurrence. It is not necessarily to be much, but just cleaning up, bathing, talking, changing clothes. Recurrence means the coming back of all symptoms, and it can be told by an unsteady pulse. The mild can recover with recuperation while the severe need to be checked on their physique if they are sthenia or asthenia. If it is asthenia, the circulation needs to be enhanced to activate the viscera, and recovery would happen once the exterior and interior are synchronized.[148]

The patient's knowledge, self-consciousness and self-control during recuperation are very important. Generally speaking, they should stay quiet and rest, without much talking or working. There are also many prescriptions listed in the back of the medical book, so that patients can find their own ways to treat themselves if problems occur, emphasizing the practicality of daily life. In addition, Chen Cunren said: "During the disease, disordered diet are likely to lead to asthenia and debilitation; proper diet provides an opportunity to change the physique from weak to strong. It is important to know the relationship between typhoid fever and diet".[149] Chen believed that failure to pay attention to food or other taboos would lead to a new disease, which would result in various "deficiency" or "damage" causing diseases, such as "asthenic consumption". He Lianchen said: "In a recurrence of febrile disease, if the symptoms of this deficiency damage also comes back, it is an indication that healthy Qi fails to overwhelm the pathogenic factors. The healthy Qi is to be promoted in order to eliminate the pathogenic factors. It is a battle between them. Only when the pathogenic factors are eradicated and the healthy Qi is preserved can the disease be cured".[150] Recuperation is a part of the treatment that can not be ignored. "Promoting healthy Qi" is even more important than the treatment itself. He Lianchen cited 24 symptoms to explain that doctors must be knowledgeable about the various symptoms that may occur to patients during recuperation, so as to understand the treatment methods. He said: "The remaining pathogens of both typhoid fever and warm diseases are all caused by the residual pathogenic factors, lack of recuperation or the ignorance

147 (Qing) Dai Tianzhang, revised by He Lianchen, Vol. 1. General Theory of Febrile Diseases.Therapies of Febrile Diseases Sequela, included in *Revised Generalizations on Febrile Diseases*, p. 69.

148 (Qing) Dai Tianzhang,revised by He Lianchen:Vol. 1. General Theory of Febrile Diseases.Therapy of Febrile Diseases Syndrome, included in *Revised Generalizations on Febrile Diseases*. p. 65.

149 Chen Cunren, Popular Medical Discourse, included in Lu Zheng (ed.), *Collection ofRare Modern Traditional Chinese.Medicine.Medical Talk,* pp. 1012.

150 (Qing) Dai Tianzhang,revised by He Lianchen,Vol. 1. General Theory of Febrile Diseases.Therapy of Febrile Diseases Syndrome,included in *Revised Generalizations on Febrile Diseases*. pp. 67–69.

of taboos."[151] The thinking based on taboos actually dominates the whole post illness recuperation. In general, these taboos and the diseases caused by their violation can be explained by various complications. In terms of treatment, it mainly focuses on "tonifying deficiency" and "clearing away heat", and the drugs or food selected are mainly of cold property.[152]

The Chinese believe that the rehabilitation of fever is not just taking medicine, but also a period of recuperation. During this period of rehabilitation, patients will experience various states. If they ignore this, many other diseases will occur, For example, Qin Bowei said, "It will take some time to recover. However, there must be three kinds of phenomena during this period, one is fragility, the other is sensitivity, and the third is the improvement of the supply mechanism, which leads to anemia, skinniness, hair falling, movement difficulties, variable body temperature, light sleep, hyperappetite, and increased sexual desire. It is advisable to keep quiet and rest, otherwise the disease will recur and deteriorate."[153] Therefore, the knowledge of Chinese medicine, which is mainly about food prohibition and some other taboos, is integrated into daily life, and the most important of them can be summarized by "resting" and "observing the rules".

In the process of recuperation, we must pay attention to the harmony between the body and the external Qi. In the *Climate Regulation Therapy*, He Lianchen explicated in the first place that "The method of climate regulation refers to keeping warm in winter and cool in summer, which is in compliance with seasons for health care... The *Taisu Sutra* says: those who are comfortable with cold won't suffer in winter nor sweat in summer. If the residence is free from the eight pathogenic factors, they can be at peace".[154] In addition to a large number of quotations from *Internal Canon*

---

[151] (Qing) Dai Tianzhang,revised by He Lianchen: Vol. 1. General Theory of Febrile Diseases. Therapies of Febrile Diseases Syndrome, included in *Revised Generalizations on Febrile Diseases*, p. 70.

[152] He Lianchen said, "The recuperation period after recovery can be in two stages: tonifying deficiency and clearing away heat. One is to nourish the spleen, and the other is to nourish the stomach. If one is suffering from Qi deficiency, there should be less grain taken after recovery, and if the circulation is stagnant, or the stool is not solid, or there is nausea and saliva, it is advisable to take the 6-ingredient combo with appropriate dosages. There are also two methods for clearing away heat: the heat at the beginning of the illness is excessive, and it is advisable to use bitter cold medicine to clear it; while the heat after a serious illness is deficient, it is advisable to use sweet cold medicine, and the difference between the two is huge. The natural Qi owes all to appetite.If there is a deficiency in body fluid, the promotion of fluid production is the tonic for the deficiency. Therefore, it is proper to combine the medicine of promoting fluid production with the medicine of relieving cold and heat, and to treat the deficiency heat after fever, such as ophiopogon japonicus, radix rehmanniae, cortex moutan, northern sea cucumber, American ginseng, fresh dendrobium, pear juice, sugarcane juice, bamboo juice, and thatch root. Zhongjing and Hejian mainly used bamboo leaf gypsum soup and Tianshui powder to clear up the heat, which is meant for the combination of sweet and cold. "(Qing) Dai Tianzhang,revised by He Lianchen, Vol. 1. General Theory of Febrile Diseases. Therapies of Febrile Diseases Syndrome, included in *Revised Generalizations on Febrile Diseases*, pp. 76–77.

[153] Qin Bowei, Practical Chinese Medicine, p. 55.

[154] He Lianchen (ed.),revised by Wang Zhipu et al., *Updated Popular Treatise on Typhoid Fever*, Cao Bingzhang's preface, p. 498.

of Medicine,[155] it also quotes the theory of "eight pathogenic factors", expounding that the taboos of external Qi and life are not to be violated.[156] It is said that every season has factors that are particularly vulnerable to certain diseases, most of which are caused by seasonal Qis. For example, "When the spring sun arises, everything sprouts. In February, when there is a swing of cold and hot, those with a potential sick heat in summer would have an outburst of the disease in spring".[157] "Summer brings out the fatal diseases. Just look at the withered grass and fallen leaves. Their juice is drained in summer, which explains why there are more diseases in summer than in other seasons".[158] As for the recuperation time in each season, it is also mostly related to food taboos and residence taboos, such as "hot as it is in summer, it is not proper to have ice water, jelly, ice cream, cold porridge, or whatever is cold, fried, fat, sweet and spicy, and do not wash your face with cold water".[159] The air of autumn is so deadly that "it is no good to eat fried beef or pork, nor chicken, raw fish, foul wine, or any food that is stale, salty, vinegary, sticky and slippery that is hard to digest. The cold food in summer would lead to dysentery and malaria in autumn".[160] In winter, "It is advised to avoid sweating so as to maintain one's Yang, and medicinal liquor is needed for nourishment. As it is getting colder, putting on cotton padded clothes,

---

[155] He Lianchen (ed.), revised by Wang Zhipu et al., *Updated Popular Treatise on Typhoid Fever*, Cao Bingzhang's preface, p. 498.

[156] According to the context of *The Essential Substance*, "eight pathogenic factors", or "eight winds", are the false pathogenic factors that harm people. Quoted from (Tang) Yang Shangshan,*The Essential Substance in the Inner Canon of the Yellow Emperor*, Vol. 28, pp. 200–202. The "eight pathogenic factors" in the *Perspectives of Typhoid Fever* by the later generations refer to "the external wind, cold, heat and dampness, and the internal hunger and indulgence. Indulgence is not satiety, but the damage is caused by idleness, which is the opposite of working. *The Inner Canon* says:" Labor warms one up, while satiety enables one's movements, which activates the blood. "It is said in the West Mountain Record:" Long time working brings peace, satiety preserves energy, and long time leisure promotes the power against stagnation." (Jin) Liu Wansu, Internal and External Pathogenic Factors, included in" *Perspectives of Typhoid Fever. Collection of Alternative Methods for Typhoid Fever*, Beijing: People's Health Publishing House, 1982, p. 7. It also says: "Most children's clothes are dried in the sun during the day and collected at night. They can't stay in the open air overnight, or the children would have the damp heat and feel restless by putting them on the next day. This is the so-called eight pathogenic factors. In the long term, the children would turn pale and skinny, suffering from stomachache, feeling feverish, crying at night, or have sick scabies. The old saying refers to it as the infantile chancre disease, that is, the clothes that stay overnight in the open air and are stained with chancre birds' droppings can make children sick. It is thus called the infantile chancre disease. This may not be true. The so-called eight pathogenic factors by the ancient scholars are being damp, hot, windy, cold, frightened, stagnant, hungry and full. " (Ming) Xu Chunfu, Collection of Children (I). Clothes Drying, included in *Ancient and Modern Medicine Vol. 88*, Beijing: People's Health Publishing House, 1991, p. 851.

[157] He Lianchen (ed.),revised by Wang Zhipu et al., *Updated Popular Treatise on Typhoid Fever*, pp. 498–499.

[158] He Lianchen (ed.), revised by Wang Zhipu et al., *Updated Popular Treatise on Typhoid Fever*, p. 499.

[159] He Lianchen (ed.), revised by Wang Zhipu et al., *Updated Popular Treatise on Typhoid Fever*, p. 499.

[160] He Lianchen (ed.), revised by Wang Zhipu et al., *Updated Popular Treatise on Typhoid Fever*, p. 499.

instead of using fire frequently to warm up, which would bring heat to the heart and cause anxiety." With excessive Yang in one's body, it is not advisable to bathe in hot water, or the forced sweat would open one's pores and the body is susceptible to external pathogenic factors. It is not recommended to go out early when there is frost, and some liquor can help in flushing the cold. It is not smart to have a lot of scallions, as it would cause the dissipation of Yang Qi.[161] In general, it is said to abide by seasonal food and daily life taboos in order to resist disease. However, most of the theories refer to the various aspects of Qi in life, but none of them involve western hygiene. It can be seen that TCM knowledge on daily recuperation during the Republic of China period was based on traditional theories.

Some people adopted western theories occasionally, as mentioned previously. They did not follow the taboos, nor contradict traditional concepts of classical medicine, belonging to the school of absorption and integration. For example, Yang Zemin explained the "cooling" method, "this is the western ice compress method, which is a cooling method for a certain part of the body. It is used for the purpose of easing the body function, preventing inflammation, and relieving pain.... The snake medicine and furuncle medicine commonly used by people are also cold drugs. They are effective as cooling methods. This is the same as using ice tablets to treat ophthalmia, stomatitis, and laryngitis"[162] to bring down fever. Ding Fubao also suggested that the head should be cooled with ice or water when the headache is severe.[163] Another example is the "ice method", which is to cure diseases that are not suitable for drinking water, and the thirst can be quenched with ice in the mouth. This method can also be used for fever, but "crystal sugar" cannot be added into ice water when the sick doesn't like a sweet taste and it is a better substitute.[164] There is also recuperation therapy. Yang said: "Those who overeat and have digestive organ damage have to keep a strict diet and eat less to recuperate. Taking medicine is of no use".[165] There was even a transference method. Yang equated it with western psychological suggestion and self hypnosis. Yang believed that sunlight-air therapy is also acceptable, though it is not found in classical medicine—"being not mentioned by the ancients".[166]

---

161 He Lianchen (ed.), revised by Wang Zhipu et al., *Updated Popular Treatise on Typhoid Fever,* p. 500.

162 Yang Zemin, 3. On Treatment (I) Therapies,*Medical Talk in Seclusion,* pp. 131–132.

163 Ding Fubao, Communication between Chinese and Western Prescriptions, p. 100.

164 Yang Zemin, 3. On Treatment (I) Therapies,*Medical Talk in Seclusion,* p. 134.

165 Yang Zemin,3. On Treatment (I) Therapies,*Medical Talk in Seclusion,* p. 132.

166 Yang Zemin,3. On Treatment (I) Therapies,*Medical Talk in Seclusion,* pp. 132–133.

9.7 The Modern Rebirth of Personal Hygiene—The Continuation and Conversion of the Body View of Qi, Blood and Essence

In addition to diet and food prohibition, we can not ignore the role of drugs. Most historians are not knowledgeable in medicine, but they have a keen sense of the social culture and body view in a specific era from the vast historical data, which presents the value of historical discussion. For febrile diseases, we must pay attention to all kinds of complications. Another kind is the complications caused by the violation of sex taboos, which is as critical as food damage. The knowledge of sex and food taboos are often the two keys to epidemic prevention.[167] In terms of sex knowledge, it is generally reflected in two ancient disease names, one is "Yin-Yang transference", and another is "labor damage". In fact, both of them involve the damage caused by sexual intercourse when the febrile disease is not cured, which is of great harm to the recuperation of the febrile disease.[168] When talking about syphilis in *Orthodox Surgery*, it was recorded that the cause of syphilis is that "when the weather changes, pathogenic spirits gather and attack", but "it is always changed by damp heat and pathogenic fire". However, "Qi infection is mild, and sex infection is severe". In the view of TCM, the infection of Qi is always mild, but if it involves the infection of sex or desire, will it aggravate the disease a lot more?[169] *Revised General Febrile Diseases* says: "In terms of sex damage, it's not as serious for a man as for a woman who could possibly die with the tongue sticking out a few inches with saliva running. For those newly recovered from febrile disease, Yin-Yang transference would occur in the first 100 days after the recovery before their strength is restored if they have

[167] For example, "For old or young, strong or weak, people with cold and hot diseases, due to deficiency or excess, often use fried loquat leaves to make soup instead of tea to purge the lung Qi, which can prevent all the pathogenic factors. In particular, they must be careful about their living style by having a good diet, keeping light tastes and controling their appetite. In summer, they should be vegetarians for 30 to 50 days,with no stimulating food and limited sex". Shaoxing Medical Association, Treatment of Damp and Warm Epidemics, included in Li Shunbao (ed.), *Complete Book of Warm Diseases*, Vol. II, p. 2100.

[168] He Lianchen said: "Yin-Yang transference of warm disease: Yin-Yang transference, for men or women, is due to sexual intercourse right after the recovery of warm disease. For a woman, who has sex with a man before the complete restoration of health, it is called Yang transference.For a man, it is called Ying transference. It is characterized by a hot body, depressed chest, heavy head, squinting eyes, tight limbs, bellyache, folded hands and feet. All lead to death. If death is not immediate, they would suffer from a stressed abdomen, depressed chest, heavy head and the feeling of limb separation,weak pulse,blood and Qi deficiency, exhaustion, trance, being unable to move in bed and need help in living, which would last no more than a few years. (21) Recurrence of warm disease due to overwork: even when recovered, the Yin and Yang are not yet harmonious. Early sexual intercourse would cause the invasion of Yin into the abdomen which ends up in cramps. It is called sex damage. "(Qing) Dai Tianzhang, revised by He Lianchen,Vol. 1. General Theory of Febrile Diseases. Therapies of Febrile Diseases Syndrome, included in *Revised Generalizations on Febrile Diseases*, p. 33.

[169] (Ming) Chen Shigong, Section 36. Syphilis,*Orthodox Surgery,*Tianjin: Tianjin Science and Technology Press, 2000, p. 219.

sex. This is the thought from Sun Simiao".[170] It can be seen that sex taboos had been around for a long time. In ancient times, the sex taboo was originally a method of health preservation and disease treatment.[171] In modern times, it fell into the areas of witchcraft and alchemy. Doctors generally only talked about sex taboos, including the discussion of febrile disease. The orthodox medical books tend to avoid the topic of sexual health preservation.

As for the diseases caused by the lack of resistance and Qi mentioned above, the recuperation of a fever is often discussed together with the body view of physical weakness and malnutrition.[172] Their relevance may be as what Chen Guofu said: "If a person is very healthy, he has some kind of resistance, which can certainly deal with ordinary diseases. It is only in the case of overeating when there is forced digestion, or in the case of being too cold or hot when the body is trying to work on its defense, that the microorganisms can take advantage to make entry into the body. In addition, there is excessive brain use, or sex indulgence that the body resistance would be too overly consumed to fight against the invasion of foreign enemies".[173] In the Chinese concept, sex can not only lead to the loss of the "essence" of the human body, but also make people weak, resulting in a constitution prone to exogenous fevers. The resistance of "individuals", including the strength of spirit and body, as well as the smoothness of blood circulation, are all elements of a resistance to germs. The weakness and fatigue of the body are always used to refer to some diseases during the Republic of China period. The most representative diseases were kidney deficiency and spermatorrhea, as well as "neurasthenia", which became a new disease in China.[174] The loss of "semen" or "vital energy" from the human body is very much feared by the Chinese. Xia Ruitang was over 65 when he married his last wife. They had no children. Xia, as a TCM doctor, believed in some personal ways to keep healthy and he never got sick. He believed in the theory of "conserving essence" and

---

[170] (Qing) Dai Tianzhang, revised by He Lianchen,Vol. 1. General Theory of Febrile Diseases.Therapy of Febrile Diseases Syndrome, included in *Revised Generalizations on Febrile Diseases*, p. 37.

[171] For the relationship between medical prescription and sexual intercourse, see Lin Fuji, A Brief Discussion on the Relationship between Early Taoism and Sexual Intercourse, *Proceedings of the Institute of Historical Language, Academia Sinica*,70.2(1999), pp. 233–300. Li Jianmin & Li Zhende, On the Medical Prescriptions for Childbirth between Han and Tang Dynasties—Also on the Origin of Gynecology and Gender Discussion, *Proceedings of the Institute of Historical Language, Academia Sinica*, 68.2 (1997), pp. 283–367.

[172] For example, Qin Bowei said: "Those who cannot fully recover often suffer from after effect, or turn from acute diseases to chronic diseases, or have complications. They are mostly weak, malnourished, and have genetic problems". Cited from his book, *Practical TCM*, p. 55.

[173] Chen Guofu, The Way of Health, included in Mr. Chen Guofu Scholarship Fund Management Committee (ed.), *Selected Works of Mr. Chen Guofu's Medical and Health Thoughts*, pp. 179–180.

[174] The doctoral thesis of Hugh L. Shapiro is quite groundbreaking: *The View from a Chinese Asylum: Defining Madness in 1930's Peking*, Ph.D. Harvard University, 1995, pp. 246–250. In addition, the significance of the transformation of modern body shape and quality of "kidney essence" can be referred to Pi Kuoli, *Body View and Ideological Transformation of Modern TCM—Tang Zonghai and the Era of Convergence of TCM and Western Medicine,* Chapter 8.

that one should not let semen leak after 65, which is very important for men's health. It can be seen that the preservation of "essence" is important for human health.

In the theory of febrile diseases, there is also an influential theory called "hidden heat". Doctors who hold this theory believe that the most powerful pathogenic factors would sometimes hibernate in the human body. If people do not keep "kidney essence" well in winter, they are likely to suffer from febrile diseases in other seasons.[175] On the contrary, if the "essence" is well preserved, one can avoid the disease.[176] Zhang Jingyue (1563–1640) once said, "Typhoid fever usually starts from those who failed to preserve essence during winter and who are hungry. If they don't preserve essence in winter, pathogenic factors will easily enter. Those who are hungry and tired are particularly vulnerable. This is why epidemics occur after a famine. The sick carry the strong epidemic Qi which is very infectious. The weak are the first to be infected and in turn become infectious, causing more sickness when it's cold in winter."[177] Zhang believed that those in need of essence are particularly vulnerable to the epidemics. Although the modern theory of "hidden heat" was sternly questioned by the bacteriology, Zhang Xichun explained that people suffering from febrile disease always seem to have a physical imbalance of cold and heat. "No preservation of essence in winter" means that there is a bad heat hidden in the body, which is easy to be triggered by exogenous Qi to induce febrile disease. This traditional theory was not antiquated due to the challenge of the bacteriology.[178]

What's more, some Chinese doctors explained why the loss of kidney essence was easy to cause exogenous diseases with the epidemic body view in the Ming

---

[175] For example, in the context of *Treatise on Typhoid Fever*, the term "hidden heat" is a kind of physical state of "cold in the human body" or "the kidney does not store essence in winter". In spring, disease pathogens release from the inside to the outside of the body, and eventually cause warm diseases. (Qing) Miao Zunyi,Survey of Febrile Diseases and Their Seasonal Variables, A Study on Febrile Disease, included in *Complete Book of Warm Diseases, Vol. I*, p. 147.

[176] Yu Chang, a doctor in the Qing Dynasty, summarized several types of epidemic warm diseases, which is the most detailed: "It is said in *Internal Canon of Medicine*: if cold damage is caused in winter, and warm disease would then show up in spring,which is a typical case. If no essence is preserved in winter, warm diseases would show up in springtime, which is another case. Still another case is cold damage being caused while no essence is being preserved in winter, and warm disease show up in spring. The above three examples are used to discuss warm disease syndrome and explore its treatment, followed by the examples of Zhongjing's three Yangs and three Yins, which are consistent. Cold damage caused in winter would have pathogenic factors hidden under the skin, which is called three Yangs in the pathogenic factors. No preservation of essence in winter and the pathogenic factor is hidden in Yin, which is called three Yins in the pathogenic factors. "(Qing) Miao Zunyi, (Shang Lun) On Warm Disease in March of Spring. Self Preface (General Idea), A Study on Warm Diseases, included in *Complete Book of Warm Diseases, Vol. I*, p. 161.

[177] (Ming) Zhang Jiebin, Miscellaneous Cases, Epidemics and Argument, *Jingyue Complete Works Part I, Vol. 13,* Shanghai: Shanghai Science and Technology Press, 1996, p. 225.

[178] Zhang Xichun said, "Most people sick with warm diseases have internal heat. When the spring sun begins to shine, they have less infected external factors and the heat suddenly turns into warm diseases. Lack of essence preservation in winter causes Yin deficiency, and the heat is accumulated in the viscera, which is activated by external sensations, same as those with internal heat". See his book: Treatment to the Spring Febrile Diseases Caused by the Cold Damage and Lack of Essence Preservation in Winter, *Chinese Medicine with Reference to the West, Part II,* pp. 458–459.

and Qing Dynasties, As Cao Bingzhang said, "From the theory of triple-energizer in *Longchuan Sketch*, it is consistent with the western theory by Tang Zonghai. Both maintain that the triple-energizers originate from the kidney. Thus when the heart is burning with desire, the essence of triple-energizers is released from the vital organs, so that the limbs can not be nourished. The membrane of triple energizers is empty and unable to protect the skin and hair, nor prevent the cold and heat pathogenic factors from invasion".[179]

This is the way to release the essence from the human body, combined with the theory of membrane origin of the epidemics, and supported by the modern physician Tang Zonghai's statement to increase the rationality of the theory. In modern times, these comprehensive body views are often used as the physical evidence of various kidney deficiency and weak constitution, while "deficiency" and "disease" will affect each other, that is, a vicious circle, in which exogenous fevers, such as cold, is also likely to lead to kidney deficiency, just like "deficiency fatigue".[180]

TCM believes that febrile disease is particularly serious for those who have kidney deficiency. Miao Xiyong said: "Those who are incurable or hard to cure with typhoid and epidemic diseases lack the vitality in lower energizer".[181] It is an important connotation of health preservation based on the prevention of kidney deficiency, which is still being maintained and emphasized in the knowledge of modern febrile diseases. For example, "One should not put the feet high up when sleeping, as it would lead to kidney deficiency in the long term, accompanied with cold feet".[182] Physical weakness will lead to vulnerability to infectious diseases, and the two are mutually causal. The treatment of extraneous diseases, of course, can not be ignored. On the factor of "kidney deficiency", Chen Cunren said: "Where the kidney is weak, the body Qi is weak and cold, the body is addicted to alcohol and lust. With greasy food casually taken, it is common to see the sick being drained out, getting skinnier each day and suffering from bad physical damage, though it is not too obvious at the beginning. Without immediate treatment, and if it comes with an exogenous disease, the case would be severe and incurable".[183] In daily life, a lot of behaviors will lead to the loss of vital energy. The busy city life, excessive brain consumption, fatigue, masturbation, spermatorrhea and the sequelae caused by improper recuperation after an exogenous fever will all lead to kidney deficiency. Liang Shiqiu once said, "It's probably true that fever is due to fire, cough to cold, phlegm to lung heat, and lumbago to kidney deficiency. A doctor should prescribe medicine even if the cause

---

[179] Cao Bingzhang, Research on the Origins of the Triple-energizer Membrane in Summer, Summary of Syndrome and Treatment of Summer Diseases, included in Lu Zheng (ed.),*Collection of Rare Modern Traditional Chinese*, p. 690.

[180] Shanghai Shen Bao Newspaper Office (ed.), *Shen Bao,* March 17, 1937, p. 2.

[181] (Ming) Miao Xiyong, The Effective Therapies of Febrile Diseases in Spring and Summer, included in *Medical Notes in the Awakening Room*. p. 9.

[182] He Lianchen (ed.), revised by Wang Zhipu et al., *Updated Treatise on Popular Typhoid Fever,* p. 503.

[183] Chen Cunren, Popular Medical Discourse, included in Lu Zheng(ed.), *Collection of Rare Modern TCM.Medical Talk*, p. 999.

is unknown, or he is not a doctor".[184] The concept of kidney deficiency, phlegm, fire, heat, wind and cold are all common pathological terms in China. In fact, various exogenous diseases are also related to kidney deficiency, which is a body concept rarely noticed by scholars studying Chinese medical history in the past.

Some researchers who studied medical advertising during the Republic of China period, including Huang Kewu, Zhang Zhejia, Zhang Zhongmin, Zhang Ning, Yang Xiangyin and Cochran Sherman, have explicated the characteristics of medical advertising in this period. In particular, the boundary between TCM and Western medicine at that time was quite vague. In order to stand out in the increasingly competitive drug market, drug dealers used various well-known traditional medical concepts, as well as the novel western body concepts to convince all possible consumers. Sex diseases, brain weakness, blood deficiency and kidney deficiency are often the major targets of these advertisements.[185] In fact, this kind of advertisement is also related to the concept of strong physical fitness in modern China. The image of a weak nation and a sick man seems to be the decadent image attached to modern Chinese people, for which there are numerous examples.[186] Some satirize the weak body of the political authorities and literati in the late Qing Dynasty, as Liang Qichao said, "The elderly are lifeless while the young are weak".[187] During the Republic of China period, Chiang Kai-shek believed that the image of "a sick man" of the weak Chinese people was a "weak and cowardly life style" developed under the long-term oppression of imperialism, which manifested itself as "unhygienic" conduct, such as stooping, loose, corrupted, lack of discipline, poor spirit and untidy clothes.[188] This "weak" image is often related to the indiscretion and indulgence of personal behavior. For example, Chen Cunren said:

> Masturbation is a bad habit among the youth, which is common nowadays… That prostitution is very popular, especially among the youth of Shanghai. It is so common to see pale and decadent young people all over. When contracting typhoid fever or febrile disease, few of them can get over it. Often, the patient would die with two or three symptoms. Those who barely recovered would suffer from impotence, premature ejaculation, and other symptoms of the sick. To cure this disease, on one hand, young people need to make the utmost

184 Liang Shiqiu, Doctors, included in *Essays of Yashe*, pp. 134–135.

185 Frank Dikotter, *Sex, Culture and Modernity in China: Medical Science and the Construction of Sexual Identities in the Early Republican Period*, London: Hurst & Co.,1995, pp. 122–145. Feng Ke expressed in his book that during the Republic of China period, nationalism was the center of national construction, and his attitude toward sex was still more supportive of strengthening management and control. In order to revive the country, individual sexuality must be managed and controlled, and new health concepts and bacterial theories be integrated. With less discussion about the country, the book directly cuts into the daily life dominated by Qi and body in TCM. There are also many intersections between the gender discourse and body view in TCM and Western medicine.

186 Yang Ruisong, Imagining National Shame: "A Sick Man of East Asia" in the History of Modern Chinese Ideology and Culture, *Journal of History of Political University*, 2005 (23), pp. 1–44.

187 Luo Jialun, Restoring the Standard of the Body Beauty Before the Tang Dynasty, *New Outlook on Life,* Taichung: Zeng Wen Publishing House, 1981, p. 35.

188 Wu Shufeng (ed.), The Archives of President Jiang Zhongzheng: A Sketch Script, Volume 6, Taipei: National History Museum, 2003, August, 19, 1929, pp. 419–420.

> determination to get rid of bad habits; on the other hand, they need to take medicine for a long time to cultivate their own health. Every winter, they may as well take nourishing medicine to make up for their lost vitality, so as to promote body growth, and cure their neurasthenia. When all diseases are completely cured, new vigor can be activated, the blood can be produced, the essence can be regenerated, and the health can be improved day by day.[189]

This unsanitary "personal" life style is mostly related to masturbation or excessive indulgence. The loss of essence and blood in the body makes it impossible to deal with a febrile disease, and weakness is presented all over. Upon the recovery, the body is weak, and various complications would easily follow. "Febrile disease can cause the loss of blood. Although the main disease is gone, when blood loss is not recovered for a long time, it would be the cause of headache, back pain, emaciation, a pale face, mental and body fatigue, energy loss and so on. Except for this, the long term loss of blood may cause the recurrence or change of the disease at any time".[190] There came a lot of tonic drugs. Bridie Andrews noticed that these blood supplement advertisements generally claimed that adequate blood is the foundation of health. Insufficient or loss of blood will lead to weakness and disease.[191] At the beginning of the twentieth century, neurasthenia was regarded as an upper class disease, which is different from a cold,[192] but in China, there is a strong causal relationship between the two. As early as the late Qing Dynasty, neurasthenia was related to the blood that nourished its normal operation, which was often ignored by researchers. Perhaps such a body view of connecting blood with nerves affects the new discussion of TCM diseases.[193] In the discussion of febrile diseases, neurasthenia is similar to the "weak" state caused by anemia, tuberculosis and exogenous diseases such as typhoid fever and malaria. It can also be treated with tonic drugs (see Fig. 9.4).[194]

The thought of tonifying the kidney to prevent exogenous fever is related to the classical medicine "labour damage", so we can find more clues from many daily drug advertisements. For example, the "Kidney Qi Pill" produced by Foci State Pharmaceutical Factory makes full use of the body theory of classical febrile diseases, and emphasizes that winter is a good time to replenish essence. Once spring comes, kidney Qi is sufficient, body and spirit are healthy, and resistance becomes stronger, which can naturally avoid "getting sick in spring" and achieve the effect of "letting go of all diseases naturally" (see Fig. 9.5).[195]

The advertisement said: "When spring comes, it is easy to make people feel nervous, and the increase of seasonal diseases and the recurrence of kidney disease

---

189 Chen Cunren, Popular Medical Discourse, included in Lu Zheng(ed.), *Collection of Rare Modern TCM.Medical Talk*, pp. 1006–1007.

190 Shanghai Shen Bao Newspaper Office (ed.), *Shen Bao,* August 23, 1936, p. 3.

191 Bridie Andrews, "Blood Disease" and the History of Chinese Medicine, "included in Yu Xinzhong (ed.), *Medical Treatment and Health since the Qing Dynasty*, p. 185.

192 See C. Harrison's pen and ink painting in 1913, quoted from Roy Porter: *A Brief History of Madness*, p. 197.

193 Editorial Department of Globe News Agency(ed.), *Pictorial Daily,* Vol. 5, p. 7.

194 Shanghai Shen Bao Newspaper Office (ed.), *Shen Bao,*March 25, 1937, p. 4.

195 Shanghai Shen Bao Newspaper Office (ed.), *Shen Bao,* January 12, 1937, p. 2.

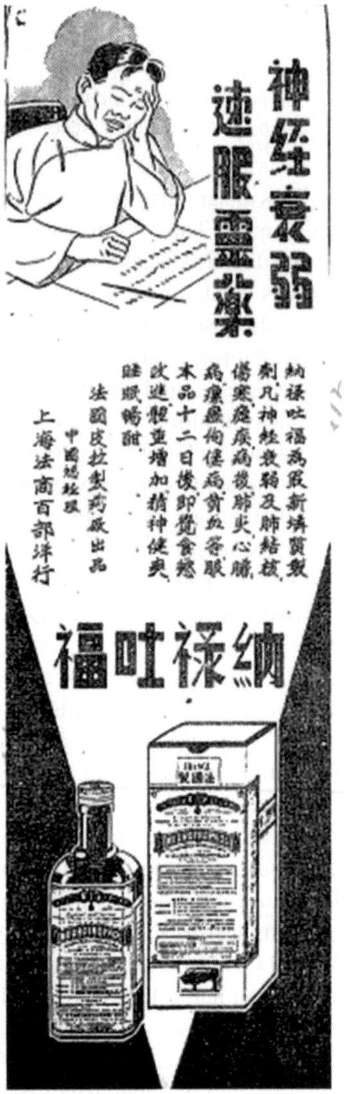

Fig. 9.4 Neurasthenia quick-acting medicine—nurotrophol

is more than other seasons."[196] This is a seasonal relationship between exogenous seasonal diseases and kidney disease. Moreover, such advertisements are always connected with sexual diseases. In fact, the logic between them is still the essence of the kidney. The drug mentioned the relationship among "endocrine", "gonad" and

[196] Shanghai Shen Bao Newspaper Office (ed.), *Shen Bao*, March 2, 1937, p. 2.

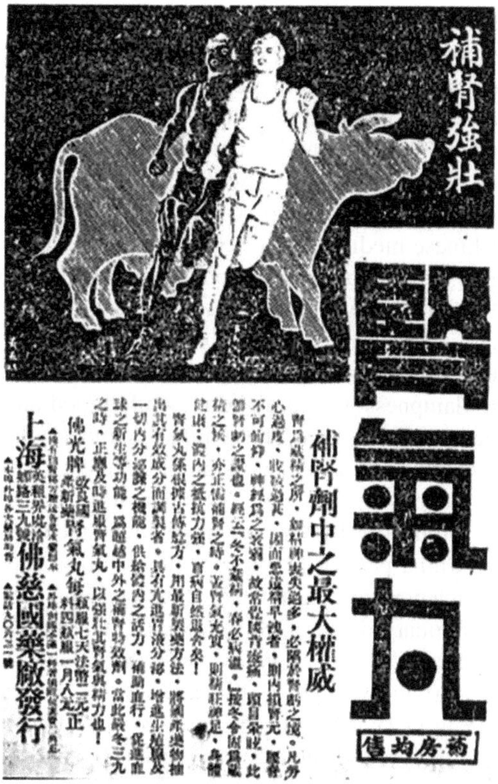

Fig. 9.5 Kidney tonifying agent—Kidney Qi Pill

kidney Qi function, which can be regarded as a broad concept of weak body, and advocates the use of drugs to regulate and supplement.[197]

Exogenous fever was often compared with bacteriology in modern Chinese medicine. For example, there was a Japanese drug named "Rendan" at that time, which emphasized that it could prevent epidemics, seasonal diseases. The advertisement said that "unhygienic" or "careless diet" would cause diseases. Fortunately, the drug had strong "stomach building power" and "bactericidal power", which could help maintain health.[198] This advertisement strengthens the absorption of gastrointestinal organs to enhance the human body's resistance to external

---

[197] Ibid. The body and medical concept of "endocrine" and "gonad" had massively invaded people's daily life in the early Republic of China period. As the context of febrile disease is still different, it is not intended to be discussed here. See Pi Kuoli, *From "Tonifying the Kidney" to "Hormone" Therapy:Anti-disease Strategies and Daily Life History during the Republic of China Period.*

[198] Shanghai Shen Bao Newspaper Office (ed.), *Shen Bao*, July 22, 1936, p. 3. In fact, at the end of the Qing Dynasty, various kinds of anti epidemic pills came out, most of which can prevent and ward off epidemics, such as the "Red Treasure Pill" and "Revitalizing Hundred Treasure Pill" from Chinese and French pharmacies. Quoted from Editorial Department of Globe News Agency(ed.), *Pictorial Daily*, Vol. 1, p. 1.

bacteria and achieve the function of "sterilization and epidemic prevention".[199] In other advertisements, we are surprised to find that the drug can promote the secretion of various good hormones, so as to enrich nutrition, and enhance or restore the resistance and physical strength of the weak.[200] Some advertisements even say that it has added "holmes" and "vitamins" as its outstanding effects.[201] The drug also brings up the relationship between "healthy body and vigorous spirit" and "preventing and controlling epidemic diseases".[202] This can be explained with the "essence" of Chinese medicine, but it was often replaced by terms such as resistance and physical strength after the Republic of China period. The opposite is the body view of "deficiency fatigue".[203] Yu Wuyan said: "According to TCM, deficiency fatigue is caused externally by indulgence and internally by seven emotions, with improper diet and uncontrolled lust. Liquor damages the lungs and stomach, which will lead to dampness and fumigation, while blood and Qi would disappear, and lust would damage the kidney. The seminal chamber will be empty, and there will be no control over lust".[204] The discussion of deficiency fatigue is mostly caused by indiscretion in daily life or ignorance of moderation.

Influenced by Western medicine in the late Qing Dynasty and the early Republic of China period, pulmonary tuberculosis was usually compared to the disease of deficiency fatigue in TCM, thus deriving the names of tuberculosis, phthisis, and pulmonary disease(all relating to "fatigue-痨"-translator's note). There were also works such as *On Pulmonary Disease* (Ge Lianfu et al. in 1914), *Guide to Tuberculosis* (Qin Bowei in 1920), and *A Study of Deficiency Fatigue* (edited by Zhu Zhensheng in 1936).[205] In the early years of the Republic of China period, the medical profession and average people believed that exogenous diseases would turn into tuberculosis if they were delayed in treatment for too long or not well nursed, such as the common concept of "a cold not being cured would turn into phthisis".[206] Many drugs for treating colds and coughs would emphasize this concept (see Fig. 9.6).[207] This is an example of uncured exogenous diseases causing internal damages, which is common in Chinese medical discourse. Moreover, the prevention and recuperation of various exogenous diseases are often related to the new drug "hormone". This kind of advertisement refers to the change of external seasons and environmental "Qi", which is an important cause of exogenous diseases, such as cold, typhoid

[199] Shanghai Shen Bao Newspaper Office (ed.), *Shen Bao*, August 16, 1936, p. 3.

[200] Shanghai Shen Bao Newspaper Office (ed.), *Shen Bao*, May 7, 1936, p. 3.

[201] Shanghai Shen Bao Newspaper Office (ed.), *Shen Bao*, July 11, 1936, p. 5.

[202] Shanghai Shen Bao Newspaper Office (ed.), *Shen Bao*, November 18, 1918, p. 3.

[203] The recuperation of exogenous febrile diseases is also closely related to kidney essence. There will be no further discussion here in order to avoid complications.

[204] Yu Wuyan, New Interpretations of the Synopsis of the Golden Treatise in Illustrated Annotations, p. 96.

[205] Deng Tietao & Cheng Zhifan, General History of Chinese Medicine · Modern History, p. 31.

[206] Lu Jinsheng, Tuberculosis, Jingjing Medical Talk, included in Shen Hongrui & Liang Xiuqing (eds.), *General Views on Chinese Medicine in China*, p. 1369.

[207] Shanghai Shen Bao Newspaper Office (ed.), *Shen Bao,* March 16, 1937, Local Supplement.

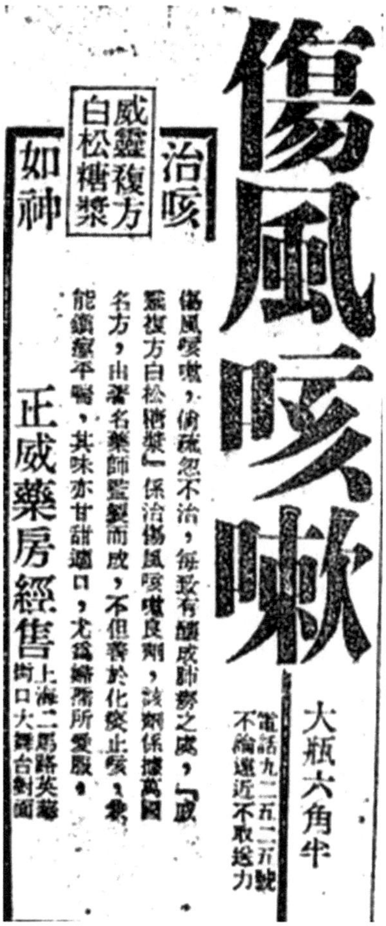

Fig. 9.6 Cold and cough medicine

fever or febrile diseases.[208] This external "Qi" often affect the secretion of human hormones, as: "In the plum season, the weather is changeable, with the abrupt turn of being cold or hot. Being affected by the weather, the hormones in human bodies are abnormal, and diseases are rampant for the loss of energy".[209] Another example is the advertisement of "German Forever Young Supplement":

Since the beginning of autumn, it has been very hot. This is the "autumn tiger" between autumn and summer. Because the climate is not normal, the endocrine function of the human body is often disordered, which hinders metabolism and nutrition, followed immediately by insomnia, fatigue, boredom, small and bloody urine. The resistance would get weaker each day, and it is easy to contract epidemics as well

[208] Shi Yiren, *Seasonal Diseases of TCM*, pp. 20–28.

[209] Shanghai Shen Bao Newspaper Office (ed.), *Shen Bao,* June 20, 1936, p. 3.

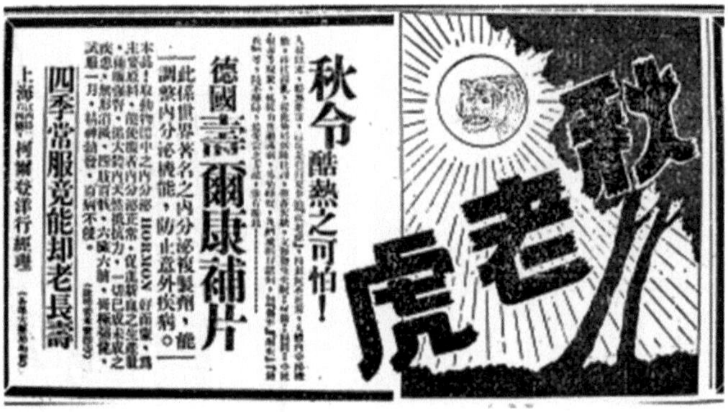

Fig. 9.7 German forever young supplement

as gastrointestinal diseases, such as "typhoid fever", "dysentery" or "malaria". It is impossible to be prevented. The most appropriate way is to take this (see Fig. 9.7).[210]

Such advertisements often equate the normality of endocrine with the power of human resistance. There are many kinds of human endocrine. As Yun Tieqiao said, there are many kinds of glands, but these discussions often point to the secretion of gonads related to the kidney, which may be greatly affected by the season and current climate, and suffer from serious epidemics. If hormone endocrine preparations are taken, the various exogenous fever diseases would be prevented.

What kind of people are vulnerable to exogenous diseases? In addition to some patients with chronic or special diseases, they can also include the elderly and children with poor resistance, which is common. Among many daily discussions in the early Republic of China period about how the loss of vital energy in the body would cause diseases, one of them was that "spermatorrhea" would lead to exogenous fever. An advertisement said that a reader named Yao Yunping wrote to the newspaper that he had a serious spermatorrhea, suffering from dizziness and cold, and was easy to catch cold. By taking "Himit Tables" and "Reproduction Pills", he felt much better. The fundamental logic of these drugs is to combine kidney essence with various health elements to create a description of drugs curing all diseases (see Fig. 9.8).[211] The readers also asked some questions about these drugs, and the doctor replied in the newspaper: this drug is a "preparation combining endocrine elements such as testicular adrenal gland, pituitary gland, thyroid gland", which is a specific drug to fundamentally solve the problem of spermatorrhea. It can be cured by five or six packs of pills. One must abstain from sex till its recovery, which is quite similar to the concept of "labor damage".[212] In some pages, it is emphasized that Reproduction Pills had been added to the drug, but it is doubtful what that is. Advertising data shows

[210] Shanghai Shen Bao Newspaper Office (ed.), *Shen Bao*, August 19, 1936, p. 4.

[211] Shanghai Shen Bao Newspaper Office (ed.), *Shen Bao,* January 6, 1936, p. 4.

[212] Q & A between Yao Yunping and Zhou Xiaohan, *Q & A on Various Spermatogenic Diseases and Treatment Methods,* August 8, 1936, p. 5.

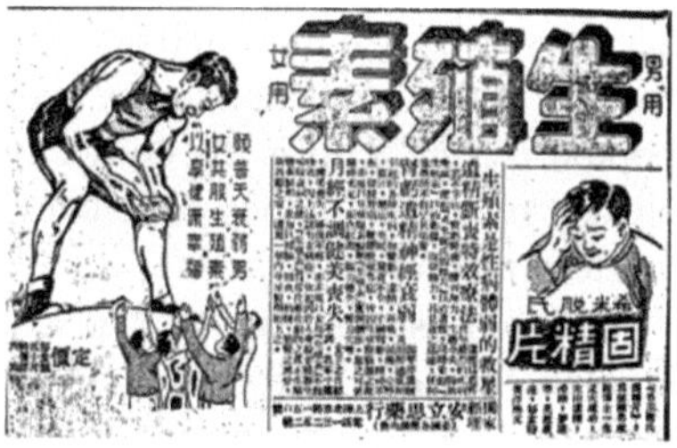

Fig. 9.8 Reproduction pills

that it is actually a comprehensive preparation of some glands. This is quite special, because most of them still use gonadal elements or hormones. Such a "hodgepodge" type of explanation may only be a propaganda.[213]

In terms of recuperation from exogenous diseases, a drug advertisement focusing on enhancing resistance declared: "(German Shouerkang Supplement) takes the endocrine hormone as the main ingredient. It can regulate human endocrine, promote the production of new blood, vitalize the brain and kidney, enhance the inherent resistance of the body, virtually eliminate all potential diseases and strengthen the four limbs and six internal organs. After taking it for one month, the patient will be vigorous and free from any diseases."[214]

In addition to taking the medicine, recuperation is needed in order to recover: "Mr.Zhao, a patient who was severely infected with an epidemic in early summer, was fortunately hospitalized and cured, but he was unable to recover for a while due to severe damage to his vitality. He was introduced by a German doctor to take 'Reproduction Pills' to recuperate his sick body. He eventually recovered and became strong after taking three packs".[215]

All of the above are the effects of hormone preparation on exogenous diseases. If an exogenous disease is not well nursed, it will enter into a state of deficiency fatigue, which is connected with the aforementioned "turning into tuberculosis". "Tuberculosis" was a disease with multiple meanings during the Republic of China period. At the beginning, it did not only refer to "pulmonary tuberculosis", which has been pointed out by many scholars. Spermatorrhea is also a kind of "consumptive disease (痨)". For example, the advertisement of the drug "Regenerating Spirit" claims that "it can effectively improve sleep and revitalize whoever suffering from extreme fragility or fatigue, preventing the occurrence of spermatorrhea during sleep." The advertisement also took advantage of the foreign brand, emphasizing that "it was invented by the famous French doctor Gabrial after a decade of research, and had

---

[213] Drugs such as "Himit Tablets" and "Reproduction Pills" are both western medicines. In addition to the selling point of being created by an Austrian physiologist, "Reproduction Pills" emphasized that it is made from the gonad material extracted from the body of "young animals" with various supplements. Quoted from Jia Zhizhong, Advice to the Young Suffering from Spermatorrhea, Shanghai Shen Bao Newspaper Office (ed.), *Shen Bao,* August 19, 1936, p. 5.

[214] Shanghai Shen Bao Newspaper Office (ed.), *Shen Bao,* August 19, 1936, p. 4.

[215] Doctor Jia Zhizhong, Neurasthenia—Aging Before Getting Old, Shanghai Shen Bao Newspaper Office (ed.), *Shen Bao,* August 8, 1936, p. 5.

been tested by ten thousand people. It is the crystallization of the study for the treatment of male kidney deficiency and spermatorrhea, which has gained the world-wide popularity".[216] This is the body culture orientation of "consumption (痨)", which is closely related to kidney deficiency and deficiency fatigue in TCM, but it is totally a western medicine.

Tuberculosis is also known as pulmonary tuberculosis, and its pathogen also involves bacteria. After the bacteria invade the lungs, they breed and multiply in the lungs, causing induration. Therefore, it has the name of pulmonary tuberculosis, which is an explanation based on the theory of bacterial pathogenicity at that time. However, since there was no effective bactericidal specific drugs, a large number of lung tonic drugs were used in daily life, all of which gave the sick the hope of recovery. These drugs are more or less related to the concept of tonifying the kidney and supplementing hormones. As Shen Zhaoquan said: "The treatment of lung disease depends on the natural and vigorous function of the human body, which enables the connective tissue to proliferate and surround the lesion, so that it can be cured. Some believed that drugs can kill tuberculosis, such as the drugs aggressively advertised. They are not only useless, but sometimes very harmful, or even deadly for lung disease...Sometimes these (bactericidal) drugs are truly effective, but it is due to the inherent strong resistance to cure lung disease naturally rather than be cured by the drugs (bactericidal)." Hormone therapy focused not only on sterilization, the most powerful statement of Western medicine then, but also on strengthening the body's resistance. He added: "Today, the most effective lung disease treatments can only be supported by human power". This "human power" that can enhance the human body's resistance is the "organ therapy" of hormones, which is a new technology in the "modern tuberculosis treatment community".

This treatment mainly aims to reverse the physiological functions destroyed by diseases and aging cells, and enhance body resistance. An advertisement line goes "It is a mixed oral liquid (Phith Weal)–by extracting the endocrine and hormone from the fresh lungs and spleens of healthy animals". In addition to the claim of being able to repair damaged lung function, this drug also claims to be able to consolidate the tissue around the lesion, harden it, and surround the "pathogenic tuberculosis bacteria", so that it can be naturally eliminated.[217] It can be seen that this hormone drug is related to the treatment of "lung" and "spleen", and should be related to the weakness of the lungs and poor appetite of patients with pulmonary tuberculosis. After taking this medicine, "the sick would feel refreshed with increased appetite, loose expectoration, less cough, and be free of hot flashes, night sweats, and blood phlegm within a few days. Taking this medicine continuously, accompanied by a general hygiene therapy, it can be completely cured in a very short time. This organ therapy had been dominant in the chemical therapeutic world since its birth, but now

[216] Shanghai Shen Bao Newspaper Office (ed.), *Shen Bao,* August 19, 1936, p. 5.

[217] Shen Zhaoquan, The Danger of Pulmonary Disease Patients, Shanghai Shen Bao Newspaper Office (ed.), *Shen Bao,* August 21, 1936, p. 5.

it is being abandoned and coming to its end".[218] At last, the advertisement claimed that the therapy would replace chemotherapy, which could also be regarded as an expectation and imagination of technological progress for the new hormone therapy when there were no ideal antibacterial drugs at that time.

9.8 "The Exotic View of Modern Health"—TCM Recuperation Period

> To compare with the health theories of other countries in the world is to seek the communication between eastern and western theories. Although European and American medical science has remarkably developed as a special discipline, more attention is paid to material and daily life care. In view of inherent health preservation theories and mental recuperation, China seems to be at a more advanced level.[219]
>
> —Shen Zongyuan: The Collection of Chinese Health Preservation Theories, 1930.

Shen Zongyuan is very confident in the "hygiene" of TCM. This chapter mainly discusses the diet, recuperation, taboos and essence nourishing of TCM, which has actually run through all possible aspects of medical history in the whole TCM exogenous febrile diseases in daily life. Chen Cunren said: "Chinese medicine is better at eliminating the cause of a disease than seeking superficial and quick effect. Therefore, it is best at regulating chronic and complex diseases. As it is free of side effects and highly toxic elements, it has no reaction even with constant intake. It can also cure complicated diseases. Therefore, Chinese medicine is good at treating mixed diseases, in expunging both the symptoms and causes, with multiplied methods".[220] This indicates the assurance of TCM recuperation knowledge. The history of TCM is thought-provoking for readers. From the perspective of "individuals", the methods of protecting the life of an individual during the Republic of China period can be quite diverse, but the most important aspects are based on the Chinese body view of Qi, blood and essence. Although they have been connected with some western medicine knowledge, the spirit behind them is still more or less based on traditional medicine.

Just like Cheng Hanzhang believed, in the early Republic of China period, Western medicine did not guide patients on how to recuperate after illness or improve their physique to fight against disease. Maybe western medicine practioners believed that these were included in public health policies. He explicated that Western medicine has

---

[218] Shen Zhaoquan, The Development of the Latest Therapy for Lung Disease—The Oral Administration of Organ Preparations is Proved to be the Most Practical. Shanghai Shen Bao Newspaper Office (ed.), *Shen Bao,* September 25, 1936, p. 4.

[219] Shen Zongyuan, et al.(ed.),Two Kinds of Chinese Traditional Health Preservation. The Collection of Chinese Health Preservation Theories, p. 79.

[220] Chen Cunren, Popular Medical Discourse, included in Lu Zheng(ed.), *Collection ofRare Modern TCM.Medical Talk*, p. 993.

the mission of guiding patients "from a scientific and moral standpoint".[221] However, we can see that many small details of daily life can not be explained from a scientific or moral perspective. In fact, the recurrence of many diseases, recuperation, and dietary taboos are related to the body language of the sick, showing a body view of keeping quiet and moderate, as well as the daily verification of medical experience. In the past research on the history of modern Chinese medicine, too much attention was paid to the "internal history" exploration of the treatment methods in the classic medical books.[222] Such important knowledge as diet therapy and recuperation was ignored, which has a strong personal feature of "self operation" of patients in daily life. Rather than relying on scientific verification, it is just the body's subtle feelings of "Qi deficiency", "spermatorrhea loss" or being attacked by external "Qi", which is used as the important pathological references. In the author's opinion, with the pressure of Western medicine and the demand for the rationalization of TCM theory, what the Chinese medicine of the Republic of China period did was not to abandon the old theory, but to constantly find out similar "relapses" from the classics, as well as to find opportunities that can practice their expertise in daily life beyond the rationality of public health. Yang Zemin believed that there were many TCM treatment methods, and medicine is only one of them. The reason was that TCM was often mild and had no immediate effect on the acute diseases or people with a weak constitution. In this case, we must attach importance to other treatment methods or supplement them with daily recuperation methods,[223] which was also a feature of modern Chinese medicine that cannot be ignored in the history of medical development.

While repeatedly interpreting classical medical books, Chinese medicine during the Republic of China period was still communicating with Western medicine, even being under its influence. For example, Chinese medicine has absorbed a lot of knowledge about nutrition and resistance, which has been transformed into the basis for explaining dietotherapy or food prohibition. On diet issues such as meat and milk after a fever, they are not completely the same as the traditional methods. With a lot taboos discussed, some views are conflicting. All of these represent that the integration of Chinese and Western medicine is not a one-way road, but a mutual and multi-dimensional interaction, which is a natural phenomenon under the modern dialogue between Chinese and Western medicine. However, many new Western medicines mostly adopt the theory of kidney deficiency and spermatorrhea loss of TCM, which has created a drug consumption culture and controversy that is both Chinese and Western. It may partially replace the knowledge pedigree[224] of TCM tonic drugs, and in a different way, it packs the concepts of Qi, blood, essence,

---

[221] Cheng Hanzhang, A Brief Introduction to Western Medicine, pp. 40–41.

[222] For example, the experiences of therapeutic methods are emphasized in Zhu Jianping (ed.), *Research on Major Innovations in Modern Chinese Medicine,* Chapter 3, Chapter 4, The framework of *General History of Chinese Medicine · Modern History* (edited by Deng Tietao and Cheng Zhifan) also emphasizes the development of clinical medicine. Others are mostly oriented to the system and educational history, with little concern for the history of daily life.

[223] Yang Zemin, 3. Discussion on Law (I) Governance, *Medical Talk in Seclusion,* p. 134.

[224] For the knowledge context of traditional "nourishing" drugs, see (Qing) Wang Ang, *Collection of Medical Prescriptions*, Tainan: No.1 Bookstore, 1986, pp. 1–32.

disease prevention, weakness prevention and other thoughts of traditional medicine with a new scientific concept, which has become a new trend and a continuation of the discussion, namely the transformation of the tonic culture within the science of exogenous febrile diseases. There's still a lot of study needed in medical history and this chapter is only limited to the topic of febrile diseases.[225] TCM during the Republic of China period emphasized multiple body expositions such as seasons, Qi and physique, while ignoring the influence of bacteriology. The theory of bacteria has also definitely become a material evidence when Chinese medicine of the Republic of China period discussed body resistance, kidney essence and recuperation after illness, which could be a demonstration of the modernity of new Chinese medicine.

[225] Zhang Ning, "The Trademark Dispute of Aspirin between China's New Pharmaceutical Industry and Bayer Pharmaceutical Factory in Germany during the Republic of China Period", *Collection of the Institute of Modern History, Academia Sinica,,* No. 59 (2008.3), pp. 193–199.

Chapter 10
Conclusion: Writing Modern Chinese History with Chinese Medicine

> China is not a country without science. In mathematics and medicine, China has a long history starting from ancient times. However, Chinese medicine is also artistic, which is an invention and evolution of human physiology. Western medicine, on the other hand, has evolved from the discovery of human physics. They are very different from each other, but they both belong to the categories of science... Today, if China were to learn from western modern science, it must have its own traditional artistry involved in the study in order to instill Chinese traditional culture to modern human art. In other words, we can't say that China has imported Western scientization, but that China has revived its own scientization, making it less prone to diseases. The cultural future of China should be remedied by our own power. It is true that we should be exposed to new western science, but we should not jeopardize our own vitality. In this way, the great goal and ideal of China's cultural evolution that began thousands of years ago can continue to strive toward becoming reality.[1]
>
> —In 1941, Qian Mu's speech at the Chongqing Central Training Corps

10.1 Review: Contribution and Limitations

In a limited space, this book describes the various confrontations, dialogues, rejections and exchanges between bacteriology and TCM since the Republic of China period. Little by little, they converged into the views and connotations of today's TCM exogenous febrile diseases. If the spread of medical history is regarded as a cultural phenomenon, the manifestation of modern Chinese medicine focusing on internal medicine and Western medicine focusing on surgery has almost become a mantra for doctors and patients.[2] In the traditional internal medical literature, the knowledge of fever and its derivatives is the largest among all branches of TCM. The development of this discipline can be regarded as a concentrated essence version of

---

[1] Qian Mu, *Evolution of Chinese Cultural Tradition, New Theory of Chinese History*, Beijing: SDX Joint Publishing Company, 2001, pp. 346–347.

[2] (Qing) Ling Huan, Extraordinary Prescriptions for Surgery, included in Qiu Qingyuan (ed.), *San San Medical Book, Vol. I* Beijing: China TCM Press, 1998, p. 250.

© Zhonghua Book Company 2026

K. Pi, *The Contest of Modern Chinese and Western Medicine*,
https://doi.org/10.1007/978-981-95-2832-5_10

the development axis of modern Chinese medicine. How can we neglect the exploration of the development of TCM history? In the past, when it comes to the TCM history of febrile diseases, we often had a general discussion on the background of its wide range or the contributions of several doctors. Scholars were not aware of what important medical literature is in this discipline, how knowledge is transformed, and how it affects daily life. The scope of research is mostly limited to the late Qing Dynasty, but less to the Republic of China period. This book attempts to carry out a multi perspective "modern history of Chinese febrile diseases" with the idea of "multi-dimensional medical history" so as to fill in some blanks.

History was originally meant to explain about its people and events in the past. On this basis, modern Chinese medicine has at least two tendencies: first, it is still necessary to review the classics.[3] This is not just a current phenomenon. Its modern thought formation is closely related to the academic characteristics of modern Chinese medicine. In the past, researchers in various schools of modern history always emphasized the influence of "westernization". In fact, it is inevitable for the study of modern Chinese history to return to classics. Perhaps as an extension of "looking at China from the periphery",[4] the history of Japanese Han medicine can also be a perspective in the study of the development of Chinese medicine in modern China.[5] The study of Japanese Han medicine had spiritually and physically enhanced Chinese medicine. The referential value of the Japanese translation of medical terms also redefined diseases in TCM.[6]

---

[3] Cao Dongyi said: "We talk about syndrome differentiation, six meridians, triple energizers, and Wei Qi Ying Xue (the four dimensional changes of a disease--the translator's note) every day. It's traditional, completely traditional! This is what Deng Tietao believed in, and the rule on which TCM was established! This is exactly why Mr. Deng, as well as a generation of famous doctors, emphasized the significance of 'reviewing the classics'. 'The holy way means the normal way, which is applicable in daily life.'" Cao Dongyi (ed.), *The Battle of TCM Heroes against SARS—SARS and the Study on the TCM Standard of Diagnosis and Treatment of Exogenous Febrile Diseases*, Beijing: Ancient Books of TCM Press, 2006, p. 104.

[4] Ge Zhaoguang, *Dwelling in China: Reconstructing the Historical Discourse on "China"*, pp. 291–309.

[5] Fukagawa Shindo. *History of the Battle between Han and Western Medicine. Battle of Politics*, Tokyo: Medical Sage Society, 1981. This chapter supplements the influence of Japanese Han medical works in China. For the practice of TCM and its scientization in Taiwan, see Liu Shiyong, Medicine, Business and Social Imagination: The Scientification of Japanese Han Medicine and Scientific Chinese Medicine in Taiwan, *Technology, Medical Treatment and Society*, 2010 (11), pp. 150–197.

[6] "The revival of Japanese Han medicine has caused a problem of belief in Chinese medicine and Western medicine in China, particularly those who currently believe in Western medicine. Recently newspapers and magazines in Japan have taken this as a focus of discussion in their publications, and famous magazines have set special columns for discussion on Royal Han medicine. Three prescriptions, for lung disease, gonorrhea and beriberi respectively, of. Japanese Han Medicine have been proved by the clinical tests of various hospitals to have magic effects. In March, Hikichi Kogoro, a medical lecturer at Imperial University of Japan and the dean of Nanyang Hall Hospital, who received his PhD in Germany, visited China together with the interpreter Dokei Takashi. They visited the TCM doctor Fei Zibin in Shanghai and Gu Yunruo, Song Airen, Gu Yuecha, Wang Wenxi and Mao Ziming in Suzhou. He said: 'I have devoted myself to medicine for more than 20 years. Since I started my business, I have made considerable achievements, but I have never stopped learning, and I returned to Germany for my internship. However, my study of the scientific

The doctors of the Republic of China period advocated the revival of ancient classics for the development of Chinese medicine. The ancient classics include not only the medical books before the Tang Dynasty, but also the classics of the epidemic febrile diseases school later. Meanwhile the relationship between the two was competitive. Until modern times, the relationship between the typhoid fever school and warm disease school was in a state of constant restructuring.[7] At the beginning of the Republic of China period, *Treatise on Typhoid Fever* was elevated to a higher status, laying the foundation for the study of TCM internal medicine (see Fig. 10.1).[8] Liu Duzhou called the book "the soul of TCM", which has its origin.[9]

This also confirms the second view, that is, why modern Chinese medicine emphasizes the integration of the essence of typhoid fever school and warm disease school. Most modern scholars studying febrile diseases believed that the two systems can not be separated. For example, the typhoid scholar Wan Yousheng once wrote *The Integration of the Typhoid Fever and Warm Disease School*,[10] which was called "one of the books required in studying typhoid fever".[11] In the Qing Dynasty, "typhoid fever" could not be regarded as a real "epidemic". For example, *Treatise on Typhoid Fever* by Zhang Zhong is meant to distinguish the diseases of the four seasons—winter, spring,

---

treatment still needs the support of Royal Han Medicine. In recent years, every introduction of new drugs has been supplemented with Chinese medicine decoction, with remarkable effects. The German medical field has established cooperative facilities of Han medicine, and many graduates of medical universities learn Han medicine to acquire knowledge. It can be inferred that there must be truth in Han medicine today, so that I came to China to investigate. 'The doctor happily came to China for knowledge exchange. He also said he would, upon his returning, organize the Han Medical Research Society in Nanyang Hall of Qingshan, with the purpose of having a great collection of world medical science, he would call for the writings from famous doctors from all over the country to publish books and newspapers. With all the distinguished experts present as members of the society, he was willing to have the cooperation work at intellectual and financial levels." It can be confirmed that there was frequent communication between Han medicine and TCM besides the knowledge transfer from medical books. Quoted from Lu Shige, The Revival of Chinese Medicine in Japan, Shige's Medical Talk, included in Shen Hongrui and Liang Xiuqing (eds.), *General Medical Views on Chinese Medicine in China*, pp. 2046–2047.

[7] Cao Dongyi, *New Theory of Febrile Disease—on the Development of TCM from the Evolution of Fever Diagnosis and Treatment*, Beijing: China TCM Press, 2008, pp. 66–69, 170–175.

[8] For example, Ye Jinqiu wrote the *Analysis of Zhongjing Theory* (1936), which was referred to as the "Complete Book of TCM Internal Medicine" in the advertisement. From the advertisement on *Spring and Autumn of the Medical World*, 1936 (120), p. 43.

[9] Expanding from the original meaning of *Treatise on Typhoid Fever*, especially in the field of internal medicine, various researches have been carried out. See Liu Shien and Mao Shaofang (ed.), *Commentaries of Contemporary Famous Doctors on Zhongjing's Typhoid Fever*, Beijing: Xueyuan Publishing House, 2008, pp. 144–145.

[10] Wan Yousheng pointed out at the beginning that although there are differences between the cold and the warm, in a broad sense, they are all included in the six Qis. This is also in line with the trend of modern febrile diseases to attach importance to the theory of generalized Qi. The concept of six Qis is the main theory used as the frame of reference to bacteriology. Wan Yousheng, *The Integration of the Typhoid Fever School and Warm Disease School*, Shanghai: Shanghai Science and Technology Press, 1988, p. 1.

[11] Meng Yongli et al. (eds.), *Modern Research and Clinical Application of Typhoid Fever*, Beijing: Xueyuan Press, 1998, p. 2.

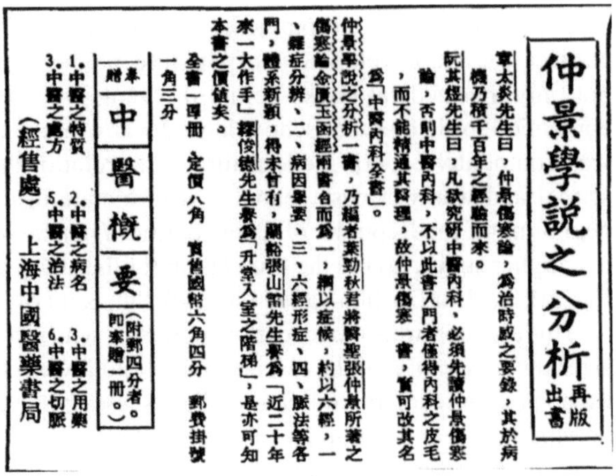
仲景學說之分析 再版出書

章太炎先生曰，仲景傷寒論，爲治時感之要錄，其於病機乃積千百年之經驗而來。

阮其煜先生曰，凡欲究研中醫內科，必須先讀仲景傷寒論，否則中醫內科，不以此書入門者僅得內科之皮毛，而不能精通其醫理，故仲景傷寒一書，實可改其名爲「中醫內科全書」。

仲景學說之分析一書，乃編者葉勁秋君將醫聖張仲景所著之傷寒論金匱玉函經兩書合而爲一，綱以症候，約以六經，一、雜症分辨、二、病因舉要、三、六經形症、四、脈法等各門，體系新穎，得未曾有，蘭谿張山雷先生譽爲「近二十年來一大作手」，釋俊德先生譽爲「升堂入室之階梯」，是亦可知本書之價值矣。

全書一厚冊 定價八角 實售國幣六角四分 郵費掛號一角三分

贈本 中醫概要 (附郵四分者。即奉贈一冊。)

1.中醫之特質 2.中醫之病名 3.中醫之用藥

3.中醫之處方 5.中醫之治法 6.中醫之切脈

(經售處) 上海中國醫藥書局

Fig. 10.1 The Republication of the *Analysis of Zhongjing Theory*

summer and autumn, that can not be incorporated into epidemics."[12] However, after the modern development process, the *Treatise on Febrile Diseases* was upgraded to a new level, not only becoming a branch of infectious diseases, but also gaining the classical status of exogenous febrile diseases". Shi Zhensheng said: "Exogenous fever is an acute infectious disease according to modern views". "It is wrong to think the *Treatise on Febrile Diseases* includes many miscellaneous diseases. Some symptoms appear to be miscellaneous diseases, but they are exactly the characteristics of various exogenous fever diseases".[13] The debate between TCM and Western medicine in modern fever studies has confirmed that the debate on typhoid and warm diseases is no longer able to confront Western theories, and must be integrated into a new category and disciplinary boundary. This shows that modern TCM infectious diseases have gradually taken shape. Before the Qing Dynasty, there was no science of exogenous febrile diseases at all. It was a consensus gradually formed after continuous discussion in modern times. In addition to the significance of "general theory", the science of epidemic febrile diseases also provides new knowledge for the discussion of infectious diseases to absorb nutrients. Therefore, in TCM infectious diseases, there are actually branches in the general theory, and even the discussion on single infectious diseases is gradually emerging.

There is no doubt that TCM can certainly cure the plague, but the treatment of infectious diseases with modern significance that being tested by bacteriology is the result of continuous dialogue between TCM and western bacteriology since the Republic of China period, the reinterpretation and the affirmation of the experience and treatment methods in classical medical books, building confidence and redefining exogenous febrile diseases. This process demonstrated the process of "re canonization" of TCM documents. Important medical books were repeatedly printed

[12] (Qing) Zhang Fengkui, additionally annotated by Ye Ziyu, The Preface to Yu Jiayan's 'Theory of Epidemics', Supplement of Ye Ping's The Complete Book of Heatstroke, included in Cao Bingzhang (eds.), *Great Achievements in Chinese Medicine*, Vol. 16 (II), p. 39.

[13] Meng Yongli et al. (eds.), *Modern Research and Clinical Application of Typhoid Fever*, p. 2.

and published during the Republic of China period in order to strengthen the internal recognition of the knowledge system of TCM warm diseases. In addition, during the Republic of China period, the typhoid fever school and warm disease school had not yet completely settled their disputes, but their views were gradually consistent, which was the general trend of academic development. Since then, whenever TCM was being faced infectious diseases, it must seek therapeutic inspiration from the classics within these two systems. Shao Yanzhi described Zhang Shou, in his *Suxuan Medical Talk* published in 1935, as being ""old but assertive as a dragon by quoting the records to suit the classics, using the western views to support Zhongjing theory and interpreting the views of Ye and Wu to unify the typhoid fever school and warm disease school".[14] It is an ideal expectation for modern medicine to integrate the schools of typhoid fever and warm diseases, as well as Western theory. Ideal and reality can not be completely equated. Although TCM in the early Republic of China period discussed scientific "academic research", it still had to face the history of the debate between the schools of typhoid fever and warm diseases. The author believes that the Chinese medicine industry was not only faced with the overwhelming classics and the internal academic debate, but also had to respond to the new bacteriology. In terms of how much Western knowledge was to be used, the opinions were so different that it led to the disorganization of the general work, and the pace of scientization, including academic research, was slowed down.

Of course, this phenomenon was accompanied by a series of influences, which determined the character of modern Chinese medicine. History is like a copper coin, which has both positive and negative sides. We can't just look at one side and forget the other side that we once owned. When TCM was moving toward modernization, it was classified into tradition unknowingly by various forces, positive and negative. Perhaps, the change of TCM is obvious to all, and many theories have been transformed. However, traditions remain unchanged, and its academic system, instead of being completely broken, still has its continuity. In 1947, Hong Guanzhi held that the education of modern Chinese medicine should not only attach importance to the establishment of research institutes, collate literature with scientific methods, but also learn to apply Western medicine, the equipment and the methods of diagnosing infectious diseases, so as to incorporate dimensions of both traditional and modern science.[15] From this book, it can be seen that "re canonization" of TCM is overwhelming, which leads to the process of TCM from absorbing the theory of bacteria, accepting some theories and debates, to eventually abandoning "most" of the experimental science of bacteria, leaving it behind and trying to find a new position from the literature instead. This can be a process of choosing and giving up. It enables modern Chinese medicine to cure infectious diseases, but it will not find a bunch of

[14] Shao Canzhi, From Zhang Zhongjing's Green Dragon Decoction to Zhang Shoufu's Clarification of Various Prescriptions, Suxuan Medical Talk, included in Lu Zheng (ed.), *Collection of Rare Modern TCM. Medical Talk*, p. 620.

[15] Hong Guanzhi, Proposals to the Education Authorities and the TCM Education Enthusiasts for the Prerequisite of TCM Education, *New TCM,* 1947, New Issue (1), p. 2.

"germicides" or use bacteriology to argue about disease names only.[16] Ever since after 1949, although the "antibacterial" of TCM was not particularly emphasized, the development of Chinese medicine in general has been changing with the national policy, and antibacterial or anti-virus turned to lead the direction of development. In 1971, Zhou Enlai instructed the Chinese Medicine Research Institute to start the research on antiviral Chinese medicine and provide funds to build a virus laboratory, which is another big change for TCM.[17] At that time, Taiwan did not seem to have large-scale funding subsidies or laboratory research on it.[18] Most modern TCM textbooks use a disease name given by Western medicine to correspond to many diseases or syndromes of TCM,[19] without "treating the bacterial causes".[20]

In the summer of 1953, Yu Wuyan treated a 24-year-old woman at No. 18, Yudeli Street, Guoyutang Street, Shanghai. She suffered from "damp warm typhoid fever" 18 days after childbirth. First, she was treated by a TCM doctor with fermented soybean and bean rolls. Then, she got injections of the advanced "bactericidal drug" penicillin from the Western medicine. With 8 injections, the treatment were still ineffective. Yu was invited to administer treatment. He was told that her condition had deteriorated rapidly. Fortunately, she was finally cured. Yu recalled:

> It can be seen that for every disease at present, if it does not heal at the beginning, it will be followed by complex variations. It is futile to rely on one or two kinds of medicines without

[16] In 1959, Pu Fuzhou did not talk much about bacteria at the "National Academic Conference on Acute Infectious Diseases" held at the Beijing Institute of TCM. He believed that patients' physical problems were the "cause". The author believes that instead of being a matter-of-fact conclusion, it is more a path "chosen" by academic development, the practical tests of daily life and the dialogue with Western medicine, involving many historical factors.

[17] Fu Hangyu, Premier Zhou Instructs Chinese Medicine Research Institutes to Do Antiviral Research, which was included in Zou Naili et al. (eds.), *The Unforgettable Forty Years,* Beijing: Ancient Chinese Medicine Publishing House, 1995, pp. 71–73.

[18] In recent years, in view of antibacterial and viral research of Chinese herbal medicine, there have been publications such as *Development of Chinese Herbal Medicine against Influenza Virus* by Lin Zhenwen, a professor in the Department of Medical Laboratory Biotechnology of China Medical University, *Development of New Chinese Herbal Medicine against Enterovirus by* Lin Yingru, a professor in the Department of TCM, and *Application of TCM in the Development of Antibacterial and Anti inflammatory* by Professor Lai Zhihe in the Department of Medicine, etc. See http://www.cmu.edu.tw/news_detail.php?Id=509 (published in 2009–10–28).

[19] The view that bacteriology is not supposed to be the basis of the discussion about the exclusive disease name is also presented in the work of "disease name comparison". Even in Taiwan, as a result of the "unification of Chinese and Western medicine", this kind of comparative work was also based on the disease names of Western medicine, accompanied by matching each disease with Chinese medicine. It is not the "one-to -one disease name" matching, which is defined as "treatment based on syndrome differentiation" rather than the spirit of "defining bacteria". Lin Zhaogeng (ed.), *A Dictionary of Chinese and Western Medical Diseases*, Vol. 1, Beijing: People's Health Publishing House, 2002, Self Preface and Introduction.

[20] As for the development method of TCM "sterilizing", there were still sporadic discussions in TCM after 1949. For example, He Yunhe once wrote the "pharmacological experiment of bacteria production and sterilization", but its theory is very primary and its accuracy is questionable. On the whole, it is at most a scientific confirmation which in no way is to weaken the status of Qi theory. See He Yunhe, *Scientific Direction of TCM*, Shanghai: Shanghai TCM Publishing House, 1954, p. 86.

> using the prescriptions with adjustments. In addition, antibiotic preparations have the function of antibacterial use. On one hand, they can interfere with the nutrition of bacteria, and on the other hand, it can control the activity of germs, have them cornered and eventually eliminated, but it can never directly kill bacteria. However, as far as prescriptions are concerned, none of them can have the definite function of excreting bacteria, which is also a disadvantage of Western medicine therapy.[21]

It can be seen that even after the invention of antibiotics, TCM still called for syndrome differentiation and treatment without relying on several specific drugs as it was very dangerous. This highlights the thinking that modern Chinese medicine did not take "sterilization" as its strength. The third chapter of this book also explains the problems of TCM in sorting out disease names, which is quite similar to what Liang Shuming said:

> When it comes to medicine, China claims to have it, but in fact it is a craft. For Western medicine prescription, one medicine is for one disease and there should be no difference made. For the skillful TCM doctors, all the expertise lies in their prescriptions. Ten doctors may have ten prescriptions, and they can be very different, as there is no standard for either the disease nor the treatment of diseases. What exactly is the disease? What is the "cause of the disease"? It is told more by personal observations than examinations! (There is no mention of "disease" in Chinese medical books.) What is the composition of a drug? How does it work? There is no need to ask. Only the terms as "the warm and the cool" are used to determine whether it (Qi) belongs to "the warm" or "the cool" by its property. Opinions differ greatly. That's why ten doctors would have ten prescriptions for the same disease. It is the spirit of science that requires an objective and shared knowledge; it is the spirit of art to ignore the rigid rules and regulations and advocates talents.[22]

In the West, science is valued while in the East, art is valued. This involves the development of culture, which is really a thorny problem for Chinese medicine. Liang believed that it was a misunderstanding that there was no mention of "disease" in Chinese medical books. It should be said that there was no mention of "disease" defined by western medicine. TCM during the Republic of China period did not develop standards and methods for testing bacteria. Although the adoption of disease names was affected by the uniformity of interpretations brought about by the bacteriological definition, it was reluctant to adopt the standard of bacteria naming, and was affected by the debate within its own academic system on its way toward "unification of disease names", which ultimately led to failure. Fortunately, due to bacteriology-based naming, Chinese medicine had a different standard and reference from its past, and a clearer scope. This is one aspect of the transformation of modern Chinese medicine that was greatly influenced by western medicine. In the Outline of the Central National Medical Center on the Arrangement of the Academic Standards of Chinese Medicine, it has been established that "the pathological changes in the new general theory are mainly based on the changes in the functional morphology of the disease, which are referred as physical signs. The theory of disease in China,

---

[21] Zhang Wenkang (ed.), *A Series of Chinese Medicine Clinicians for A Century. Yu Wuyan*, Beijing: China TCM Press, 2001, pp. 18–19.

[22] Liang Shuming, *East-West Culture and Philosophy*, Taipei: Taiwan Commercial Press, 2002, p. 34.

which is the most detailed and feasible, is divided into six meridians, which are called Qi-based in terms of Zhong Jing's *Treatise on Febrile Diseases.* The ancient and the present syndromes should be taken into consideration with the variables in general pathology, along with all other theories, establishing a different disease theory."[23] The essence of this outline is to achieve the goal of unification and standardization by systematizing and classifying the disciplines.[24] The premise is that we must try our best to provide a new statement based on Zhang Zhongjing's classical theory with reference to the Western classification of diseases.

Shi Yiren summarized the history of the collision between Chinese and Western medicine since modern times, and believed that "Chinese medicine focuses on the imbalance of the human body Qi, not on one's physical situation and the change of properties during a disease". The author has discussed the controversy of Chinese and Western medicine in his master's thesis,[25] but only limited to physiology. This book further discusses the controversy of pathology. Generally speaking, "Qi" is still the main criterion for explaining pathology in TCM. Shi said: "(Chinese medicine) regards all diseases as the result of imbalanced Qi. The regulation of it would fix the problem and cure the disease". What Shi said about "focusing on function instead of the physical situation is the characteristic and treatment method of TCM" is consistent with the main line of the development of modern Chinese medicine.[26]

In his early years, Gu Jiegang, a modern scholar, wrote the preface for the book *Extensive Learning*, which said: "Scholars should share their learning with the world without limiting it to one country nor one family. Those who identify their scholars with a country or a school can only be regarded as the learning of history but not as true learning. If they take the study of history as learning, their minds will be confined to ancient books. The ancient books remain unchanged, and their learning will not move forward".[27] The knowledge of modern Chinese medicine may have changed from private learning to public school learning, which can be discussed and commented by many. Not sticking to ancient books is the bottom line for the knowledge of a discipline, which is truly needed. Fortunately, since the introduction of western medicine bacteriology into China, TCM has never strongly rejected the theory of bacteria, but incorporated it into the new curriculum. From a practical point of view, TCM explains the physical changes of bacteria in the human body with various toxins. Taking bacteria as a biological role, it emphasizes that "bacteria are in the air"—bacteria cannot grow without external factors such as air, season, temperature and moisture—and then puts bacteriology into the category of Qi theory,

[23] Secretariat of the Central Chinese Medical Center, Outline of TCM Academic Standards Compiled by the Central Chinese Medical Center Approved by the Academic Sorting Committee in the Meeting of October 29, 2021, *Chinese Medicine Bulletin*, Vol. 1 (2), 1932 (11), pp. 2–3.

[24] Secretariat of the Central Chinese Medical Center, Record of the Preparatory Meeting of the Central Chinese Medical Center, *Chinese Medicine Bulletin*, Vol. 1 (2), 1932 (11), p. 8.

[25] Pi Kuoli, *Body View and Ideological Transformation of Modern TCM—Tang Zonghai and the Era of Convergence of TCM and Western Medicine*, pp. 404–418.

[26] Shi Yiren, *Shi's Internal Canon of Medicine*, p. 21.

[27] Gu Jiegang, *Walking on the Road of History—the Author's Own Account*, p. 35.

which is the historical model of the convergence of modern Chinese Qi theory and Western medicine bacteria theory.

In the part of Qi theory, there are not many discussions about the five movements and six Qis, which may be related to "what they (new medicine) reject is the theory of five movements, six Qis, Yin and Yang, and five elements, rather than the quintessence of Chinese medicine such as rhubarb and licorice". What many anti-Chinese medicine scholars opposed was a theory rather than the efficacy of herbal medicine.[28] However, modern Chinese medicine kept the basis of the theory of Qi, that is, it still carried out a dialogue on the basis of the external sense of "six Qis", the seasonal Qi and bacteriology. Zhang Taiyan's "theory of bacteria based on ancient views" mentioned in the article is very representative. He responded to bacteriology by mixing ancient knowledge of natural history, biology and medicine. Japanese Han medicine strongly supported TCM to classify the sweat method, detoxification and other therapies in the classics as "sterilization", which had more or less strengthened the confidence of Chinese medicine in the discussion. The two ways to acquire the knowledge of "sterilization", in addition to absorbing the theory of Western medicine bacteriology, were no more than discussing the possibility of "sterilization" from the perspective of typhoid and warm disease systems on body diseases and the mechanism of drug treatment. This is where they found the ways to kill bacteria.

Sean Hsiang-Lin Lei analyzed the significance of the scientific integration of TCM into the national public health system, which was a very important transformation during the Republic of China period. The so-called public health, including systems, regulations and insurance matters, is in fact a complete copy of the experiences of Europe, America and Japan. It is not a product of China. What was China thinking? This book gives further analyzes to the issue that TCM still needed to face the pressure of reforming the classics in addition to the scientific debate. Although it did not use bacteriological experimental methods and pathological expositions, TCM still continued to play an important role in the daily life of ordinary people. Without being able to intervene with an abundance of "public" health affairs, TCM had learned a lot from the West its cleaning and hygiene measures, and achieved a selective health modernity based on the integration of Chinese and Western medicine. There was a set of clean and sanitary mechanisms behind bacteriology. Although it had more or less affected the Chinese people's view of health, most of the theories that modern Chinese medicine really absorbed were based on the more primary "miasma theory" of Western medicine, in which both Chinese and Western medicine had expressed their loathing of the rotten and the filth. Even though personal hygiene is often portrayed as the key of public health, it often involves the introspection due to the lack of state laws, regulations or government effectiveness. During the Republic of China period, the so-called hygiene or prevention of infections still paid attention to individual behaviors, including the contact among the individuals, or individuals and groups, and focused on personal health, health preservation and disease prevention.

[28] Zhuang Zhaoxiang, Changes in the Study of Materia Medica (1941), included in Guo Zhengzhao, et al. (eds.), *Collection of Chinese Scientific and Technological Civilization,* Taipei: Shepherd Boy Publishing House, 1978, p. 562.

In the era of low efficiency in the country and the uneven distribution of regional health resources, it had indeed strengthened the view of personal hygiene (health preservation).[29]

In contrast to the appeal of Western medicine for diagnosis and treatment in hospitals, TCM can still play a role in health preservation, epidemic prevention, daily recuperation and other functions in the family or where medical treatment is not popular. Much knowledge of recuperation, dietotherapy and daily taboos also come from classical medical books. If we seek "scientific evidence" in everything, I am afraid that many customs and taboos coming from experience in daily life will not be proved and must be abandoned. Both Chapter 1 and Chapter 6 of this book discuss the personal hygiene laws of TCM, which contain a lot of feasibility in daily life. TCM and Western medicine share the common ground in their discussions on daily health preservation, diet and physical fitness. Even though Chinese medicine was influenced by western nutriology later, it still retained certain characteristics, which also confirmed that there was a strong connection between the upper level (doctors) and theoretical knowledge of Chinese medicine in the lower society.

More to be desired from the book is that the "multi-dimensional medical history" cannot cover all the history of fever and all the pathological treatises. The author believes that there are stories to be discovered about the treatment and definition of many infectious diseases during the Republic of China period, and the history of individual infectious diseases can be further studied in the future. In addition, modern history material is vast and still needs to be further updated. As long as this book is aiming at the definition and discussion of the name of exogenous febrile diseases in TCM and Western medicine, the debate of "Qi" and "bacteria" can not be avoided. Moreover, most of the research we see now is based on the definition of Western medicine, rather than the discussion of TCM context. To understand the latter, it is necessary to carry out a multi-level discussion on the literature, historical development and characteristics of the foundation of TCM febrile diseases during the Republic of China period, which is also the modest contribution of the book, serving as the "basic project" to construct the infectious disease history of "TCM style".

[29] Sean Hsiang-Lin Lei's research has presented an important tendency: at many times, the most important concern of political leaders during the Republic of China period was not the large-scale construction of the medical system, but a sense of disgust and awakening at the "personal" level. The country under the rule of the Nationalist Party may not be able to promote large-scale public health construction, but the discussion of personal hygiene involved a personal transformation plan that was conducive to the formation of the nation. Sun Yat-sen, Chen Guofu, and Chiang Kai-shek all participated in and tried to introduce this personal hygiene exposition and feeling. See Sean Hsiang-Lin, *Why Hygiene Is Not Protecting Life—Alternative Hygiene, Self and Diseases in the Period of the Republic of China period,* Taiwan Social Research Quarterly, No. 54 (2004.06), pp. 41.

10.2 West Wind and East Wind—History of Culture from the Perspective of Traditional Medicine

Yang Zhiyi, a TCM doctor, said in 1936, "The establishment of any academic school that has lasted for a long time is definitely to be valued". ① Many traditional Chinese schools in modern times are truly valuable and passing them down is no easy job. Even if the "re canonization" as mentioned in this book is not a logical trend, the process behind it is actually very complicated. When the "TCM Abolition Act" came out in 1929, a TCM doctor named Lei Ji wrote a letter listing the reasons why Chinese medicine should not be abolished at once. As a result, the reply from the Ministry of Health gave him a firm negative response.

It is a smattering of knowledge to hold that "for Chinese medicine, the disease is caused by pathogenic Qi, while for Western medicine it is caused by bacteria", as stated in the letter. There is even the thinking that bacteria is caused by pathogenic factors, and there would be no bacteria without pathogenic factors, which is totally wrong and lacks the common sense of biology. The test of the meat mentioned in the original letter, however, proves that although the cooked meat is sterilized, if the meat itself or the meat container is not completely sterilized, the bacteria that have not been killed can still develop, which indicates that this is not enough to prove the existence of pathogenic factors. The doctor had no knowledge of bacteriology except the word "bacteria". According to medical science, the causes of diseases are very complex, and not all of them are caused by microorganisms. Microorganisms have numerous types, and not all of them can cause diseases. Without this common sense, his argument was nothing but the occurrence of bacteria, which is meaningless and worthless. The proposal was undoubtedly dismissed.[30]

This reply is tantamount to saying that the "Qi theory" opposite to bacteriology is nonsense from the standpoint of the state. As for the complexity of microbiology, it is not a science that can be understood by the empty talk of TCM. Many examples in cultural circles are cited in the book. Finally, there is Chen Duxiu's statement. He believed that modern Chinese people must pay equal attention to science and human rights if they want to break away from ignorance.

Some doctors don't know science, they don't understand the structure of the human body, nor can they analyze drug properties, and they never heard about infectious bacteria and toxins. What they know about is nothing but that the theory of the five elements can overcome cold and heat, and regulate Yin and Yang by using the ancient prescriptions. Its technique is almost the same as that of an archer. The most magical thing is "Qi", which is about the same as the mystery of devilish alchemy. Looking

[30] "Proposal for the Cancellation of the TCM Abolition Act (I)", file number 001130006001143a46a" from "National Government" file in "National History Museum". The official document was signed by Xue Dubi, the Civil Service Office of the National Government. He was not a strong advocate of TCM abolition. The official letter only represents the tough attitude of the central health administration. See Wei Jiahong, *National Government and TCM* (Zhongli, Master's Thesis of History Institute of the "Central University", 1998), pp. 52–61. A relatively new research reference: *Transplantation and Transcendence: Medical Administration of TCM during the Republic of China Period,* Beijing: China TCM Press, 2007, Chapter 3.

all over the universe, I can by no means find out where "Qi" is from. To eradicate all this thinking without common sense and a belief based on nothing is the only way to adhere to science. In explaining the truth, science seeks for proof. Compared with what we think as being arbitrary, this is a slow process, but every step is steady, nothing like the illusion of flying without actually taking even one step.[31]

Both the legitimacy of national laws and regulations, as well as the rationality of scientific development go against the fallacy of the theory of Qi in TCM. Is modern Chinese medicine faced with sticking to its traditional theory or choosing to join in the camp of Western medicine by dumping the theory of Qi? Is it the only choice of Chinese medicine to give way and abandon the theory of Qi? At that time, the dilemma of TCM was quite similar to the swing and "dichotomy" shown by intellectuals in many areas at the beginning of the Republic of China period.[32] Qian Mu once said, "Of eastern and western culture, it's been an issue perplexing all Chinese for nearly a century as which wins over the other or which is more superior than the other. I am one of those who have also been trapped all my life by this issue".[33] I'm afraid it is very difficult to make a decision to turn to western culture immediately, especially for intellectuals who are influenced by traditional culture. Zhou Mingzhi pointed out that Hu Shi's vacillation in many aspects was due to an inferiority complex or anxiety in the face of western values, which prompted him to return to the traditional and seek self-respect as a Chinese. Zhou defined this mentality as: "the internal assimilation of the old and the new"—they look to the West while not being able to completely abandon the tradition,[34] and their swing "from West to East" was actually looking for an outlet for modernity. In other words, we can observe from another perspective that in addition to legality and science, TCM also represents inherently the character of traditional culture. This was unfavorable for Chinese medicine in the process of scientific development, but the future was still unknown at the time.

---

[31] Chen Duxiu, Caution to the Youth, *New Youth,* 1915 (1:1), p. 6.

[32] Zhang Hao, *The Exploration of the Times,* Taipei: Lianjing Publishing House, 2004, pp. 136–137.

[33] Qian Mu, *Memoirs of Parents in My 80s. Memories of Teachers and Friends*, p. 46.

[34] Zhou Mingzhi, *Hu Shi and the Choice of Modern Chinese Intellectuals,* Guilin: Guangxi Normal University Press, 2005, p. 209. In addition, to discuss the tangle and variability of interests and ideals between intellectuals and complex interpersonal networks and politics, see R. Keith Schoppa, translated by Zhou Wubiao, *Blood Road-The Mystery of Shen Dingyi (Xuanlu) in Revolutionary China*, Nanjing: Jiangsu People's Publishing House, 1999. Another example is that Kang Lvdao used psychoanalysis in the early stage to speculate that "inconsistent" behavior of Liang Qichao might be due to his "circulatory depression". In fact, "contradiction" was the common problem of the intellectuals in the early Republic of China period. See his paper: The Contradictory Liang Qichao: A Psychological Interpretation, *Sinology Research* 3.1 (1985.06), pp. 185–198. Huang Kewu once commented on the legacy of the Chinese intellectual and ideological circles brought by the contradictory forces: "The creative dialogues and the spirit of self-conscious introspection in ideological circles brought about by the debate between the two sides of for-against 'May 4th' (The New Cultural Movement in 1919-the translator's note), is the enlightenment of modern China". Quoted from his paper: Where the Soul Goes—Rethinking of Liang Qichao and Confucianism China and Its Modern Destiny, included in Zheng Dahua & Zou Xiaozhan (ed.), *Thinkers and Modern Chinese Thought*, Beijing: Social Science Literature Press, 2005, pp. 91–114.

TCM during the Republic of China period inherited a body view that was understood according to the content and theory of classical medical books. To create a discourse "out of nothing", a convincing new interpretation must be developed with reference to the relevant books of bacteriology according to the doctors' study of classical medicine. It is precisely what modern Japanese Han medicine did in modern times. When discussing the possibility of TCM sterilization, Tang Ben's inspiration came not only from Japanese Han medicine research, but also from ancient Chinese medical classics. For Western medicine, with the rapid progress of science and technology, "classics" cannot be ever lasting. Ancient medical books do not need to be read and annotated repeatedly. In terms of culture, the traditions carried by Western medical science are not as profound as TCM. Modern Western medicine relies on experiments to study bacteria, while TCM relies on classical medicine to understand the knowledge of "six Qis", which is fundamentally different. "Qi" represents the property of matter, such as the taste and taboos of food, the way of recuperation and the spatial characteristics. Understanding this set of knowledge is of great help to understand the Chinese-style disease discourse, and has a daily practical nature close to body feelings. It is not only an illusory philosophical discourse, but also a basic "element" of western science.[35] Although some doctors advocated abolishing "Qi" and sorting out TCM classics with scientific methods, the method was still to distinguish the relationship between pharmacology and treatment based on the treatment symptoms and curative effects in TCM literature. It is difficult to avoid the question of "Qi" in such sorting and research methods.[36] Zhang Taiyan once said: "The skills in medical practice are similar to the strategies in a war. They are acquired by keen observations. It is not a philosophy, but the adaptability according to difference circumstances".[37] In 1936, Tang Shenxuan took Zhang Taiyan's views as "a perfect combination of heaven and earth. How can it be achieved without his years of accumulation ?"[38] Medicine is based on the principle of change, which must be experienced personally. Theory is only an introduction, and the specific principle needs to be verified by clinical experiences. Therefore, modern Chinese medicine has been worried about adopting Western medicine the most, namely the acceptance of a whole set of knowledge systems of technical operation and the explanation of diseases behind Western medicine and bacteriology, including the use of western textbooks. It is quite difficult to carry out TCM while being faced with the question of how much classical medical theory can be preserved.

In the exploration of modern academic transformation, all disciplines, including medicine, have been actually faced with a "two-way reflection". That is, the response to new theories or western learning and the reflection on the positioning of traditional

---

[35] Yabuuti Kiyosi, translated by Liang Ce et al., *China, Science and Civilization*, Taipei: Shu Xin Press, 1989, pp. 24–25.

[36] Ye Juquan, My Views on the Study of Chinese Medical Literature, *Spring and Autumn of the Medical World*, 1936 (118), p. 5.

[37] Zhang Nianchi, *My Grandfather Zhang Taiyan*, Shanghai: Shanghai People's Publishing House, 2011, p. 107.

[38] Zhang Nianchi, *My Grandfather Zhang Taiyan*, p. 113.

learning in the new era, or the reproduction of the value of classical medical books through western science, as Luo Xieyuan from Sichuan once admired, "... is quite a pleasure to see the diseases buried in the ancient papers for thousands of years finally be revealed to the world!"[39] Although the real collation didn't take place until after the 1950s,[40] its general ideology and development can be seen during the Republic of China period, which had been important in the TCM history for a century, and will continue to be explored in the future. The example of Yun Tieqiao in the book can well illustrate the attitude of the TCM school,[41] showing an awkward and tense relationship among bacteria, disease names and its own academic study. He insisted on responding to the crisis that TCM was about to lose the power to define the names of the diseases by taking the position of the six Qis, four seasons or syndrome differentiation, but in fact he could not be free of pressure in the era of "learning bacteria theory". In general, what Yun could do was to find out any possibility of unifying and defining diseases based on *Treatise on Typhoid Fever* by ignoring the main body of the theory of bacteria. In fact, various "sterilization" methods were also inspired from various pharmacology and classics. For example, "sweating" may focus on the classics of typhoid fever, and "detoxification" may focus on the discussion of warm disease or epidemics. The discussion of fever in Chinese medicine during the Republic of China period was not only about the significance of "sterilization", otherwise it cannot explain why Chinese medicine had not moved toward the development of bactericides, nor re-considered the treatment in this direction. In addition to the lack of laboratories and scientific methods, it is more important that Chinese medicine, even if it has fungicides, should observe the limits of the Qi theory, because Chinese medicine is based on the cold or hot "Qi", instead of bacteria, in the treatment. Modern Chinese medicine, based on the integrity of "Qi theory" and body view, adopted an argumentative and highly selective attitudes toward western bacteriology. Studying TCM with the science of Western medicine will indeed make TCM too westernized, which was also the doubt of Chinese medicine during the Republic of China period that "if it is westernized, it will no longer be TCM".

The study of modern medical history cannot be based on the perspectives of TCM or Western medicine, new or old and if it is scientific or not. Modern TCM doctors have continuously adopted the disease discourse of Western medicine, but still studied ancient classics in the classroom. They read *Treatise on Typhoid Fever*, without talking much about "typhoid fever" with patients. This is a very interesting phenomenon. He Yunhe said, "In 1929, Zhang Taiyan set up the Shanghai Chinese Medical College, which was the first Chinese medical school formally based on modern medicine. The courses in the school were prescribed by Lu Yuanlei. Basic medicine, such as biology, chemistry, anatomy and physiology, all adopted modern

---

[39] Luo Xieyuan, On the Invention of Microbiology in Chinese Medicine, *Modern TCM,* Vol. 2, 1941 (01), p. 22.

[40] Pi Kuoli, *The Development of TCM in Shanghai (1950–1965)—An Investigation Centered on the People's Daily.*

[41] In Chapter 5, it is called "two-way (the West and China) introspection in the modern academic transformation".

medical courses. The applied disciplines were mainly based on the original TCM ones, and focused on the experience of *Treatise on Typhoid Fever*".[42] Probably the same is true of the basic courses of modern Chinese medicine. In 1935, the courses of Suzhou National Medical School, even the three-year study period, had western medicine bacteria and anatomy as compulsory courses in the first year, while the Department of TCM Internal Medicine had them scheduled in the second year, with more class hours. This initiated the study mode of the "West over China".[43] However, this experience needed to be put into clinical practice, while the technology of medical sterilization and surgery were not applied yet, which featured modern Chinese medicine academics. Even if inevitably influenced by the West, the "traditional" boundaries of modern disciplines were rarely as complete as those of TCM. This study is practically significant as well as functional. We should constantly remind modern Chinese medicine that "wisdom and classics of sages and sages of all dynasties" were not understandable to every doctor during the Republic of China period. When reviewing these assets, we should not forget that Western medicine was still very alien to many TCM doctors. The exploration of this history is not only for its historical significance, but also for the enlightenment of clinical treatment. How can one doubt the production of innovative ideas in the review of the ancient by studying the medical history documents?

This is the interesting part of the history of modern Chinese medicine. There is no need to discuss the "westernization" of modern Chinese learning. This old framework will prevent us from seeing the whole picture of modern Chinese history because it has only a single perspective. Many people may question whether this is an "anti science" position. In terms of historical research, there can't be only a single-line discussion, just as what Dorothy Ko proposed for a breakthrough in the framework of the "May 4th Historical Outlook" (the new cultural movement in 1919-translator's note).[44] The author shares the view that: if we maintain the "May 4th Historical Outlook" to question if Chinese medicine is scientific, or why Chinese medicine is not scientific, we will never find the feasibility of TCM in modern multicultural history and in modern daily life. Even if we explore the part affected by Western medicine, we can't know what kind of protection and compromise TCM had made during that time. What's more, for most Chinese people, life is not composed of only science, but also involves nature and culture. Culture and history don't have to develop in just one track.

Although "science" occupied the main part of the intellectual transformation during the Republic of China period, the power of "tradition" was liberated from the shackles of cultural inferiority and self-inspection caused by foreign aggression, and gradually showed its true value. Qian Mu once criticized western science as nearly

---

42 Zhang Nianchi, *My Grandfather Zhang Taiyan*, p. 111.

43 Suzhou Periodical Office of TCM, *Suzhou Journal of TCM*, 1935 (07), pp. 17–19.

44 Dorothy Ko, translated by Miao Yanwei, *Footbinding:The Rise and Fall of the Worship for Golden Lotus*, Nanjing: Jiangsu People's Publishing House, 2009, Preface, pp. 1–13.

"destroying human nature while pursuing materialism",[45] which may be similar to Yumoto's theory of the test tube being equivalent to the human body. Mao Zedong said in 1957, "Now I feel that the international situation has got to a new turning point. There are two winds in the world: the east wind and the west wind. There is a Chinese proverb: either the east wind prevails over the west wind, or the west wind prevails over the east wind. I think the current situation is characterized by the east wind prevailing over the west wind".[46] Mao Zedong was very optimistic about the development of Chinese socialism, which can overcome western imperialism. It is probably the hope that China can find its own way without being interfered and suppressed by the West. For the leaders of that generation, science was important, but tradition should not be abandoned, For example, Chiang Kai-shek said, "I hope equal attention should be given to the significant learning of China from the old days, as much as to the new science and learning. The knowledge in the old books of China is very profound".[47] "In the past, we were so dedicated to the foreign learnings instead of learning our culture. We forgot our own essence, and lost our inherent virtue and spirit, which stopped us from saving the country and completing the revolutionary cause. Now if we don't wake up early, we would be in danger of national subjugation and extinction if this continues".[48] It may reflect this concern about the loss of traditional culture. TCM after the 1930s caught the tide of nationalism and took advantage of the trend of "renaissance and national revival", just to ride on the train of traditional academic renewal and autonomy. This tendency cannot be ignored by modern medical history scholars.[49]

Where would "modern" China be led to? For nearly a hundred years, everyone has been trying to seek answers for this question. Qian Mu, who was cured of typhoid fever by TCM, said[50]: "Chinese culture has always focused on the humanities. It takes more seriously the specific synthesis than the abstract generalization. Due to

[45] Qian Mu, Communication between China and the West and Cultural Renewal, *Introduction to the History of Chinese Culture*, p. 228.

[46] Central Committee Literature Research Office of the Communist Party of China (ed.), *Mao Zedong's Manuscripts since the Founding of the People's Republic of China*, Vol. 6, Beijing: Central Literature Publishing House, 1992, p. 630.

[47] Xiu Zhouhuan (ed.), *President Jiang Zhongzheng's Archives: A Brief Draft,* Vol. 9, Taipei: National History Museum, January 12, 1931, 2006, pp. 363–364.

[48] Gao Mingfang (ed.), *President Jiang Zhongzheng's Archives: A Brief Draft,* Vol. 18, January 8, 1933, p. 66.

[49] Chen Wujiu, Problems in the System of TCM? *Spring and Autumn of the Medical World*, 1937 (121), pp. 5–6.

[50] Qian Mu recalled this experience: "When I was at home during the summer vacation, I suddenly became infected with typhoid fever and was almost killed by the medicine. Ten miles away, there was a famous doctor Shen, whose father and elder brother were admired. I went to see him many times, and I got better.... My mother took care of me by staying at my bedside morning and night. She slept in her clothes, no fanning in summer and got little sleep. Not until after two months, could I gradually have thin porridge. Before dawn, my mother boarded the house and took the home-made pickled melon. In another ten days, I started eating rice. "I guess Qian's mother was knowledgeable about the ways of "fasting" for typhoid fever. Quoted from Qian Mu, *Memoirs of Parents in My 80s. Memories of Teachers and Friends,* p. 31.

this reason, it often leaves room for the new and opens for the changes and integration at any time. This is the Chinese people's strength, being open, comprehensive, absorbent and flexible. If we hold that the evolution of the humanities can use and control natural science, it is not a problem that Chinese traditional culture can accommodate the modern western scientific civilization. Not only can it tolerate, but it can also assimilate and update. This is our hope for the future of China's new cultural era."[51] The concern of the literati was the same. The leaders of the modern state also made the statements on the future of China. When talking about the expectation of "national medicine", Chiang Kai-shek said: "The Central State Medical Center was established in Beijing yesterday. This is an important matter for the progress of Chinese medicine from the stand point of consolidation. I can see the great efforts made."[52] Mao Zedong said: "Chinese medicine is a great treasure, which should be explored and improved."[53] Obviously this is based on the inherent concern for traditional culture. From a historical perspective, science is not necessarily the only concern. The argument that science and technology should blow the west wind and culture should blow the east wind should be a neutralization acceptable to all scholars concerned with the development of Chinese history.

Of so many TCM books, it needs to be discussed in detail and proved with time in regard to how to sort them out and what standards to use from the cultural point of view. Zhang Guohua, a TCM doctor, said:

> Chinese medicine has been popular. What people don't feel happy about it is that each disease is interpreted differently by different doctors, and there comes the criticism against each other, which is not the same as that of Western medicine that is governed by a system. In order to improve TCM, it is urgent to plan for a unified system. However, how can it be possible to plan for a unified system? There is a reason why it is difficult to seek unity. The metaphysics is the way while physics is the implement. The implement is crude while its way is exquisite. The way of TCM is also the way of metaphysics. There is a great disparity among doctors. Western medicine only seeks form and quality, while Chinese medicine is deeply concerned with Qi functions. This is why it is easy for Western medicine to form a system, while for TCM, it is difficult. The question is: can't TCM be unified? It is said: it is necessary to first establish a unified medical system before the development of a unified academic system. It's to be based on the principle of *Materia Medica, Inner Canon, Classics on Medical Problems, and Golden Collection.* As for what schools to follow in view of external syndromes or internal syndromes, what books are to be studied for all other kinds of miscellaneous syndromes, it is to be explored in the long run. Pick up the essence and discard the dross, make the annotations concise by keeping the essentials, so that no regrets are left in all departments and the unified medicine study is established. The later generations can take it as the standard, with simple practice and speculations, and eventually draw up

---

[51] Qian Mu, Communication between China and the West and Cultural Renewal, *Introduction to the History of Chinese Culture*, p. 221.

[52] Gao Sulan, *The Archives of President Jiang Zhongzheng: A Sketch Script: Vol. 10*, March 18, 1931, p. 283.

[53] In 1954, Mao Zedong said, "We often emphasize partially on the shortcomings of TCM without seeing that it is one of the precious cultural heritages of China". Wang Zhenrui, *A Historical Review of the Integration of Chinese and Western Medicine*, Shijiazhuang: Hebei Education Press, 2002, pp. 50–51.

a medical integration, which will be known to the world, and will always be the orthodox school of medicine.[54]

Western medicine focuses on form and quality while TCM focuses on Qi, which is the most complex and difficult to form a unified standpoint, but Zhang believed that it is still necessary to start from traditional medical books. Shi Yiren said: "Although cholera and acne were widely spread in ancient China, the treatment methods were different and could not be unified. Diphtheria, dysentery, malaria, typhus, scarlet fever and other symptoms and treatment methods were also different. Although there are some records in ancient books about intestinal fever and relapsing fever, the names had not been determined, and the treatment methods were disorganized; pestis and meningitis are missing in the ancient medical books. All of the above present us with the necessity for the work of compilation."[55] This is the biggest challenge of modern Chinese medicine in the theory of exogenous fever. How to study the diseases and treatments buried in the ancient papers for thousands of years is a subject that modern Chinese medicine and even future Chinese medicine should explore.

In terms of the opinions of scholars and doctors during the Republic of China period, this book covers all aspects of TCM in addition to the "TCM Abolition Act". Talking about his serious illness, Zhang Taiyan once said, "In my early life, I have been diligent in learning but did not have much interest in Taoism. When reading the medical classics, I was quite confused. With a lot of suffering during my middle age, I began to seek the Mahayana scripture along with Lao and Zhuang. In my later years, I extended my readings to the two Chengs, Chen, and Wang, acquiring a lot of knowledge. Though being achieved and living in peace, I have been anxious day and night whenever an epidemic occurs, fearing that I may not survive. Then I started to work on the medical classics". Zhang also dabbled in western learning. In his later years, starting from his own practice with reference to the culture in general, he saw the essence of the medical classics as a way of medical research.[56] Zhang regarded his study of medical classics as a personal reading experience, from reading to clinical practice, rather than shaking test tubes and peering through microscopes. However, "convergence" basically is still the way of modern Chinese medicine. In addition, Qian Mu said that the Chinese people have a "neutral" character,[57] which

[54] Zhang Guohua, Why It Is Difficult for TCM to a Have a Unified System, The Change of Medicine, included in Lu Zheng (ed.), *Collection of Rare Modern TCM. Medical Talk*, p. 257.

[55] Shi Yiren, *Chinese Epidemiology*, Preface, p. 1.

[56] Zhang Nianchi, *My Grandfather Zhang Taiyan,* Shanghai: Shanghai People's Publishing House, 2011, pp. 105–106.

[57] Qian Muyan, "As China started its development of science as that being done in the West, would the Chinese cultural tradition be damaged or destroyed? This question is quite important. In my opinion, China's cultural tradition will never be damaged by the introduction and development of modern western science, because Chinese traditional culture has always been happy to accept foreign elements and keep its original methods intact. This is not only due to the leniency of Chinese character, but also due to the unique neutralizing character of the traditional Chinese culture, making the absorption and integration possible in many ways. " He also cited religious thought as an example: "Confucianism can tolerate Jesuit, but Jesuit cannot tolerate Confucianism. In the late Ming and early Qing Dynasties, the Chinese people could accept Matteo Ricci, but the western churches

absorbs western science without damaging traditional culture. The course of modern Chinese medicine can prove this view to some extent.

Wang Fansen had a lot of insightful discussions on modern tradition and anti-traditional thoughts. He believed that "conservative" and "retro" are two different ideological trends. The former is simply loyal to the current tradition, while the so-called "retro" in modern Chinese medicine is to transcend and sublate the pure tradition and accumulate more reform momentum.[58] Therefore, TCM during the Republic of China period had to merge with western culture, and we can not reject all western influences with cultural arrogance. "Tradition" and "retro" are not necessarily in conflict with "westernization". In fact, the two were mutually affected. Traditional learning has definitely incorporated some elements of the West. Zhang Taiyan once summarized the strengths of Chinese and Western medicine, respectively: "The shape of viscera and blood vessels, which people could not understand when they first learned anatomy, should be judged by Western medicine". "If the viscera are occluded by disease, Western medicine has the better treatment than TCM". "Among the diseases TCM can do better than Western medicine in treatment, typhoid fever should be the first".[59] It can be seen that it was still of value for TCM study of fever, and TCM at that time did not limited itself by the self-righteous cultural barriers. "Bacteria" is a science that connects the pathology of Western medicine, while "Qi" is another science that connects the TCM. Before finding a way of communication that could truly satisfy both Chinese and Western medicine, TCM abolition had been the key note of Western medicine, while what TCM could do was nothing but relying on its efficacy and culture established in the classical medical books.

10.3 Medical History and National History from the Perspective of "Multi-dimensional Medical History Research"

The "multi-dimensional medical history" proposed in this book is a methodological attempt. The final review here is just made as a summary with some observations. First, this concept tries to find a balance between "generalization" and "specialization". It is unnecessary to define "specialization". As for "generalization", scholars during the Republic of China period attached great importance to the method of studying history. He Bingsong (1890–1946) said: "Since the abolition of the imperial examination and the establishment of schools in the late Qing Dynasty, it is quite urgent for ordinary students and the general public to learn from Chinese and

rejected him. That's the difference". This actually contains the differences between Chinese and Western cultural views. Quoted from his publication: Communication between China and the West and Cultural Renewal, *Introduction to the History of Chinese Culture*, p. 221.

[58] Wang Fansen, *The Pedigree of Modern Chinese Thought and Learning*, Shijiazhuang: Hebei Education Press, 2001, pp. 91–148.

[59] Zhang Nianchi, *My Grandfather Zhang Taiyan*, p. 108.

foreign general history. However, in the past 20 years, the works of Western general history have made considerable achievements, but there are few compilations of Chinese general history that can be compatible with the modern historical perspective. Why?"[60] In fact, today's historiography tends to study minor problems. It has been "specialized" rather than "general". *The Outline of National History* is still an irreplaceable compulsory reading in the university classroom. It can be seen that the concept of general history advocated by scholars since the early Republic of China period had little progress.[61] As long as "generalization" is required, the important historical facts must be collected in the field of modern history. But what is "important"? Zhang Yinlin (1905–1942) shared the very objective views that can be used for reference. First of all, the "multi-dimensional medical history" must be able to explain what aspects of modern Chinese medicine has changed and what its course is. This is the "standard for the origins of the current situation". Secondly, in view of the trend of "re canonization" of this book, it can explain the "standard of cultural value" of modern Chinese medicine history and the close relationship between the writing of traditional books and cultural values. As for Zhang's "standard of novelty", the selected data of this book is not yet complete, but as Liu Xianxin (1896–1932), a scholar in the early Republic of China period, said: "Reading the history, observing the changes, and examining the relationship among the events, is just like threading copper coins. It is necessary to have a summary of the results first, so as to prepare for the deduction. It is also a shortcut. However, there is still a lot of information that is not limited to one person, nor to be put in one book. The compilation can include many significant events. Scholars can draw inferences from the details and make the summaries".[62] This book sketches the main stance of medical history, which is the controversy between "Qi" and "bacteria" between modern Chinese and Western medicine. Let it be known that, there are some areas left unexplored, such as the health history and practices in some poor areas, which is the blind spot under this framework.

As for the integration of internal and external history emphasized in the introduction, there are also responses in this book. We should pay as much attention to the theoretical responses of TCM as to the propagation and practice of Qi and bacteria in daily life, as well as the cognition of pathology and disease names in different societies and cultural contexts. "Multi-dimensional medical history" focuses on understanding the relationship between fever and bacteriology in TCM—it is impossible to deal with the problems of individual infectious diseases one by one, except for the case of typhoid fever which is more representative. In addition, there is still much to explore about the daily practice and recuperation culture of exogenous fevers in TCM. What covered in this book is just the part that was less concerned in the past.

---

[60] He Bingsong, A New Interpretation of General History, included in Liu Yinsheng et al. (eds.), *Collected Works of He Bingsong*, Beijing: Commercial Press, 1996, p. 77.

[61] Sang Bing, *Scholars and Academics in the Late Qing and Republic of China Period*, Beijing: Zhonghua Publishing House, 2008, pp. 49–58.

[62] Liu Xianxin, Introduction to History, *Liu Xianxin's Academic Essays: Literary Handouts,* Guilin: Guangxi Normal University Press, 2007, p. 234.

Liang Qichao once appealed the internal history be done by science and technology experts, and external history be undertaken by historians. He cited the history of astronomy as an example, "For example, the records of astronomy, from the *Records of the Grand Historian · On Astronomy* to *A History of the Ming Dynasty · Astronomical Records,* are all about the constellations and equations, which belongs to the scope of astronomy and should not be included in history. As far as other aspects are concerned, such as when the culminant star was discovered, when the leap, or the procession of the equinoxes were invented, and even the discrimination of stars and planets, the debate over the canopy or ellipsoid earth theories, the inference of the ecliptic and the equator, are all the results of Chinese people's continuous efforts, and the manifestation of their activities is in the scope of history. So astronomy is one thing, and the history of astronomy is another."[63] Although the author is no expert on the history of astronomy, if we are not willing to pursue any areas of the internal history by skipping the professional issues and cutting out this part of historical events to the science and technology (internal history) specialists, then how will historians expand the field of historical data and research horizons? What's more, either the medical history of western bacteriology or Chinese medicine has its own scientific and technological context in a particular society. It is hard to separate "internal history" and "external history" in a clear-cut way.

The interesting part of Chinese medical history is that Chinese medicine is rooted in the classical perception of the characteristics of Qi in daily life and the pathological phenomena it triggers,[64] which are confirmed by the experience of one's life. TCM can be taken as a part of human literature. Qian Mu said: "The characteristics of culture and history are called the 'succession' or 'continuity', which are established and can not be changed. This unchangeable feature is also called life or spirit. The life and spirit of a nation's culture and history take shape from its special environment, special problems, special efforts, and special achievements, and become a special mechanism… This historicity means that it evolves in accordance with the continuation of the problems in reality. The problems vary in accordance with the actual situations of different regions and individuals."[65] The TCM experimental field can be seen in the personal body perception and daily life constructed by specific cultural history. It won't make sense if the history of TCM is only regarded as or cut into pure scientific history or internal history.

As early as 1927, Liu Xianxin wrote the *Compendium of Archaeological Folklore*, which included many items of the "new social history" that came out later. Of course, medical history can also be found in the *Compendium*: medical divination, astrology and boxing are classified as "acrobatics". In addition, the item of "Local Customs" in the list of the Beijing University Custom Survey attached to the book also lists

---

[63] Liang Qichao, *Methodologies of Chinese History Research*, Shanghai: Zhonghua Book Company, 1936, p. 30.

[64] The body sense of color, smell, wind, etc. can be seen in Masahisa Kuriyama, translated by Chen Xinhong, *The Language of the Body—A Study of the Mystery of the Body from the Perspective of Chinese and Western Cultures*, Chapters 4 and 6.

[65] Qian Mu, *The Outline of National History*, Taipei: Taiwan Commercial Press, 1995, p. 911.

the items of "Hygiene Vs Filth", including food, clothing, residence and bathing. Liu did not take these as "folk customs" to be ignored. Instead, he believed that the study of history is the "human study", that is, "history, culture and science all aim at values, in a rational sense. Value is determined by human beings". Liu has marked the annotation of "health and disease" in the section of "Human Constitution".[66] If we study the history of TCM with the mentality of "folk" history, it is obviously the history of the lower level rather than the mainstream.[67] The historians of the Republic of China period put the research of medical history into the fields of folk custom research, cultural history and special history. Folk customs, as it is referred, doesn't mean it is to be taken slightly. Liu Xianxin said: "The so-called customs of ordinary people refer to the street life of people, which is as important as the study of academia and politics. It is common for everything to follow a general rule". It goes with the saying, "a survey of a society is a study of its customs".[68] As for the monographs of special history, the most representative is probably what Liang Qichao said "it is the doctors' job to study Chinese medicine and the treatment; it is the historians' job to describe the inventions and progress of medicine in various eras". It is the so-called "new sovereignty (special history) in the old territory (traditional history)".[69] Special history has been greatly influenced by western historiography since the early Republic of China period.[70] Although many scholars expressed their alertness and solutions to the fragmentation of historiography, they are mostly happy to see its success. They only needed to put forward a number of methods to focus on a scope without exploring further details. For example, Lv Simian maintained that scholars should expand the categories of history, and should be able to "highlight the main points to make it more readable".[71]

The purpose of the author's perspective of "multi-dimensional medical history" was to seek some integration between specialized internal history and the concerned issues of historians, enhance the connotation and scope of the national history discourse, to prevent the successors from being deterred by the emphasis on "special history". It's up to the readers to give their assessment. Liang Qichao said, "Old historians were not aware of this difference, so their accounts often intruded into the boundaries of various areas of science. The science descriptions were vague, and their historical texts were dull and complicated, making it impossible to read. Their writings continuously focus on the accounts beyond history, which should be their

[66] Liu Xianxin, Sequel, *Liu Xianxin's Academic Essays: Literary Handouts,* Guilin: Guangxi Normal University Press, 2007, pp. 193, 197, 243.

[67] Jiang Shaoyuan, *Folk Customs and Superstitions,* Beijing: Beijing Publishing House, 2003, pp. 121–166.

[68] Gu Jiegang, *Contemporary Chinese Historiography*, Shanghai: Shanghai Ancient Books Publishing House, 2006, pp. 86–87.

[69] Liang Qichao, *Methodologies of Chinese History Research*, p. 30. For example, Liu Xianxin cited the French historian's *Classification of Historical Facts* to illustrate that the first item "State of Matters" includes research on human body, race, anatomy, physiology, pathology, life and death.

[70] Liu Xianxin, Introduction to History, *Liu Xianxin's Academic Essays: Literary Handouts,* pp. 225–226.

[71] Lv Simian, *Methods of Historical Research*, Taipei: Wunan Publishing House, 2002, pp. 43–44.

initial task. The departure from it would only make readers fight through thousands of volumes in vain, in the way of chasing after wind. This can serve as an enlightenment for the historians of today. They can be more committed to what is within historical category than what is beyond historical category".[72] There are areas too specialized to be dealt with in this book from a historical perspective, such as the experiments of bacteriology and the history of bacteriology in Western medicine in China. The author believes that they are more complex than the history of TCM, and with limited time and space of the book, it can only be left to the efforts of others.

As national history, modern history in the past emphasized China's modernization, with modernization and westernization as the main body, while less attention was given to the trend and strength of classicalization. Now there are more calls for studying history from the perspective of Chinese history or China-oriented history. To understand the modern transformation of various disciplines, we must give it a more in-depth exploration. Qian Mu said, "As for the westernization of the Chinese people at that time, they were ashamed of themselves and did not dare to discuss it recklessly… The essence of four to five thousand years of Chinese history and traditional culture was not outstandingly presented. It seems that in the future pursuit of academic research, it is necessary to have a general understanding and grasp of Chinese culture, starting from the origin of all disciplines".[73] If the history of TCM is not based on the deep concern of culture, what could be the way out for the development of TCM? It would probably end up being a matter of internal history. It's like the fact that a TCM doctor who abandons classical Chinese medicine is no longer a TCM doctor. The TCM history starting from classic medical books and theories is the perspective of this book in understanding the history of Chinese medicine.

---

[72] Liang Qichao said, "In the future, historians should, on one hand, divide their categories into the specialties of various sciences, so as to promote the development of autonomy without encroaching on their authorities; while on the other hand, they should consider themselves as the governor of the general system, organizing all the knowledge and various activities". For details, see his book, *Methodologies of Chinese History Research*, p. 31.

[73] Qian Mu, 20. *Settling Down in Taiwan, Memoirs of Parents in My 80s. Memories of Teachers and Friends*, p. 348.

Correction to: The Contest of Modern Chinese and Western Medicine

Correction to:
K. Pi, *The Contest of Modern Chinese and Western Medicine*,
https://doi.org/10.1007/978-981-95-2832-5

The original version of this book was inadvertently published with incorrect name of the book author which has now been changed from "Guoli Pi" to "Kuoli Pi" as per the author's passport. Also, the line "Sponsored by Chinese Fund of Humanities and Social Sciences" has been included on the copyright page. The book has been updated with the changes.

The updated version of this book can be found at
https://doi.org/10.1007/978-981-95-2832-5

© Zhonghua Book Company 2026

K. Pi, *The Contest of Modern Chinese and Western Medicine*,
https://doi.org/10.1007/978-981-95-2832-5_11

Appendix I

The Chinese era is the symbol that the Chinese calendar uses for recording and naming years. The ten Heavenly Stems are: jia, yi, bing, ding, wu, ji, geng, xin, ren, gui. The twelve Earthly Branches are: zi, chou, yin, mou, chen, si, wu, wei, shen, you, xu, hai. After observing the lunar month, the ancients found that the moon always waxes and wanes roughly 12 times a year, and two lunar months account for about 60 days.So the order of the ten Heavenly Stems and the order of the twelve Earthly Branches are properly matched in turn. In terms of recording date, 60 years is considered to be a full-time cycle. The Chinese era chronology was first invented in ancient times and is still in use now.

Appendix for the Ten Heavenly Stems and the Twelve Earthly Branches

Chia 甲	I 乙	Ping丙	Ting丁	Mou 戊	Chi 己	keng 庚	hsin辛	Jen 壬			
Tzu 子	cho丑	yin寅	mao卯	ch'en 辰	Ssu 巳	Wu 午	wei未	shen申	yu酉	hsu戌	hai亥

© Zhonghua Book Company 2026

K. Pi, *The Contest of Modern Chinese and Western Medicine*,
https://doi.org/10.1007/978-981-95-2832-5

Appendix II

Appendix for the Five Watches

In ancient China, there was also a method to divide the night into five periods, called five watches, as follows:

1st Watch	19:00–21:00
2nd Watch	21:00–23:00
3rd Watch	23:00–01:00
4th Watch	01:00–03:00
5th Watch	03:00–05:00

© Zhonghua Book Company 2026

K. Pi, *The Contest of Modern Chinese and Western Medicine*,
https://doi.org/10.1007/978-981-95-2832-5

MIX
Papier aus verantwortungsvollen Quellen
Paper from responsible sources
FSC® C105338

If you have any concerns about our products,
you can contact us on
ProductSafety@springernature.com

In case Publisher is established outside the EU,
the EU authorized representative is:
Springer Nature Customer Service Center GmbH
Europaplatz 3, 69115 Heidelberg, Germany

Printed by Libri Plureos GmbH
in Hamburg, Germany